Reference Manual for Magnetic Resonance Safety, Implants, and Devices: 2012 Edition

Frank G. Shellock, Ph.D.

Adjunct Clinical Professor of Radiology and Medicine
Keck School of Medicine
University of Southern California

Director of MRI Studies of Biomimetic MicroElectronic
Systems (BMES) Implants, National Science Foundation
BMES Engineering Research Center
University of Southern California

Adjunct Professor of Clinical Physical Therapy, Division of
Biokinesiology and Physical Therapy, School of Dentistry
University of Southern California

Founder
Institute for Magnetic Resonance
Safety, Education, and Research

President
Shellock R & D Services, Inc.
Los Angeles, California

Biomedical Research Publishing Group
Los Angeles, CA

Made in the United States of America

Library of Congress Cataloging-in-Publication Data

Shellock, Frank G.

    Reference Manual for Magnetic Resonance Safety, Implants, and Devices: 2012 Edition

Frank G. Shellock

      p. cm.

    Includes bibliographical references.

    ISBN-10, 0-9746410-8-1; ISBN-13, 978-0-9746410-8-9

    1. Magnetic resonance imaging—Complications—Handbooks, manuals, etc. 2. Metals in medicine—Magnetic properties—Handbooks, manuals, etc. 3. Implants, Artificial—Magnetic properties—Handbooks, manuals, etc. I. Title.

    [DNLM: 1. Magnetic Resonance Imaging—contraindications—handbooks. 2. Nuclear Magnetic Resonance—handbooks. 3. Metals—handbooks. 4. Implants]

Disclaimer

This textbook was designed to provide a desk reference for radiologists, MRI technologists, facility managers, MRI physicists, MRI researchers, and others. The information is current through the publication date of this textbook. MRI users are advised to check with the manufacturer of a given implant or device to obtain the most recent information prior to performing an MRI procedure on a patient with an implant or device in question. The content of this book is designed for general informational purposes only and is not intended to be nor should it be construed to be technical or medical advice or opinion on any specific facts or circumstances.

The author and publisher of this work disclaim any liability for the acts of any physician, individual, group, or entity acting independently or on behalf of any organization that utilizes information for a medical procedure, activity, service, or other situation through the use of this textbook.

The content of this book makes no representations or warranties of any kind, expressed or implied, as to the information content, materials or products, included in this book. The author and publisher assume no responsibilities for errors or omissions that may include technical or other inaccuracies, or typographical errors. The author and publisher of this work specifically disclaim all representations and warranties of any kind, expressed or implied, as to the information, content, materials, or products included or referenced in this textbook.

The author and publisher disclaim responsibility for any injury and/or damage to persons or property from any of the methods, products, instructions, or ideas contained in this publication.

The author and publisher disclaim liability for any damages of any kind arising from the use of the book, including but not limited to direct, indirect, incidental, punitive and/or consequential damages.

The information and comments provided in this book are not intended to be technical or medical recommendations or advice for individuals or patients. The information and comments provided herein are of a general

DEDICATION

To Jaana,

A truly extraordinary person,
a gentle soul, and kindred spirit.

You are forever in my heart.

Contents

Acknowledgements

As always, I am indebted to Sam Valencerina, B.S., R.T. (R)(MR), MRI Clinical Coordinator and Manager, University of Southern California, University Hospital, Los Angeles, CA, for his exceptional MRI capabilities and most professional assistance in the evaluation of implants and devices. I am particularly grateful to Alexa L. Carrington for completing the arduous task of proof reading this textbook. Special thanks to Mr. Mark Bass for his talented contributions that permit the timely publication of this textbook each year.

Preface

Welcome to the *tenth version* of the **Reference Manual for Magnetic Resonance Safety, Implants, and Devices.** Magnetic resonance (MR) procedures continue to expand with regard to usage and complexity. Patient management and safety issues are important aspects of this diagnostic modality. Because MR technology continuously evolves, it is necessary to update, revise, and add to the safety topics in this textbook in consideration of the latest information.

This annually-revised textbook series is a comprehensive resource that includes guidelines and recommendations for safety based on the latest peer-reviewed articles, labeling information from device manufacturers, as well as documents developed by professional organizations including the International Society for Magnetic Resonance in Medicine (ISMRM), the American College of Radiology (ACR), the Food and Drug Administration (FDA), the National Electrical Manufacturers Association (NEMA), the International Electrotechnical Commission (IEC), the Medical Devices Agency (MDA), and the International Commission on Non-Ionizing Radiation Protection (ICNIRP).

Section I presents safety guidelines, recommendations, and information for patient management in the MRI environment. Similar to prior editions, the content for **Section I** was carefully reviewed and updated, as needed. **Section II** provides the latest information for implants, devices, and materials tested for safety in the MR environment. **"The List"** continues to grow and contains data for thousands of objects.

The use of 3-Tesla MR systems for brain, musculoskeletal, body, cardiovascular, and other applications has become routine in many clinical settings. Because prior investigations that determined safety for implants and devices used mostly MR systems operating at 1.5-Tesla or less, it is crucial to perform *in vitro* testing at 3-Tesla to characterize MRI issues for implants, especially with regard to magnetic field interactions and, in certain cases, to assess MRI-related heating as well as alterations in the operational or functional aspects of these devices. Therefore, investigations from our group and others have evaluated MRI issues for implants and devices at 3-Tesla. This information is presented in herein.

Healthcare professionals are advised to review the terminology developed by the American Society for Testing and Materials (ASTM) International, which is currently applied to implants and devices, thus, replacing terms that were often confusing or misused. The terms, *MR Safe*, *MR Conditional*, and *MR Unsafe* are explained in this textbook. Notably, this terminology has not been applied *retrospectively* to implants and devices that previously received Food and Drug Administration (FDA) approved labeling using the terms "*MR safe*" or "*MR compatible*". Therefore, this should be understood to avoid undue confusion regarding the matter of labeling for "older" vs. "newer" implants, or for those items that have recently undergone MRI evaluations.

In addition, with regard to labeling, there is often confusion about the term "highest spatial gradient magnetic field" as it is applied to the MRI information for a given implant or device. Therefore, an explanation of this term is provided in the updated version of this textbook.

Appendix III, *Websites for Biomedical Companies*, lists company websites. This section has been further expanded to include additional companies to help MRI healthcare professionals access the latest safety information for implants and devices.

Because of the continued concern pertaining to the use of MRI contrast agents and the association with nephrogenic systemic fibrosis (NSF), this textbook provides a discussion that includes several open questions and issues. In addition, websites and links are provided to allow MRI healthcare professionals to access and review the latest information on this important topic.

Frank G. Shellock, Ph.D.

Celebrating more than 25 Years of Service to the MRI Community

SECTION I

Guidelines and Recommendations for MR Safety

Bioeffects of Static Magnetic Fields

The introduction of magnetic resonance (MR) technology as a clinical imaging modality in the early 1980s is responsible for a substantial increase in human exposure to strong static magnetic fields. Most MR systems in use today operate at fields ranging from 0.2- to 3-Tesla. According to the latest guidelines from the U.S. Food and Drug Administration, clinical MR systems using static magnetic fields up to 8.0-Tesla are considered a "non-significant risk" for adult patients. The exposure of research subjects to fields above this level requires approval of the research protocol by an Institutional Review Board and the informed consent of the subjects.

Currently, the most powerful MR system used for human subjects operates at 9.4-Tesla, but there are plans to develop even higher field strength scanners. Several investigations now describe physiologic findings obtained in human subjects, including volunteers, patients, and workers relative to exposures to the 9.4-Tesla MR system. For the short-term exposures experienced by volunteers and patients, no readily demonstrated health risks were identified. However, a study conducted to evaluate sensory symptoms and vestibular function in workers exposed to the 9.4-Tesla MR system revealed that all participants noted sensory symptoms related to the exposure. The investigators concluded that, while the workers experienced sensory symptoms, it is unclear whether long-term vestibular damage or other changes occur. The higher rates of vestibular changes may argue for improved worker surveillance and exposure control.

With respect to short-term exposures, the available information that pertains to the effects of static magnetic fields on biological tissues is extensive. Investigations include studies on alterations in cell growth and morphology, cell reproduction and teratogenicity, DNA structure and gene expression, pre- and post-natal reproduction and development, blood brain barrier permeability, nerve activity, cognitive function and behavior, cardiovascular dynamics, hematological indices, temperature regulation, circadian rhythms, immune responsiveness, neurological processing of visual and auditory information, and other biological processes. The majority of these studies concluded that exposures to static magnetic fields produce no substantial or harmful bioeffects. Although there have been reports of potentially injurious effects of static magnetic fields on isolated cells or organisms, no effect has been verified or firmly established as a scientific fact. The documented serious injuries and few fatalities that have occurred with MR system magnets were in association with the inadvertent introduction or presence of ferromagnetic objects (e.g., oxygen tanks, wheelchairs, aneurysm clips, etc.) into the MR environment.

Regarding the effects of long-term exposures to static magnetic fields, there are several physical mechanisms of interaction between tissues and static magnetic fields that could theoretically lead to pathological changes in human subjects. However, quantitative analysis of these mechanisms indicates that they are below the threshold of significance with respect to long-term, adverse bioeffects.

Presently, the peer-reviewed literature does not contain carefully controlled studies that support the absolute safety of chronic exposure to powerful magnetic fields. With the increased clinical use of interventional MR procedures, there is a critical need for such investigations. In addition, although there is no evidence for a cumulative effect of magnetic field exposure on health, further studies of the exposed populations (MR healthcare professionals, patients that undergo repeat studies, interventional MR users, etc.) will help establish guidelines for occupational and patient exposures to powerful static magnetic fields.

REFERENCES

Atkinson IC, et al. Safety of human MRI at static fields above the FDA 8 T guideline: sodium imaging at 9.4 T does not affect vital signs or cognitive ability. J Magn Reson Imaging. 2007;26:1222-7.

Atkinson IC, et al. Vital signs and cognitive function are not affected by 23-sodium and 17-oxygen magnetic resonance imaging of the human brain at 9.4 T. J Magn Reson Imaging. 2010;32:82-7.

Besson J, et al. Cognitive evaluation following NMR imaging of the brain. Journal of Neurology, Neurosurgery, and Psychiatry 1984;47:314-316.Brockway J, Bream P. Does memory loss occur after MR imaging? Journal of Magnetic Resonance Imaging 1992;2:721-728.

Brody A, et al. Induced alignment of flowing sickle erythrocytes in a magnetic field: A preliminary report. Investigative Radiology 1985;20:560-566.

Brody A, et al. Preservation of sickle cell blood flow pattern(s) during MR imaging: An *in vivo* study. American Journal of Roentgenology 1988; 151:139-141.

Budinger TF. Nuclear magnetic resonance (NMR) in vitro studies: known thresholds for health effects. J Comput Assisted Tomog 1981;5:800-811.

Cavin ID, et al. Thresholds for perceiving metallic taste at high magnetic field. J Magn Reson Imaging. 2007;26:1357-61.

Chakeres DW, de Vocht F. Static magnetic field effects on human subjects related to magnetic resonance imaging. Prog Biophys Mol Biol 2005;87:255-265.

de Vocht F, et al. Acute neurobehavior effects of exposure, health complaints and cognitive performance among employees of an MRI scanners manufacturing department. Journal of Magnetic Resonance Imaging 2006;23:197-204.

de Vocht F, et al. Acute neurobehavior effects of exposure to static magnetic fields: analysis of exposure-response relations. Journal of Magnetic Resonance Imaging 2006;23:291-297.

de Vocht F, et al. Cognitive effects of head-movements in stray fields generated by a 7 Tesla whole-body MRI magnet. Bioelectromagnetics. 2007;28:247-55.

Feychting M. Health effects of static magnetic fields--a review of the epidemiological evidence. Prog Biophys Mol Biol. 2005;87:241-6.

Franco G, et al. Focusing ethical dilemmas of evidence-based practice in SMF-exposed MRI-workers: a qualitative analysis. Int Arch Occup Environ Health. 2010;83:417-21.

Fuentes MA, et al. Analysis and measurements of magnetic field exposures for healthcare workers in selected MR environments. IEEE Trans Biomed Eng. 2008;55:1355-64.

Glover PM, et al. Magnetic-field-induced vertigo: a theoretical and experimental investigation. Bioelectromagnetics. 2007;28:349-61.

Hartwig V, et al. Biological effects and safety in magnetic resonance imaging: a review. Int J Environ Res Public Health. 2009;6:1778-98.

Heinrich A, et al. Effects of static magnetic fields on cognition, vital signs, and sensory perception: A meta-analysis. J Magn Reson Imaging. 2011;34:758–763.

Hong CZ, Shellock FG. Short-term exposure to a 1.5 Tesla static magnetic field does not effect somato-sensory evoked potentials in man. Magnetic Resonance Imaging 1989;8:65-69.

Hsieh CH, et al. Deleterious effects of MRI on chondrocytes. Osteoarthritis Cartilage. 2008;16:343-51.

International Electrotechnical Commission (IEC), Medical Electrical Equipment, Particular requirements for the safety of magnetic resonance equipment for medical diagnosis, International Standard IEC 60601-2-33, 2002.

International Commission on Non-Ionizing Radiation Protection (ICNIRP) Statement, Medical magnetic resonance procedures: protection of patients. Health Physics 2004;87:197-216.

Innis NK, et al. Behavioral effects of exposure to nuclear magnetic resonance imaging: II. Spatial memory tests. Magnetic Resonance Imaging 1986;4:281-284.

Kannala S, et al. Occupational exposure measurements of static and pulsed gradient magnetic fields in the vicinity of MRI scanners. Phys Med Biol. 2009;54:2243-57.

Kangarlu A, et al. Cognitive, cardiac, and physiological safety studies in ultra high field magnetic resonance imaging. Magn Reson Imaging 1999;17:1407-1416.

Karpowicz J, et al. Exposure to static magnetic field and health hazards during the operation of magnetic resonance scanners. Med Pr. 2011;62:309-21.

Karpowicz J, Gryz K. Health risk assessment of occupational exposure to a magnetic field from magnetic resonance imaging devices. Int J Occup Saf Ergon. 2006;12:155-67.

Kay H, Herfkens R, Kay B. Effect on magnetic resonance imaging on Xenopus Laevis embryogenesis. Magnetic Resonance Imaging 1988; 6:501-506.

Laszlo J, Gyires K. 3 T homogeneous static magnetic field of a clinical MR significantly inhibits pain in mice. Life Sci. 2009;84:12-7.

Muller S, Hotz M. Human brainstem auditory evoked potentials (BAEP) before and after MR examinations. Magnetic Resonance in Medicine 1990;16:476-480.

Ossenkopp KP, et al. Behavioral effects of exposure to nuclear magnetic resonance imaging: I. Open-field avoidance behavior an passive avoidance learning in rats. Magnetic Resonance Imaging 1986;4:275-280.

Patel M, et al. Pilot study investigating the effect of the static magnetic field from a 9.4-T MRI on the vestibular system. J Occup Environ Med. 2008;50:576-83.

Prasad N, Wright D, Ford J, Thornby J. Safety of 4-T MR imaging: Study of effects on developing frog embryos. Radiology 1990;174:251-253.

Sakurai T, Terashima S, Miyakoshi J. Effects of strong static magnetic fields used in magnetic resonance imaging on insulin-secreting cells. Bioelectromagnetics. Bioelectromagnetics. 2009;30:1-8.

Schenck JF. Health effects and safety of static magnetic fields. In: Shellock FG, ed. Magnetic resonance procedures: health effects and safety. Boca Raton, FL: CRC Press, 2001; pp. 1-30.

Schenck JF. Safety of strong, static magnetic fields. J Magn Reson Imaging 2000;12:2-19.

Schenck JF, et al. Human exposure to 4.0-Tesla magnetic fields in a whole-body scanner. Medical Physics 1992;19:1089-1098.

Schlamann M, et al. Exposure to high-field MRI does not affect cognitive function. J Magn Reson Imaging. 2010;31:1061-6.

Schlamann M, et al. Short term effects of magnetic resonance imaging on excitability of the motor cortex at 1.5T and 7T. Acad Radiol. 2010;17:277-81.

Schwartz J, Crooks L. NMR imaging produces no observable mutations or cytotoxicity in mammalian cells. American Journal of Roentgenology 1982;139:583-585.

Schwenzer NF, et al. Do static or time-varying magnetic fields in magnetic resonance imaging (3.0 T) alter protein-gene expression?-A study on human embryonic lung fibroblasts. J Magn Reson Imaging. 2007;26:1210-5.

Schwenzer NF, Bantleon R, Maurer B, et al. In vitro evaluation of magnetic resonance imaging at 3.0 Tesla on clonogenic ability, proliferation, and cell cycle in human embryonic lung fibroblasts. Invest Radiol. 2007;42:212-217.

Shellock FG, Crues JV. MR procedures: biologic effects, safety, and patient care. Radiology, 2004;232:635-652.

Shellock FG, Schaefer DJ, Crues JV. Exposure to a 1.5 Tesla static magnetic field does not alter body and skin temperatures in man. Magnetic Resonance in Medicine 1989;1:371-375.

Shellock FG, Schaefer DJ, Gordon CJ. Effect of a 1.5 Tesla static magnetic field on body temperature of man. Magnetic Resonance in Medicine 1986;3:644-647.

Short W, et al. Alteration of human tumor cell adhesion by high-strength static magnetic fields. Investigative Radiology 1991;27:836-840.

Silva AK, Silva EL, Egito ES, Carrico AS. Safety concerns related to magnetic field exposure. Radiat Environ Biophys. 2006;45:245-52.

Simmons A, Hakansson K. Magnetic resonance safety. Methods Mol Biol. 2011;711:17-28.

Tomasi DG, Wang R. Induced magnetic field gradients and forces in the human head in MRI. J Magn Reson Imaging. 2007;26:1340-5.

Toyomaki A, Yamamoto T. Observation of changes in neural activity due to the static magnetic field of an MRI scanner. J Magn Reson Imaging. 2007;26:1216-21

U.S. Department of Health and Human Services, Food and Drug Administration, Center for Devices and Radiological Health, Guidance for Industry and FDA Staff. Criteria for Significant Risk Investigations of Magnetic Resonance Diagnostic Devices, July 14, 2003.

Valiron O, et al. Cellular disorders induced by high magnetic fields. Journal of Magnetic Resonance Imaging 2005;22:334-340.

Vaughan T, et al. 9.4-T human MRI: preliminary results. Magn Reson Med. 2006;56:1274-1282.

Vecchia P, Hietanen M, et al. Guidelines on limits of exposure to static magnetic fields. International Commission on Non-Ionizing Radiation Protection. Health Physics 2009;96:504-14.

Vogl T, et al. Influence of magnetic resonance imaging on evoked potentials and nerve conduction velocities in humans. Investigative Radiology 1991; 26:432-437.

Von Klitzing L. Do static magnetic fields of NMR influence biological signals? Clin Phys Physiol Meas 1986;7:157-160.

Weintraub MI, et al. Biologic effects of 3 Tesla (T) MR imaging comparing traditional 1.5-T and 0.6-T in 1,023 consecutive outpatients. J Neuroimaging. 2007;17:241-5.

Weiss M, et al. Bioeffects of high magnetic fields: A study using a simple animal model. Magnetic Resonance Imaging 1992;10:689-694.

Yamaguchi-Sekino S, et al. Biological effects of electromagnetic fields and recently updated safety guidelines for strong static magnetic fields. Magn Reson Med Sci. 2011;10:1-10.

Yuh WTC, Ehrhardt JC, Fisher DJ, Shields RK, Shellock FG. Phantom limb pain induced in amputee by strong magnetic fields. J Magn Reson Imaging 1992;2:221-223.

Zaremba LA. FDA guidance for magnetic resonance system safety and patient exposures: current status and future considerations. In: Shellock FG, ed. Magnetic resonance procedures: health effects and safety. Boca Raton, FL: CRC Press, 2001; pp. 183-196.

Bioeffects of Gradient Magnetic Fields

During magnetic resonance (MR) procedures, gradient or time-varying magnetic fields may stimulate nerves or muscles in patients by inducing electrical fields. This topic has been thoroughly reviewed by Bencsik et al., Schaefer et al., Nyenhuis et al., and Bourland et al. The potential for interactions between gradient magnetic fields and biological tissues is dependent on a variety of factors including the fundamental field frequency, the maximum flux density, the average flux density, the presence of harmonic frequencies, the waveform characteristics of the signal, the polarity of the signal, the current distribution in the body, the electrical properties, and the sensitivity of the cell membrane.

GRADIENT MAGNETIC FIELD-INDUCED STIMULATION

Several investigations have characterized MR system-related, gradient magnetic field-induced stimulation in human subjects. At sufficient exposure levels, peripheral nerve stimulation is perceptible as "tingling" or "tapping" sensations. At gradient magnetic field exposure levels from 50% to 100% above perception thresholds, patients may become uncomfortable or experience pain. At extremely high levels, cardiac stimulation is a concern. However, the induction of cardiac stimulation requires exceedingly large gradient fields that are more than an order of magnitude greater than those used currently by commercially available MR systems.

With regard to gradient magnetic fields, the U.S. Food and Drug Administration considers that MR procedures using rates of change (dB/dt) sufficient to produce severe discomfort or painful nerve stimulation a significant risk. These safety standards for gradient magnetic fields associated with present-day MR systems appear to adequately protect patients from potential hazards or injuries.

Interestingly, studies performed in human subjects have indicated that anatomical sites of peripheral nerve stimulation vary depending on the activation of a specific gradient (i.e., x-, y- or, z-gradient). For example, stimulation sites for x-gradients included the bridge of the nose, left side of the thorax, iliac crest, left thigh, buttocks, and the lower back. Stimulation sites for y-gradients included the scapula, upper arms, shoulder, right side of the thorax, iliac crest, hip, hands, and upper back. Stimulation sites for z-gradients included the scapula, thorax, xyphoid, abdomen, iliac crest, and upper and lower back. Peripheral nerve stimulation sites were typically found at bony prominences. According to Schaefer et al., since bone is less conductive than the surrounding tissue, it may increase current densities in narrow regions of tissue between the bone and the skin, resulting in lower nerve stimulation thresholds than expected.

REFERENCES

Abart J, et al. Peripheral nerve stimulation by time-varying magnetic fields. Journal of Computer Assisted Tomography 1997; 21:532–538.

Bencsik M, Bowtell R, Bowley R. Electric fields induced in the human body by time-varying magnetic field gradients in MRI: numerical calculations and correlation analysis. Phys Med Biol. 2007;52:2337-53.

Bourland JD, Nyenhuis JA, Schaefer DJ. Physiologic effects of intense MRI gradient fields. Neuroimaging Clin North Am 1999; 9:363–377.

Budinger TF, et al. Physiological effects of fast oscillating magnetic field gradients. Journal of Computer Assisted Tomography 1991;15:609–614.

Cohen MS, Weisskoff R, Kantor H. Sensory stimulation by time varying magnetic fields. Magn Reson 1990;14:409–414.

de Vocht F, et al. Exposure to alternating electromagnetic fields and effects on the visual and visuomotor systems. Br J Radiol. 2007;80:822-8.

Doherty J, Whitman G, Robinson M, et al. Changes in cardiac excitability and vulnerability in NMR fields. 1985;20:129-135.

Ehrhardt JC, et al. Peripheral nerve stimulation in a whole-body echo-planar imaging system. J Magn Reson Imaging 1997;7:405–409.

Feldman RE, Hardy CJ, et al. Experimental determination of human peripheral nerve stimulation thresholds in a 3-axis planar gradient system. Magn Reson Med. 2009;62:763-70.

Fuentes MA, et al. Analysis and measurements of magnetic field exposures for healthcare workers in selected MR environments. IEEE Trans Biomed Eng. 2008;55:1355-64.

Glover PM. Interaction of MRI field gradients with the human body. Phys Med Biol. 2009;54:R99-R115.

Glover PM, Eldeghaidy S, Mistry TR, Gowland PA. Measurement of visual evoked potential during and after periods of pulsed magnetic field exposure. J Magn Reson Imaging. 2007;26:1353-6.

Ham CLG, Engels JML, van de Weil GT, Machielsen A. Peripheral nerve stimulation during MRI: effects of high gradient amplitudes and switching rates. J Magn Reson Imaging 1997;7:933–937.

Hartwig V, et al. Biological effects and safety in magnetic resonance imaging: a review. Int J Environ Res Public Health. 2009;6:1778-98.

Irnich W, Schmitt F. Magnetostimulation in MRI. Magn Reson Med 1995;33:619–623.

International Commission on Non-Ionizing Radiation Protection (ICNIRP) Statement, Medical magnetic resonance procedures: protection of patients. Health Physics 2004;87:197-216.

Kannala S, et al. Occupational exposure measurements of static and pulsed gradient magnetic fields in the vicinity of MRI scanners. Phys Med Biol. 2009;54:2243-57.

Kangarlu A, Tang L, Ibrahim TS. Electric field measurements and computational modeling at ultrahigh-field MRI. Magn Reson Imaging. 2007;25:1222-1226.

King KF, Schaefer DJ. Spiral scan peripheral nerve stimulation. J Magn Reson Imaging 2000; 12:164-170.

Li Y, et al. Numerically-simulated induced electric field and current density within a human model located close to a z-gradient coil. J Magn Reson Imaging. 2007;26:1286-95.

Mansfield P, Harvey PR. Limits to neural stimulation in echo-planar imaging. Magn Reson Med 1993; 29:746–758.

Nyenhuis JA, Bourland J, Kildishev AV, Schaefer DJ. Health effects and safety of intense gradient fields. In: Shellock FG, ed. Magnetic resonance procedures: health effects and safety. Boca Raton, FL: CRC Press, 2001; 31-54.

Nyenhuis JA, Bourland JD, Schaefer DJ. Analysis from a stimulation perspective of magnetic field patterns of MR gradient coils. J Appl Phys 1997;81:4314–4316.

Schaefer DJ, Bourland JD, Nyenhuis JA. Review of patient safety in time-varying gradient fields. J Magn Reson Imaging 2000; 12:20-29.

Schwenzer NF, Bantleon R, et al. Do static or time-varying magnetic fields in magnetic resonance imaging (3.0 T) alter protein-gene expression? A study on human embryonic lung fibroblasts. J Magn Reson Imaging. 2007;26:1210-5.

Shellock FG, Crues JV. MR procedures: biologic effects, safety, and patient care. Radiology, 2004;232:635-652.

U.S. Department of Health and Human Services, Food and Drug Administration, Center for Devices and Radiological Health, Guidance for Industry and FDA Staff. Criteria for Significant Risk Investigations of Magnetic Resonance Diagnostic Devices, July 14, 2003.

Vogt FM, et al. Increased time rate of change of gradient fields: Effect on peripheral nerve stimulation at clinical MR imaging. Radiology 2004;233:548-554.

Weintraub MI, et al. Biologic effects of 3 Tesla (T) MR imaging comparing traditional 1.5-T and 0.6-T in 1,023 consecutive outpatients. J Neuroimaging. 2007;17:241-5.

Bioeffects of Radiofrequency Fields

The majority of the radiofrequency (RF) power transmitted for MR imaging or spectroscopy (including carbon decoupling, fast spin echo pulse sequences, magnetization transfer contrast pulse sequences, etc.) procedures is transformed into heat within the patient's tissue as a result of resistive losses. Not surprisingly, the bioeffects associated with exposure to RF radiation are related to the thermogenic aspects of this electromagnetic field.

Prior to 1985, there were no reports concerning the thermophysiologic responses of human subjects exposed to RF radiation during MR procedures. Since then, many investigations have characterized the thermal effects of MR procedure-related heating.

SPECIFIC ABSORPTION RATE

Thermoregulatory and other physiologic changes that a human subject exhibits in response to exposure to RF radiation are dependent on the amount of energy that is absorbed. The dosimetric term used to describe the absorption of RF radiation is the specific absorption rate (SAR). SAR is the mass normalized rate at which RF power is coupled to biological tissue and is typically indicated in units of watts per kilogram (W/kg). The relative amount of RF radiation that an individual encounters during an MR procedure is designated as the whole-body-averaged SAR. Other SAR levels relative to the body part exposed or peak SAR level (i.e., the amount in one gram of tissue) may also be reported by the MR system.

Measurements or estimates of SAR are not trivial, particularly in human subjects. There are several methods of determining this parameter for the purpose of RF energy dosimetry. The SAR that is produced during an MR procedure is a complex function of numerous variables including the frequency (i.e., determined by the strength of the static magnetic field of the MR system), the type of RF pulse used (e.g., 90° vs. 180° pulse), the repetition time, the type of transmit RF coil used, the volume of tissue contained within the transmit RF coil, the configuration of the anatomical region exposed, as well as other factors.

With regard to RF energy, the U.S. Food and Drug Administration currently indicates that MR procedures that exceed certain SAR values may pose significant risks (please refer to **Appendix I** to review these values).

THERMOPHYSIOLOGIC RESPONSES TO MR PROCEDURE-RELATED HEATING

Thermophysiologic responses to MR procedure-related heating depend on multiple physiologic, physical, and environmental factors. These include the duration of exposure, the rate at which energy is deposited, the response of the patient's thermoregulatory system, the presence of an underlying health condition, and the ambient conditions within the MR system.

In regards to temperature regulation in human subjects, when exposed to a thermal challenge, the human body loses heat by means of convection, conduction, radiation, and evaporation. Each mechanism is responsible to a varying degree for heat dissipation, as the body attempts to maintain thermal homeostasis. If the thermoregulatory effectors are not capable of totally dissipating the heat load, an accumulation or storage of heat occurs along with an elevation in local and/or overall tissue temperatures.

Various health conditions may affect an individual's ability to tolerate a thermal challenge including cardiovascular disease, hypertension, diabetes, fever, old age, and obesity. In addition, medications including diuretics, beta-blockers, calcium blockers, amphetamines, and sedatives can alter thermoregulatory responses to a heat load. Certain medications have a synergistic effect with RF radiation with respect to tissue heating. The environmental conditions (i.e., ambient temperature, relative humidity, and airflow) that exist in the MR system will also affect tissue temperature changes associated with RF energy-induced heating.

The first study of human thermal responses to RF radiation-induced heating during an MR procedure was conducted by Schaefer et al. Temperature changes and other physiologic parameters were assessed in volunteer subjects exposed to a relatively high, whole-body-averaged SAR (approximately 4.0-W/kg). The data indicated that there were no excessive temperature elevations or other deleterious physiologic consequences related to exposure to RF energy.

Several studies were subsequently conducted involving volunteer subjects and patients undergoing MR procedures, with the intent of obtaining information that would be applicable to patients typically encountered in the MR setting. These investigations demonstrated that changes in body temperatures were relatively minor (i.e., less than 0.6 degrees C). While there was a tendency for statistically significant increases in skin temperatures to occur, these were of no serious physiological consequences.

Interestingly, various studies reported a poor correlation between body temperature and skin temperature changes versus whole-body-averaged SARs associated with clinical MR procedures. These findings are not surprising considering the range of thermophysiologic responses that are possible in human subjects relative to a given SAR level. For example, as previously indicated, an individual's thermoregulatory system can be greatly impacted by the presence of an underlying condition or medication that can impair the ability to dissipate heat.

An extensive investigation by Shellock et al. was conducted in volunteer subjects exposed to MR examinations performed at a whole-body-averaged SAR of 6.0-W/kg. To date, this is the highest level of RF energy that human subjects have been exposed to in association with MR procedures. Tympanic membrane temperature, six different skin temperatures, heart rate, blood pressure, oxygen saturation, and skin blood flow were monitored. The findings indicated that an MR procedure performed at a whole body averaged SAR of 6.0-W/kg can be physiologically tolerated by an individual with normal thermoregulatory function.

VERY-HIGH FIELD MR SYSTEMS

Many MR systems now operate at a static magnetic field strength of 3-Tesla, several operate at 4-Tesla and 7-Tesla, and one at 9.4-Tesla. These very-high-field MR systems are capable of depositing RF power that exceed those associated with a 1.5-Tesla MR system. Therefore, investigations are needed to characterize thermal responses in human subjects to determine potential thermogenic hazards associated with the use of these powerful MR devices, especially since frequency related differences likely exist. To date, several investigations have been conducted to address MR procedure-related heating performed using very-high-field MR systems.

REFERENCES

Atalar E. Radiofrequency safety for interventional MRI procedures. Acad Radiol. 2005;12:1149-1157.

Boss A, Graf H, Berger A, et al. Tissue warming and regulatory responses induced by radio frequency energy deposition on a whole-body 3-Tesla magnetic resonance imager. J Magn Reson Imaging. 2007;26:1334-9.

Bottomley PA. Turning up the heat on MRI. J Am Coll Radiol. 2008;5:853

Bottomley PA, Edelstein WA. Power deposition in whole body NMR imaging. Med Phys 1981;8: 510-512.

Budinger TF. Nuclear magnetic resonance (NMR) in vitro studies: known thresholds for health effects. J Comput Assisted Tomog 1981;5:800-811.

Collins CM. Numerical field calculations considering the human subject for engineering and safety assurance in MRI. NMR Biomed. 2009;22:919-26.

Collins CM, Wang Z. Calculation of radiofrequency electromagnetic fields and their effects in MRI of human subjects. Magn Reson Med. 2011;65:1470-82.

Drinkwater BL, Horvath SM: Heat tolerance and aging. Med Sci Sport Exer 1979;11:49-55.

Gorny KR, et al. Calorimetric calibration of head coil SAR estimates displayed on a clinical MR scanner. Phys Med Biol. 2008;53:2565-76.

Gowland PA, De Wilde J. Temperature increase in the fetus due to radio frequency exposure during magnetic resonance scanning. Phys Med Biol. 2008;53:L15-8.

Hand JW, Li Y, et al. Prediction of specific absorption rate in mother and fetus associated with MRI examinations during pregnancy. Magn Reson Med. 2006;55:883-893.

Hand JW, et al. Numerical study of RF exposure and the resulting temperature rise in the foetus during a magnetic resonance procedure. Phys Med Biol. 2010;55:913-30.

Hartwig V, et al. Biological effects and safety in magnetic resonance imaging: a review. Int J Environ Res Public Health. 2009;6:1778-98.

International Commission on Non-Ionizing Radiation Protection (ICNIRP) Statement, Medical magnetic resonance procedures: protection of patients. Health Physics 2004;87:197-216.

International Electrotechnical Commission (IEC), Medical Electrical Equipment, Particular requirements for the safety of magnetic resonance equipment for medical diagnosis, International Standard IEC 60601-2-33, 2002.

Kangarlu A, Shellock FG, Chakeres D. 8.0-Tesla MR system: Temperature changes associated with radiofrequency-induced heating of a head phantom. J Magn Reson Imaging 2003;17:220-226.

Kangarlu A, Ibrahim TS, Shellock FG. Effects of coil dimensions and field polarization on RF heating inside a head phantom. Magnetic Resonance Imaging 2005;23:53-60.

Kenny WL. Physiological correlates of heat intolerance. Sports Med 1985;2:279-286.

Kikuchi S, et al. Temperature elevation in the fetus from electromagnetic exposure during magnetic resonance imaging. Phys Med Biol. 2010;55:2411-26.

Jauchem JR. Effects of drugs on thermal responses to microwaves. Gen Pharmacol 1985;16:307-310.

Neufeld E, et al. Analysis of the local worst-case SAR exposure caused by an MRI multi-transmit body coil in anatomical models of the human body. Phys Med Biol. 2011;56:4649-59.

Oh S, et al. Experimental and numerical assessment of MRI-induced temperature change and SAR distributions in phantoms and in vivo. Magn Reson Med. Magn Reson Med. 2010;63:218-23.

Rowell LB. Cardiovascular aspects of human thermoregulation. Circ Res 1983;52:367-379.

Schaefer DJ. Health effects and safety of radiofrequency power deposition associated with magnetic resonance procedures. In: Shellock FG, ed. Magnetic resonance procedures: health effects and safety. Boca Raton, FL: CRC Press, 2001;55-74.

Shellock FG. Radiofrequency energy-induced heating during MR procedures: a review. J Magn Reson Imaging 2000;12:30-36.

Shellock FG, Crues JV. MR procedures: biologic effects, safety, and patient care. Radiology 2004;232:635-652.

Shellock FG, Crues JV. Temperature, heart rate, and blood pressure changes associated with clinical MR imaging at 1.5-T. Radiology 1987;163:259-262.

Shellock FG, Crues JV. Corneal temperature changes associated with high-field MR imaging using a head coil. Radiology 1988;167:809-811.

Shellock FG, Crues JV. Temperature changes caused by clinical MR imaging of the brain at 1.5 Tesla using a head coil. Am J Neuroradiol 1988;9:287-291.

Shellock FG, Rothman B, Sarti D. Heating of the scrotum by high-field-strength MR imaging. Am J Roentgenol 1990;154:1229-1232.

Shellock FG, Schatz CJ. Increases in corneal temperature caused by MR imaging of the eye with a dedicated local coil. Radiology 192;185:697-699.

Shellock FG, Schaefer DJ. Radiofrequency energy-induced heating during magnetic resonance procedures: laboratory and clinical experiences In: Shellock FG, ed. Magnetic resonance procedures: health effects and safety. Boca Raton, FL: CRC Press, 2001;75-96.

Shellock FG, Schaefer DJ, Crues JV. Alterations in body and skin temperatures caused by MR imaging: Is the recommended exposure for radiofrequency radiation too conservative? Br J Radiol 1989; 62:904-909.

Shellock FG, Schaefer DJ, Kanal E. Physiologic responses to MR imaging performed at an SAR level of 6.0 W/kg. Radiology 1994;192:865-868.

Shrivastava D, Hanson T, et al. Radiofrequency heating at 9.4T: in vivo temperature measurement results in swine. Magn Reson Med. 2008;59:73-8.

Shrivastava D, et al. Radio frequency heating at 9.4T (400.2 MHz): in vivo thermoregulatory temperature response in swine. Magn Reson Med. 2009;62:888 95.

Shrivastava D, et al. Radiofrequency heating in porcine models with a "large" 32 cm internal diameter, 7 T (296 MHz) head coil. Magn Reson Med. 2011;66:255-63.

Shuman WP, et al. Superficial and deep-tissue increases in anesthetized dogs during exposure to high specific absorption rates in a 1.5-T MR imager. Radiology 1988;167:551-554.

Stuchly MA, Abrishamkar H, Strydom ML. Numerical Evaluation of Radio Frequency Power Deposition in Human Models during MRI. Conf Proc IEEE Eng Med Biol Soc. 2006;1:272-275.

U.S. Department of Health and Human Services, FDA, CDRH, Guidance for Industry and FDA Staff. Criteria for Significant Risk Investigations of Magnetic Resonance Diagnostic Devices, July 14, 2003.

Wang Z, Lin JC, Vaughan JT, Collins CM. Consideration of physiological response in numerical models of temperature during MRI of the human head.J Magn Reson Imaging. 2008;28:1303-1308.

Weintraub MI, Khoury A, Cole SP. Biologic effects of 3 Tesla (T) MR imaging comparing traditional 1.5-T and 0.6-T in 1,023 consecutive outpatients. J Neuroimaging. 2007;17:241-5.

Acoustic Noise
and MR Procedures*

Various types of acoustic noise are produced during the operation of an MR system. Problems associated with acoustic noise for patients and healthcare professionals include annoyance, verbal communication difficulties, heightened anxiety, temporary hearing loss and, in extreme cases, the potential for permanent hearing impairment.

Acoustic noise may pose a particular problem to specific patient groups. For example, patients with psychiatric disorders may become confused or suffer from increased anxiety as the result of exposure to loud noise. Sedated patients may experience discomfort in association with high noise levels.

In addition, neonates may have adverse reactions to acoustic noise. Reeves MJ, et al. (2010) recently conducted a study to address this issue. The findings suggested that exposure of the fetus to 1.5-T MR imaging during the second and third trimesters of pregnancy is not associated with an increased risk of substantial neonatal hearing impairment or cochlear injury.

HEARING AND THE IMPACT OF ACOUSTIC NOISE

The human ear is a highly sensitive wide-band receiver, with the typical frequency range for normal hearing being between 20-Hz to 20,000-Hz. The ear does not tend to judge sound powers in absolute terms, but assesses how much greater one power is than another. The logarithmic decibel scale, dB, is used when referring to sound power.

Noise is defined in terms of frequency spectrum (in Hz), intensity (in dB), and time duration. Noise can be steady-state, intermittent, impulsive, or explosive. Transient hearing loss may occur following exposure to loud noise, resulting in a temporary threshold shift (i.e., a shift in the audible threshold).

With regard to acoustic noise associated with MR imaging, Brummett et al. reported temporary shifts in hearing thresholds in 43% of the patients scanned without ear protection or with improperly fitted earplugs. Recovery from the effects of noise occurs in a relatively short period of time. However, if the noise insult is particularly severe, full recovery can take up to several weeks. If the noise is sufficiently injurious, a permanent threshold shift at specific frequencies may occur.

MRI-RELATED ACOUSTIC NOISE

The gradient magnetic field is the main source of acoustic noise associated with an MR procedure. This noise occurs during the rapid alterations of currents within the gradient coils. These currents, in the presence of the strong static magnetic field of the MR system, produce significant (Lorentz) forces that act upon the gradient coils. Acoustic noise, manifested as loud tapping, knocking, chirping, squeaking sounds, or other sounds is produced when the forces cause motion or vibration of the gradient coils as they impact against their mountings which, in turn, flex and vibrate.

Alteration of the gradient output (rise time or amplitude) by modifying MR imaging parameters causes the acoustic noise to vary. Noise tends to be enhanced by decreases in section thickness, field of view, repetition time, and echo time. In addition to dependence on imaging parameters, acoustic noise is dependent on the MR system hardware, construction, and the surrounding environment. Furthermore, noise characteristics have a spatial dependence. For example, noise levels can vary by as much as 10 dB as a function of patient position within the bore of the MR system. The presence and size of the patient may also affect the level of acoustic noise.

CHARACTERISTICS OF MR SYSTEM-RELATED ACOUSTIC NOISE

Gradient magnetic field-induced noise levels have been measured during a variety of pulse sequences for MR systems with static magnetic field strengths ranging from 0.35 to 4-Tesla. For example, Hurwitz et al. reported that the MR imaging-related sound levels varied from 82 to 93 dB on the A-weighted scale and from 84 to 103 dB on the linear scale.

Later studies performed using a variety of MR parameters including "worst-case" pulse sequences that applied multiple gradients simultaneously (e.g., three-dimensional, fast gradient echo techniques) reported that these are among the loudest sequences, with acoustic noise levels that ranged from 103 to 113 dB (peak) on the A-weighted scale.

Additional studies measured acoustic noise generated by echo planar imaging (EPI) and fast spin echo sequences. Echo planar sequences tend to have extremely fast gradient switching times and high gradient amplitudes. Shellock et al. reported high levels of noise ranging from 114 to 115 dBA on two different high field strength (1.5-Tesla) MR systems tested during EPI sequences with parameters selected to represent "worst-case" protocols. At 3-Tesla, Hattori et al. recorded sound levels that ranged from 126 to 131 dB on a linear scale, recommending the use of both earplugs and headphones for ear protection relative to the use of 3-Tesla MR systems when certain pulse sequences are used.

ACOUSTIC NOISE AND PERMISSIBLE LIMITS

In general, acoustic noise levels recorded in the MR environment have been below the maximum limits permitted by the Occupational Safety and Health Administration of the United States. This is particularly the case when one considers that the duration of exposure is an important factor that determines the effect of noise on hearing.

The U.S. Food and Drug Administration released guidelines for acoustic noise levels that should not be exceeded in association with the operation of MR systems, as follows (please refer to **Appendix I**):

Sound Pressure Level - Peak unweighted sound pressure level greater than 140 dB. A-weighted root mean square (rms) sound pressure level greater than 99 dBA with hearing protection in place.

While the acoustic noise levels recommended for patients undergoing MR procedures on an infrequent and short-term basis may appear to be somewhat conservative, they are deemed appropriate when one considers that individuals with underlying health conditions may have problems with noise at certain levels or frequencies. Acoustic noise produced during MR procedures represents a potential risk to such patients. As previously mentioned, the possibility exists that substantial gradient magnetic field-induced noise may produce hearing problems in patients who are susceptible to the damaging effects of loud noises.

The exposure of staff and other healthcare workers in the MR environment is also a concern (e.g., those involved in interventional MR procedures or who remain in the room for patient management reasons). Accordingly, if loud noises exist in the MR environment, staff members should routinely wear ear protection if they remain in the room during the operation of the scanner. In the United Kingdom, guidelines issued by the Department of Health recommend hearing protection be worn by staff exposed to an average of 85 dB over an eight hour day.

ACOUSTIC NOISE CONTROL TECHNIQUES

Passive noise control. The simplest and least expensive means of preventing problems associated with acoustic noise during MR procedures is routinely use disposable earplugs or headphones. Earplugs, when properly used, can abate noise by 10 to 30 dB, which is usually an adequate amount of sound attenuation for the MR environment. The use of earplugs typically provides a sufficient decrease in acoustic noise that, in turn, is capable of preventing hearing problems. Therefore, for MR systems that generate substantial acoustic noise, patients should be required to wear these protective devices.

Unfortunately, passive noise control methods suffer from a number of limitations. For example, these devices hamper verbal communication with patients during the operation of the MR system. Additionally, standard earplugs are often too large for the ear canal of adolescents and infants. Importantly, passive noise control devices provide non-uniform noise attenuation over the hearing range. While high frequencies may be well attenuated, attenuation is often poor at low frequencies. This is problematic because, for certain pulse sequences, the low frequency range is where the peak MR imaging-related acoustic noise is generated.

Active Noise Control (ANC). A significant reduction in the level of acoustic noise caused by MR procedures has been accomplished using active noise cancellation. Controlling noise from a particular source by introducing "anti-phase noise" to interfere destructively with the noise source is not a new idea with regard to MR systems. For example, in 1989, Goldman et al. combined passive noise control and an active noise control system (i.e. an active system built into a headphone) to achieve an average noise reduction of approximately 14 dB.

Advances in digital signal processing technology allow efficient active noise control systems to be realized at a moderate cost. The anti-noise system involves a continuous feedback loop with continuous sampling of the sounds in the noise environment so that the gradient magnetic field-induced noise is attenuated. It is possible to attenuate the pseudo-periodic scanner noise while allowing the transmission of vocal communication or music to be maintained.

"Quiet" Pulse Sequences. Several investigators have described the development of "quite" pulse sequences which substantially decrease acoustic noise and are acceptable for MR imaging and functional MRI examinations. These techniques are particularly interesting insofar as they may be utilized even with echo planar imaging sequences.

OTHER SOURCES OF MR SYSTEM-RELATED ACOUSTIC NOISE

RF hearing. When the human head is subjected to pulsed radiofrequency (RF) radiation at certain frequencies, an audible sound perceived as a click, buzz, chirp, or knocking noise may be heard. This acoustic phenomenon is referred to as "RF hearing", "RF sound" or "microwave hearing".

Thermoelastic expansion is believed to be responsible for the production of RF hearing, whereby there is absorption of RF energy that produces a minute temperature elevation (i.e., approximately 1×10^{-6} degrees C) over a brief time period in the tissues of the head. Subsequently, a pressure wave is induced that is sensed by the hair cells of the cochlea via bone conduction. In this manner, a pulse of RF energy is transferred into an acoustic wave within the human head and sensed by the hearing organs.

With specific reference to the operation of MR scanners, RF hearing has been found to be associated with frequencies ranging from 2.4- to 170-MHz. The gradient magnetic field-induced acoustic noise that occurs during an MR procedure is significantly louder than the sounds associated with RF hearing. Therefore, noises produced by this RF auditory phenomenon are effectively masked and not perceived by patients. Currently, there is no evidence of any detrimental health effect related to the presence of RF hearing.

Noise From Subsidiary Systems. Patient comfort fans and cryogen reclamation systems associated with superconducting magnets of MR systems are the main sources of ambient acoustic noise found in the MR environment. Acoustic noise produced by these subsidiary systems is considerably less than that caused by gradient magnetic fields.

REFERENCES

Bandettini PA, et al. Functional MRI of brain activation induced by scanner acoustic noise. Magn Reson Med 1998;39:410-416.

Brummett RE, Talbot JM, Charuhas P. Potential hearing loss resulting from MR imaging. Radiology 1988;169:539-540.

Bowtell RW, Mansfield PM. Quiet transverse gradient coils: Lorentz force balancing designs using geometric similitude. Magn Reson Med 1995;34:494-497.

Chaplain GBB. Anti-noise: the Essex breakthrough. Chart Mech Engin 1983;30:41-47.

Chen CK, Chiueh TD, Chen JH. Active cancellation system of acoustic noise in MR imaging. IEEE Trans Biomed Engin 1999;46:186-190.

Cho ZH, et al. Analysis of acoustic noise in MRI. Magn Reson Imaging 1997;15:815-822.

Counter SA, Olofsson A, Grahn, Borg E. MRI acoustic noise: sound pressure and frequency analysis. J Magn Reson Imaging 1997;7:606-611.

Elliott SJ, Nelson Active noise control. IEEE Sign Proceed Magn 1983;12-35.

Elder JA. Special senses. In: United States Environmental Protection Agency, Health Effects Research Laboratory. Biological Effects of Radio frequency Radiation. EPA-600/8-83-026F, Research Triangle Park, 1984; pp. 570-571.

Goldman AM, Gossman WE, Friedlander PC. Reduction of sound levels with anti-noise in MR imaging. Radiology 1989;173:549-550.

Hall DA, et al. Acoustic, psychophysical, and neuroimaging measurements of the effectiveness of active cancellation during auditory functional magnetic resonance imaging. J Acoust Soc Am. 2009;125:347-59.

Hattori Y, Fukatsu H, Ishigaki T. Measurement and evaluation of the acoustic noise of a 3 Tesla MR scanner. Nagoya J Med Sci. 2007;69:23-28.

Hedeen RA, Edelstein WA. Characteristics and prediction of gradient acoustic noise in MR imagers. Magn Reson Med 1997;37:7-10.

Hurwitz R, Lane SR, Bell RA, Brant-Zawadzki MN. Acoustic analysis of gradient-coil noise in MR imaging. Radiology 1989;173:545-548.

International Commission on Non-Ionizing Radiation Protection (ICNIRP) Statement, Medical magnetic resonance procedures: protection of patients. Health Physics 2004;87:197-216.

Leithner K, et al. Psychological reactions in women undergoing fetal magnetic resonance imaging. Obstet Gynecol. 2008;111(2 Pt 1):396-402.

Mansfield PM, Glover PM. Beaumont J Sound generation in gradient coil structures for MRI. Magn Reson Med 1998;39:539-550.

Mansfield PM, et al. Active acoustic screening: design principles for quiet gradient coils in MRI. Meas Sci Technol 1994;5:1021-1025.

McJury MJ. Acoustic noise levels generated during high field MR imaging. Clinical Radiology 1995;50:331-334.

McJury M. Acoustic Noise and Magnetic Resonance Procedures. In: Magnetic Resonance Procedures: Health Effects and Safety. FG Shellock, Editor, CRC Press, Boca Raton, FL, 2001.

McJury M, Blug A, Joerger C, Condon B, Wyper D. Acoustic noise levels during magnetic resonance imaging scanning at 1.5 T. Brit J Radiol 1994;413-415.

McJury M, Shellock FG. Acoustic noise and MR procedures: A review. J Magn Reson Imaging 2000;12:37-45.

McJury M, et al. The use of active noise control (ANC) to reduce acoustic noise generated during MRI scanning: some initial results. Magn Reson Imaging 1997;15:319-322.

Melnick W. Hearing loss from noise exposure. In: Harris CM, ed. Handbook of Noise Control. New York: McGraw-Hill, 1979; pp. 2.

Miller LE, Keller AM. Regulation of occupational noise. In: Harris CM, ed. Handbook of noise control. New York: McGraw-Hill, 1979; pp. 1-16.

Moelker A, et al. Verbal communication in MR environments: effect of MR system acoustic noise on understanding. Radiology 2004;232:107-113.

Moelker A, Pattynama PM. Acoustic noise concerns in functional magnetic resonance imaging. Human Brain Mapping 2003;20:123-141.

More SR, Lim TC, Li M, Holland CK, Boyce S, Lee J-H. Acoustic noise characteristics of a 4 Tesla MRI scanner. Journal of Magnetic Resonance Imaging 2006;23:388-397.

Peelle JE, et al. Evaluating an acoustically quiet EPI sequence for use in fMRI studies of speech and auditory processing. Neuroimage. 2010;52:1410-9.

Philbin MK, Taber KH, Hayman LA. Preliminary report: changes in vital signs of term newborns during MR. Am J Neuroradiol 1996;17:1033-6.

Quirk ME, Letendre AJ, Ciottone RA, Lingley JF. Anxiety in patients undergoing MR imaging. Radiology 1989;170:464-466.

Reeves MJ, et al. Neonatal cochlear function: measurement after exposure to acoustic noise during in utero MR imaging. Radiology. 2010;257:802-9.

Robinson DW. Characteristics of occupational noise-induced hearing loss. In: Effects of Noise on Hearing. Henderson D, Hamernik RP, Dosjanjh DS, Mills JH, Editors. Raven Press, New York, 1976; pp. 383-405.

Roschmann P. Human auditory system response to pulsed radio frequency energy in RF coils for magnetic resonance at 2.4 to 170 MHz. Magn Reson Med 1991;21:197-215.

Ruckhäberle E, et al. In vivo intrauterine sound pressure and temperature measurements during magnetic resonance imaging (1.5 T) in pregnant ewes. Fetal Diagn Ther. 2008;24:203-10.

Schmitter S, Bock M. Acoustic noise-optimized verse pulses. Magn Reson Med. 2010 [Epub ahead of print]

Segbers M, et al. Shaping and timing gradient pulses to reduce MRI acoustic noise. Magn Reson Med. 2010;64:546-53.

Shellock FG, Kanal E. Policies, guidelines, and recommendations for MR imaging safety and patient management. J Magn Reson Imaging 1991;1:97-101.

Shellock FG, Morisoli SM, Ziarati M. Measurement of acoustic noise during MR imaging: Evaluation of six "worst-case" pulse sequences. Radiology 1994;191:91-93.

Shellock FG, et al. Determination of gradient magnetic field-induced acoustic noise associated with the use of echo planar and three-dimensional fast spin echo techniques. J Magn Reson Imaging 1998;8:1154-1157.

Strainer JC, et al. Functional MR of the primary auditory cortex: an analysis of pure tone activation and tone discrimination. Am J Roentgenol 1997;18:601-610.

Tomasi DG, Ernst T. Echo planar imaging at 4 Tesla with minimal acoustic noise. J Magn Reson Imaging 2003;128-130.

Ulmer JL, et al. Acoustic echo planar scanner noise and pure tone hearing thresholds: the effects of sequence repetition times and acoustic noise rates. J Comp Assist Tomogr 1998;22:480-486.

U.S. Department of Health and Human Services, Food and Drug Administration, Center for Devices and Radiological Health, Radiological Devices Branch, Division of Reproductive, Abdominal, and Radiological Devices, Office of Device Evaluation. Guidance for Industry and FDA Staff. Criteria for significant Risk Investigations of Magnetic Resonance Diagnostic Devices, July 14, 2003.

Body Piercing Jewelry

Ritual or decorative body piercing is extremely popular as a form of self-expression. Different types of materials are used to make body piercing jewelry including ferromagnetic and nonferromagnetic metals, as well as non-metallic materials. The presence of body piercing jewelry that is made from ferromagnetic or conductive material of a certain shape may present a problem for a patient referred for a magnetic resonance (MR) procedure or an individual in the MR environment.

Risks include uncomfortable sensations from movement or displacement that may be mild-to-moderate depending on the site of the body piercing and the ferromagnetic qualities of the jewelry (e.g., mass, degree of magnetic susceptibility, etc.). In extreme cases, serious injuries may occur. In addition, for body piercing jewelry made from electrically conducting material, there is a possibility of MRI-related heating that could cause excessive temperature increases and burns.

Because of potential safety issues, metallic body piercing jewelry should be removed prior to entering the MR environment. However, patients or individuals with body piercings are often reluctant to remove their jewelry. Therefore, if it is not possible to remove metallic body piercing jewelry, the patient or individual should be informed regarding the potential risks. In addition, if the body piercing jewelry is made from ferromagnetic material, some means of stabilization (e.g., application of adhesive tape or bandage) should be used to prevent movement or displacement.

To avoid potential heating of body piercing jewelry made from conductive materials, it is recommended to use gauze, tape, or other similar material to wrap the jewelry in such a manner as to insulate it (i.e., prevent contact) from the underlying skin. The patient should be instructed to immediately inform the MR system operator if heating or other unusual sensation occurs in association with the body piercing jewelry.

According to Muensterer (2004), even temporary or short-term piercing jewelry removal may lead to closure of the subcutaneous tract. Therefore, temporary replacement with a nonmetallic spacer may be indicated. This can be accomplished using the following procedure, as it was applied to umbilical piercing jewelry: (1) Disinfect the piercing and umbilical area with 70% isopropyl alcohol, (2) Open the piercing jewelry by removing the bead from the bar, (3) Place the tip of a tight-fitting intravenous catheter (14 or 16 gauge, without the needle) over the threaded tip of the bar, (4) Advance the intravenous catheter caudally, pushing the piercing out of the skin tract, and (5) Remove the jewelry and leaving the intravenous catheter in the subcutaneous skin tract as a spacer. After the intervention (or MRI examination), reinserted the umbilical piercing jewelry by following the described steps in reverse. Piercing jewelry located in other areas on the body may be replaced for MR examinations in the same way, with minor modifications. Of course, the above procedure must only be accomplished under the guidance and direction of a physician.

REFERENCES

Armstrong ML, Elkins L. Body art and MRI. Am J Nurs. 2005;105:65-6.

Deboer S, Seaver M, Angel E, Armstrong M. Puncturing myths about body piercing and tattooing. Nursing. 2008;38:50-54.

Laumann AE, Derick AJ. Tattoos and body piercings in the United States: a national data set. J Am Acad Dermatol. 2006;55:413-21.

Muensterer OJ. Temporary removal of navel piercing jewelry for surgery and imaging studies. Pediatrics. 2004;114:e384-6.

Shellock FG. MR safety and body piercing jewelry. Signals, No. 45, Issue 2, pp. 7, 2003.

Claustrophobia, Anxiety, and Emotional Distress in the MR Environment*

For certain patients that undergo magnetic resonance (MR) examinations, the experience may be associated with emotional distress. Referring physicians, radiologists, and MRI technologists can best manage affected patients by understanding the etiology of the problem and knowing the appropriate maneuver or intervention to implement in order to counter-act the condition.

The experience of "psychological distress" in the MR environment includes all subjectively unpleasant experiences attributable to the procedure. Distress for the patient can range from mild anxiety that can be handled with simple reassurance, to a more serious panic attack that may require psychiatric intervention or medication. Severe psychological reactions to MR examinations are characterized by the rapid onset of at least four of the following: nausea, paresthesias, palpitations, chest pain, faintness, dyspnea, choking sensation, sweating, trembling, vertigo, depersonalization, and fear of losing control or dying.

Many symptoms of a panic attack mimic over-activity of the sympathetic nervous system, prompting concern that catecholamine responses may precipitate cardiac arrhythmias or ischemia in susceptible patients. However, to date, this has not been observed in the clinical MR setting. Nevertheless, for a medically unstable patient, it is advisable to have physiologic monitoring and support readily available.

In the mildest form, distress is the normal amount of anxiety that a person may experience when undergoing a diagnostic procedure. Moderate distress, severe enough to be described as a dysphoric psychological reaction, has been reported by as many as 65% of the patients examined by MR imaging. The most severe forms of psychological distress described by patients include anxiety, claustrophobia, or panic attacks.

Claustrophobia is a disorder characterized by the marked, persistent, and excessive fear of enclosed spaces. In such affected individuals, exposure to an enclosed space such as that found with certain MR systems, almost invariably provokes an immediate anxiety response that, in its most extreme form, is indistinguishable from the panic attack described above.

The actual incidence of distress in the MR environment is highly variable across studies due to differences in outcome measures used to describe this phenomenon. Some investigatons indicated that as many as 20% of the individuals attempting to undergo MR procedures can't complete the exams secondary to serious distress such as claustrophobia or other unwanted sensations. In contrast, other investigations have reported that as few as 0.7% of individuals have incomplete or failed MR procedures due to distress.

THE IMPACT OF EMOTIONAL DISTRESS

Patient distress can contribute to adverse outcomes for the MR procedure. These adverse outcomes include unintentional exacerbation of patient distress, a compromise in the quality and, thus, the diagnostic aspects of the imaging study and decreased efficiency of the MRI facility due to delayed, prematurely terminated, or cancelled studies. Patient compliance during an MR procedure, such as the ability to remain in the MR system and to hold still long enough to complete the study, is of paramount importance to achieve a diagnostically acceptable examination. If a good quality study can't be obtained, the patient may require an invasive procedure in place of the inherently safer MR examination. Thus, for the distressed patient unable to undergo an MR procedure, there may be clinical, medico-legal, and economic related implications.

Increasing pressure to use MR system time efficiently to cover the costs of this expensive diagnostic imaging equipment puts greater stress on both staff and patients. The ability of referring physicians, radiologists, and MRI technologists to detect patient distress at the earliest possible time, to discover the source of the distress, and to provide appropriate intervention can greatly improve patient comfort, the quality of imaging, and efficiency of the facility.

FACTORS THAT CONTRIBUTE TO DISTRESS

Many factors contribute to distress experienced by certain patients undergoing MR procedures. Most commonly cited are concerns about the physical environment of the MR system. Also well documented is the anxiety associated with the underlying medical problem necessitating the MR examination. Certain individuals, such as those with psychiatric illnesses, may be predisposed to suffer greater distress.

The physical environment of the MR system is clearly one important source of distress. Sensations of apprehension, tension, worry, claustrophobia, anxiety, fear, and panic attacks have been directly attributed to the confining dimensions of the MR system. For example, for some scanners, the patient's "line of sight" may be three to ten inches from the inside of the MR system, prompting feelings of uncontrolled confinement and detachment.

Similar distressing sensations have been attributed to other aspects of the MR environment including the prolonged duration of the examination, the acoustic noise, the temperature and humidity within the MR system, and the stress related to restriction of movement. Additionally, being inside of the scanner may produce a feeling of sensory deprivation, which is also known to be a precursor of anxiety states.

Adverse psychological reactions are sometimes associated with MR procedures simply because the examination may be perceived by the patient as a "dramatic" medical test with an associated uncertainty of outcome, such that there may be fear of the presence of disease or other condition. In fact, any type of diagnostic procedure can produce anxiety for the patient.

MR systems that have an architecture that utilizes a vertical magnetic field offer a more open design that is presumed to reduce the frequency of distress associated with MR procedures. The latest versions of these "open" MR systems, despite having static magnetic field strengths of 0.3-Tesla or lower, have improved technology (i.e., faster gradient fields, optimized surface coils, etc.) that permit acceptable image quality for most types of standard, diagnostic imaging procedures. The latest generation of high-field-strength (1.5-Tesla and 3-Tesla) MR systems have shorter and wider bore configurations that likely mitigate feelings of being enclosed or being overly confined. In fact, Hunt et al. (2011) reported that the use of a 1.5-Tesla, wide-short-bore scanner increased the examination success rate in patients with claustrophobia and substantially reduced the need for anesthesia-assisted MRI examinations, even when claustrophobia was severe.

In 1993, a specially designed, low-field-strength (0.2-Tesla) MR system (Artoscan, Lunar Corporation/General Electric Medical Systems, Madison, WI and Esaote, Genoa, Italy) became commercially available for MR imaging of extremities. The use of this dedicated extremity MR system provides an accurate, reliable, and relatively inexpensive means (i.e., in comparison to the use of a whole-body MR system) of evaluating musculoskeletal abnormalities. In fact, the utilization of this extremity MR system to assess musculoskeletal pathology is an acceptable alternative to whole-body MR systems since the diagnostic capabilities for evaluation of the knee, shoulder, and other extremities has been reported to be comparable to mid- or high-field-strength MR systems.

The architecture of the extremity MR system has no confining features or other aspects that would typically create patient-related problems. This is because only the body part that requires imaging is placed inside the bore of the magnet during the MR examination. One research study reported that 100% of the MR examinations that were initiated were completed without being interrupted or cancelled for patient-related problems. The unique design of the extremity MR system is believed to have contributed to the successful completion of the MR procedures in the patients of this study.

Patients with pre-existing psychiatric disorders may be at greater risk for experiencing distress in the MR environment. Accordingly, patients with pre-existing conditions should be identified prior to MR examinations to implement anxiety-minimizing efforts (see below). Patients with other psychiatric illnesses such as depression and any illness complicated by thought dysfunction, such as schizophrenia or manic-depressive disorder, may also be at increased risk for distress in the MR environment.

Patients with psychiatric illnesses may, under normal circumstances, be able to tolerate the MR environment without a problem, as is clear from the thousands of subjects who participate in clinical neuroimaging and functional MRI research studies each year. However, the increased stress due to their medical illness or fear of medical illness can exacerbate their psychiatric symptoms to such an extent that they may have difficulty complying with MR procedures.

TECHNIQUES TO MINIMIZE PATIENT DISTRESS

Various procedures exist to minimize distress or anxiety in patients undergoing MR procedures (Table 1). Some measures should be employed for all examinations, while others may be required only if the patient experiences distress due to the factors described above.

Table 1. Techniques to manage patients with distress associated with MR procedures.

1) Prepare and educate the patient concerning specific aspects of the MR procedure (e.g., MR system dimensions, gradient noise, intercom system, constant presence of the MRI technologist, etc.).
2) Allow an appropriately screened relative or friend to remain with the patient during the MR examination.
3) Maintain verbal, visual, and/or physical contact with the patient during the MR procedure.

4) Use an appropriate stereo system to provide music to the patient.
5) Use an appropriate video monitor or goggles to provide a visual distraction to the patient.
6) Use a virtual reality environment system to provide audio and visual distraction.
7) Place the patient prone for the examination.
8) Position the patient feet-first instead of head-first into the MR system.
9) Use mirrors or prism glasses to redirect the patient's line of sight.
10) Use a blindfold so that the patient is not aware of the surroundings.
11) Use bright lights inside of the MR system.
12) Use a fan inside of the MR system.
13) Use vanilla scented oil or other aroma therapy.
14) Use relaxation techniques such as controlled breathing or mental imagery.
15) Use systematic desensitization.
16) Use medical hypnosis.
17) Use a sedative or other similar medication.

For All Patients Undergoing MR Procedures

Referring clinicians should take time to explain the reason for the MR procedure and what he/she expects to learn from the results with respect to the implications for treatment and prognosis. The single most important step is to educate the patient about the aspects of the MR examination that may be challenging or difficult. This includes conveying, in terms that are understandable to the patient, the internal dimensions of the MR system, the level of gradient magnetic field-induced acoustic noise to expect, and the estimated time duration of the examination.

Studies have documented a decrease in the incidence of premature termination of MR examinations when patients were provided with detailed information about the procedures. Accordingly, patients should be provided with an appropriate brochure or video presentation supplemented by a question and answer session with an MR-trained healthcare professional prior to the examination.

Many details of patient positioning in the MR system can increase comfort and, thus, minimize distress. Taking time to ensure comfortable positioning with sufficient padding and blankets to alleviate undue discomfort or pain is also important. Adequate ear protection should be provided routinely to decrease acoustic noise from the MR system, as needed (i.e., this is typically not required for low-field-strength MR scanners). Demonstration of the two-way intercom system, "squeeze ball", or other monitoring technique to reassure the patient that the MR staff is readily available during the examination is vital for proper patient management.

For Mildly-to-Moderately Distressed Patients

If a patient continues to experience distress after the afore-mentioned measures are implemented, additional interventions are required. Frequently, all that is necessary to successfully complete an MR examination is to allow an appropriately screened relative or friend to remain with the patient. A familiar person in the MR system room will often help an anxious patient develop an increased sense of security. If a supportive companion is not present, a staff member can maintain contact with the patient during the examination to decrease psychological distress.

Placing the patient prone so that the opening of the MR system can be seen will provide a sensation of being in a device that is more spacious. As such, prone positioning can alleviate the "closed-in" feelings frequently associated with being supine. Unfortunately, prone positioning may not be practical or appropriate if the patient has certain underlying medical conditions (e.g., shortness of breath, the presence of chest tubes, wearing a cervical fixation device, etc.). Another method of positioning the patient that may help is to place the individual feet-first instead of head-first into the scanner.

Mirrors or prism glasses can be used to permit the patient to maintain a vertical view of the outside of the MR system in order to minimize phobic responses. Using a blindfold or "eye pillow" (e.g., small pillow containing flax seeds) so that the patient is unaware of the close surroundings has also been suggested to be an effective technique for enabling anxious patients to successfully undergo MR procedures.

The environment of the MR system may be changed to optimize the management of apprehensive patients. For example, the presence of higher lighting levels tends to make most individuals feel less anxious. Therefore, the use of bright lights at either end and inside of the MR system can produce a less imposing environment for the patient. Using a fan inside of the scanner to increase airflow will also help reduce the sensation of confinement. In addition, aroma therapy (e.g., placing a cotton pad moistened with a few drops of lemon, vanilla, or cucumber oil in the MR system) can help reduce distress by providing the patient with a pleasant, olfactory stimulation.

Specialized systems that transmit music or audio communication through headphones have been developed specifically for use with MR systems. Reports have indicated that these devices successfully reduced symptoms of anxiety in patients during MR procedures. Furthermore, it is possible to provide visual stimulation to the patient via monitors or special goggles. Use of visual stimuli to distract patients tends to reduce distress. Finally, a system may be used to provide a calming virtual reality environment for the patient that may likewise serve as an acceptable means of audio and visual distraction from the MR procedure (this device is frequently used for functional MRI studies).

For Severely Distressed or Claustrophobic Patients

Patients who are at high risk for severe distress in the MR environment and can be identified as such by their referring clinician or by the scheduling MR staff person should be offered the opportunity to have pre-MR procedure behavioral therapy. MR procedures conducted in patients that previously refused or were unable to tolerate the MR environment have been reported to be successfully managed using relaxation techniques, systematic desensitization, and medical hypnosis.

In the majority of MRI facilities, patients severely affected by claustrophobia, anxiety, or panic attacks in response to MR procedures usually need sedation when attempts to counteract their distress fail. Using a short-acting sedative or an anxiolytic medication may be the only means of managing a patient with a high degree of anxiety. However, the use of sedatives in patients prior to and during MR procedures may not be required in all instances, nor is it always practical.

Importantly, the use of sedation in the MR environment requires special preparation involving several important patient management considerations. For example, the time when the patient is administered the medication for optimal effect prior to the examination must be considered along with the possibility that an adverse reaction may occur. The use of acceptable monitoring equipment operated by appropriately trained and experienced healthcare professionals is required to ensure patient safety. In addition, provisions should be available for an area to permit adequate recovery of the patient after an MR procedure that involves sedation.

[*Portions of this content were excerpted with permission from Gollub RL and Shellock FG. Claustrophobia, Anxiety, and Emotional Distress in the Magnetic Resonance Environment. In, Magnetic Resonance Procedures: Health Effects and Safety. FG Shellock, Editor, CRC Press, Boca Raton, FL, 2001. Reviewed and updated 2012.]

REFERENCES

Adamietz B, Cavallaro A, et al. Tolerance of magnetic resonance imaging in children and adolescents performed in a 1.5 Tesla MR scanner with an open design Rofo. 2007;179:826-831.

Bangard C, et al. MR imaging of claustrophobic patients in an open 1.0T scanner: motion artifacts and patient acceptability compared with closed bore magnets. Eur J Radiol. 2007;64:152-7.

Bigley J, et al. Neurolinguistic programming used to reduce the need for anaesthesia in claustrophobic patients undergoing MRI. 2010;83(986):113-7.

Dewey M, et al. Claustrophobia during magnetic resonance imaging: cohort study in over 55,000 patients. J Magn Reson Imaging. 2007;26:1322-7.

Eshed I, et al. Claustrophobia and premature termination of magnetic resonance imaging examinations. J Magn Reson Imaging. 2007;26:401-404.

Gollub RL, Shellock FG. Claustrophobia, Anxiety, and Emotional Distress in the Magnetic Resonance Environment. In, Magnetic Resonance Procedures: Health Effects and Safety. FG Shellock, Editor, CRC Press, Boca Raton, FL, 2001.

Harris LM, Cumming SR, Menzies RG. Predicting anxiety in magnetic resonance imaging scans. International Journal of Behavioral Medicine 2004;11:1-7.

Hunt CH, et al. Wide, short bore magnetic resonance at 1.5 T: Reducing the failure rate in claustrophobic patients. Clin Neuroradiol. 2011 May 20. [Epub ahead of print]

McGuinness TP. Hypnosis in the treatment of phobias: a review of the literature. Am J Clin Hypnosis 1984;26:261.

Murphy KJ, Brunberg JA. Adult claustrophobia, anxiety and sedation in MRI. Magnetic Resonance Imaging 1997;15:51.

Sarji SA, Abdullah BJ, Kumar G, et al. Failed magnetic resonance imaging examinations due to claustrophobia. Australas Radiol 1998;42:293.

Shellock FG, Kanal E. Policies, guidelines, and recommendations for MR imaging and patient management. J. Magn. Reson. Imaging 1991;1:97.

Shellock FG, Stone KR, Resnick D, et al. Subjective perceptions of MRI examinations performed using an extremity MR system. Signals 2000;32:16.

Spouse E, Gedroyc WM. MRI of the claustrophobic patient: interventionally configured magnets. Br J Radiol. 2000;73:146-151.

Thorpe S, Salkovskis PM, Dittner A. Claustrophobia in MRI: the role of cognitions. Magn Reson Imaging. 2008;26:1081-8.

Weinreb J, et al. Magnetic resonance imaging: improving patient tolerance and safety. American Journal of Roentgenology 1984;143:1285.

Wollman DE, et al. Tolerance of MRI procedures by the oldest old. Magn Reson Imaging. 2004;22:1299-304.

Epicardial Pacing Leads and Intracardiac Pacing Leads*

Although there is a theoretical risk that MRI examinations in patients with retained temporary *epicardial* leads (which consist of electrically conductive materials) could lead to cardiac excitation or thermal injury, such retained leads which are relatively short in length, usually do not form large loops, and are generally not believed to pose a significant hazard during MRI procedures.

Hartnell et al. reported on 51 patients with retained temporary epicardial pacing wires who underwent clinical MRI procedures. Of those patients examined with electrocardiographic monitoring, no arrhythmias were noted, and for all patients, no symptoms suggestive of arrhythmia or other cardiac dysfunction were identified (although the anatomic region examined and the RF energies used in the examinations were not specifically described). To date, there is no report of complications associated with performing MRI in a patient with retained epicardial leads.

By comparison, an *ex vivo* study of temporary *intracardiac*, transvenous pacing leads reported temperature increases of up to 63.1 degrees C. Preliminary results of an investigation confirmed that even unconnected temporary transvenous pacing (as well as permanent pacing) leads can undergo high temperature increases at 1.5-Tesla. In a chronic-pacemaker animal model undergoing an MRI examination at 1.5-Tesla, temperature increases of up to 20 degrees C were measured, although pathological and histological examination did not demonstrate heat-induced damage of the myocardium. The MRI conditions that generated such elevated lead temperatures included the use of the body RF coil to transmit RF energy over the area of the intracardiac pacing lead (e.g., an MRI examination of the chest/thorax).

Currently, to the best of our knowledge (i.e., the Consensus Group: Levine GN, Gomes AS, Arai AE, Bluemke DA, Flamm SD, Kanal E, Manning WJ, Martin ET, Smith JM, Wilke N, Shellock FG) there are no studies assessing the safety of temporary pacemakers (lead and external pulse generator). Unlike permanent devices, temporary pacemakers use unfixed leads that are more prone to movement, longer leads that may be more prone to induction of lead currents, and a less sophisticated pulse generator, which makes these devices more susceptible to electromagnetic interference.

Thus, patients with retained temporary *epicardial* pacing wires are believed to be able to safely undergo MRI procedures. Importantly, these patients do not need to be routinely screened for the presence of such wires before scanning. Because of the possible risks involved with temporary-pacemaker external pulse generators, such pulse generators should not be allowed in the MRI environment.

By comparison, scanning patients with temporary *intracardiac* pacing leads (without the pulse generator) is not recommended, although lead heating might be minimized or avoided by scanning anatomic regions above (e.g., head/brain) or below (e.g., lower extremities) the cardiac pacing leads. Furthermore, because the harsh electromagnetic environment associated with the MR system can alter the operation of an external pulse generator or damage it, it may not be possible to reliably pace the patient during the MRI examination, which makes the issue of scanning a patient with a temporary intracardiac, transvenous lead irrelevant in most cases.

Abandoned Intracardiac Pacing Leads

Over the lifetime using a cardiac pacemaker, an intracardiac pacing lead may be "abandoned" and replaced due to lead fracture, insulation breaks, dislodgement, or other failures and abnormalities in pacing or sensing. An abandoned lead is disconnected from the pulse generator and, during certain MR operating conditions, it may undergo substantial heating, as reported by Langman et al. (2011). Until further studies can define safe-scanning conditions for abandoned intracardiac pacing leads, MRI healthcare professionals should be aware of the higher risk of RF-induced lead tip heating.

[Portions of this section are excerpted with permission from Levine GN, Gomes AS, Arai AE, Bluemke DA, Flamm SD, Kanal E, Manning WJ, Martin ET, Smith JM, Wilke N, Shellock FG. Safety of magnetic resonance imaging in patients with cardiovascular devices: an American Heart Association scientific statement from the Committee on Diagnostic and Interventional Cardiac Catheterization. Circulation 2007;116:2878-2891. Reviewed and revised, 2012.]

REFERENCES

Achenbach S, et al. Effects of magnetic resonance imaging on cardiac pacemakers and electrodes. Am Heart J 1997;134:467-473.

Bottomley PA, Kumar A, et al. Designing passive MRI-safe implantable conducting leads with electrodes. Med Phys 2010;37:3828-43.

Dempsey MF, Condon B, Hadley DM. Investigation of the factors responsible for burns during MRI. J Magn Reson Imaging. 2001;13:627–631.

Hartnell GG, et al. Safety of MR imaging in patients who have retained metallic materials after cardiac surgery. Am J Roentgenol. 1997;168:1157–1159.

Langman DA, et al. Abandoned pacemaker leads are a potential risk for patients undergoing MRI. Pacing Clin Electrophysiol. 2011 Jul 28. [Epub ahead of print]

Langman DA, et al. Pacemaker lead tip heating in abandoned and pacemaker-attached leads at 1.5 Tesla MRI. J Magn Reson Imaging. 2011;33:426-31.

Levine GN, et al. Safety of magnetic resonance imaging in patients with cardiovascular devices: an American Heart Association scientific statement from the Committee on Diagnostic and Interventional Cardiac Catheterization. Circulation 2007;116:2878-2891.

Luechinger R, et al. In vivo heating of pacemaker leads during magnetic resonance imaging. Eur Heart J. 2005;26:376-383.

Shellock FG, Valencerina S, Fischer L. MRI-related heating of pacemaker at 1.5- and 3-Tesla: Evaluation with and without pulse generator attached to leads. Circulation 2005;112;Supplement II:561.

Extremity MR System

In 1993, a specially designed, low-field-strength (0.2-Tesla MR system, Artoscan, Lunar Corporation Madison, WI and General Electric Medical Systems, Milwaukee, WI/Esaote, Genoa, Italy) MR system became commercially available for MR imaging of extremities. This MR system uses a small-bore permanent magnet to image feet, ankles, knees, hands, wrists, and elbows.

The ergonomic design of the extremity scanner is such that the body part of interest is placed inside the magnet bore, with the patient positioned in a seated position or supine (i.e., depending on the body part that is imaged). The entire extremity MR system has a built-in radiofrequency shield and multiple body-part-specific extremity coils.

A major advantage of this particular extremity MR system is that it can be sited in a relatively small space (e.g., approximately 100 square feet) without the need for a special power source, magnetic field shielding, or radiofrequency shielding. Of note is that MR imaging using the extremity MR system has been demonstrated to provide a sensitive, accurate, and reliable assessment of various forms of musculoskeletal pathology.

Because of the unique design features of the extremity MR system (which includes a low-field-strength static magnetic field with a relatively small fringe field) and in consideration of how patients are positioned for MR procedures using this device (i.e., only the body part imaged is placed within the magnet bore while the rest of the body remains outside), it may be possible to safely image patients with aneurysm clips, even if they are made from ferromagnetic materials. Furthermore, it may be possible to perform extremity MR imaging in patients with cardiac pacemakers or implantable cardioverter defibrillators (ICDs). Therefore, investigations were conducted to specifically evaluate these safety issues.

PATIENTS WITH FERROMAGNETIC ANEURYSM CLIPS

A study was performed to assess magnetic field interactions for a variety of aneurysm clips exposed to the 0.2-Tesla extremity MR system. Twenty-two different aneurysm clips were evaluated including those made from nonferromagnetic, weakly ferromagnetic, and ferromagnetic materials (e.g., a Heifetz aneurysm clip made from 17-7PH and a Yasargil, Model FD aneurysm clip). The results indicated that none of the aneurysm clips displayed substantial magnetic field interactions in association with exposure to the 0.2-Tesla extremity MR system.

Due to the design features of the extremity MR system and in consideration of how patients are positioned during the use of this scanner (i.e., the head does not enter the magnet bore), it is considered safe to perform MR imaging in patients with the specific aneurysm clips evaluated for magnetic field interactions. These findings effectively permit an important diagnostic imaging modality to be used to evaluate patients with suspected musculoskeletal abnormalities using the Artoscan Extremity MR system.

Various studies have reported that patients with Heifetz (17-7PH) and Yasargil, Model FD aneurysm clips (i.e., two of the clips evaluated in the study using the Artoscan scanner) should not undergo MR imaging using MR systems with conventional designs because of the strong attraction shown by these implants, which poses a substantial hazard to patients.

PATIENTS WITH CARDIAC PACEMAKERS AND IMPLANTABLE CARDIOVERTER DEFIBRILLATORS

In general, patients with cardiac pacemakers and implantable cardioverter defibrillators (ICDs), especially if the devices are older models (i.e., pre-1996), are generally not permitted to undergo MR procedures. However, due to the design of the 0.2-Tesla Artoscan extremity MR system it may be possible to safely perform MR examinations in patients with these devices under certain conditions.

Since the magnetic fringe field of the extremity MR system is contained in close proximity to the 0.2-Tesla magnet and this scanner has an integrated Faraday cage, only the patient's examined extremity is exposed to electromagnetic fields when a procedure is performed. Notably, it is not possible for the MR system's gradient or RF electromagnetic fields to induce currents in a pacemaker or ICD because the patient's thorax (i.e., where the pacemaker or ICD is typically implanted) remains outside of the bore of the MR system.

Ex vivo experiments were conducted to assess MRI issues for seven different cardiac pacemakers and seven different implantable cardioverter defibrillators manufactured by Medtronic, Inc. (Minneapolis, MN), as follows:

Device	Name	Model
Pacemaker	Elite II	7086
Pacemaker	Thera D	7944
Pacemaker	Thera D	7960I
Pacemaker	Thera DR	7962i
Pacemaker	Thera SR	8940
Pacemaker	Kappa	400
Pacemaker	Kappa	700
ICD	PCD	7217D
ICD	Jewel	7219D
ICD	Jewel Plus	7220C
ICD	Micro Jewel	7221Cx
ICD	Micro Jewel II	7223Cx
ICD	Prototype	7250G
ICD	Prototype	7271

Magnetic field interactions were assessed relative to the 0.2-Tesla static magnetic field of the extremity MR system. Additionally, the cardiac pacemakers and implantable cardioverter defibrillators were operated with various lead systems attached while immersed in a tank containing physiologic saline (i.e., this apparatus was used to simulate the thorax). This *in vitro* experimental set-up was oriented in parallel and perpendicular positions relative to the closest part of the MR system to mimic patients undergoing MR procedures using this extremity scanner.

MR studies were performed on a phantom using T1-weighted, spin echo and gradient echo pulse sequences. Various functions of the pacemakers and ICDs were evaluated before, during, and after MR imaging. The results indicated that magnetic field interactions did not present problems for the devices and the activation of the pacemakers and ICDs did not substantially affect image quality. Importantly, the operation of the extremity MR system produced no alterations in the function of the cardiac pacemakers and ICDs. Therefore, in consideration of these data and in view of how patients are positioned during MR procedures using the Artoscan extremity MR system, it should be safe to perform examinations in patients with the specific cardiac pacemakers and implantable cardioverter defibrillators evaluated in this study.

REFERENCES

Ahn JM, Sartoris DJ, Kank HS, Resnick D. Gamekeeper thumb: comparison of MR arthrography with conventional arthrography and MR imaging in cadavers. Radiology 1998;206:737-744.

Barile A, et al. The use of a "dedicated" MRI system in the evaluation of knee joint diseases. Clinical MRI 1995;5:79-82.

Franklin PD, Lemon RA, Barden HS. Accuracy of imaging the menisci on an in-office, dedicated, magnetic resonance imaging extremity system. Am J Sports Med 1998;25:382-388.

Kersting-Sommerhoff B, Hof N, Lenz M, Gerhardt P. MRI of peripheral joints with a low-field dedicated system: a reliable and cost-effective alternative to high-field units? Eur Radiol 1996;6:561-565.

Maschicchi C. Dedicated MR system and acute trauma of the musculo-skeletal system. Eur J Radiol 1996;22:7-10.

Peterfy CG, Roberts T, Genant HK. Dedicated extremity MR imaging: an emerging technology. Radiol Clin North Am 1997;35:1-20.

Shellock FG. Magnetic Resonance Procedures: Health Effects and Safety. CRC Press, LLC, Boca Raton, FL, 2001.

Shellock FG, Bert, JM, Fritts HM, Gundry C, Easton R, Crues JV. Evaluation of the rotator cuff and glenoid labrum using a 0.2-Tesla, extremity MR system: MR results compared to surgical findings. Journal of Magnetic Resonance Imaging 2001;14:763-770.

Shellock FG, Crues JV. Aneurysm clips: Assessment of magnetic field interaction associated with a 0.2-T extremity MR system. Radiology 1998;208:407-409.

Shellock FG, O'Neil M, Ivans V, Kelly D, O'Connor M, Toay L, Crues JV. Cardiac pacemakers and implantable cardiac defibrillators are unaffected by operation of an extremity MR system. Am J Roentgenol 1999;72:165-17.

Shellock FG, Stone K, Crues JV. Development and clinical applications of kinematic MRI of the patellofemoral joint using an extremity MR system. Med Sci Sport Exerc 1999;31:788-791.

Shellock FG, Mullen M, Stone K, Coleman M, Crues JV. Kinematic MRI evaluation of the effect of bracing on patellar positions: qualitative assessment using an extremity MR system. Journal of Athletic Training 2000;35:44-49.

Guidelines for the Management of the Post-Operative Patient Referred for a Magnetic Resonance Procedure*

There is often confusion regarding the issue of performing a magnetic resonance (MR) procedure during the post-operative period in a patient with a metallic implant or device. Studies have supported that, if a metallic object is a "passive implant" (i.e., there is no electronically- or magnetically-activated component associated with the operation of the device) and it is made from nonferromagnetic material, the patient may undergo an MR procedure immediately after implantation using an MR system operating at 1.5-Tesla or less (or, the field strength that was used to test the device, including 3-Tesla). In fact, there are several reports that describe placement of vascular stents, coils, filters, and other implants using MR-guided procedures that include the use of high-field-strength (1.5- and 3-Tesla) MR systems. Additionally, a patient or individual with a nonferromagnetic, passive implant is allowed to enter the MR environment associated with a scanner operating at 1.5-Tesla (or, the field strength that was used to test the device, including 3-Tesla) or less immediately after its implantation.

For an implant or device that exhibits "weakly magnetic" qualities, it may be necessary to wait a period of six weeks after implantation before performing an MR procedure or allowing the individual or patient to enter the MR environment. For example, certain intravascular and intracavitary coils, stents, and filters designated as "weakly magnetic" become firmly incorporated into tissue a minimum of six weeks following placement. In these cases, retentive or counter-forces provided by tissue ingrowth, scarring, granulation or other mechanisms serve to prevent these objects from presenting risks or hazards to patients or individuals in the MR environment.

However, patients with implants or devices that are "weakly magnetic" but rigidly fixed in the body (e.g., bone screws, other orthopedic implants, or other devices) may be studied immediately after implantation. Specific information pertaining to the recommended post-operative waiting period may be found in the labeling or product insert for an implant or device.

Special Note: If there is any concern regarding the integrity of the tissue with respect to its ability to retain the implant or object in place or the implant cannot be properly identified, the patient or individual should not be exposed to the MR environment.

[*The document, **Guidelines for the Management of the Post-Operative Patient Referred for a Magnetic Resonance Procedure,** was developed by the Institute for Magnetic Resonance Safety, Education, and Research (IMRSER) and published with permission. Reviewed and updated 2012.]

REFERENCES

Ahmed S, Shellock FG. Magnetic resonance imaging safety: implications for cardiovascular patients. Journal of Cardiovascular Magnetic Resonance 2001;3:171-181.

Bueker A, et al. Real-time MR fluoroscopy for MR-guided iliac artery stent placement. J Magn Reson Imaging 2000;12:616-622.

http://www.IMRSER.org; website for the Institute for Magnetic Resonance Safety, Education, and Research

Manke C, Nitz WR, Djavidani B, et al. MR imaging-guided stent placement in iliac arterial stenoses: A feasibility study. Radiology 2001;219:527-534.

Rutledge JM, et al. Safety of magnetic resonance immediately following Palmaz stent implant: a report of three cases. Catheter Cardiovasc Interv 2001;53:519-523.

Sawyer-Glover A, Shellock FG. Pre-MRI procedure screening: recommendations and safety considerations for biomedical implants and devices. J Magn Reson Imaging 2000;12:92-106.

Shellock FG. Guidelines for the Management of the Post-Operative Patient Referred for a Magnetic Resonance Procedure. Signals, No. 47, Issue 3, pp. 14, 2003.

Shellock FG. Magnetic Resonance Procedures: Health Effects and Safety. CRC Press, LLC, Boca Raton, FL, 2001.

Shellock FG, Cosendai G, Park S-M, Nyenhuis JA. Implantable microstimulator: magnetic resonance safety at 1.5-Tesla. Investigative Radiology 2004;39:591-594.

Shellock FG, Crues JV. MR procedures: biologic effects, safety, and patient care. Radiology, 2004;232:635-652.

Spuentrup E, et al. Magnetic resonance-guided coronary artery stent placement in a swine model. Circulation 2002;105:874-879.

Teitelbaum GP, et al. MR imaging artifacts, ferromagnetism, and magnetic torque of intravascular filters, stents, and coils. Radiology 1988;166:657-664.

Teitelbaum GP, et al. Ferromagnetism and MR imaging: safety of cartoid vascular clamps. Am J Neuroradiol 1990;11:267-272.

Teitelbaum GP, Ortega HV, Vinitski S, et al. Low artifact intravascular devices: MR imaging evaluation. Radiology 1988;168:713-719.

Teitelbaum GP, et al. Evaluation of ferromagnetism and magnetic resonance imaging artifacts of the Strecker tantalum vascular stent. Cardiovasc Intervent Radiol 1989;12:125-127.

Guidelines for Screening Patients for MR Procedures and Individuals for the MR Environment

The establishment of thorough and effective screening procedures for patients and other individuals is one of the most critical components of a program that guards the safety of all those preparing to undergo magnetic resonance (MR) procedures or those needing to enter the MR environment. An important aspect of protecting patients and individuals from MR system-related accidents and injuries involves an understanding of the risks associated with the various implants, devices, accessories, and other objects that may cause problems in this setting. This requires constant attention and diligence to obtain information and documentation about these objects in order to provide the safest MR setting possible.

In addition, because most MR-related incidents have been due to deficiencies in screening methods and/or the lack of properly controlling access to the MR environment (especially with regard to preventing personal items and other potentially problematic objects from entering the MR system room), it is crucial to set up procedures and guidelines to prevent such incidents from occurring.

Magnetic Resonance (MR) Procedure Screening for Patients

Certain aspects of screening patients for MR procedures may take place during the scheduling process. These activities should be conducted by a healthcare worker specially trained in MR-safety (i.e., trained to understand the potential hazards and issues associated with the MR environment and MR procedures and to be familiar with the information contained on the screening forms for patients and individuals). While scheduling the patient, it may be ascertained if the patient has an implant or device that may be contraindicated or requires special attention for the MR procedure (e.g., a ferromagnetic aneurysm clip, pacemaker, neurostimulation system, etc.) or if there is a condition that needs careful consideration (e.g., the patient is pregnant, has a disability, history of renal failure, metallic foreign body, etc.). Preliminary screening helps to prevent scheduling patients that may be inappropriate candidates for MR examinations.

After preliminary screening, the patient must undergo comprehensive screening in preparation for the MR examination. Comprehensive screening involves the use of a printed form to document the screening procedure, a review of the information on the screening form, and a verbal interview to verify the information on the form and to allow for discussion of concerns that the patient may have. An MR-safety trained healthcare professional must conduct this important aspect of patient screening.

The screening form entitled, *Magnetic Resonance (MR) Procedure Screening Form for Patients* was created in conjunction with the Medical, Scientific, and Technology Advisory Board and the Corporate Advisory Board of the Institute for Magnetic Resonance Safety, Education, and Research (IMRSER) **(Figure 1)**. A "downloadable" version of this form may be obtained from the web sites, www.IMRSER.org and www.MRIsafety.com. This form is also available in Spanish **(Figure 2**, Translated by Olga Fernandez-Flygare, M.S., Brain Mapping Center, UCLA School of Medicine, Los Angeles, CA and Maelesa Rachele Oriente-Padilla', Loyola-Marymount University, Los Angeles, CA).

Page one of the screening form requests general patient-related information (name, age, sex, height, weight, etc.) as well as information regarding the reason for the MR examination and/or symptoms that may be present. Pertinent information about the patient is required not only to ensure that the medical records are up-to-date, but also in the event that the MRI facility needs to contact the referring physician for additional information regarding the examination or to verify the patient's medical condition.

The form requests information regarding a prior surgical procedure to help determine if there may be an implant or device present that could create a problem. Information is also requested pertaining to prior diagnostic imaging studies that may be helpful to review for assessment of the patient's condition.

Next, questions are posed to determine if there are issues that should be discussed with the patient prior to permitting entry to the MR environment. For example, information is requested regarding any problem with a previous MR examination, an injury to the eye involving a metallic object, or injury from a metallic foreign body. Questions are posed to obtain information about current or recently taken medications as well as the presence of drug allergies. There are also questions asked to assess past and present medical conditions that may affect the MR procedure or the use of an MRI contrast agent.

Important Information: MRI Contrast Agents and Nephrogenic Systemic Fibrosis (NSF). The American College of Radiology (ACR) Contrast Committee and the Subcommittee for MR Safety members recommend pre-screening patients prior to the administration of Gadolinium-Based MR Contrast Agents (GBMCA), as follows:

A recent (e.g., last 6 weeks) Glomerular Filtration Rate (GFR) assessment be reviewed for patients with a history of:

- Renal disease (including solitary kidney, renal transplant, renal tumor)
- Age >60 years old
- History of hypertension
- History of diabetes
- History of severe hepatic disease/liver transplant/pending liver transplant. For patients in this category, *only*, it is recommended that the patient's GFR assessment be nearly contemporaneous with the MR examination for which the GBMCA is to be administered.

Please review the latest information for the management of patients with underlying health conditions associated with NSF, including:

www.acr.org

www.fda.gov/Drugs/DrugSafety/ucm223966.htm

www.fda.gov/NewsEvents/Newsroom/PressAnnouncements/ucm225286.htm

www.acr.org/SecondaryMainMenuCategories/quality_safety/contrast_manual.aspx

www.acr.org/SecondaryMainMenuCategories/quality_safety/contrast_manual/Nephrogenic SystemicFibrosis.aspx

In consideration of the above, questions are posed to the patient to determine if there are conditions that may need to be considered relative to the use of MRI contrast agents and the issue of NSF. For more information on this topic, refer to the section entitled, **MRI Contrast Agents and Nephrogenic Systemic Fibrosis (NSF)***.

At the bottom of page one, there is a section for female patients that poses questions that may impact MR procedures. For example, questions regarding the date of the last menstrual period, pregnancy, or late menstrual period are included. A definite or possible pregnancy must be identified prior to permitting the patient into the MR environment so that the risk vs. the benefit of the MR procedure can be considered and discussed with the patient. MR examinations should only be performed in pregnant patients to address important clinical questions. MR facilities should have a clearly defined procedure to follow in the event that the patient has a possible or confirmed pregnancy.

Questions pertaining to the date of the last menstrual period, use of oral contraceptives or hormonal therapy, and fertility medication are necessary for female patients undergoing MR procedures that are performed to evaluate breast disease or for OB/GYN applications, as these may alter tissue contrast on MR imaging. An inquiry about breastfeeding is included in case the administration of MRI contrast media is being considered for use in nursing mothers.

Page 2 of the form has the following statement at the top of the page: **"WARNING: Certain implants, devices, or objects may be hazardous to you and/or may interfere with the MR procedure (i.e., MRI, MR angiography, functional MRI, MR spectroscopy). <u>Do not enter</u> the MR system room or MR environment if you have any question or concern regarding an implant, device, or object. Consult the MRI Technologist or Radiologist BEFORE entering the MR system room. The MR system magnet is ALWAYS on."**

Next, there is a section that lists various implants, devices, and objects to identify anything that could be hazardous to the patient undergoing the MR procedure or that may produce an artifact that could interfere with the interpretation of the MR examination. In general, these items are arranged on the checklist in order of the relative hazard or risk (e.g., aneurysm clip, cardiac pacemaker, implantable cardioverter defibrillator, electronic implant, etc.), followed by items that may produce imaging artifacts that could be problematic for the interpretation of the MR procedure. Additionally, questions are posed to determine if the patient has a breathing problem, movement disorder, or claustrophobia.

Figures of the human body are included on the second page of the form as a means of showing the location of any object inside of or on the body. This information allows the patient to indicate the approximate position of an object that may be hazardous or that could interfere with the interpretation of the MR procedure as a result of producing an artifact.

Page 2 of the screening form also has an *Important Instructions* section that states: **"Before entering the MR environment or MR system room, you must remove <u>all</u> metallic objects including hearing aids, dentures, partial plates, keys, beeper, cell phone, eyeglasses, hair pins, barrettes, jewelry, body piercing jewelry, watch, safety pins,**

paperclips, money clip, credit cards, bank cards, magnetic strip cards, coins, pens, pocket knife, nail clipper, tools, clothing with metal fasteners, & clothing with metallic threads. Please consult the MRI Technologist or Radiologist if you have any question or concern BEFORE you enter the MR system room."

Finally, there is a statement that indicates hearing protection is "advised or required" to prevent possible problems or hazards related to acoustic noise. In general, this should not be an option for a patient undergoing an MR procedure on a high-field-strength MR system. Alternatively, it may be unnecessary for a patient to use hearing protection if undergoing an MR procedure on a low-field-strength MR system.

Importantly, undergoing previous MR procedures without incidents does not guarantee a safe subsequent MR examination. Various factors (e.g., the field strength of the MR system, the orientation of the patient, the orientation of a metallic implant or object, etc.) can substantially change the scenario. Thus, a written screening form must be completed each time a patient prepares to undergo an MR examination.

With the use of any type of written questionnaire, limitations exist related to incomplete or incorrect answers provided by the patient. For example, there may be difficulties associated with patients who are impaired with respect to their vision, language fluency, or level of literacy. Therefore, an appropriate accompanying family member or other individual (e.g., referring physician) should be involved in the screening process to verify any information that may impact patient safety. Versions of this form should also be available in other languages, as needed (i.e., specific to the demographics of the MRI facility).

In the event that the patient is comatose or unable to communicate, the written screening form should be completed by the most qualified individual (e.g., physician, family member, etc.) who has knowledge about the patient's medical history and present condition. If the screening information is inadequate, it is advisable to look for surgical scars on the patient and/or to obtain plain films of the skull and/or chest to search for implants that may be hazardous in the MR environment (e.g., aneurysm clips, cardiac pacemakers, neurostimulation systems, etc.).

Following completion of the *Magnetic Resonance (MR) Procedure Screening Form for Patients*, an MR-safety trained healthcare professional must review the form's content. Next, a verbal interview must be conducted by the MR-safety trained healthcare professional to verify the information on the form and to allow discussion of any question or concern that the patient may have. This provides a mechanism for clarification and confirmation of the answers to the questions posed to the patient so that there is no miscommunication regarding important MR safety issues. In addition, because the patient may not be fully aware of the medical terminology used for a particular implant or device, it is imperative that this particular information on the form be discussed during the verbal interview.

After the comprehensive screening procedure is completed, a patient that is transferred by a stretcher, gurney, or wheelchair to the MR system room should be checked thoroughly for metallic objects such as ferromagnetic oxygen tanks, monitors, sand bags with metal shot, or other objects that could pose a hazard. Obviously, only nonferromagnetic stretchers, gurneys, wheelchairs and accessories should be allowed into the MR system room.

Magnetic Resonance (MR) Environment Screening for Individuals

Before any non-patient individual (e.g., MRI technologist, physician, relative, visitor, allied healthcare professional, maintenance worker, custodial worker, fire fighter, security officer, etc.) is allowed into the MR environment, he or she must be screened by an MR-safety trained healthcare professional. Proper screening for individuals involves the use of a printed form to document the procedure, a review of the information on the form, and a verbal interview to verify the information on the form and to allow discussion of any question or concern that the individual may have before being permitted into the MR environment.

Important Note: If for any reason the individual undergoing screening may need to enter the MR system and, thus, become exposed to the electromagnetic fields used for an MR procedure, this person must be screened using the *Magnetic Resonance (MR) Procedure Screening Form for Patients.*

In general, magnetic resonance (MR) screening forms were developed with patients in mind and, therefore, tend to pose many questions that are inappropriate or confusing to other individuals that may need to enter the MR environment. Therefore, a screening form was created specifically for individuals that need to enter the MR environment and/or MR system room. This form, entitled, *Magnetic Resonance (MR) Environment Screening Form for Individuals* was developed in conjunction with the Medical, Scientific, and Technology Advisory Board and the Corporate Advisory Board of the Institute for Magnetic Resonance Safety, Education, and Research (IMRSER) (**Figure 3**). A "downloadable" version of this form may be obtained from the web sites, www.IMRSER.org and www.MRIsafety.com.

At the top of this form, the following statement is displayed: **"The MR system has a very strong magnetic field that may be hazardous to individuals entering the MR environment or MR system room if they have certain metallic, electronic, magnetic, or mechanical implants, devices, or objects. Therefore, all individuals are required to fill out this form BEFORE entering the MR environment or MR system room. Be advised, the MR system magnet is ALWAYS on."**

The screening form for individuals requests general information (name, age, address, etc.) and poses important questions to determine if there are possible problems or issues that should be discussed with the individual prior to permitting entry to the MR environment.

A warning statement is also provided on the form, as follows: **"WARNING: Certain implants, devices, or objects may be hazardous to you in the MR environment or MR system room. Do not enter the MR environment or MR system room if you have any question or concern regarding an implant, device, or object."**

In addition, there is a section that lists implants, devices, and objects to identify the presence of an object that may be hazardous to an individual in the MR environment (e.g., an aneurysm clip, cardiac pacemaker, implantable cardioverter defibrillator (ICD), electronic or magnetically activated device, metallic foreign body, etc).

Finally, there is an *Important Instructions* section on the form that states: **"Remove all metallic objects before entering the MR environment or MR system room including hearing aids, beeper, cell phone, keys, eyeglasses, hair pins, barrettes, jewelry (including body piercing jewelry), watch, safety pins, paperclips, money clip, credit cards, bank cards, magnetic strip cards, coins, pens, pocket knife, nail clipper, steel-toed boots/shoes, and tools. Loose metallic objects are especially prohibited in the MR system room and MR environment. Please consult the MRI Technologist or Radiologist if you have any question or concern BEFORE you enter the MR system room."**

The proper use of this written form along with thorough verbal screening of the individual by an MR safety trained healthcare worker will prevent accidents and injuries in the MR environment.

[*The screening forms, *Magnetic Resonance (MR) Procedure Screening Form For Patients* and *Magnetic Resonance (MR) Environment Screening Form for Individuals* were developed in conjunction with the Institute for Magnetic Resonance Safety,

Education, and Research (IMRSER) and published with permission. Reviewed and updated 2012.]

REFERENCES

Kanal E, Barkovich AJ, Bell C, et al. ACR guidance document for safe MR practices: 2007. AJR Am J Roentgenol. 2007;188:1447-1474.

Sawyer-Glover A, Shellock FG. Pre-Magnetic Resonance Procedure Screening, In: Magnetic Resonance Procedures: Health Effects and Safety, FG Shellock, Editor, CRC Press, LLC, Boca Raton, FL, 2001.

Sawyer-Glover A, Shellock FG. Pre-MRI procedure screening: recommendations and safety considerations for biomedical implants and devices. J Magn Reson Imaging 2000;12: 92-106.

Shellock FG. New recommendations for screening patients for suspected orbital foreign bodies. Signals, No. 36, Issue 4, 2001, pp. 8-9.

Shellock FG. Biomedical implants and devices: assessment of magnetic field interactions with a 3.0-Tesla MR system. J Magn Reson Imaging 2002;16:721-732.

Shellock FG. MR safety update 2002: Implants and devices. Journal of Magnetic Resonance Imaging 2002;16:485-496.

Shellock FG, Crues JV. Commentary. MR safety and the American College of Radiology White Paper. American Journal of Roentgenology 2002;178:1349-1352.

Shellock FG, Crues JV. MR procedures: biologic effects, safety, and patient care. Radiology, 2004;232:635-652.

Shellock FG, Kanal E. Policies, guidelines, and recommendations for MR imaging safety and patient management. J Magn Reson Imaging 1991;1:97-101.

Shellock FG, Kanal E. Policies, guidelines, and recommendations for MR imaging safety and patient management. J Magn Reson Imaging 1991;1: 97-101.

Shellock FG, Kanal E. Magnetic Resonance: Bioeffects, Safety, and Patient Management. Second Edition, Lippincott-Raven Press, New York, 1996.

Shellock FG, Kanal E. SMRI Report. Policies, guidelines and recommendations for MR imaging safety and patient management. Questionnaire for screening patients before MR procedures. J Magn Reson Imaging 1994;4:749-751, 1994.

Shellock FG, Spinazzi A. MRI Safety Update: 2008, Part 2, Screening patients for MRI. American Journal of Roentgenology 2008;191:12-21.

www.acr.org; the website for the American College of Radiology
www.IMRSER.org; website for the Institute for Magnetic Resonance Safety, Education, and Research

Figure 1. Magnetic Resonance (MR) Procedure Screening Form For Patients (Developed in conjunction with the Institute for Magnetic Resonance Safety, Education, and Research, www.IMRSER.org).

MAGNETIC RESONANCE (MR) PROCEDURE SCREENING FORM FOR PATIENTS

Date ___/___/___   Patient Number _____

Name _____ Age _____ Height _____ Weight _____
        Last name   First name   Middle Initial

Date of Birth ___/___/___   Male ☐ Female ☐   Body Part to be Examined _____
             month day year

Address _____   Telephone (home) (____) ____-____

City _____   Telephone (work) (____) ____-____

State _____ Zip Code _____

Reason for MRI and/or Symptoms _____

Referring Physician _____   Telephone (____) ____-____

1. Have you had prior surgery or an operation (e.g., arthroscopy, endoscopy, etc.) of any kind?   ☐ No   ☐ Yes
   If yes, please indicate the date and type of surgery:
   Date ___/___/___   Type of surgery _____
   Date ___/___/___   Type of surgery _____
2. Have you had a prior diagnostic imaging study or examination (MRI, CT, Ultrasound, X-ray, etc.)?   ☐ No   ☐ Yes
   If yes, please list: Body part   Date   Facility
   MRI   _____ ___/___/___ _____
   CT/CAT Scan   _____ ___/___/___ _____
   X-Ray   _____ ___/___/___ _____
   Ultrasound   _____ ___/___/___ _____
   Nuclear Medicine _____ ___/___/___ _____
   Other   _____ ___/___/___ _____

3. Have you experienced any problem related to a previous MRI examination or MR procedure?   ☐ No   ☐ Yes
   If yes, please describe: _____
4. Have you had an injury to the eye involving a metallic object or fragment (e.g., metallic slivers, shavings, foreign body, etc.)?   ☐ No   ☐ Yes
   If yes, please describe: _____
5. Have you ever been injured by a metallic object or foreign body (e.g., BB, bullet, shrapnel, etc.)?   ☐ No   ☐ Yes
   If yes, please describe: _____
6. Are you currently taking or have you recently taken any medication or drug?   ☐ No   ☐ Yes
   If yes, please list: _____
7. Are you allergic to any medication?   ☐ No   ☐ Yes
   If yes, please list: _____
8. Do you have a history of asthma, allergic reaction, respiratory disease, or reaction to a contrast medium or dye used for an MRI, CT, or X-ray examination?   ☐ No   ☐ Yes
9. Do you have anemia or any disease(s) that affects your blood, a history of renal (kidney) disease, renal (kidney) failure, renal (kidney) transplant, high blood pressure (hypertension), liver (hepatic) disease, a history of diabetes, or seizures?   ☐ No   ☐ Yes
   If yes, please describe: _____

For female patients:
10. Date of last menstrual period: ___/___/___   Post menopausal?   ☐ No   ☐ Yes
11. Are you pregnant or experiencing a late menstrual period?   ☐ No   ☐ Yes
12. Are you taking oral contraceptives or receiving hormonal treatment?   ☐ No   ☐ Yes
13. Are you taking any type of fertility medication or having fertility treatments?   ☐ No   ☐ Yes
    If yes, please describe: _____
14. Are you currently breastfeeding?   ☐ No   ☐ Yes

WARNING: Certain implants, devices, or objects may be hazardous to you and/or may interfere with the MR procedure (i.e., MRI, MR angiography, functional MRI, MR spectroscopy). <u>Do not enter</u> the MR system room or MR environment if you have any question or concern regarding an implant, device, or object. Consult the MRI Technologist or Radiologist BEFORE entering the MR system room. The MR system magnet is ALWAYS on.

Please indicate if you have any of the following:

☐ Yes ☐ No   Aneurysm clip(s)
☐ Yes ☐ No   Cardiac pacemaker
☐ Yes ☐ No   Implanted cardioverter defibrillator (ICD)
☐ Yes ☐ No   Electronic implant or device
☐ Yes ☐ No   Magnetically-activated implant or device
☐ Yes ☐ No   Neurostimulation system
☐ Yes ☐ No   Spinal cord stimulator
☐ Yes ☐ No   Internal electrodes or wires
☐ Yes ☐ No   Bone growth/bone fusion stimulator
☐ Yes ☐ No   Cochlear, otologic, or other ear implant
☐ Yes ☐ No   Insulin or other infusion pump
☐ Yes ☐ No   Implanted drug infusion device
☐ Yes ☐ No   Any type of prosthesis (eye, penile, etc.)
☐ Yes ☐ No   Heart valve prosthesis
☐ Yes ☐ No   Eyelid spring or wire
☐ Yes ☐ No   Artificial or prosthetic limb
☐ Yes ☐ No   Metallic stent, filter, or coil
☐ Yes ☐ No   Shunt (spinal or intraventricular)
☐ Yes ☐ No   Vascular access port and/or catheter
☐ Yes ☐ No   Radiation seeds or implants
☐ Yes ☐ No   Swan-Ganz or thermodilution catheter
☐ Yes ☐ No   Medication patch (Nicotine, Nitroglycerine)
☐ Yes ☐ No   Any metallic fragment or foreign body
☐ Yes ☐ No   Wire mesh implant
☐ Yes ☐ No   Tissue expander (e.g., breast)
☐ Yes ☐ No   Surgical staples, clips, or metallic sutures
☐ Yes ☐ No   Joint replacement (hip, knee, etc.)
☐ Yes ☐ No   Bone/joint pin, screw, nail, wire, plate, etc.
☐ Yes ☐ No   IUD, diaphragm, or pessary
☐ Yes ☐ No   Dentures or partial plates
☐ Yes ☐ No   Tattoo or permanent makeup
☐ Yes ☐ No   Body piercing jewelry
☐ Yes ☐ No   Hearing aid
(Remove before entering MR system room)
☐ Yes ☐ No   Other implant _____
☐ Yes ☐ No   Breathing problem or motion disorder
☐ Yes ☐ No   Claustrophobia

Please mark on the figure(s) below
the location of any implant or metal
inside of or on your body.

RIGHT   LEFT   LEFT   RIGHT

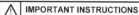 **IMPORTANT INSTRUCTIONS**

Before entering the MR environment or MR system room, you must remove <u>all</u> metallic objects including hearing aids, dentures, partial plates, keys, beeper, cell phone, eyeglasses, hair pins, barrettes, jewelry, body piercing jewelry, watch, safety pins, paperclips, money clip, credit cards, bank cards, magnetic strip cards, coins, pens, pocket knife, nail clipper, tools, clothing with metal fasteners, & clothing with metallic threads.

Please consult the MRI Technologist or Radiologist if you have any question or concern BEFORE you enter the MR system room.

NOTE: You may be advised or required to wear earplugs or other hearing protection during the MR procedure to prevent possible problems or hazards related to acoustic noise.

I attest that the above information is correct to the best of my knowledge. I read and understand the contents of this form and had the opportunity to ask questions regarding the information on this form and regarding the MR procedure that I am about to undergo.

Signature of Person Completing Form: _____   Date ____/____/____
                                                                   Signature

Form Completed By: ☐ Patient ☐ Relative ☐ Nurse _____
                                                          Print name   Relationship to patient

Form Information Reviewed By: _____
                                               Print name   Signature

☐ MRI Technologist   ☐ Nurse   ☐ Radiologist   ☐ Other _____

Figure 2. Magnetic Resonance (MR) Procedure Screening Form For Patients: Spanish Version.

CUESTIONARIO PREVIO A ESTUDIO CON RESONANCIA MAGNÉTICA (MR)
PARA PACIENTES

Fecha ____/____/____   Número de paciente _____

Nombre _____   Edad _____ Altura _____ Peso _____
Apellido   Primer Nombre   Segundo Nombre

Fecha de nacimiento ____/____/____   Varón☐ Hembra☐   Parte del cuerpo a ser examinada _____
Mes Día Año

Dirección _____   Teléfono (domicilio) (____) ____-____

Ciudad _____   Teléfono (trabajo) (____) ____-____

Provincia _____   Código Postal _____

Motivo para el estudio de MRI y/o síntomas _____

Médico que le refirió _____   Teléfono (____) - _____

1. Anteriormente, ¿le han hecho alguna cirugía u operación (e.g., artroscopía, endoscopía, etc.) de cualquier tipo? ☐ No ☐ Sí
Si respondió afirmativamente, indique la fecha y que tipo de cirugía:
Fecha ____/____/____ Tipo de cirugía _____
Fecha ____/____/____ Tipo de cirugía _____
2. Anteriormente, ¿le han hecho algún estudio o exámen de diagnóstico (MRI, CT, Ultrasonido, Rayos-X, etc.)? ☐ No ☐ Sí
Si respondió afirmativamente, descríbalos a continuación:
Parte del Cuerpo	Fecha	Lugar/Institución
MRI	/ /	
CT/CAT	/ /	
Rayos-X	/ /	
Ultrasonido	/ /	
Medicina Nuclear	/ /	
Otro,	/ /	
3. ¿Ha tenido algún problema relacionado con estudios ó procedimientos anteriores con MR? ☐ No ☐ Sí
Si respondió afirmativamente, descríbalos: _____
4. ¿Se ha golpeado el ojo con un objeto ó fragmento metálico (e.g., astillas metálicas, virutas, objeto extraño, etc.)? ☐ No ☐ Sí
Si respondió afirmativamente, describa el incidente: _____
5. ¿Ha sido alcanzado alguna vez por un objeto metálico u objeto extraño (e.g. perdigones, bala, metralla, etc.)? ☐ No ☐ Sí
Si respondió afirmativamente, describa el incidente: _____
6. ¿Esta actualmente tomando ó ha recientemente tomado algún medicamento o droga? ☐ No ☐ Sí
Si respondió afirmativamente, indique el nombre del medicamento: _____
7. ¿Es Ud. alérgico/a a algún medicamento? ☐ No ☐ Sí
Si respondió afirmativamente, indique el nombre del medicamento: _____
8. ¿Tiene historia de asma, reacción alérgica, enfermedad respiratoria, ó reacción a contrastes ó tinturas usados en MRI, CT, ó Rayos-X? ☐ No ☐ Sí
9. ¿Tiene anemia u otra enfermedad que afecte su sangre, algún episodio de enfermedad de riñón, fracaso de riñón,
un transplante de riñón, hipertensión, la historia de la diabetes, relativo al hígado ó de ataques epilépticos?
Si respondió afirmativamente, descríbalos: _____ ☐ No ☐ Sí

Para los pacientes femeninos:
10. Fecha de su último periodo menstrual: ____/____/____   En la menopausia? ☐ No ☐ Sí
11. ¿Está embarazada ó tiene retraso con su periodo menstrual? ☐ No ☐ Sí
12. ¿Está tomando contraceptivos orales ó recibiendo tratamiento hormonal? ☐ No ☐ Sí
13. ¿Está tomando algún tipo de medicamento para la fertilidad ó recibiendo tratamientos de fertilidad? ☐ No ☐ Sí
Si responde afirmativamente, descríbalos a continuación: _____
14. ¿Está amamantado a su bebé? ☐ No ☐ Sí

Translated with permission 5/05 Olga Fernandez-Flygare, M.S., Brain
Mapping Center, UCLA School of Medicine, Los Angeles, CA

ADVERTENCIA: Ciertos implantes, dispositivos, u objetos pueden ser peligrosos y/o pueden interferir con el procedimiento de resonancia magnética (es decir, MRI, MR angiografía, MRI funcional, MR espectroscopía). **No entre** a la sala del escáner de MR o a la zona del laboratorio de MR si tiene alguna pregunta o duda relacionadas con un implante, dispositivo, u objeto. Consulte con el técnico o radiólogo de MRI ANTES de entrar a la sala del escáner de MR. **Recuerde que el imán del sistema MR está SIEMPRE encendido.**

Por favor indique si tiene alguno de los siguientes:

☐ Sí ☐ No Pinza(s) de aneurisma
☐ Sí ☐ No Marcapasos cardíaco
☐ Sí ☐ No Implante con desfibrilador para conversión cardíaca (ICD)
☐ Sí ☐ No Implante electrónico ó dispositivo electrónico
☐ Sí ☐ No Implante ó dispositivo activado magnéticamente
☐ Sí ☐ No Sistema de neuroestimulación
☐ Sí ☐ No Estimulador de la médula espinal
☐ Sí ☐ No Electrodos ó alambres internos
☐ Sí ☐ No Estimulador de crecimiento/fusión del hueso
☐ Sí ☐ No Implante coclear, otológico, u otro implante del oído
☐ Sí ☐ No Bomba de infusión de insulina ó similar
☐ Sí ☐ No Dispositivo implantado para infusión de medicamento
☐ Sí ☐ No Cualquier tipo de prótesis (ojo, peneal, etc.)
☐ Sí ☐ No Prótesis de válvula cardíaca
☐ Sí ☐ No Muelle ó alambre del párpado
☐ Sí ☐ No Extremidad artificial ó prostética
☐ Sí ☐ No Malla metálica (stent), filtro, ó anillo metálico
☐ Sí ☐ No Shunt (espinal ó intraventricular)
☐ Sí ☐ No Catéter y/u orificio de acceso vascular
☐ Sí ☐ No Semillas ó implantes de radiación
☐ Sí ☐ No Catéter de Swan-Ganz ó de termodilución

☐ Sí ☐ No Parche de medicamentos (Nicotina, Nitroglicerina)
☐ Sí ☐ No Cualquier fragmento metálico ó cuerpo extraño
☐ Sí ☐ No Implante tipo malla
☐ Sí ☐ No Aumentador de tejidos (e.g. pecho)
☐ Sí ☐ No Grapas quirúrgicas, clips, ó suturas metálicas
☐ Sí ☐ No Articulaciones artificiales (cadera, rodilla, etc.)
☐ Sí ☐ No Varilla de hueso/coyuntura, tornillo, clavo, alambre, chapas, etc.
☐ Sí ☐ No Dispositivo intrauterino (IUD), diafragma, ó pesario
☐ Sí ☐ No Dentaduras ó placas parciales
☐ Sí ☐ No Tatuaje ó maquillaje permanente
☐ Sí ☐ No Perforación (piercing) del cuerpo
☐ Sí ☐ No Audífono *(Quíteselo antes de entrar a la sala del escáner de MR)*
☐ Sí ☐ No Otro implante_____
☐ Sí ☐ No Problema respiratorio ó desorden del movimiento
☐ Sí ☐ No Claustrofobia

Por favor marque en la imagen de abajo la localización de cualquier implante o metal en su cuerpo.

DERECHA   IZQUIERDA   DERECHA

⚠ **¡AVISO IMPORTANTE!**

Antes de entrar a la zona de MR ó a la sala del escáner de MR, tendrá que quitarse todo objeto metálico incluyendo audífono, dentaduras, placas parciales, llaves, beeper, teléfono celular, lentes, horquillas de pelo, pasadores, todas las joyas (incluyendo "body piercing"), reloj, alfileres, sujetapapeles, clip de billetes, tarjetas de crédito ó de banco, toda tarjeta con banda magnética, monedas, plumas, cuchillos, corta uñas, herramientas, ropa con enganches de metal, y ropa con hilos metálicos.

Por favor consulte con el Técnico de MRI ó Radiólogo si tiene alguna pregunta o duda ANTES de entrar a la sala de escáner de MR.

NOTA: Es posible se le pida usar auriculares u otra protección de sus oídos durante el procedimiento de MR para prevenir problemas ó riesgos asociados al nivel de ruido en la sala del escáner de MR.

Atestiguo que la información anterior es correcta según mi mejor entender. Leo y entiendo el contenido de este cuestionario y he tenido la oportunidad de hacer preguntas en relación a la información en el cuestionario y en relación al estudio de MR al que me voy a someter a continuación.

Firma de la persona llenando este cuestionario: _____   Fecha___/___/___
                                                                        Firma

Cuestionario lleno por: ☐Paciente ☐Pariente ☐Enfermera _____   _____
                                                                  Nombre en letra de texto   Relación con el paciente

Información revisada por: _____   _____
                                      Nombre en letra de texto   Firma
☐ Técnico de MRI   ☐Enfermera   ☐ Radiólogo   ☐ Otro _____

Translated with permission Olga Fernandez-Fygare, M.S., Brain Mapping Center, UCLA School of Medicine, Los Angeles, CA

Figure 3. Magnetic Resonance (MR) Environment Screening Form for Individuals (Developed in conjunction with the Institute for Magnetic Resonance Safety, Education, and Research, www.IMRSER.org).

MAGNETIC RESONANCE (MR) ENVIRONMENT SCREENING FORM FOR INDIVIDUALS*

The MR system has a very strong magnetic field that may be hazardous to individuals entering the MR environment or MR system room if they have certain metallic, electronic, magnetic, or mechanical implants, devices, or objects. Therefore, all individuals are required to fill out this form BEFORE entering the MR environment or MR system room. Be advised, the MR system magnet is ALWAYS on.

*NOTE: If you are a patient preparing to undergo an MR examination, you are required to fill out a different form.

Date ___/___/___   Name _____   Age _____
    month   day   year   Last Name   First Name   Middle Initial

Address _____   Telephone (home) (____) ____-_____

City _____   Telephone (work) (____) ____-_____

State _____   Zip Code _____

1. Have you had prior surgery or an operation (e.g., arthroscopy, endoscopy, etc.) of any kind?   ☐ No ☐ Yes
   If yes, please indicate date and type of surgery: Date ___/___/___ Type of surgery _____
2. Have you had an injury to the eye involving a metallic object (e.g., metallic slivers, foreign body)?   ☐ No ☐ Yes
   If yes, please describe: _____
3. Have you ever been injured by a metallic object or foreign body (e.g., BB, bullet, shrapnel, etc.)?   ☐ No ☐ Yes
   If yes, please describe: _____
4. Are you pregnant or suspect that you are pregnant?   ☐ No ☐ Yes

⚠ **WARNING:** Certain implants, devices, or objects may be hazardous to you in the MR environment or MR system room. Do not enter the MR environment or MR system room if you have any question or concern regarding an implant, device, or object.

Please indicate if you have any of the following:
☐ Yes ☐ No Aneurysm clip(s)
☐ Yes ☐ No Cardiac pacemaker
☐ Yes ☐ No Implanted cardioverter defibrillator (ICD)
☐ Yes ☐ No Electronic implant or device
☐ Yes ☐ No Magnetically-activated implant or device
☐ Yes ☐ No Neurostimulation system
☐ Yes ☐ No Spinal cord stimulator
☐ Yes ☐ No Cochlear implant or implanted hearing aid
☐ Yes ☐ No Insulin or infusion pump
☐ Yes ☐ No Implanted drug infusion device
☐ Yes ☐ No Any type of prosthesis or implant
☐ Yes ☐ No Artificial or prosthetic limb
☐ Yes ☐ No Any metallic fragment or foreign body
☐ Yes ☐ No Any external or internal metallic object
☐ Yes ☐ No Hearing aid
          (Remove before entering the MR system room)
☐ Yes ☐ No Other implant _____

⚠ **IMPORTANT INSTRUCTIONS**

Remove all metallic objects before entering the MR environment or MR system room including hearing aids, beeper, cell phone, keys, eyeglasses, hair pins, barrettes, jewelry (including body piercing jewelry), watch, safety pins, paperclips, money clip, credit cards, bank cards, magnetic strip cards, coins, pens, pocket knife, nail clipper, steel-toed boots/shoes, and tools. Loose metallic objects are especially prohibited in the MR system room and MR environment.

Please consult the MRI Technologist or Radiologist if you have any question or concern BEFORE you enter the MR system room.

I attest that the above information is correct to the best of my knowledge. I have read and understand the entire contents of this form and have had the opportunity to ask questions regarding the information on this form.

Signature of Person Completing Form: _____   Date ___/___/___
                                Signature

Form Information Reviewed By: _____   _____
                            Print name   Signature

☐ MRI Technologist   ☐ Radiologist   ☐ Other _____

Guidelines to Prevent Excessive Heating and Burns Associated with Magnetic Resonance Procedures*

Magnetic resonance (MR) imaging is a relatively safe diagnostic modality. However, damaged radiofrequency coils, physiologic monitors, electronically-activated devices, and external accessories or objects made from conductive materials have caused excessive heating, resulting in burn injuries to patients undergoing MR procedures. Heating of implants and similar devices may also occur, but this tends to be problematic primarily for objects made from conductive materials that have elongated shapes or that form loops of a certain diameter. For example, excessive MRI-related heating has been reported for leads, guidewires, certain types of catheters (e.g., catheters with thermistors or other conducting components), and certain external fixation or cervical fixation devices.

In the United States, many incidents of excessive heating have been reported in patients undergoing MR procedures that were unrelated to equipment problems or the presence of conductive external or internal implants or materials [review of data files from U.S. Food and Drug Administration, Center for Devices and Radiological Health, Manufacturer and User Facility Device Experience Database, MAUDE, http://www.fda.gov/cdrh/maude.html and U.S. Food and Drug Administration, Center for Devices and Radiological Health, Medical Device Report, http://www.fda.gov/CDRH/mdrfile.html]. In a review of the MAUDE data base for a 10 year period, Hardy and Weil (2010) (medical device reviewers for the FDA) indicated that 419 thermal injuries were associated with MRI.

These incidents included first, second, and third degree burns that were experienced by patients. In many of these cases, the reports indicated that the limbs or other body parts of the patients were in direct contact with transmit body radiofrequency (RF) coils or other transmit RF coils of the MR systems. In other cases, skin-to-skin contact points were suspected to be responsible for these injuries, however, the exact mechanism responsible for these incidents is unknown.

MR systems require the use of RF pulses to create the MR signal. This RF energy is transmitted through free space from the transmit RF coil to the patient. When conducting materials are placed within the RF field, a concentration of electrical currents sufficient to cause excessive heating and tissue damage may occur. Therefore, only devices with carefully designed current paths can be made safe for use during MR procedures. Simply insulating conductive material (e.g., wire or lead) or separating it from the patient may not be sufficient to prevent excessive heating or burns from occurring for some devices.

Furthermore, certain elongated shapes (i.e., depending on the length and the transmit RF frequency) exhibit the phenomenon of "resonance" that increases their propensity to concentrate RF currents. At the operating frequencies of present day MR systems, conducting loops of tens of centimeters in size can create problems and, therefore, must be avoided, unless high impedance techniques are used to limit the RF current. Importantly, even loops that include small gaps separated by insulation may still conduct currents.

To prevent excessive heating and possible burns in association with MR procedures, the following guidelines are recommended:

1) Prepare the patient for the MR procedure by ensuring that there are no unnecessary metallic objects contacting the patient's skin (e.g., drug delivery patches with metallic components, jewelry, necklaces, bracelets, key chains, etc.).

2) Prepare the patient for the MR procedure by using insulation material (i.e., appropriate padding) to prevent skin-to-skin contact points and the formation of "closed-loops" from touching body parts.

3) Insulating material (minimum recommended thickness, 1-cm) should be placed between the patient's skin and transmit RF coil that is used for the MR procedure (alternatively, the transmit RF coil itself should be padded). There should be no direct contact between the patient's skin and the transmit RF body coil of the MR system. This may be accomplished by having the patient place his/her arms over his/her head or by using elbow pads or foam padding between the patient's tissue and the transmit RF body coil of the MR system. This is especially important for MR examinations that use the transmit RF body coil or other large RF coils for transmission of RF energy.

4) Use only electrically conductive devices, equipment, accessories (e.g., ECG leads, electrodes, etc.), and materials that have been thoroughly tested and determined to be safe or otherwise acceptable for MR procedures.

5) Carefully follow specific MR safety or MR conditional criteria and recommendations for implants made from electrically-conductive materials (e.g., bone fusion stimulators, neurostimulation systems, cardiac pacemakers, cochlear implants, etc.).

6) Before using electrical equipment, check the integrity of the insulation and/or housing of all components including surface RF coils, monitoring leads, cables, and wires. Preventive maintenance should be practiced routinely for such equipment.

7) Remove all non-essential electrically conductive materials from the MR system prior to the MR procedure (i.e., unused surface RF coils, ECG leads, EEG leads, cables, wires, etc.).

8) Keep electrically conductive materials that must remain in the MR system from directly contacting the patient by placing thermal and/or electrical insulation between the conductive material and the patient.

9) Keep electrically conductive materials that must remain within the transmit body RF coil or other transmit RF coil of the MR system from forming conductive loops. Note: The patient's tissue is conductive and, therefore, may be involved in the formation of a conductive loop, which can be circular, U-shaped, or S-shaped.

10) Position electrically conductive materials to prevent "cross points". A cross point is the point where a cable crosses another cable, where a cable loops across itself, or where a cable touches either the patient or sides of the transmit RF coil more than once. Even the close proximity of conductive materials with each other should be avoided because cables and RF coils can capacitively-couple (without any contact or crossover) when placed close together.

11) Position electrically conductive materials (e.g., cables, wires, etc.) to exit down the center of the MR system, *not* along the side of the MR system or close to the transmit RF body coil or other transmit RF coil.

12) Do not position electrically conductive materials across an external metallic prosthesis (e.g., external fixation device, cervical fixation device, etc.) or similar device that is in direct contact with the patient.

13) Allow only properly trained individuals to operate devices (e.g., monitoring equipment) in the MR environment.

14) Follow all manufacturer instructions for the proper operation and maintenance of physiologic monitoring or other similar electronic equipment intended for use during MR procedures.

15) Electrical devices that do not appear to be operating properly during the MR procedure should be removed from the patient immediately.

16) Closely monitor the patient during the MR procedure. If the patient reports sensations of heating or other unusual sensation, discontinue

the MR procedure immediately and perform a thorough assessment of the situation.

17) RF surface coil decoupling failures can cause localized RF power deposition levels to reach excessive levels. The MR system operator will recognize such a failure as a set of concentric semicircles in the tissue on the associated MR image or as an unusual amount of image non-uniformity related to the position of the transmit RF coil.

The adoption and regular practice of these guidelines will ensure that patient safety is maintained, especially as more conductive materials and electronically-activated devices are used in association with MR procedures.

[*The document, Guidelines to Prevent Excessive Heating and Burns Associated with Magnetic Resonance Procedures, was developed by the Institute for Magnetic Resonance Safety, Education, and Research (IMRSER) and published with permission. Reviewed and updated 2012.]

REFERENCES

Bashein G, Syrory G. Burns associated with pulse oximetry during magnetic resonance imaging. Anesthesiology 1991;75:382-3.

Brown TR, Goldstein B, Little J. Severe burns resulting from magnetic resonance imaging with cardiopulmonary monitoring. Risks and relevant safety precautions. Am J Phys Med Rehabil 1993;72:166-7.

Chou C-K, et al. Absence of radiofrequency heating from auditory implants during magnetic resonance imaging. Bioelectromagnetics 1997;44:367-372.

Diaz F, Tweardy L, Shellock FG. Cervical fixation devices: MRI issues at 3-Tesla. Spine 2010;35:411-5

Dempsey MF, Condon B. Thermal injuries associated with MRI. Clin Radiol 2001;56:457-65.

Dempsey MF, Condon B, Hadley DM. Investigation of the factors responsible for burns during MRI. J Magn Reson Imaging 2001;13:627-631.

ECRI, Health Devices Alert. A new MRI complication? Health Devices Alert May 27, pp. 1, 1988.

ECRI. Thermal injuries and patient monitoring during MRI studies. Health Devices Alert 1991;20: 362-363.

ECRI. Hazard Report. Patients can be burned by damaged MRI AV entertainment systems. Health Devices. 2008;37:379-80

Finelli DA, Rezai AR, Ruggieri PM, Tkach JA, Nyenhuis JA, Hrdlicka G, Sharan A, Gonzalez-Martinez J, Stypulkowski PH, Shellock FG. MR imaging-related heating of deep brain stimulation electrodes: In vitro study. Am J Neuroradiol 2002;23:1795-1802.

Haik J, Daniel S, et al. MRI induced fourth-degree burn in an extremity, leading to amputation. Burns. 2009;35:294-6.

Hall SC, Stevenson GW, Suresh S. Burn associated with temperature monitoring during magnetic resonance imaging. Anesthesiology 1992;76:152.

Hardy PT 2nd, Weil KM. A review of thermal MR injuries. Radiol Technol. 2010;81:606-9.

Heinz W, Frohlich E, Stork T. Burns following magnetic resonance tomography study. (German) Z Gastroenterol 1999;37:31-2.

http://www.IMRSER.org; website for the Institute for Magnetic Resonance Safety, Education, and Research

International Commission on Non-Ionizing Radiation Protection (ICNIRP) Statement, Medical magnetic resonance procedures: protection of patients. Health Physics 2004;87:197-216.

International Electrotechnical Commission (IEC), Medical Electrical Equipment, Particular requirements for the safety of magnetic resonance equipment for medical diagnosis. International Standard IEC 60601-2-33, 2002.

Jacob ZC, et al. MR imaging-related electrical thermal injury complicated by acute carpal tunnel and compartment syndrome: case report. Radiology. 2010;254:846-50.

Johnston T, et al. Intraoperative MRI: safety. Neurosurg Clin N Am. 2009;20:147-53.

Jones S, Jaffe W, Alvi R. Burns associated with electrocardiographic monitoring during magnetic resonance imaging. Burns 1996;22:420-421.

Kainz W. MR heating tests of MR critical implants. J Magn Reson Imaging. 2007;26:450-1

Kanal E, Barkovich AJ, Bell C, et al. ACR guidance document for safe MR practices: 2007. AJR Am J Roentgenol. 2007;188:1447-1474.

Kanal E, Shellock FG. Burns associated with clinical MR examinations. Radiology 1990;175: 585.

Kanal E, Shellock FG. Policies, guidelines, and recommendations for MR imaging safety and patient management. J Magn Reson Imaging 1992;2:247-248.

Karoo RO, Whitaker IS, Garrido A, Sharpe DT. Full-thickness burns following magnetic resonance imaging: a discussion of the dangers and safety suggestions. Plast Reconstr Surg. 2004;114:1344-1345.

Keens SJ, Laurence AS. Burns caused by ECG monitoring during MRI imaging. Anaesthesia 1996;51:1188-9.

Kim LJ, et al. Scalp burns from halo pins following magnetic resonance imaging. Case Report. Journal of Neurosurgery 2003;99:186.

Knopp MV, et al. Unusual burns of the lower extremities caused by a closed conducting loop in a patient at MR imaging. Radiology 1996;200:572-5.

Knopp MV, et al. Safety considerations to avoid current-induced skin burns in MRI procedures. (German) Radiologe 1998;38:759-63.

Kugel H, et al. Hazardous situation in the MR bore: induction in ECG leads causes fire. Eur Radiol 2003;13:690-694.

Lange S, Nguyen QN. Cables and electrodes can burn patients during MRI. Nursing. 2006;36:18.

Mattei E, et al. Temperature and SAR measurement errors in the evaluation of metallic linear structures heating during MRI using fluoroptic probes. Phys Med Biol. 2007;52:1633-46.

Nakamura T, et al. Mechanism of burn injury during magnetic resonance imaging (MRI)-simple loops can induce heat injury. Front Med Biol Eng 2001;11:117-29

Newcombe VF, et al. Potential heating caused by intraparenchymal intracranial pressure transducers in a 3-tesla magnetic resonance imaging system using a body radiofrequency resonator: assessment of the Codman MicroSensor Transducer. J Neurosurg. 2008;109:159-64.

Nyenhuis JA, et al. Heating near implanted medical devices by the MRI RF-magnetic field. IEEE Trans Magn 1999;35:4133-4135.

Rezai AR, Finelli D, Nyenhuis JA, Hrdlick G, Tkach J, Ruggieri P, Stypulkowski PH, Sharan A, Shellock FG. Neurostimulator for deep brain stimulation: Ex vivo evaluation of MRI-related heating at 1.5-Tesla. Journal of Magnetic Resonance Imaging 2002;15:241-250.

Ruschulte H, Piepenbrock S, Munte S, Lotz J. Severe burns during magnetic resonance examination. Eur J Anaesthesiol. 2005;22:319-320.

Schaefer DJ. Safety aspects of radio-frequency power deposition in magnetic resonance. MRI Clinics of North America 1998;6:775-789.

Shellock FG. Magnetic Resonance Procedures: Health Effects and Safety. CRC Press, LLC, Boca Raton, FL, 2001.

Shellock FG. Radiofrequency-induced heating during MR procedures: A review. Journal of Magnetic Resonance Imaging 2000;12: 30-36.

Shellock FG. Guest Editorial. Comments on MRI heating tests of critical implants. Journal of Magnetic Resonance Imaging 2007;26:1182-1185.

Shellock FG, Crues JV. MR procedures: biologic effects, safety, and patient care. Radiology, 2004;232:635-652.

Shellock FG, Slimp G. Severe burn of the finger caused by using a pulse oximeter during MRI. American Journal of Roentgenology 1989;153:1105.

Smith CD, et al. Health effects of induced electrical fields: implications for metallic implants. In: Shellock FG, ed. Magnetic resonance procedure: health effects and safety. Boca Raton, FL: CRC Press, 2001; 393-414.

U.S. Food and Drug Administration, Center for Devices and Radiological Health (CDRH), Medical Device Report (MDR) (http://www.fda.gov/CDRH/mdrfile.html).

U.S. Food and Drug Administration, Center for Devices and Radiological Health (CDRH), Manufacturer and User Facility Device Experience Database, MAUDE, (http://www.fda.gov/cdrh/maude.html).

Yamazaki M, et al. Investigation of local heating caused by closed conducting loop at clinical MR imaging: Phantom study. Nippon Hoshasen Gijutsu Gakkai Zasshi. 2008;20;64:883-5.

Infection Control In the MRI Environment*

The magnetic resonance (MR) imaging environment is a complex and potentially dangerous setting with respect to issues involving infection control, particularly because custodial personnel and routine cleaning equipment are not permitted to enter this area without adhering to strict policies and procedures. Importantly, cleaning the MR system room is often the responsibility of the MR system operator, who is rarely trained or certified in infection control. Therefore, it is unreasonable to believe that the MRI environment, especially the MR system and associated accessories (e.g., inside the bore of the scanner, surface coils, the positioning pads/sponges, patient management devices, etc.), can be cleaned safely and effectively by untrained personnel. This important task requires specialized written procedures and training.

Patients with serious infections typically undergo diagnostic imaging during the course of their treatment. There is frequently a lack of special procedures for managing highly contagious patients, particularly at outpatient imaging centers and mobile MR scanners. Contagious patients may simply be placed on the MR system table and scanned, while the next patient, possibly an immunosuppressed child with a sprained knee, is put on the table directly after this infected patient without properly cleaning the table, pads, and sponges. Obviously, this is a serious situation that deserves attention. Therefore, all MRI facilities must take appropriate action to ensure that the MR environment is not a site for exposing patients and healthcare workers to microorganisms that are capable of causing infectious diseases.

At many MRI centers, there is a misconception that merely placing a clean sheet over the scanner table, without actually cleaning the mattress between patients, will prevent the spread of infectious agents. Of note is that placing clean sheets on a contaminated surface may contaminate the sheets and pose further infectious risk when the sheets are handled. Of further concern is that very few MRI facilities clean inside of the bore of the MR system on a regular basis. Positioning pads and sponges may only be cleaned once a day.

There is also the issue of potentially spreading infectious agents by direct or indirect contact among the imaging staff and patients within the imaging department or center. For MR systems in mobile facilities, ensuring proper hygiene is often more difficult, since these sites may not have a sink or running water. Therefore, hand-washing between patients as well as using hand sanitizer regularly is of crucial importance.

Another overlooked area is presence of torn or frayed positioning pads, sponges, and scanner table mattresses used in association with MRI examinations. Once the covering material has been breached, the surfaces of these items cannot be properly cleaned and should be immediately removed and replaced. It is well known that, if disinfected, a smooth surface can be repeatedly used without problems. However, for items with a porous surface (e.g., those made from "spongy" materials), the presence of infectious agents, including Methicillin-resistant Staphylococcus aureus, MRSA, can be detected even after performing disinfection. Thus, porous surfaces made of such materials cannot be adequately cleaned and disinfected.

Protecting patients and staff takes a concerted effort by all parties involved in the MRI facility. There is no question that infection control has not received the attention that it deserves and there is a growing concern that at least some of the spread of infectious agents could be coming from outpatient imaging centers and radiology departments in hospitals.

The following recommendations are provided for MRI facilities to address infection control standards that are used throughout the healthcare industry:

Recommendations for Infection Control in the MRI Environment

1) Have a written infectious control policy to include cleaning procedures for the MRI environment, as well as a cleaning schedule, and have it posted throughout the center.
2) Implement a mandatory hand-washing / hand-sanitizing procedure between each patient not only for MRI healthcare workers, but also for others who come into contact with patients.
3) Clean the MR scanner table, inside the bore of the MR system, and other items that come into contact with a patient. Infection control experts recommend that this be done between patients.
4) Clean all positioning pads and sponges with an approved disinfectant. Infection control experts recommend cleaning after each patient.

5) Periodically inspect the pads with a magnifying glass, particularly at the seams, to identify fraying or tearing. Replace the pads, as needed.

6) Use pillows with a waterproof covering that is designed to be surface wiped. Replace pillows when this barrier is compromised.

7) Promptly remove body fluids and then disinfect all contaminated areas.

8) If the patient has an open wound or history of infection, especially related to MRSA, gloves and gowns must be worn by all staff members coming into contact with the patient. These barriers must be removed before touching other areas not coming into contact with the patient (e.g., door knobs, scanner console, computer keyboards, etc.).

9) The scanner table, positioning sponges, and pads should be completely cleaned with disinfectant before the next patient is scanned, if this procedure is not already being performed between each patient. For patients with any known infectious process, add 10-15 minutes to the scheduled scan time to ensure that there is enough time to thoroughly clean the room and patient-related surfaces.

10) All furniture should be periodically cleaned. Ideal surfaces are those that are waterproof, nonporous, and easy to clean. Infection control experts recommend that such cleaning be performed between patients.

[Content excerpted with permission for content provided by Peter Rothschild, M.D. Louisville, KY. Reviewed and updated 2012.]

REFERENCES

Brennan PJ, Abrutyn E. Developing policies and guidelines. Infec Control Hosp Epidemiol 1995; 16:512-517.

CNA. MRSA Alert: MRI infection creates new "superbug" concerns. AlertBulletin. Issue 4, 09, www.CNA.com/healthpro

Datta R, Huang SS. Risk of infection and death due to methicillin-resistant Staphylococcus aureus in long-term carriers. Clin Infect Dis. 200815;47:176-81.

Guidelines for Environmental Infection Control and Healthcare Facilities Recommendations of CDC and Healthcare Infection Control Practices Advisory Committee (HICPAC) 2003. This is available from the Center for Disease Control and Prevention, www.cdc.gov

Haley RW, et al. The efficacy of infection surveilliance and control programs in preventing nosocomial infections in US hospitals. Am J Epidemiology 1985;121:182-205.

Huang SS, Datta R, Platt R. Risk of acquiring antibiotic-resistant bacteria from prior room occupants. Arch Intern Med. 2006;166:1945-51.

Huang SS, et al. Impact of routine intensive care unit surveillance cultures and resultant barrier precautions on hospital-wide methicillin-resistant Staphylococcus aureus bacteremia. Clin Infect Dis. 2006;43:971-8.

Lawton, RM, et al. Prepackaged hand hygiene educational tools facilitate implementation. Am J Infection Control 2006; 34: 152-154.

Oie S, et al. Contamination of environmental surfaces by Staphylococcus aureus in a dermatological ward and its preventive measures. J Hosp Infect. 1998;40:135-40.

Pulgliese G, et al. Development and implementation of infection control policies and procedures. In: Mayhill CG. Hospital Epidemiology and Infection Control. 2nd Ed. Philadelphia: Lippincott, Williams and Wilkins, 1999:1357-1366.

Shiomori T, et al. Evaluation of bedmaking-related airborne and surface methicillin-resistant Staphylococcus aureus contamination. J Hosp Infect. 2002;50:30-5.

Yokoe DS, Classen, D. Improving patient safety through infection control: A new healthcare imperative. 2008;29:S3-S11.

Magnetic Resonance Imaging: Information for Patients*

What is magnetic resonance imaging (MRI)?

MRI, or magnetic resonance imaging, is a means of "seeing" inside of the body in order for doctors to find certain diseases or abnormal conditions. MRI does not rely on the type of radiation (i.e., ionizing radiation) used for an x-ray or computed tomography (CT). The MRI examination requires specialized equipment that uses a powerful, constant magnetic field, rapidly changing local magnetic fields, radiofrequency energy, and dedicated equipment including a powerful computer to create very clear pictures of internal body structures.

During the MRI examination, the patient is placed within the MR system or "scanner". The powerful, constant magnetic field aligns a tiny fraction of subatomic particles called protons that are present in most of the body's tissues. Radiofrequency energy is applied to cause these protons to produce signals that are picked up by a receiver within the scanner. The signals are specially characterized using the rapidly changing, local magnetic field and computer-processed to produce images of the body part of interest.

What is MRI used for?

MRI has become the preferred procedure for diagnosing a large number of potential problems in many different parts of the body. In general, MRI creates pictures that can show differences between healthy and unhealthy tissue. Doctors use MRI to examine the brain, spine, joints (e.g., knee, shoulder, wrist, and ankle), abdomen, pelvic region, breast, blood vessels, heart and other body parts.

Is MRI safe?

To date, over 400 million patients have had MRI examinations. MRI has been shown to be extremely safe as long as proper safety precautions are taken. In general, the MRI procedure produces no pain and causes no known short-term or long-term tissue damage of any kind.

The powerful magnetic field of the scanner can attract certain metallic objects that are "ferromagnetic", causing them to move suddenly and with great force towards the center of the MR system. This may pose a risk to the patient or anyone in the path of the object. Therefore, great care is taken to prevent ferromagnetic objects from entering the MR system room. It is vital that you remove metallic objects in advance of an MRI examination, including watches, jewelry, and items of clothing that have metallic threads or fasteners.

The MRI facility has a screening procedure that, when carefully followed, will ensure that the MRI technologist and radiologist knows about the presence of metallic implants and materials so that special precautions can be taken (see below). In some unusual cases, the examination may be cancelled because of concern related to a particular implant or device. For example, if an MRI is ordered, it may be cancelled if the patient has a ferromagnetic aneurysm clip because of the risk of dislodging the clip from the blood vessel. Also, the magnetic field of the scanner can damage an external hearing aid or cause a heart pacemaker to malfunction. If you have a bullet, shrapnel, or similar metallic fragment in your body there is a potential risk that it could change position, possibly causing injury.

How to prepare for the MRI examination.

There's no special preparation necessary for the MRI examination. Unless your doctor specifically requests that you not eat or drink anything before the exam, there are no food or drink restrictions. Continue to take any medication prescribed by your doctor unless otherwise directed.

You won't be allowed to wear anything metallic during the MRI examination, so it would be best to leave watches, jewelry or anything made from metal at home. Even some cosmetics contain small amounts of metals, so it is best to not wear make-up.

In order to prevent metallic objects from being attracted by the powerful magnet of the MR system, you may receive a gown (which is advisable) to wear during your examination. Items that need to be removed before entering the MR system room include:

- Purse, wallet, money clip, credit cards, other cards with magnetic strips
- Electronic devices such as beepers or cellular phones
- Hearing aids
- Metallic jewelry, watches
- Pens, paper clips, keys, nail clippers, coins
- Hair barrettes, hairpins
- Any article of clothing that has a metallic zipper, buttons, snaps, hooks, under-wires, or metallic threads
- Shoes, belt buckles, safety pins

Before the MRI procedure, you will be asked to fill out a screening form asking about anything that might create a health risk or interfere with the examination. You will also undergo an interview by a member of the MRI facility to ensure that you understand the questions on the form. Even if you have undergone an MRI procedure before at this or another facility, you will still be asked to complete an MRI screening form.

Examples of items or things that may create a health hazard or other problem during an MRI exam include:

- Pacemaker
- Implantable cardioverter defibrillator (ICD)
- Neurostimulation system
- Aneurysm clip
- Metallic implant
- Implanted drug infusion device
- Foreign metal objects, especially if in or near the eye
- Shrapnel or bullet
- Permanent cosmetics or tattoos
- Dentures/teeth with magnetic keepers
- Other implants that involve magnets
- Medication patch (i.e., transdermal patch) that contains metallic foil

Check with the MRI technologist or radiologist at the MRI facility if you have questions or concerns about any implanted object or health condition that could impact the MRI procedure. This is particularly important if you have undergone surgery involving the brain, ear, eye, heart, or blood vessels.

Important Note: If you are pregnant or think that you could be pregnant, you must notify your physician and the radiologist or the MRI technologist at the MRI facility prior to the MRI procedure.

Before entering the MR system room, any friend or relative that might be allowed to accompany you will be asked questions to ensure that he or she may safely enter the room and will likewise be instructed to remove all metallic objects. Additionally, this individual will need to fill out a screening form.

What is the MRI examination like?

The MRI examination is performed in a special room that houses the MR system or "scanner". You will be escorted into the room by a staff member of the MRI facility and asked to lie down on a comfortably padded table that gently glides you into the scanner.

In order to prepare for the MRI examination, you may be required to wear earplugs or headphones to protect your hearing because, when certain scanners operate, they may produce loud noises. These loud noises are normal and should not worry you.

For some MRI studies, a contrast agent called "gadolinium" may be injected into a vein to help obtain a clearer picture of the body part that is undergoing examination. At some point during the procedure, a nurse or MRI technologist will slide the table out of the scanner to inject the contrast agent. This is typically done through a small needle connected to an intravenous line that is placed in an arm or hand vein. A saline solution will drip through the intravenous line to prevent clotting until the contrast agent is injected at some point during the exam. Unlike contrast agents used in x-ray studies, MRI contrast agents do not contain iodine and, therefore, rarely cause allergic reactions or other problems.

The most important thing for you to do is to relax and remain still. Most MRI exams take between 15 to 45 minutes to complete depending on the body part imaged and how many images are needed, although some may take 60 minutes or longer. You'll be told ahead of time how long your scan is expected to take.

You will be asked to remain perfectly still during the time the imaging takes place, but between sequences some minor movement may be allowed. The MRI technologist will advise you, accordingly.

When the MRI procedure begins, you may breathe normally, however, for certain examinations it may be necessary for you to hold your breath for a short period of time.

During your MRI examination, the MR system operator will be able to speak to you, hear you, and observe you at all times. Consult the MR system operator if you have any questions or feel anything unusual.

When the MRI procedure is over, you may be asked to wait until the images are examined to determine if more images are needed. After the scan, you have no restrictions and can go about your normal activities.

Once the entire MRI examination is completed, the pictures will be reviewed by a radiologist, a specially-trained physician who is able to interpret the images for your doctor. The radiologist will send your doctor a report. You should contact your doctor to go over your results and discuss your next step.

DISCLAIMER

This information is provided for the sole purpose of educating you as to the basics of the MRI examination. You should rely on your physician, a radiologist, or an MRI technologist for specific information about your own examination.

[*Developed in conjunction with the Safety Committee of the International Society for Magnetic Resonance in Medicine, www.ISMRM.org. Reviewed and updated 2012.]

Metallic Foreign Bodies and Screening

A patient or individual with a history of being injured by a metallic foreign body such as a bullet, shrapnel, or other metallic object should be thoroughly screened and evaluated prior to admission to the area of the MR system. This is particularly important because serious injury may occur as a result of movement or dislodgment of the metallic foreign body as it is attracted by the powerful static magnetic field. In addition, excessive heating may occur, although this tends to happen only if the object is made from conductive material and has an elongated shape or forms a loop of a certain diameter.

The relative risk of injury is dependent on the ferromagnetic properties of the foreign body, the geometry and dimensions of the object, the strength of the static magnetic field, and the strength of the spatial gradient magnetic field of the MR system. Additionally, the potential for injury is related to the amount of force with which the object is "fixed" or retained within the tissue (i.e., counter-force or retention force from scarring or encapsulation may prevent migration of the metal) and whether or not it is positioned in or adjacent to a sensitive site of the body such as vital neural, vascular, or soft tissue structure.

The use of plain film radiography is the technique of choice recommended to detect metallic foreign bodies for individuals and patients prior to admission to the MR environment. This includes screening for the presence of metallic orbital foreign bodies (see **Metallic Orbital Foreign Bodies and Screening**). The sensitivity of plain film radiography is considered to be sufficient to identify any metal object with a mass large enough to present a hazard to an individual or patient in the MR environment.

REFERENCES

Boutin RD, et al. Injuries associated with MR imaging: survey of safety records and methods used to screen patients for metallic foreign bodies before imaging. Am J Roentgenol 1994;162:189.

Dempsey MF, Condon B, Hadley DM. Investigation of the factors responsible for burns during MRI. J Magn Reson Imaging 2001;13:627-631.

Elster AD, et al. Patient screening prior to MR imaging: a practical approach synthesized from protocols at 15 U.S. medical centers. Am J Roentgenol 1994;162:195.

International Commission on Non-Ionizing Radiation Protection (ICNIRP) Statement, Medical magnetic resonance procedures: protection of patients. Health Physics 2004;87:197-216.

Jarvik JG, Ramsey JG. Radiographic screening for orbital foreign bodies prior to MR imaging: Is it worth it? Am J Neuroradiol 2000;1:245.

Eshed I, Kushnir T, et al. Is magnetic resonance imaging safe for patients with retained metal fragments from combat and terrorist attacks? Acta Radiol. 2010;51:170-4.

Mani, RL. In search of an effective screening system for intraocular metallic foreign bodies prior to MR - An important issue of patient safety. Am J Neuroradiol 1988;9:1032.

Murphy KJ, Burnberg JA. Orbital plain film as a prerequisite for MR imaging: is a known history of injury sufficient screening criteria? Am J Roentgenol 1996;167:1053.

Otto PM, et al. Screening test for detection of metallic foreign objects in the orbit before magnetic resonance imaging. Invest Radiol 1992;27:308-311.

Seidenwurm DJ, et al. Cost utility analysis of radiographic screening for an orbital foreign body before MR imaging. Am J Neuroradiol 2000;21:426.

Shellock FG. Magnetic Resonance Procedures: Health Effects and Safety. CRC Press, LLC, Boca Raton, FL, 2001.

Shellock FG, Crues JV. MR procedures: biologic effects, safety, and patient care. Radiology, 2004;232:635-652.

Shellock FG, Kanal E. SMRI Safety Committee. Policies, guidelines, and recommendations for MR imaging safety and patient management. J Magn Reson Imaging 1991;1:97-101.

Williams S, et al. Ferrous intraocular foreign bodies and magnetic resonance imaging. Am J Ophthalmology 1998;105:398.

Zhang Y, et al. Tiny ferromagnetic intraocular foreign bodies detected by magnetic resonance imaging: a report of two cases. J Magn Reson Imaging. 2009;29:704-7.

Metallic Orbital Foreign Bodies and Screening

The case report in 1986 by Kelly et al. regarding a patient that sustained an orbital injury from a metallic foreign body led to substantial controversy regarding the procedure required to screen patients prior to MR procedures. Notably, this incident is the only serious eye-related injury that has occurred in the MR environment (i.e., based on a review of the peer-reviewed literature). In consideration of this, the policy of performing radiographic screening for orbital foreign bodies in patients or individuals simply because of a history of occupational exposure to metallic fragments must be reconsidered.

A study by Seidenwurm et al. (2000) evaluated the practical aspects and cost-effectiveness of using a clinical versus radiographic technique to initially screen patients for orbital foreign bodies before MR procedures. The cost of screening was determined on the basis of published reports, disability rating guides, and a practice survey. A sensitivity analysis was performed for each variable. For this analysis, the benefits of screening were avoidance of immediate, permanent, nonameliorable, or unilateral blindness.

The findings of Seidenwurm et al. support the fact that the use of clinical screening before radiography increases the cost-effectiveness of foreign body screening by an order of magnitude (i.e., assuming base case ocular foreign body removal rates). From a clinical screening standpoint for a metallic foreign body located in the orbit, asking the patient "Did a doctor get it all out?" serves this purpose.

Seidenwurm et al. implemented the following policy with regard to screening patients with suspected metallic foreign bodies, "If a patient reports injury from an ocular foreign body that was subsequently removed by a doctor or that resulted in negative findings on any examination, we perform MR imaging…Those persons with a history of injury and no subsequent negative eye examination are screened radiographically." Of note is that Seidenwurm et al. performed more than 100,000 MRI procedures under this protocol without incident.

Thus, an occupational history of exposure to metallic fragments, by itself, is insufficient to mandate radiographic orbital screening. Therefore, guidelines for foreign body screening should be based on this information and because radiographic screening before MR procedures on the basis of occupational exposure alone is neither clinically necessary nor cost-effective.

Clinical Screening Protocol. The procedure to follow with regard to patients with suspected metallic orbital foreign bodies involves asking them if they had an ocular injury. If they sustained an ocular injury, they are asked whether they had a medical examination at the time of the injury and whether they were told by the examining doctor, "It's all out." If they did not have an injury, if they were told their ophthalmologic examination was normal, and/or if the foreign body was removed entirely at the time of the injury, then they can proceed to MR imaging.

Radiographic Screening Protocol. Based on the results of the clinical screening protocol, patients are screened radiographically if they sustained an ocular injury related to a metallic foreign object and they were told that the eye examination revealed that the foreign body was not removed. In such a case, the MRI examination is postponed and the patient is scheduled for screening radiography.

In the event that the removal of the entire metallic foreign body cannot be verified or if there is insufficient information to confirm that there is no metallic foreign body present, screening radiography should be used prior to MRI.

SCREENING ADOLESCENTS FOR METALLIC ORBITAL FOREIGN BODIES

A case report by Elmquist and Shellock (1996) illustrates that special precautions are needed for screening adolescent patients prior to MR procedures. This article described an incident in which a 12-year-old patient accompanied by his parent completed all routine screening procedures prior to MR imaging of the lumbar spine. The patient and parent provided negative answers to all questions regarding prior injuries by metallic objects and the presence of metallic foreign bodies.

While entering the MR system room, the adolescent patient appeared to be anxious about the examination. He was placed in a feet-first, supine position on the MR system table and prepared for the procedure. As the patient was moved slowly toward the opening of a 1.5-Tesla MR system, he complained of a pressure sensation in his left eye. The MRI technologist immediately removed the patient from the MR environment.

Once again, the patient was questioned regarding a previous eye injury. The patient denied sustaining such an injury. Despite that patient's response, a metallic foreign body in the orbit was suspected. Therefore, plain film radiographs of the orbits were obtained and revealed a metallic foreign body in the left orbit. The patient and parent were counseled regarding the implications of future MR procedures with respect to the possibility of significant eye injury related to movement or dislodgment of the metallic object. This case demonstrates that routine safety protocols may be insufficient for adolescents referred for MR procedures. Accordingly, it is recommended to provide adolescents with additional screening that includes private counseling about the hazards associated with the MR environment.

REFERENCES

Boutin RD, et al. Injuries associated with MR imaging: survey of safety records and methods used to screen patients for metallic foreign bodies before imaging. Am J Roentgenol 1994;162:189.

Elmquist C, Shellock FG, Stoller D. Screening adolescents for metallic foreign bodies before MR procedures. J Magn Reson Imaging 1996;5:784.

Elster AD, et al. Patient screening prior to MR imaging: a practical approach synthesized from protocols at 15 U.S. medical center. Am J Roentgenol 1994;162:195.

Jarvik JG, Ramsey JG. Radiographic screening for orbital foreign bodies prior to MR imaging: Is it worth it? Am J Neuroradiol 2000;21:245.

Kanal E, Barkovich AJ, et al. ACR guidance document for safe MR practices: 2007. AJR Am J Roentgenol. 2007;188:1447-1474.

Kelly WM, et al. Ferromagnetism of intraocular foreign body causes unilateral blindness after MR study. Am J Neuroradiol 1986;7: 243.

Mani RL. In search of an effective screening system for intraocular metallic foreign bodies prior to MR - An important issue of patient safety. Am J Neuroradiol 1988;9:1032.

Murphy KJ, Brunberg JA. Orbital plain film as a prerequisite for MR imaging: is a known history of injury sufficient screening criteria? Am J Roentgenol 1996;167:1053.

Seidenwurm DJ, et al. Cost utility analysis of radiographic screening for an orbital foreign body before MR imaging. Am J Neuroradiol 2000;21: 426.

Shellock FG. New recommendations for screening patients for suspected orbital foreign bodies. Signals, No. 36, Issue 4, pp. 8-9, 2001.

Shellock FG, Kanal E. SMRI Safety Committee. Policies, guidelines, and recommendations for MR imaging safety and patient management. J Magn Reson Imaging 1991;1:97-101.

Williams S, et al. Ferrous intraocular foreign bodies and magnetic resonance imaging. Am J Opthalmol 1998;05:398.

Zhang Y, et al. Tiny ferromagnetic intraocular foreign bodies detected by magnetic resonance imaging: a report of two cases. J Magn Reson Imaging. 2009;29:704-7.

Monitoring Patients in the MR Environment

Conventional monitoring equipment and accessories were not designed to operate in the harsh magnetic resonance (MR) environment that utilizes electromagnetic fields that can adversely affect or alter the operation of these devices. Fortunately, physiologic monitors and other patient support devices have been developed or specially-modified to perform properly in this setting.

MR healthcare professionals must consider the ethical and medico-legal ramifications of providing proper patient care that includes identifying patients that require monitoring in the MR setting and following a proper protocol to ensure their safety by using appropriate equipment, devices, and accessories. The early detection and treatment of complications that may occur in high-risk, critically-ill, sedated, or anesthetized patients undergoing MR procedures can prevent relatively minor problems from becoming life-threatening situations.

GENERAL POLICIES AND PROCEDURES

Monitoring during an MR examination is indicated whenever a patient requires observations of vital physiologic parameters due to an underlying health problem or is unable to respond or alert the MRI technologist or other healthcare professional regarding pain, respiratory problem, cardiac distress, or difficulty that might arise during the procedure. In addition, a patient should be monitored if there is a greater potential for a change in physiologic status during the MR exam. **Table 1** summarizes the patients that may require monitoring during MR procedures. Besides patient monitoring, various support devices and accessories may be needed for use in high-risk patients to ensure safety.

Because of the widespread use of MRI contrast agents and the potential for adverse effects or idiosyncratic reactions to occur, it is prudent to have monitoring equipment and accessories readily available for the proper management and support of patients who may experience side-effects. This is emphasized because adverse events, while extremely rare, may be serious or life threatening.

In 1992, the Safety Committee of the Society for Magnetic Resonance Imaging first published guidelines and recommendations concerning the monitoring of patients during MR procedures. This information indicates that all patients undergoing MR examinations should be visually and/or verbally (e.g., intercom system) monitored, and that patients who are sedated, anesthetized, or are unable to communicate must be physiologically monitored and supported by the appropriate means.

Importantly, guidelines issued by the Joint Commission on Accreditation of Healthcare Organizations (JCAHO) indicate that patients receiving sedatives or anesthetics require monitoring during administration and recovery from these medications. Other professional organizations, including the American Society of Anesthesiologists (ASA), similarly recommend the need to monitor certain patients using proper equipment and techniques.

Table 1. Patients that require monitoring and support during MR procedures.

- Physically or mentally unstable patients.
- Patients with compromised physiologic functions.
- Patients who are unable to communicate.
- Neonatal and pediatric patients.
- Sedated or anesthetized patients.
- Patients undergoing MR-guided interventional or intraoperative procedures.
- Critically-ill or high-risk patients.
- Patients who may have a reaction to an MRI contrast agent or medications.

SELECTION OF PARAMETERS TO MONITOR

The proper selection of the specific physiologic parameters that should be monitored during the MR procedure is crucial for patient safety. Various factors must be considered including the patient's medical history, present condition, the use of medication and possible side effects, as well as aspects of the MR procedure to be performed. For example, if the patient requires general anesthesia during the MR procedure, monitoring multiple physiologic parameters is required. Policies and procedures for the management of the patient in the MR environment should be comparable to those used in the operating room or critical care setting, especially with respect to monitoring and support requirements. Specific recommendations for physiologic monitoring of patients during MR examinations should be developed in consideration of "standard of care" issues as well as in consultation with anesthesiologists and other similar healthcare specialists. Notably, the Society of Anesthesiologists Task Force on Anesthetic Care for Magnetic Resonance Imaging recently presented a practice advisory on anesthetic care for patients undergoing MRI.

PERSONNEL INVOLVED IN PATIENT MONITORING

Only healthcare professionals with appropriate training and experience should be permitted to monitor and manage patients during MR procedures. The healthcare professional must be experienced with the operation of the monitoring equipment and accessories used in the MR environment and should be able to recognize equipment malfunctions, device problems, and recording artifacts. Furthermore, this individual should be well-versed in screening patients for conditions that may complicate the procedure. For example, patients with asthma, congestive heart failure, obesity, obstructive sleep apnea, and other conditions are at increased risk for having problems during sedation or anesthesia. Also, the healthcare professional must be able to identify and manage adverse events using appropriate equipment and procedures.

Policies and procedures must be implemented to continue physiologic monitoring and management of the patient by trained personnel after the MR procedure is performed. This is especially needed for a patient recovering from the effects of a sedative or general anesthesia.

The monitoring of physiologic parameters and management of the patient during an MR procedure may be the responsibility of one or more individuals depending on the level of training for the healthcare professional and in consideration of the condition, medical history, and procedure that is to be performed for the patient. These individuals include anesthesiologists, nurses, MRI technologists, or radiologists.

EMERGENCY PLAN

The development, implementation, and regular practice of an emergency plan that addresses and defines the activities, use of equipment, and other pertinent issues related to a medical emergency are important for patient safety. For example, a plan needs to be developed for handling patients if there is the need to remove them from the MR system room to perform cardiopulmonary resuscitation. Obviously, taking necessary equipment such as a cardiac defibrillator, intubation instruments, or other similar devices near the MR system could pose a substantial hazard to the patients and healthcare workers if these are not safe for use in the MR environment. Healthcare professionals who are members of the cardiopulmonary resuscitation (i.e., "code blue") team must be trained to conduct their activities in the MR setting.

For out-patient or mobile MR facilities, it is necessary to educate outside emergency personnel (e.g., paramedics, firefighters, etc.) regarding the potential hazards associated with the MR environment. Typically, MRI facilities not affiliated with or in close proximity to a hospital must contact paramedics to handle medical emergencies and to transport patients to the hospital for additional care. Therefore, personnel responsible for summoning the paramedics, notifying the hospital, and performing other integral activities must be designated beforehand to avoid problems and confusion during an actual emergent event.

TECHNIQUES AND EQUIPMENT USED TO MONITOR AND SUPPORT PATIENTS

Physiologic monitoring and support of patients is not a trivial task in the MR environment. The types of equipment for patient monitoring and support must be considered carefully and utilized properly to ensure the safety of both patients and MR healthcare professionals.

Several potential problems and hazards are associated with the performance of patient monitoring and support in the MR environment. Physiologic monitors and accessories that contain ferromagnetic components (e.g., transformers, outer casings, etc.) can be strongly attracted by the static magnetic field used of the MR system, posing a serious "missile" or projectile hazard to patients and healthcare workers.

Necessary or critical devices that have ferromagnetic components should be permanently fixed to the floor or tethered to the wall and properly labeled with warning information to prevent them from being moved too close to the MR system. All personnel involved with MR procedures should be aware of the importance of the placement and use of the equipment, especially with regard to the hazards of moving portable equipment too close to the MR system to prevent serious missile-related and other accidents.

Electromagnetic fields associated with the MR system can significantly effect the operation of conventional monitoring equipment, especially those with displays that involve electron beams (i.e., CRTs). In addition, the monitoring equipment, itself, may emit spurious noise that, in turn, produces artifacts on the MR images.

Physiologic monitors that contain microprocessors or other similar components may "leak" and produce electromagnetic interference that can substantially alter MR images. To prevent adverse interactions between the MR system and physiologic monitors, RF-shielded cables, RF filters, special outer RF-shielded enclosures, or fiber-optic techniques can be utilized to prevent image-related or other problems in the MR environment.

During the operation of MR systems, electrical currents may be generated in the conductive materials of monitoring equipment that are used as part of the interface to the patient. These currents can be of sufficient magnitude to cause excessive heating and thermal injury to the patient. Serious burns have occurred in association with MR procedures that were directly attributed to the utilization of monitoring devices. These injuries were related to the use of electrocardiographic lead wires, plethysmographic gating systems, pulse oximeters, and other types of monitoring equipment comprised of wires, cables, or similar components made from conductive materials. Therefore, it is important to follow the instructions and recommendations from the manufacturers with regard to the use of the devices in the MR environment. Fortunately, modern-day physiologic monitoring devices utilize fiber-optic techniques to prevent many of the afore-mentioned issues that exist with "hard-wire" cables, wires, and patient-monitor interfaces.

MONITORING EQUIPMENT AND SUPPORT DEVICES

This section describes the physiologic parameters that may be assessed in patients during MR examinations using appropriate monitoring equipment for the MR environment. In addition, various devices and accessories that are useful for the support and management of patients are presented.

Electrocardiogram and Heart Rate

Monitoring the patient's electrocardiogram (ECG) in the MR environment is particularly challenging because of the inherent distortion of the ECG waveform that occurs using MR systems operating at high field strengths. This effect is observed as blood, a conductive fluid, flows through the large vascular structures in the presence of the static magnetic field of the MR system. The resulting induced biopotential is seen primarily as an augmented T-wave amplitude, although other non-specific waveform-changes are also apparent on the ECG. Since altered T-waves or ST segments may be associated with cardiac disorders, static magnetic field-induced ECG-distortions may be problematic for certain patients. For this reason, it may be necessary to obtain a baseline recording of the ECG prior to placing the patient inside the MR system along with a recording obtained immediately after the MR procedure to determine the cardiac status of the patient.

Additional artifacts caused by the static, gradient, and RF fields of the MR system can severely distort the ECG, making observation of morphologic changes and detection of arrhythmias difficult. ECG artifacts that occur in the MR environment may be decreased substantially by implementing several simple techniques that include, the following:

- Use ECG electrodes that have minimal metal or those recommended by the manufacturer
- Select electrodes and cables that contain nonferromagnetic metals
- Place the limb electrodes in close proximity to one another
- Position the line between the limb electrodes and leg electrodes parallel to the magnetic field flux lines
- Maintain a small area between the limb and leg electrode
- Twist or braid the ECG leads
- Position the area of the electrodes near or in the center of the MR system

The use of proper ECG electrodes (i.e., those tested and deemed to be acceptable for patients by the monitoring equipment manufacturer) is required to ensure patient safety and proper recording of the ECG in the MR environment. Accordingly, ECG electrodes have been specially developed for use during MR procedures to protect the patient from potentially hazardous conditions. These ECG electrodes were also designed to reduce imaging artifacts.

Fiber-optic ECG recording techniques may be used to prevent burns during MR examinations. For example, one such fiber-optic system acquires the ECG waveform using a special transceiver that resides in the MR system bore along with the patient and is located near the ECG electrodes. A module digitizes and optically encodes the ECG waveform and transmits it to the monitor using a fiber-optic cable. The use of this fiber-optic ECG technique eliminates the potential for burns associated with hard-wired ECG systems by removing the conductive patient cable and the "antenna effect" that are typical responsible for excessive heating.

Besides using an ECG monitor, the patient's heart rate may be determined continuously during the MR procedure using other acceptable devices including a photoplethysmograph and a pulse oximeter. A noninvasive, heart rate and blood pressure monitor (see section below) can also be utilized to obtain intermittent or semi-continuous recordings of heart rate during the MR examination.

Blood Pressure

Conventional, manual sphygmomanometers may be adapted for use during MR procedures. This is typically accomplished by lengthening the tubing from the cuff to the device so that the mercury column and other primary components may be positioned an acceptable distance (e.g., at 200 gauss or higher fringe field level) from the MR system. Blood pressure measuring devices that incorporate a spring-gauge may be adversely affected by magnetic fields, causing them to work erroneously in the MR setting. Therefore, spring-gauge blood pressure devices should undergo pre-clinical testing before being used to monitor patients.

A blood pressure monitor that uses the oscillometric method may be utilized to obtain semi-continuous recordings of systolic, diastolic, and mean blood pressures as well as pulse rate. These devices can record systemic blood pressure in adult, pediatric, and neonate patients, selecting the appropriate blood pressure cuff size for the subject. However, the intermittent inflation of the blood pressure cuff by an automated, noninvasive blood pressure monitor may disturb lightly sedated patients, especially infants or neonates, causing them to move and disrupt the MR procedure. For this reason, the use of a noninvasive blood pressure monitor may not be the best instrument to conduct physiologic monitoring in every patient.

Respiratory Rate and Apnea

Because respiratory depression and upper airway obstruction are frequent complications associated with the use of sedatives and anesthetics, monitoring techniques that detect a decrease in respiratory rate, hypoxemia, or airway obstruction should be used during the administration of these drugs. This is particularly important in the MR environment because visual observation of the patient's respiratory efforts is often difficult.

Respiratory rate monitoring can be performed during MR procedures by various techniques. The impedance method that utilizes chest leads and electrodes (similar to those used to record the ECG) may be used to monitor respiratory rate. This technique of recording respiratory rate measures a difference in electrical impedance induced between the leads that correspond to changes in respiratory movements. Unfortunately, the electrical impedance method of assessing respiratory rate tends to be inaccurate in pediatric patients because of the small volumes and associated motions of the relatively small thorax.

Respiratory rate may also be monitored using a rubber bellows placed around the patient's thorax or abdomen (i.e., for "chest" or "belly" breathers). The bellows is attached to a pressure transducer that records body movements associated with inspiration and expiration. However, the bellows monitoring technique, like the electrical impedance method, is only capable of recording body movements associated with respiratory efforts. Therefore, these respiratory rate monitoring techniques do not detect apneic episodes related to upper airway obstruction (i.e., absent airflow despite respiratory effort) and, therefore, may not provide sufficient sensitivity for assessing patients during MR procedures. For this reason, assessment of respiratory rate and identification of apnea should be accomplished using more appropriate monitoring devices.

Respiratory rate and apnea may be monitored during MR procedures using an end-tidal carbon dioxide monitor or a capnometer. These devices measure the level of carbon dioxide during the end of the respiratory cycle (i.e., end-tidal carbon dioxide). Additionally, capnometers provide quantitative data with respect to end-tidal carbon dioxide that is important for determining certain aspects of gas exchange in patients. The waveform provided on the end-tidal carbon dioxide monitors is also useful for assessing whether the patient is having difficulties breathing. The interface between the patient for the end-tidal carbon dioxide monitor and capnometer is a nasal or oro-nasal cannula that is made from plastic. This interface prevents potential adverse interactions between the monitor and the patient during an MR examination.

Oxygen Saturation

Oxygen saturation is a crucial variable to measure in sedated and anesthetized patients. This physiologic parameter is measured using pulse oximetry, a monitoring technique that assesses the oxygenation of tissue. Additionally, the patient's heart rate may be calculated by measuring the frequency that pulsations occur as the blood moves through the vascular bed. Thus, a pulse oximeter can be used to determine oxygen saturation and pulse rate on a continuous basis by measuring the transmission of light through a vascular site such as the ear lobe, finger-tip, or toe. Notably, anesthesiologists consider the use of pulse oximetry to be the standard practice for monitoring sedated or anesthetized patients.

Commercially-available, specially-modified pulse oximeters that have hard-wire cables have been used to monitor sedated patients during MR procedures with moderate success. Unfortunately, these pulse oximeters tend to work intermittently during the operation of the MR system, primarily due to interference from the gradient and/or radio frequency electromagnetic fields. Of greater concern is the fact that pulse oximeters with hard-wire cables have been responsible for many patient burn injuries during MRI examinations, presumably as a result of excessive current being induced in the conductive cables.

Pulse oximeters have been developed that use fiber-optic technology to obtain and transmit the physiologic signals from the patient. These devices operate without interference by the electromagnetic fields used for MR procedures. Several different fiber-optic pulse oximeters are commercially available for use in the MR environment.

Temperature

There are several reasons to monitor body and/or skin temperatures during MR procedures. These include recording temperatures in neonates with inherent problems retaining body heat (a tendency that is augmented during sedation or anesthesia), in patients during MR procedures that use high levels of RF power, and in patients with underlying conditions that impair their ability to dissipate heat.

Skin and body temperatures may be monitored during MR procedures using a variety of techniques. However, it should be noted that the use of hard-wire, thermistor or thermocouple-based techniques to record temperatures in the MR environment typically cause artifacts or erroneous measurements due to direct heating of the temperature probes. A more appropriate, effective and easier technique of recording temperatures during MR examinations is with the use of a fluoroptic thermometry system. Notably, monitoring skin temperature, alone, is insufficient to ensure patient safety as this parameter does not provide proper information relative to deep body or core temperature. (See section in this textbook entitled, "**Monitoring Body Temperature During MRI**".)

The fluoroptic monitoring system has several important features that make it particularly useful for temperature monitoring during MR procedures. For example, this device incorporates fiber-optic probes that are small but efficient in carrying optical signals over long paths, it provides noise-free applications in electromagnetically hostile environments, and has fiber-optic components that will not pose a risk to patients.

Multi-Parameter Physiologic Monitoring Systems

In certain cases, it is necessary to monitor several different physiologic parameters simultaneously in patients undergoing MR examinations. While several different stand-alone units may be used to accomplish this task, the most efficient means of recording multiple parameters is by utilizing a monitoring system that permits the measurement of different physiologic functions such as heart rate, respiratory rate, blood pressure, and oxygen saturation.

Currently, there are a number of multi-parameter patient monitoring systems that are acceptable for use in the MRI environment, even in the 3-Tesla setting. Typically, these devices are designed with components positioned within the MR system room and incorporate special circuitry to substantially reduce the artifacts that effect the recording of ECG and other physiologic variables, making them also useful for the performance of "gated" MR procedures.

Ventilators

Devices used for mechanical ventilation of patients typically contain mechanical switches, microprocessors, and ferromagnetic components that may be adversely effected by the electromagnetic fields used by MR systems. Ventilators that are activated by high pressure oxygen and controlled by the use of fluidics (i.e., no requirements for electricity) may still have ferromagnetic parts that can malfunction as a result of interference from MR systems.

Ventilators have been modified or specially-designed for use during MR procedures performed in adult as well as neonatal patients. These devices tend to be constructed from non-ferromagnetic materials and have undergone pre-clinical evaluations to ensure that they operate properly in the MR environment, without producing artifacts on MR images.

Some ventilators only operate properly and are approved at a "safe" distance from the MR system due to the presence of ferromagnetic parts, including batteries. Thus, these devices are labeled "MR Conditional' and the conditions for use must be followed carefully. Therefore, it is advisable to permanently fix these ventilators to the floor or tether them to prevent missile-related accidents. Furthermore, these devices must be properly labeled with warning information to prevent them from being moved too close to the MR system. Healthcare workers should be trained regarding the specific MR conditional aspects of these ventilators.

Additional Devices and Accessories

A variety of devices and accessories are often necessary for support and management of high-risk or sedated patients in the MR setting. Gurneys, oxygen tanks, gas regulators, stethoscopes, suction devices, infusion pumps, power injectors, and other similar devices and accessories shown to be acceptable for the MR environment may be obtained from various manufacturers and distributors. Additionally, there are gas anesthesia systems available that were designed for use in patients undergoing MR procedures.

SEDATION

Whenever sedatives are used, it is imperative to perform physiologic monitoring to ensure patient safety. In addition, it is important to have the necessary equipment readily available in the event of an emergency. These requirements should also be followed for patients undergoing sedation in the MR environment.

There is controversy regarding who should be responsible for performing sedation of patients in the MR setting. (For the sake of discussion, the terms "sedation" and "anesthesia" are used interchangeably since they are actually part of the same continuum.) Obviously, there are medical, regulatory, administrative, and financial issues to be considered.

In general, for patients with conditions that complicate sedation procedures, a nurse under the direction of an anesthesiologist or a specially trained radiologist may be responsible for preparing, sedating, monitoring, and recovering these cases. However, for patients with serious medical or other unusual problems, it is advisable to utilize anesthesia consultation to properly manage these individuals before, during, and after MR procedures.

In addition, the MRI facility should establish policies and guidelines for patient preparation, monitoring, sedation, and management during the post-sedation recovery period. These policies and guidelines should be based on standards established by the American Society of Anesthesiologists (ASA), the American College of Radiology (ACR), the American Academy of Pediatrics Committee on Drugs (AAP-COD), and the Joint Commission on Accreditation of Healthcare Organizations (JCAHO).

Practice Guidelines for Sedation and Anesthesia from the American Society of Anesthesiologists indicate that an trained healthcare professional must be present that is responsible for monitoring the patient if a sedative or anesthetic agent is used. Furthermore, the following aspects of patient monitoring must be performed:

1) Visual monitoring
2) Assessment of the level of consciousness
3) Evaluation of ventilatory status
4) Evaluation of oxygen status assessed via the use of pulse oximetry
5) Determination of hemodynamic status via the use of blood pressure monitoring and electrocardiography if significant cardiovascular disease is present in the patient

Healthcare professionals must be able to recognize complications of sedation such as hypoventilation and airway obstruction as well as be able to establish a patent airway for positive-pressure ventilation.

Patient Preparation

Special patient screening must be conducted to identify conditions that may complicate sedation in order to properly prepare the patient for the administration of a sedative. This screening procedure should request important information from the patient that includes the following: major organ system disease (e.g., diabetes, pulmonary, cardiac, or hepatic disease), prior experience or adverse reactions to sedatives or anesthetics, current medications, allergies to drugs, and a history of alcohol, substance, or tobacco abuse.

In addition, the "nothing by mouth" (NPO) interval for the patient must be determined to reduce the risk of aspiration during the procedure. The ASA "Practice Guidelines Regarding Preoperative Fasting" recommend a minimum NPO periods of two hours for clear liquids, four hours for breast milk, six hours for infant formula, and six hours for a "light meal". The NPO period is extremely important because sedatives may depress the patient's gag reflex.

Administration of Sedation

A thorough discussion of sedation techniques especially with regard to the use of various pharmacologic agents is outside the scope of this monograph. Therefore, interested readers are referred to the excellent, comprehensive review of this topic written by Reinking Rothshild (2000), A review of more recent peer-reviewed papers on this topic is also recommended.

Documentation

During the use of sedation, written records must be maintained that indicate the patient's vital signs as well as the name, dosage, and time of administration for all drugs that are given to the patient. The use of a time-based anesthesia-type record, such as that recommended by Reinking Rothschild (2000), is the best means of maintaining written documentation for sedation of patients in the MR environment.

Post-Sedation Recovery

After sedation, the medical care of the patient must continue. This is especially important for pediatric patients because certain medications have relatively long half-lives (e.g., chloral hydrate, pentobarbitol, etc.). Therefore, an appropriate room with monitoring and emergency equipment must be available to properly manage these patients.

Prior to allowing the patient to leave the MRI facility, the patient should be alert, oriented, and have stable vital signs. In addition, a responsible adult should accompany the patient home. Written instructions that include an emergency telephone number should be provided to the patient.

REFERENCES

American College of Radiology, ACR standard for the use of intravenous conscious sedation, and ACR standard for pediatric sedation/analgesia. In, 1998 ACR Standards, Reston, VA, American College of Radiology 1998; pp. 123.

American Academy of Pediatrics Committee on Drugs, Guidelines for monitoring and management of pediatric patients during and after sedation for diagnostic and therapeutics procedures. Pediatrics 1992;89:1100.

American Academy of Pediatrics; American Academy of Pediatric Dentistry, Guidelines for monitoring and management of pediatric patients during and after sedation for diagnostic and therapeutic procedures: an update. Pediatrics. 2006;118:2587-602.

A Report by the ASA Task Force on Sedation and Analgesia by Non-Anesthesiologists. Practice guidelines for sedation and analgesia by non-anesthesiologists. Anesthesiology 1996;84:459.

Dalal PG, et al. Sedation and anesthesia protocols used for magnetic resonance imaging studies in infants: provider and pharmacologic considerations. Anesth Analg. 2006;103:863-8.

De Sanctis Briggs V. Magnetic resonance imaging under sedation in newborns and infants: a study of 640 cases using sevoflurane. Paediatr Anaesth. 2005;15:9-15.

Gooden CK. Anesthesia for magnetic resonance imaging. Curr Opin Anaesthesiol. 2004;17:339-42.

Greenberg KL, Weinreb J, Shellock FG. "MR conditional" respiratory ventilator system incident in a 3-T MRI environment. Magn Reson Imaging. 2011 Aug 18. [Epub ahead of print]

Henrichs B, Walsh RP. Intraoperative magnetic resonance imaging for neurosurgical procedures: anesthetic implications. AANA J. 2011;79:71-7.

Holshouser B, Hinshaw DB, Shellock FG. Sedation, anesthesia, and physiologic monitoring during MRI. J Magn Reson Imaging 1993;3:553-558.

Johnston T, et al. Intraoperative MRI: safety. Neurosurg Clin N Am. 2009;20:147-53.

Kanal E, Shellock FG. Policies, guidelines, and recommendations for MR imaging safety and patient management. Patient monitoring during MR examinations. J Magn Reson Imaging 1992;2:247.

Kanal E, Shellock FG. Patient monitoring during clinical MR imaging. Radiology 1992;185:623.

Kanal E, Barkovich AJ, Bell C, et al. ACR guidance document for safe MR practices: 2007. AJR Am J Roentgenol. 2007;188:1447-1474.

McArdle C, et al. Monitoring of the neonate undergoing MR imaging: Technical considerations. Radiology 1986;159:223.

McClain CD, et al. Anesthetic concerns for pediatric patients in an intraoperative MRI suite. Curr Opin Anaesthesiol. 2011 Aug 11. [Epub ahead of print]

Reinking Rothschild D. Chapter 5, Sedation for open magnetic resonance imaging. In, Open MRI, P. A. Rothschild and D. Reinking Rothschild, Editors, Lippincott, Williams and Wilkins, Philadelphia, 2000, pp. 39.

Practice advisory on anesthetic care for magnetic resonance imaging: a report by the Society of Anesthesiologists Task Force on Anesthetic Care for Magnetic Resonance Imaging. Anesthesiology. 2009;110:459-79.

Schulte-Uentrop L, Goepfert MS. Anaesthesia or sedation for MRI in children. Curr Opin Anaesthesiol. 2010;23:513-7.

Serafini G, et al. Anesthesia for MRI in the paediatric patient. Minerva Anestesiol. 2005;71:361-6.

Shellock FG, Kanal E. Magnetic Resonance: Bioeffects, Safety, and Patient Management. Second Edition, Lippincott-Raven Press, New York, 1996.

Shellock FG. Chapter 11, Patient monitoring in the MR environment. In: Magnetic Resonance Procedures: Health Effects and Safety. CRC Press, Boca Raton, FL, 2001, pp. 217-241.

Monitoring Body Temperature During MRI

Introduction

Magnetic resonance imaging (MRI) has been an important diagnostic imaging modality for almost 30 years. Advancements in technology and imaging protocols have contributed to the growth of MRI applications and expanded the demographic of patient populations from neonates to high-risk patients. The use of sedation or anesthesia is necessary for certain MRI examinations, especially for pediatric or critically-ill patients (1). Importantly, the volume of pediatric patients undergoing MRI or computed tomography (CT) procedures under sedation or anesthesia has grown at an annual rate of 8% - 9% (2). This monograph focuses on the need to monitor body temperature in patients during MRI and discusses the sites to record temperature based on efficacy and stability of the measurement, as well as the response time (i.e., the temporal resolution) during temperature fluctuations.

Monitoring Patients in the MRI Environment

Conventional monitoring equipment and accessories were not designed to operate in the harsh MRI environment that utilizes electromagnetic fields that can adversely affect or alter the operation of these devices (3). Fortunately, various monitors and other patient support devices have been developed to perform properly during MRI procedures.

MRI healthcare professionals must consider the ethical and medico-legal ramifications of providing proper patient care that includes identifying patients that require monitoring in the MRI setting and following a proper protocol to ensure their safety by using appropriate equipment, devices, and accessories (3). The early detection and treatment of complications that may occur in high-risk, critically-ill, sedated, or anesthetized patients undergoing MRI examinations can prevent relatively minor issues from becoming life-threatening situations.

General Policies and Procedures

Patients undergoing MRI examinations while under sedation or general anesthesia require the same standard of care that is provided in operating rooms and intensive care units (ICU)(4, 5). This involves monitoring vital physiological parameters including the electrocardiogram (ECG), oxygen saturation, blood pressure, end tidal carbon dioxide (CO_2), and body temperature (6, 7). The use of sedation or anesthesia is necessary for certain MRI examinations, especially for pediatric or critically-ill patients (3, 8). Importantly, children represent the largest group requiring sedation for MRI exams (3, 8). Sedation is used on children to minimize discomfort, motion and anxiety during the procedure (8, 9). The American Academy of Pediatrics and the American College of Radiology have published guidelines for monitoring children and adults during sedation (8, 10). The vital signs that must be monitored include the heart rate, blood pressure, respiratory rate, oxygen saturation, blood oxygenation, and body temperature (8).

Because of the widespread use of MRI contrast agents and the potential for adverse effects or idiosyncratic reactions to occur, it is prudent to have appropriate monitoring equipment and accessories readily available for the proper management and support of patients who may experience side-effects. This is emphasized because adverse events, while extremely rare, may be serious or life threatening. In addition, patients may have adverse reactions to other medications while undergoing MRI procedures.

In 1992, the Safety Committee of the Society for Magnetic Resonance Imaging published guidelines and recommendations concerning the monitoring of patients during MRI procedures (11). This information indicates that all patients undergoing MRI examinations should be visually (e.g., using a camera system) and/or verbally (e.g., intercom system) monitored, and that patients who are sedated, anesthetized, or are unable to communicate should be physiologically monitored and supported by the appropriate means.

Injuries and fatalities have occurred in association with MRI examinations. These may have been prevented with the proper use of monitoring equipment and devices (3, 4, 11). Notably, guidelines issued by the Joint Commission on Accreditation of Healthcare Organizations (JCAHO) indicate that patients receiving sedatives or anesthetics require monitoring during administration and recovery from these medications (12). Other professional organizations similarly recommend the need to monitor certain patients using proper equipment and techniques (5, 6, 8, 9, 13).

Why Monitor Body Temperature?

In human subjects, "deep" body or core temperature is regulated between 36 and 38 degrees C by the hypothalamus and continuously fluctuates due to diurnal, internal, and external factors (14). Importantly, the regulation of body temperature is suppressed by anesthesia and generally results in patients becoming hypothermic (15, 16). Side-effects of a decrease in body temperature can range from hypovolemia, myocardial ischemia, cardiac arrhythmia, pulmonary edema, decreased cerebral blood flow in cases of mild hypothermia, to mortality related to extreme hypothermia (17).

Additionally, some patients may experience malignant hyperthermia, which is a rare life-threatening condition that is usually triggered by exposure to certain drugs used for general anesthesia. In susceptible individuals, these drugs can induce a drastic and uncontrolled increase in skeletal muscle oxidative metabolism, which overwhelms the body's capacity to supply oxygen, remove carbon dioxide, and regulate body temperature. Malignant hyperthermia can eventually lead to circulatory collapse and death if not quickly identified and treated.

The anesthesiologist or nurse anesthetist may not be able to clearly visualize or have close access to the patient during the MRI procedure due to the design of the MR system. The anesthesiologist or nurse anesthetist may not be in the immediate proximity of the patient during the MRI procedure due to the design of the MR system. Therefore, it is imperative to continuously monitor the body temperature and provide real time information to the anesthesia healthcare professional. It is also important that the measurement site has clinical relevance and a relatively "fast" response time to any fluctuation in body temperature because the anesthesiologist or nurse anesthetist is unable to visualize the discoloration of the patient skin in cases of sudden temperature changes.

Measuring Body Temperature During an MRI

The accuracy and efficacy of the measurement of body temperature has been a topic of discussion for many years (14, 18, 20). The measurement of temperature in a human subject is affected by the following factors (14, 21):

- The site of measurement (e.g., skin, oral, esophagus, rectal, pulmonary artery, hypothalamus, bladder, tympanic membrane, axillary area).
- Environmental conditions (temperature and humidity).
- The measurement technique (e.g., mercury thermometer, electronic thermometer, thermistor probe or catheter, thermocouple-based probe, infrared radiation readers, fiber optic method).

The most accurate body temperature is measured at the hypothalamus, but this site is not accessible by any practical means. Therefore, a "deep" body site that directly reflects the temperature "sensed" by the hypothalamus will provide clinically relevant information (14). For example, sites that provide high levels of accuracy and correlation to deep body temperature are pulmonary artery blood, urinary bladder, the esophagus, and rectum (18, 19, 22). However, the temporal resolution for each site varies, which can dramatically impact the ability to recognize clinically important changes that may require prompt patient management (14, 18).

When monitoring temperature during MRI, the decision on which body site to use should be based on accuracy as well as accessibility. There may be limitations on the type of equipment available for temperature measurements in the MR system room (3, 8, 23). For example, hard wire thermistor or thermocouple-based sensors are prone to measurement errors due to electromagnetic interference (EMI) and may introduce artifacts in the MR images (3). Fiber optic sensors (i.e., fluoroptic thermometry) are optimally used to record temperatures in the MRI environment because they safe and unaffected by EMI (3).

In the MRI setting, anesthesiologists, nurse anesthetists, and clinicians may be feel that they are limited to measure "surface" temperatures, such as those in the skin, axilla, and groin. However, these temperature measurement sites are very problematic insofar as they do not properly reflect "deep" body temperature and exhibit considerable temporal differences when changes occur. Another option is to use a minimally invasive measurement technique to record temperature in the rectum or esophagus.

While a so-called "surface" temperature site (i.e., skin, axilla, and groin) tends to be used for temperature recordings during MRI mainly because of the ease of obtaining the measurement with currently available equipment, this method does not provide an accurate representation of body temperature and is susceptible to substantial variations and erroneous information relative to the "deep" body temperature due to the specific site selected for temperature probe placement, patient movement, and environmental conditions (14, 19, 20)

Importantly, recording skin or surface temperature during MRI can be influenced by the level of the patient's perspiration due to RF heating and the use of blankets or air circulation from the fan in the bore of the MR system. Additionally, investigations have demonstrated that peripheral vasoconstriction resulting from skin surface cooling decreases the surface temperature measurement without influencing the core or deep body temperature (24).

In contrast, core or "deep" body temperature measurements require additional set up time and are minimally invasive but provide a more accurate representation of the body temperature (14). The two most prevalent core temperature measurement sites used during MRI procedures are the rectum and esophagus.

Rectal temperature measurements are highly accurate and usually within 0.6 degrees C of the deep body temperature (14). The main drawback to this temperature measurement site is associated with a lag or delay in the temporal response to changing body temperature due to the presence of thermal inertia from the intervening tissues (i.e., between the rectum and hypothalamus). This temporal delay may also be caused by the presence of feces and poor blood supply in the rectum (14, 25). A clinical investigation reported that the rectal temperature substantially lagged in response to changes in body temperature (25). The lack of temporal resolution can expose the patient to a hypothermic or hyperthermic condition for an extended period without it being recognized by the clinician. Also, special care must be taken when placing a rectal temperature probe in neonatal or pediatric patient to prevent perforation and infection (14, 25).

Esophageal temperature measurements provide a high level of accuracy and good temporal correlation to deep body temperature due to the close proximity to the aorta, a deep body site (20). In addition to the accuracy, the temperature recorded in the esophagus is responsive to fluctuations in body temperature and readily tracks changes compared to rectal or surface temperature measurement sites (14, 25). The only caveat is that the accuracy of measuring temperature in the esophagus is directly related to the proper positioning of the temperature sensor (14, 19). Airflow in the trachea can impact the measured temperature if the probe is not inserted deep enough into the esophagus. The recommended placement of the temperature sensor is in the lower one-third of the esophagus for an accurate core temperature measurement (14).

Monitoring Body Temperature During MRI: Recommendations

In consideration of the available temperature measurement sites that may be monitored during MRI, especially with regard to which site provides the most accurate information along with the best temporal resolution, the temperature of the esophagus will provide the most acceptable and clinically relevant information. Furthermore, esophageal temperature is insensitive to ambient air circulation and patient perspiration during the MRI examination and has the added benefit of fast response time to temperature fluctuations in the deep body compared to the measurement of temperature in the rectum. The current availability of temperature probes and recording equipment properly designed for use in the MRI setting, permits the monitoring of body temperature in the esophagus, which provides physiologic information that is vital to patient care.

[Excerpted with permission from Thacker V, Shellock FG. Monitoring Body Temperature During MRI.]

REFERENCES

(1) Schulte-Uentrop L, Goepfert MS. Anaesthesia or sedation for MRI in children. Curr Opin Anaesthesiol. 2010;23:513-7.

(2) Watchel RE, Dexter F, Dow AJ. Growth rates in pediatric diagnostic imaging and sedation. Anesthesia and Analgesia 2009;108:1616-1621.

(3) Shellock FG. Chapter 11, Patient Monitoring in the MRI Environment. In: Magnetic Resonance Procedures: Health Effects and Safety. CRC Press, Boca Raton, FL, 2001, pp. 217-241.

(4) Kanal E, Shellock, FG. Patient monitoring during clinical MR imaging. Radiology 1992;185:623.

(5) Practice Advisory on Anesthetic Care for Magnetic Resonance Imaging, Anesthesiology 2009;110:459–79

(6) Standards For Basic Anesthetic Monitoring (Approved By The ASA House of Delegates on October 21, 1986, And Last Amended On October 25, 2005)

(7) Holshouser, B., Hinshaw, D. B., and Shellock, F. G. Sedation, anesthesia, and physiologic monitoring during MRI. J Magn Reson Imaging 1993;3:553-558.

(8) American Academy of Pediatrics; American Academy of Pediatric Dentistry, Cote CJ, Wilson S; Work Group on Sedation. Guidelines for monitoring and management of pediatric patients during and after sedation for diagnostic and therapeutic procedures: an update. Pediatrics. 2006;118:2587-602.

(9) Kanal E, Barkovich AJ, et al. ACR guidance document for safe MR practices: 2007. AJR Am J Roentgenol. 2007;188:1447-1474.

(10) American College of Radiology, ACR standard for the use of intravenous conscious sedation, and ACR standard for pediatric sedation/analgesia. In, 1998 ACR Standards, Reston, VA, American College of Radiology 1998.

(11) Kanal E, Shellock, FG. Policies, guidelines, and recommendations for MR imaging safety and patient management. Patient monitoring during MR examinations. J Magn Reson Imaging 1992;2:247.

(12) Joint Commission on Accreditation of Healthcare Organizations. Sedation and anesthesia care standards. Oakbrook Terrace, IL:2003.

(13) Dalal PG, et al. Sedation and anesthesia protocols used for magnetic resonance imaging studies in infants: provider and pharmacologic considerations. Anesth Analg. 2006;103:863-8.

(14) Knies RC. Temperature Measurement in Acute Care: The Who, What, Where, When, Why, and How? Web Article http://enw.org/Research-Thermometry.htm (Accessed June 24, 2011)

(15) Michiaki Y. Anesthesia and Body Temperature: Temperature Regulation under General Anesthesia Combined with Epidural Anesthesia. Journal of Clinical Anesthesia 2000; 24:1416-1424.

(16) Takashi M. Anesthesia and Body Temperature: General Anesthesia and Thermoregulation. Journal of Clinical Anesthesia 2000; 24:1408-1415.

(17) Schubert A. Side Effects of Mild Hypothermia. Journal or Neurological Anesthesiology 1995, Vol 7, No. 2, Page 139-147

(18) Lilly JK, Boland JP, Zekan S. Urinary Bladder temperature Monitoring: A new Index of Body Core Temperatures, Critical Care Medicine 1980;8:742-744

(19) Lefrant J –Y, et al. Temperature Measurement in intensive care patients: comparison of urinary bladder, esophageal, rectal, axillary, and inguinal methods versus pulmonary artery core method. Intensive care Med 2003; 29:414-418 .

(20) Robinson J, Charlton J, Seal R, Spady D, Joffres MR. Esophageal, rectal, axillary, tympanic, and pulmonary artery temperatures during cardiac surgery. Canadian Journal of Anesthesiology 1998;45:317-323.

(21) Takashi A. Anesthesia and Body Temperature: interoperative monitoring of body temperature and its significance. Journal of Clinical Anesthesia, 2000;24:1432-1443.

(22) Shellock FG, Rubin SA. Simplified and highly accurate core temperature measurements. Med Prog Technol.1982;8:187-8.

(23) Gooden CK. Anesthesia for magnetic resonance imaging. Curr Opin Anaesthesiol. 2004;17:339-42.

(24) Wilson TE, et al. Skin surface cooling elicits peripheral and visceral vasoconstriction in humans. Journal of Applied Physiology 2007;103:1257-1262.

(25) Newsham KR, et al. Comparison of rectal and tympanic thermometry: Discussion. Southern Medical Journal 2002; 95, 804-810.

MRI Contrast Agents and Adverse Reactions*

Adverse Reactions to Gadolinium-Based Contrast Media*

Gadolinium chelates have been approved for parenteral use since the late 1980s. Although these agents can be differentiated on the basis of stability, viscosity, and osmolality, they cannot be differentiated on the basis of efficacy. Gadolinium chelates are extremely well tolerated by the vast majority of patients in whom they are injected. Acute adverse reactions are encountered with a lower frequency than is observed after administration of iodinated contrast media.

Adverse Reactions

The frequency of all acute adverse events after an injection of 0.1 or 0.2 mmol/kg of gadolinium chelate ranges from 0.07% to 2.4%. The vast majority of these reactions are mild, including coldness at the injection site, nausea with or without vomiting, headache, warmth or pain at the injection site, paresthesias, dizziness, and itching. Reactions resembling an "allergic" response are very unusual and vary in frequency from 0.004% to 0.7%. A rash, hives, or urticaria are the most frequent of this group, and very rarely there may be bronchospasm. Severe, life-threatening anaphylactoid or nonallergic anaphylactic reactions are exceedingly rare (0.001% to 0.01%). In an accumulated series of 687,000 doses there were only 5 severe reactions. In another survey based on 20 million administered doses there were 55 cases of severe reactions. Fatal reactions to gadolinium chelate agents occur but are extremely rare.

Gadolinium chelates administered to patients with acute renal failure or severe chronic kidney disease can result in a syndrome of nephrogenic systemic fibrosis (NSF). (See the Chapter on NSF) (www.acr.org/SecondaryMainMenuCategories/quality_safety/contrast_m anual/NephrogenicSystemicFibrosis.aspx)

Risk Factors

The frequency of acute adverse reactions to gadolinium contrast media is about 8 times higher in patients with a previous reaction to gadolinium-based contrast media. Second reactions to gadoliniumbased media (GBCM) can be more severe than the first. Persons with asthma and various other allergies, including to other medications or foods are also at greater risk, with reports of adverse reaction rates as high as 3.7%. Although there is no cross-reactivity, patients who have had previous allergic-like reactions to iodinated contrast media are also in this category.

In the absence of any widely accepted policy for dealing with patients with prior contrast reactions (especially to gadolinium-based media) and the need for subsequent exposure to magnetic resonance (MR) agents, it does seem prudent to at least take precautions in a patient who previously had a reaction to GBCM. It should be determined if gadolinium-based contrast medium is necessary, if a different brand could be used, and if 12 to 24 hours of premedication with corticosteroids and antihistamines could be initiated. This administration is particularly applicable in patients who had prior moderate to severe reactions.

Nephrotoxicity

Gadolinium agents are considered to have no nephrotoxicity at approved dosages for MR imaging. MR with gadolinium has been used instead of contrastenhanced CT in those at risk for developing worsening renal failure if exposed to iodinated contrast media. However, in view of the risk of NSF in patients with severe renal dysfunction, this practice should only be considered after reviewing the recommendations for use of gadolinium-based contrast in this group of patients.

Gadolinium agents are radiodense and can be used for opacification in CT and angiographic examinations instead of iodinated radiographic contrast media. However, there is controversy about whether gadolinium contrast media are less nephrotoxic at equally attenuating doses. Caution should be used in extrapolating the lack of nephrotoxicity of intravenous (IV) gadolinium at MR dosages to its use for angiographic procedures, including direct injection into the renal arteries. No assessment of gadolinium versus iodinated contrast nephrotoxicity by randomized studies of equally attenuating doses is currently available. Initially, radiographic use of high doses of gadolinium agents was proposed as an alternative to nephrotoxic iodinated contrast media in patients with renal insufficiency. However, because of the risk of NSF following gadolinium-based contrast material administration, especially in patients with acute renal failure or severe chronic kidney disease, and because of the unknown nephrotoxicity of high doses of gadolinium agents, use of these contrast media for conventional angiography is no longer recommended.

The Safety of Gadolinium-Based Contrast Media (GBCM) in Patients With Sickle Cell Disease

Early in vitro research dealing with the effects of MRI on red blood cells (erythrocytes) suggested that fully deoxygenated sickle erythrocytes align perpendicularly to a magnetic field. It was hypothesized that this alignment could further restrict sickle erythrocyte flow through small vessels and, thus conceivably could promote vaso-occlusive complications in sickle cell patients (1). The further supposition that the IV administration of GBCM might potentiate sickle erythrocyte alignment, thereby additionally increasing the risk of vaso-occlusive complications, is mentioned in the FDA package inserts (as of 2009) for two GBCM approved for use in the United States (gadoversetamide (OptiMARK, Mallinckrodt) and gadoteridol (Prohance, Bracco Diagnostics)).

To the best of our knowledge and noted in a review (2) of the literature, there has been no documented in vivo vaso-occlusive complication directly related to the IV administration of a GBCM in a sickle cell disease patient. Several small scientific studies (3–5) of patients with sickle cell have employed MR imaging with GBCM without reported adverse effects. In addition, a review (2) of the literature fails to provide evidence for clinically significant hemolysis following the IV administration of GBCM in sickle cell disease patients.

Therefore, it is our opinion that any special risk to sickle cell patients from IV administered GBCM at currently approved dosages must be extremely low, and there is no reason to withhold these agents from patients with sickle cell disease. However, as in nonsickle cell disease patients, GBCM should be administered only when clinically indicated.

Treatment of Acute Adverse Reactions

Treatment of moderate or severe acute adverse reactions to gadolinium-based contrast media is similar to that for moderate or severe acute reactions to iodinated contrast media.

In any facility where contrast media are injected, it is imperative that personnel trained in recognizing and handling reactions and the equipment and medications to do so be on site or immediately available. Most MR facilities take the position that patients requiring treatment should be taken out of the imaging room immediately and away from the magnet so that none of the resuscitative equipment becomes a magnetic hazard.

Extravasation

The incidence of extravasation in one series of 28,000 doses was 0.05%. Laboratory studies in animals have demonstrated that both gadopentetate dimeglumine and gadoteridol are much less toxic to the skin and subcutaneous tissues than are equal volumes of iodinated contrast media. The small volumes typically injected for MR studies limit the chances for a compartment syndrome. For these reasons the likelihood of a significant injury resulting from extravasated MR contrast media is extremely low. Nonionic MR contrast media are less likely to cause symptomatic extravasation than hypertonic agents such as gadopentate dimeglumine.

Serum Calcium Determinations

Some gadolinium-based MR contrast media interfere with total serum calcium values as determined with some calcium assay methods. It should be emphasized that these MR contrast media do not cause actual reductions in serum calcium, only that the contrast media interferes with the test, leading to falsely low serum calcium laboratory values. In one report by Brown and associates (6), calcium levels measured by only one of three different assays (the orthocresolphthalein assay) showed a temporary decrease for just two of four studied gadolinium-based contrast media, the length and severity of which closely mirrored the concentration of the measured gadolinium-based media in blood. Specifically, this decrease was seen after injection of gadoversetamide and gadodiamide, but not with gadopentetate dimeglumine or gadoteridol.

Off-Label Usage

Radiologists commonly use contrast media for a clinical purpose not contained in the labeling and thus commonly use contrast media off-label. By definition, such usage is not approved by the Food and Drug Administration. However, physicians have some latitude in using gadolinium chelates off label as guided by clinical circumstances, as long as they can justify such usage in individual cases. Examples include MR angiography, cardiac applications, and pediatric applications in patients younger than two years of age. In addition, no gadolinium chelate is approved in the United States for use in a power injector.

REFERENCES

1. Brody AS, Sorette MP, Gooding CA, et al. AUR memorial Award. Induced alignment of flowing sickle erythrocytes in a magnetic field. A preliminary report. *Invest Radiol* 1985; 20:560–566.
2. Kanal E, Shellock FG, Talagala L. Safety considerations in MR imaging. *Radiology* 1990; 176:593–606.

3. Umans H, Haramati N, Flusser G. The diagnostic role of gadolinium enhanced MRI in distinguishing between medullary bone infarct and osteomyelitis. *Magn Reson Imaging* 2000; 18:255–262.
4. Westwood MA, Shah F, Anderson LJ, et al. Myocardial tissue characterization and the role of chronic anemia in sickle cell cardiomyopathy. *J Magn Reson Imaging* 2007; 26:564–568.
5. Zimmerman RA. MRI/MRA evaluation of sickle cell disease of the brain. *Pediatr Radiol* 2005; 35:249–257.
6. Brown JJ, Hynes MR, Wible JH, Jr. Measurement of serum calcium concentration after administration of four gadolinium- based contrast agents to human volunteers. *AJR Am J Roentgenol* 2007; 189:1539–1544.

Suggested Reading *(Articles that the Committee recommends for further reading on this topic are provided here.)*

7. Broome DR, Girguis MS, Baron PW, Cottrell AC, Kjellin I, Kirk GA. Gadodiamide-associated nephrogenic systemic fibrosis: why radiologists should be concerned. *AJR Am J Roentgenol* 2007; 188:586–592.
8. Cochran ST, Bomyea K, Sayre JW. Trends in adverse events after IV administration of contrast media. *AJR Am J Roentgenol* 2001; 176:1385–1388.
9. Cohan RH, Ellis JH, Garner WL. Extravasation of radiographic contrast material: recognition, prevention, and treatment. *Radiology* 1996; 200:593–604.
10. Cohan RH, Leder RA, Herzberg AJ, et al. Extravascular toxicity of two magnetic resonance contrast agents. Preliminary experience in the rat. *Invest Radiol* 1991; 26:224–226.
11. Goldstein HA, Kashanian FK, Blumetti RF, Holyoak WL, Hugo FP, Blumenfield DM. Safety assessment of gadopentetate dimeglumine in U.S. clinical trials. *Radiology* 1990; 174:17–23.
12. Haustein J, Laniado M, Niendorf HP, et al. Triple-dose versus standard-dose gadopentetate dimeglumine: a randomized study in 199 patients. *Radiology* 1993; 186:855–860.
13. Jordan RM, Mintz RD. Fatal reaction to gadopentetate dimeglumine. *AJR Am J Roentgenol* 1995; 164:743–744.
14. Kanal E, Barkovich AJ, Bell C, et al. ACR guidance document for safe MR practices: 2007. *AJR Am J Roentgenol* 2007; 188:1447–1474.
15. Kuo PH, Kanal E, Abu-Alfa AK, Cowper SE. Gadoliniumbased MR contrast agents and nephrogenic systemic fibrosis. *Radiology* 2007; 242:647–649.
16. Lin J, Idee JM, Port M, et al. Interference of magnetic resonance imaging contrast agents with the serum calcium measurement technique using colorimetric reagents. *J Pharm Biomed Anal* 1999; 21:931–943.
17. McAlister WH, McAlister VI, Kissane JM. The effect of Gd-dimeglumine on subcutaneous tissues: a study with rats. *AJNR Am J Neuroradiol* 1990; 11:325–327.

18. Murphy KJ, Brunberg JA, Cohan RH. Adverse reactions to gadolinium contrast media: a review of 36 cases. *AJR Am J Roentgenol* 1996; 167:847–849.

19. Murphy KP, Szopinski KT, Cohan RH, Mermillod B, Ellis JH. Occurrence of adverse reactions to gadolinium-based contrast material and management of patients at increased risk: a survey of the American Society of Neuroradiology Fellowship Directors. *Acad Radiol* 1999; 6:656–664.

20. Nelson KL, Gifford LM, Lauber-Huber C, Gross CA, Lasser TA. Clinical safety of gadopentetate dimeglumine. *Radiology* 1995; 196:439–443.

21. Niendorf HP, Brasch RC. Gd-DTPA tolerance and clinical safety. In: Brasch RC, Drayer BP, Haughton VM, et al, ed. *MRI Contrast Enhancement in the Central Nervous System: A Case Study Approach*. New York, NY: Raven; 1993:11–21.

22. Niendorf HP, Haustein J, Cornelius I, Alhassan A, Clauss W. Safety of gadolinium-DTPA: extended clinical experience. *Magn Reson Med* 1991; 22:222–228; discussion 229–232.

23. Nyman U, Elmstahl B, Leander P, Nilsson M, Golman K, Almen T. Are gadolinium-based contrast media really safer than iodinated media for digital subtraction angiography in patients with azotemia? *Radiology* 2002; 223:311–318; discussion 328–319.

24. Olukotun AY, Parker JR, Meeks MJ, Lucas MA, Fowler DR, Lucas TR. Safety of gadoteridol injection: U.S. clinical trial experience. *J Magn Reson Imaging* 1995; 5:17–25.

25. Omohundro JE, Elderbrook MK, Ringer TV. Laryngospasm after administration of gadopentetate dimeglumine. *J Magn Reson Imaging* 1992; 2:729–730.

26. Runge VM. Safety of approved MR contrast media for intravenous injection. *J Magn Reson Imaging* 2000; 12:205–213.

27. Runge VM. Safety of magnetic resonance contrast media. *Top Magn Reson Imaging* 2001; 12:309–314.

28. Runge VM, Bradley WG, Brant-Zawadzki MN, et al. Clinical safety and efficacy of gadoteridol: a study in 411 patients with suspected intracranial and spinal disease. *Radiology* 1991; 181:701–709.

29. Salonen OL. Case of anaphylaxis and four cases of allergic reaction following Gd-DTPA administration. *J Comput Assist Tomogr* 1990; 14:912–913.

30. Shellock FG, Hahn HP, Mink JH, Itskovich E. Adverse reaction to intravenous gadoteridol. *Radiology* 1993; 189:151–152.

31. Spinosa DJ, Kaufmann JA, Hartwell GD. Gadolinium chelates in angiography and interventional radiology: a useful alternative to iodinated contrast media for angiography. *Radiology* 2002; 223:319–325; discussion 326–317.

32. Takebayashi S, Sugiyama M, Nagase M, Matsubara S. Severe adverse reaction to iv gadopentetate dimeglumine. *AJR Am J Roentgenol* 1993; 160:659.

33. Tardy B, Guy C, Barral G, Page Y, Ollagnier M, Bertrand JC. Anaphylactic shock induced by intravenous gadopentetate dimeglumine. *Lancet* 1992; 339:494.

34. Thomsen HS. Nephrogenic systemic fibrosis: A serious late adverse reaction to gadodiamide. *Eur Radiol* 2006; 16:2619–2621.

35. Tishler S, Hoffman JC, Jr. Anaphylactoid reactions to i.v. gadopentetate dimeglumine. *AJNR Am J Neuroradiol* 1990; 11:1167; discussion 1168–1169.

36. Weiss KL. Severe anaphylactoid reaction after i.v. Gd-DTPA. *Magn Reson Imaging* 1990; 8:817–818.

37. Witte RJ, Anzai LL. Life-threatening anaphylactoid reaction after intravenous gadoteridol administration in a patient who had previously received gadopentetate dimeglumine. *AJNR Am J Neuroradiol* 1994; 15:523–524.

MRI Contrast Agents and Breast Feeding Mothers*

Administration of Contrast Media to Breast-Feeding Mothers*

Administration of either an iodinated or a gadolinium-based contrast media occasionally is indicated for an imaging study on a woman who is breast-feeding. Both the patient and the patient's physician may have concerns regarding potential toxicity to the infant from contrast media that is excreted into the breast milk.

The literature on the excretion into breast milk of iodinated and gadolinium-based contrast media and the gastrointestinal absorption of these agents from breast milk is very limited however, several studies have shown that (1) less than 1% of the administered maternal dose of contrast medium is excreted into breast milk; and (2) less than 1% of the contrast medium in breast milk ingested by an infant is absorbed from the gastrointestinal tract. Therefore, the expected dose of contrast medium absorbed by an infant from ingested breast milk is extremely low.

Iodinated X-ray Contrast Media (Ionic and Nonionic)

Background
The plasma half-life of intravenously administered iodinated contrast medium is approximately 2 hours, with nearly 100% of the media cleared from the bloodstream within 24 hours. Because of its low lipid solubility, less than 1% of the administered maternal dose of iodinated contrast medium is excreted into the breast milk in the first 24 hours (1, 2). Because less than 1% of the contrast medium ingested by the infant is absorbed from its gastrointestinal tract (3), the expected dose absorbed by the infant from the breast milk is less than 0.01% of the intravascular dose given to the mother. This amount represents less than 1% of the recommended dose for an infant undergoing an imaging study, which is 2 mL/kg. The potential risks to the infant include direct toxicity and allergic sensitization or reaction, which are theoretical concerns but have not been reported.

Recommendation
Mothers who are breast-feeding should be given the opportunity to make

an informed decision as to whether to continue or temporarily abstain from breast-feeding after receiving intravascularly administered iodinated contrast media. Because of the very small percentage of iodinated contrast medium that is excreted into the breast milk and absorbed by the infant's gut, we believe that the available data suggest that it is safe for the mother and infant to continue breast-feeding after receiving such an agent. If the mother remains concerned about any potential ill effects to the infant, she may abstain from breast-feeding for 24 hours with active expression and discarding of breast milk from both breasts during that period. In anticipation of this, she may wish to use a breast pump to obtain milk before the contrast study to feed the infant during the 24-hour period following the examination.

Gadolinium-Based Contrast Agents

Background
Gadolinium compounds are safe and useful as magnetic resonance imaging contrast media. Although free gadolinium is neurotoxic, when complexed to one of a variety of chelates it is safe for use in most adults and children. These hydrophilic gadolinium chelate agents have pharmacokinetic properties very similar to those of iodinated X-ray contrast media. Like iodinated contrast media, gadolinium contrast media have a plasma half-life of approximately 2 hours and are nearly completely cleared from the bloodstream within 24 hours.

Less than 0.04% of the intravascular dose given to the mother is excreted into the breast milk in the first 24 hours (4–6). Because less than 1% of the contrast medium ingested by the infant is absorbed from its gastrointestinal tract (7), the expected dose absorbed by the infant from the breast milk is less than 0.0004% of the intravascular dose given to the mother. Even in the extreme circumstance of a mother weighing 150 kg and receiving a dose of 0.2 mmol/ kg, the absolute amount of gadolinium excreted in the breast milk in the first 24-hours after administration would be no more than 0.012 mmol. Thus, the dose of gadolinium absorbed from the gastrointestinal tract of a breast-feeding infant weighing 1,500 grams or more would be no more than 0.00008 mmol/kg, or 0.04% (four ten-thousandths) of the permitted adult or pediatric (2 years of age or older) intravenous dose of 0.2 mmol/kg. The potential risks to the infant include direct toxicity (including toxicity from free gadolinium, because it is unknown how much, if any, of the gadolinium in breast milk is in the unchelated form) and allergic sensitization or reaction, which are theoretical concerns but have not been reported.

Recommendation

Review of the literature shows no evidence to suggest that oral ingestion by an infant of the tiny amount of gadolinium contrast medium excreted into breast milk would cause toxic effects (8). We believe, therefore, that the available data suggest that it is safe for the mother and infant to continue breast-feeding after receiving such an agent.

If the mother remains concerned about any potential ill effects, she should be given the opportunity to make an informed decision as to whether to continue or temporarily abstain from breast-feeding after receiving a gadolinium contrast medium. If the mother so desires, she may abstain from breast-feeding for 24 hours with active expression and discarding of breast milk from both breasts during that period. In anticipation of this, she may wish to use a breast pump to obtain milk before the contrast study to feed the infant during the 24-hour period following the examination.

REFERENCES

1. Ilett KF, Hackett LP, Paterson JW, McCormick CC. Excretion of metrizamide in milk. *Br J Radiol* 1981; 54:537–538.

2. Johansen JG. Assessment of a non-ionic contrast medium (Amipaque) in the gastrointestinal tract. *Invest Radiol* 1978; 13:523–527.

3. Kubik-Huch RA, Gottstein-Aalame NM, Frenzel T, et al. Gadopentetate dimeglumine excretion into human breast milk during lactation. *Radiology* 2000; 216:555–558.

4. Nielsen ST, Matheson I, Rasmussen JN, Skinnemoen K, Andrew E, Hafsahl G. Excretion of iohexol and metrizoate in human breast milk. *Acta Radiol* 1987; 28:523–526.

5. Rofsky NM, Weinreb JC, Litt AW. Quantitative analysis of gadopentetate dimeglumine excreted in breast milk. *J Magn Reson Imaging* 1993; 3:131–132.

6. Schmiedl U, Maravilla KR, Gerlach R, Dowling CA. Excretion of gadopentetate dimeglumine in human breast milk. *AJR Am J Roentgenol* 1990; 154:1305–1306.

7. Weinmann HJ, Brasch RC, Press WR, Wesbey GE. Characteristics of gadolinium-DTPA complex: a potential NMR contrast agent. *AJR Am J Roentgenol* 1984; 142:619-624.

8. Hylton NM. Suspension of breast-feeding following gadopentetate dimeglumine administration. *Radiology* 2000; 216:325–326.

MRI Contrast Agents and Pregnant Patients*

Administration of Contrast Media to Pregnant or Potentially Pregnant Patients

Studies of low-molecular weight water-soluble extracellular substances such as iodinated diagnostic and gadolinium-based magnetic resonance (MR) contrast media in pregnancy have been limited, and their effects on the human embryo or fetus are incompletely understood. Iodinated diagnostic contrast media have been shown to cross the human placenta and enter the fetus in measurable quantities (1, 2). A standard gadolinium-based MR contrast medium has been shown to cross the placenta in primates and appear within the fetal bladder within 11 minutes after intravenous administration (3). It must be assumed that all iodinated and gadolinium-based contrast media behave in a similar fashion and cross the blood-placental barrier into the fetus.

After entering the fetal blood stream, these agents will be excreted via the urine into the amniotic fluid and be subsequently swallowed by the fetus (4). It is then possible that a small amount will be absorbed from the gut of the fetus and the rest eliminated back into the amniotic fluid, the entire cycle being repeated innumerable times.

In the study in primates, placental enhancement could be detected up to 2 hours following the intravenous (IV) administration of gadopentetate dimeglumine. When gadopentetate dimeglumine was injected directly into the amniotic cavity, it was still conspicuous at 1 hour after administration (3). There are no data available to assess the rate of clearance of contrast media from the amniotic fluid.

Iodinated X-Ray Contrast Media (Ionic and Nonionic)

Diagnostic iodinated contrast media have been shown to cross the human placenta and enter the fetus when given in usual clinical doses. In-vivo tests in animals have shown no evidence of either mutagenic or teratogenic effects with low-osmolality contrast media (LOCM). No adequate and well-controlled teratogenic studies of the effects of these media in pregnant women have been performed.

In conjunction with the existing ACR policy for the use of ionizing radiation in pregnant women, we recommend that all imaging facilities should have polices and procedures to attempt to identify pregnant patients prior to the performance of any examination involving ionizing radiation to determine the medical necessity for the administration of iodinated contrast media. If a patient is known to be pregnant, both the potential radiation risk and the potential added risks of contrast media should be considered before proceeding with the study.

While it is not possible to conclude that iodinated contrast media present a definite risk to the fetus, there is insufficient evidence to conclude that they pose no risk. Consequently, the Committee on Drugs and Contrast Media recommends the following:

A. The radiologist should confer with the referring physician and document in the radiology report or the patient's medical record the following:

1) That the information requested cannot be acquired without contrast administration or via another image modality (e.g., ultrasonography).

2) That the information needed affects the care of the patient and fetus *during the pregnancy.*

3) That the referring physician is of the opinion that it is not prudent to wait to obtain this information until after the patient is no longer pregnant.

B. It is recommended that pregnant patients undergoing a diagnostic imaging examination with ionizing radiation and iodinated contrast media provide informed consent to document that they understand the risk and benefits of the procedure to be performed and the alternative diagnostic options available to them (if any), and that they wish to proceed.

Gadolinium-Based Contrast Agents

It is known that gadolinium-based MR contrast media cross the human placenta and into the fetus when given in clinical dose ranges. No adequate and well-controlled teratogenic studies of the effects of these media in pregnant women have been performed. A single cohort study of 26 women exposed to gadolinium chelates during the first trimester of pregnancy showed no evidence of teratogenesis or mutagenesis in their progeny.

Gadolinium chelates may accumulate in the amniotic fluid and remain there for an indefinite period of time, with potential dissociation of the toxic free gadolinium ion from the chelate; the significance of this exposure to the fetus is uncertain, and its potential association with nephrogenic systemic fibrosis (NSF) in the child or mother is unknown. Therefore, gadolinium chelates should not be routinely used in pregnant patients.

The ACR Guidance Document for Safe MR Practices (2) also covers use of MR contrast media in pregnant patients, and its recommendations are consistent with those in this Manual. See also the preceding Chapter on NSF (www.acr.org/SecondaryMainMenuCategories/quality_safety/contrast_m anual/NephrogenicSystemicFibrosis.aspx)

Because it is unclear how gadolinium-based contrast agents will affect the fetus, these agents should be administered only with extreme caution. Each case should be reviewed carefully and gadolinium-based contrast agent administered only when there is a potential overwhelming benefit to the patient or fetus that outweighs the possible risk of exposure of the fetus to free gadolinium ions. The radiologist should confer with the referring physician and document the following in the radiology report or the patient's medical record:

1) That information requested from the MR study cannot be acquired without the use of IV contrast or by using other imaging modalities.

2) That the information needed affects the care of the patient and fetus *during the pregnancy.*

3) That the referring physician is of the opinion that it is not prudent to wait to obtain this information until after the patient is no longer pregnant.

It is recommended that the pregnant patient undergoing an MR examination provide informed consent to document that she understands the risk and benefits of the MR procedure to be performed, and the alternative diagnostic options available to her (if any), and that she wishes to proceed.

REFERENCES

1. Dean PB. Fetal uptake of an intravascular radiologic contrast medium. *Rofo* 1977; 127:267–270.

2. Kanal E, Barkovich AJ, Bell C, et al. ACR guidance document for safe MR practices: 2007. *AJR Am J Roentgenol* 2007; 188:1447–1474.

3. Moon AJ, Katzberg RW, Sherman MP. Transplacental passage of iohexol. *J Pediatr* 2000; 136:548-549.

4. Panigel M, Wolf G, Zeleznick A. Magnetic resonance imaging of the placenta in rhesus monkeys, Macaca mulatta. *J Med Primatol* 1988; 17:3–18.

Suggested Reading *(Articles that the Committee recommends for further reading on this topic are provided here.)*

5. De Santis M, Straface G, Cavaliere AF, Carducci B, Caruso A. Gadolinium periconceptional exposure: pregnancy and neonatal outcome. *Acta Obstet Gynecol Scand* 2007; 86:99–101.

6. Donandieu AM, Idee JM, Doucet D, et al. Toxicologic profile of iobitridol, a new nonionic low-osmolality contrast medium. *Acta Radiol Suppl* 1996; 400:17–24.

7. Etling N, Gehin-Fouque F, Vielh JP, Gautray JP. The iodine content of amniotic fluid and placental transfer of iodinated drugs. *Obstet Gynecol* 1979; 53:376–380.

8. Heglund IF, Michelet AA, Blazak WF, Furuhama K, Holtz E. Preclinical pharmacokinetics and general toxicology of iodixanol. *Acta Radiol Suppl* 1995; 399:69–82.

9. Kelleher J, Feczko PJ, Radkowski MA, Griscom NT. Neonatal intestinal opacification secondary to transplacental passage of urographic contrast medium. *AJR Am J Roentgenol* 1979; 132:63–65.

10. Morisetti A, Tirone P, Luzzani F, de Haen C. Toxicological safety assessment of iomeprol, a new X-ray contrast agent. *Eur J Radiol* 1994; 18 Suppl 1:S21–31.

11. Webb JA, Thomsen HS, Morcos SK. The use of iodinated and gadolinium contrast media during pregnancy and lactation. *Eur Radiol* 2005; 15:1234–1240.

MRI Contrast Agent: MultiHance Frequently Asked Questions

QUESTION: How does the safety profile of MultiHance compare to the other currently available gadolinium-based contrast agents.

ANSWER: The safety profile of MultiHance is similar to that of the other approved gadolinium agents. As stated in the American College of Radiology Manual on Contrast Media, gadolinium-containing contrast media are extremely well tolerated by the vast majority of patients in whom they are injected. Clinical studies have been performed comparing the safety profiles of other gadolinium-based contrast agents and MultiHance. In these studies the frequency and type of adverse reactions seen after the two agents were similar.

QUESTION: Do the container closure or formulation of MultiHance contain latex?

ANSWER: No.

QUESTION: Since the MultiHance package insert contains a contra-indication for use in patients with known allergic or hypersensitivity reactions to gadolinium or any other ingredient, can we use MultiHance in patients who developed a sensitivity reaction such as hives after administration of another gadolinium-based contrast agent?

ANSWER: No. It is advisable to seek a different modality anytime a patient exhibits sensitivity to a component of a drug. However, please note that this type of a statement is made in all of the gadolinium agent package inserts. It is contained in the contraindications section of the last two agents approved by the FDA (MultiHance and OptiMARK) and it is contained in the warnings section of the earlier approved agents (ProHance, Magnevist, and Omniscan). There is no evidence that adverse reactions are more frequent or more serious with the more recently approved agents.

QUESTION: Should breastfeeding be discontinued after administration of MultiHance?

ANSWER: The MultiHance package insert suggests that breastfeeding be discontinued for approximately 24 hours after administration of MultiHance. There is similar language in the package inserts of the other approved gadolinium contrast agents.

QUESTION: Is there any information about the safe use of MultiHance for MR arthrography procedures?

ANSWER: Currently there is no literature describing MultiHance use for MR arthrography. This is not an approved indication for any gadolinium contrast agent, however numerous protocols for this procedure have been published.

QUESTION: Is there any information available about the use of MultiHance in patients with renal impairment?

ANSWER: The MultiHance package insert CLINICAL PHARMACOL-OGY section contains a sub-section entitled "Pharmacokinetics in Special Populations. Renal Impairment" stating that: "the overall extent of elimination of gadobenate was not influenced by impaired renal function. Also, no differences were noted in patients with renal impairment in the rate and type of adverse events reported compared with healthy volunteers, and no deterioration in renal function was observed in this population following the administration of MULTIHANCE. Therefore, dosage adjustment is not recommended". These recommendations are based on studies with MultiHance conducted in patients with varying degrees of renal impairment and in patients on hemodialysis.

QUESTION: For what indications has MultiHance been studied that are not contained in the package insert?

ANSWER: Liver Imaging, Magnetic Resonance Angiography (MRA), Body/MRA, Breast Imaging, MRI/Acute Myocardial Infarction, CNS Imaging in pediatric patients.

QUESTION: Why doesn't MultiHance have a pediatric imaging indication in the U.S.?

ANSWER: No safety concerns have been raised about the use of MultiHance in children. In fact, MultiHance is approved for use in pediatric patients in Canada. To date, the safety and efficacy of MultiHance has been evaluated in 174 children between the age of 6 months and 16 years. In addition, the pharmacokinetics of MultiHance in children was studied in 25 subjects. This can be compared to the 173 patients that were enrolled in clinical trials with Omniscan. The safety profile of MultiHance in children was found to be equal to that of Magnevist and the pharmacokinetics were found to be similar to those in adult patients. The FDA has requested that a larger population of children be studied before granting the pediatric indication in the US. The manufacturer of MultiHance (Bracco Diagnostics Inc.) decided to launch the product for adults in the U.S. while obtaining the additional requested data in pediatric patients.

QUESTION: The package insert states that once MultiHance is filled into a plastic syringe, it should be used immediately. Is there a reason that is specific to MultiHance that would require this precaution?

ANSWER: There are no data that suggests that MultiHance acts any differently than the other gadolinium-based contrast agents when exposed to plastic syringes. In fact, the OptiMARK package insert contains the same statement. The FDA now requires that this precaution be placed in the IV administered contrast agent labeling. The reason for the statement is that it is possible for extractable contaminants to leach from the plastic used to make the syringe. Unless there is stability data for all commercially available plastic syringes that proves otherwise, the precaution is required. The Magnevist package insert contains the statement "After Magnevist injection is drawn into the syringe the solution should be used immediately." The ProHance and Omniscan package inserts contain this statement as well. This statement is found in the PRECAUTIONS –General section of these package inserts.

QUESTION: Can MultiHance be double dosed as is sometimes done with ProHance or Omniscan?

ANSWER: Currently MultiHance is approved in the U.S. at a dose of 0.1 mmo/kg body weight. Due to the higher relaxivity of MultiHance it may not be necessary to give higher doses in certain applications. Several reports in the literature describe the use of dosages greater than that indicated in the DOSAGE AND ADMINISTRATION section of the MultiHance package insert. In a comprehensive safety assessment published in 2000, Kirchin and colleagues found no increase in the rate of adverse events in patients given higher doses of MultiHance.

QUESTION: What is the potential for MultiHance interaction with drugs which undergo a similar hepatobiliary elimination?

ANSWER: Following IV injection, Gd-BOPTA, the active ingredient of MultiHance, is internalized by hepatocytes through a passive mechanism (simple diffusion though the hepatocyte cell membrane) and a small percentage is actively excreted via the ATP-dependent export pump for anionic conjugates MRP2 (multidrug resistance-associated protein 2, also known as multi-specific organic anion transport system, cMOAT), located in the apical membranes of hepatocytes. MRP2 functions as the major exporter of organic anions from the liver into the bile, such as conjugated bilirubin. Gd-BOPTA, even in patients with reduced liver function, had no impact on the elimination of conjugated bilirubin, although conjugated bilirubin can be only eliminated by the MRP2.

The following drugs with substantial hepatic excretion via the MRP2 and a narrow therapeutic window have been used in combination with MultiHance in clinical trials: daunorubicin, doxorubicin, epirubicin, glyburide (glibenclamide), tamoxifen, taxol, and taxotere. The most frequent concomitant use was of glyburide (43 patients). No adverse events suggestive of hypoglycemia, cholestatic jaundice, agranulocytosis, or aplastic and/or hemolytic anemia (indicative of overdosing of glyburide) were observed. The magnitude of the changes in conjugated bilirubin in these patients was negligible and similar to that observed in patients who did not take drugs competing for the MRP2. No adverse events suggestive of increased blood levels of the anthracyclines or the taxanes (cardiac toxicity, bone marrow depression), nor of increased blood levels of tamoxifen (flushes, nausea, vomiting, or thromboembolic complications) were noted. No other serious clinical adverse events or significant ECG and laboratory abnormalities were reported for these patients. Out of approximately 1.3 million patients exposed to MultiHance to date, no data suggest that Gd-BOPTA interferes with the uptake or metabolism of any drug or biological agent.

This may be explained by the fact that: a) only single administrations of MultiHance are used; b) a small percentage of the injected dose of Gd-BOPTA (0.6-4%) is excreted into the bile; c) most drugs competing for the the MRP2 can also be eliminated by other liver transporters (e.g., MDR1, MRP1, and BCRP); d) MRP2 is not only expressed on the hepatocytes, but also on enterocytes of the proximal small intestine, and proximal renal tubular cells; e) anthracyclines and taxanes lead to overexpression of MDR1, MRP1 and MRP2 in hepatic and non-hepatic tissues, like cancer tissues, small intestine, kidney, and others. In view of the available data, MultiHance is not expected to interfere with the elimination of drugs with a narrow therapeutic window which are excreted via the MRP2 pathway, nor to affect the course of treatment with these drugs.

QUESTION: Can anaphylactic reactions occur in patients who are hypersensitive to benzyl alcohol?

ANSWER: Hypersensitivity to benzyl alcohol is mainly described in the literature in the form of contact dermatitis following external administration (delayed-type dermatitis). No one has ever shown a correlation between a contact allergy (delayed type, cell-mediated) to benzyl alcohol and systemic reactions (immediate type, not cell-mediated) following parenteral administration. Important: benzyl alcohol is present in many drug formulations, has been administered in millions and millions of people, but the literature reports only 3 reports of possible hypersensitivity following parenteral administration, and none of them was an anaphylactic or anaphylactoid reaction.

Hypersensitivity to gadolinium chelates is more frequent and much more clinically important than possible hypersensitivity to benzyl alcohol.

Serious and life threatening hypersensitivity reactions to gadolinium chelates are well documented and may occur with any gadolinium agent. Such documentation for benzyl alcohol is difficult if not impossible to find. Vials of MultiHance may contain only minute traces of benzyl alcohol.

QUESTION: Does MultiHance affect colorimetric assays for serum calcium?

ANSWER: No. It is well known that some gadolinium chelates, notably gadodiamide (Omniscan) and gadoversetamide (OptiMARK), may interfere with the colorimetric determination of serum calcium or other metal or metabolites. The mechanism of this interference appears to be related to the propensity of the agent to de-chelate once injected. According to Bracco Diagnostics Inc., the manufacturer of MultiHance, this agent has been thoroughly evaluated for potential interference in colorimetric assay tests in two separate batteries of test and no interference was demonstrated. The assays tested included: Albumin (BCG method), Alkaline Phosphatase (AP), Bilirubin (total) (DPD method), Calcium (O-CPC method), Chloride, Cholesterol (CHOD-PAP method), Creatine kinase (CK) (NAC-activated) Creatinine, Glucose, Glutamate oxalacetate transaminase (GOT or ASAT), Glutamate phosphate transinase (GPT or ALAT), Iron (ferrozin-method), Lactate dehydrogenase (LDH) (optimized UV test), Phosphate (direct phosphomolybdate method), Sodium/potassium, Total proteins (Biuret method), Triglycerides (GPO-PAP method), and Urea.

REFERENCES

Shellock FG, Parker JR, Pirovano G, Shen N, Venetianer C, Kirchin MA, Spinazzi A. Safety characteristics of gadobenate dimeglumine: Clinical experience from intra- and interindividual comparison studies with gadopentate dimeglumine. Journal of Magnetic Resonance Imaging 2006;24:1378-1285.

Shellock FG, Parker J, Spinazzi A. Safety of gadobenate dimeglumine: summary of findings from clinical studies and post-marketing surveillance. Investigative Radiology 2006;41:500-509.

MRI Contrast Agents and Nephrogenic Systemic Fibrosis (NSF)*

Definition

Even if the first cases of nephrogenic systemic fibrosis (NSF) were identified in 1997, and the first published report of 14 cases appeared in 2000 [1], NSF has only recently received great attention, especially because of its possible association with exposure to gadolinium-based contrast agents (GBCAs). "Nephrogenic" does not mean that the disease is caused by factors originating in the kidney, but that NSF has been observed only in patients with chronic kidney disease, while "systemic" emphasizes the systemic nature of this fibrosing disorder [2]. It was previously known as "Nephrogenic Fibrosing Dermopathy", since its most prominent and visible effects are observed in the skin, where the histopathologic findings closely parallel those observed in wound healing reactions [1, 3, 4, 5]. The nomenclature of the disease has been changed to NSF based on autopsy case reports of individual NSF patients that have reported variable degrees of myocardial, pericardial, and pleural fibrosis, along with the involvement of nerves and skeletal muscles [6, 7, 8]. The disease is progressive and can be associated with a fatal outcome. There is still no definitive cure.

Diagnosis

NSF cannot be detected using a single diagnostic test. A confident diagnosis can usually be reached through the combination of a good clinical history, a good physical exam and the histopathologic examination of a biopsy specimen of involved skin. The main elements that should guide physicians in the diagnostic process are the clinical presentation in the setting of severe renal insufficiency and, more important, confirmatory cutaneous histopathologic findings [9].

So far, NSF has been observed only in patients with acute or chronic severe renal insufficiency (glomerular filtration rate, GFR, <30 mL/min/1.73m^2), or acute renal insufficiency of any severity due to the hepato-renal syndrome or in the perioperative liver transplantation period [9]. The majority of patients with NSF have a GFR <15 mL/min and are receiving (or have received) either hemodialysis, peritoneal dialysis, or both [9].

The skin changes can mimic progressive systemic sclerosis with a predilection for the extremity involvement that can extend to the torso. It has not been reported to occur on the face, palms, or soles. Unlike scleroderma, NSF usually spares the face. Skin lesions usually begin with swelling, progressing to erythematous papules and coalescing hyperpigmented, browny plaques with *peau d'orange* surface. Peripheral irregular fingerlike or ameboid projections may be present along with islands of sparing. Bullae and nodules have also been reported. The skin involvement is often symmetrical and bilateral. Upon eye examination, new onset of white-yellow scleral plaques with dilated capillary loops may be seen in patients less than 45 years of age [1, 4, 9, 10].

The involved skin and subcutis usually becomes markedly thickened and hardened, with a wooden consistency to palpation. The induration characteristically involves the distal extremities first, gradually proceeding to involve the proximal extremities to the level of the mid-thigh and mid-upper arms [1, 9, 10]. The involvement of the skin and subcutis overlying joints often causes a decrease in function of the hands and feet first, and then of more proximal joints in affected extremities, with elbows angled inwards and downwards and the body stooped over. Pedal plantar flexion may be sufficiently severe, making walking difficult or impossible. Joint contractures may develop very rapidly, with patients becoming wheelchair bound days to weeks after NSF starts, so that patients may become wheelchair dependent [9, 10].

If renal function is restored, the skin lesions may stabilize or even regress [9]. Occasional patients (estimated at less than 5%) have rapidly progressive, fulminant NSF, associated with an accelerated loss of mobility, and often severe pain [9, 10].

Patients with NSF may complain of itching and sharp pain. Itching and pain may be localized in the affected areas, in the rib cage or hips. Loss of appetite and muscle weakness are commonly described [9, 10].

When the above noted signs and symptoms are observed in patients with severe renal insufficiency, a biopsy should be performed to obtain specimens of involved skin.

Histologically, NSF is characterized by dermal fibrosis [11]. There is always an increased number of fibrocytes, that are CD34 and procollagen I positive when stained immunohistochemically [11]. This dual positivity is characteristic of so-called "circulating fibrocytes," mesenchymal stem cells of bone marrow origin that participate in wound repair [11, 12].

In early lesions of NSF, collagen bundles may be quite narrow, with abundant edema fluid and/or mucin separating them. Procollagen I positivity is already present, but noted inconspicuously in the perinuclear cytoplasm of the bland dermal fibrocytes. In more advanced disease, collagen bundles become thicker (still generally maintaining clefts of separation between their neighbors) and the cytoplasm of the fibrocytes becomes plump and intensely procollagen I positive [13]. The dermis is always involved by the histopathological pattern noted above, while the epidermis is not typically affected by NSF, although some degree of basilar pigmentation and epidermal acanthosis may be noted in advanced disease [13]. The subcutaneous septa are markedly widened. In these deeper NSF foci, the widened septa are collagenized in the same manner as described above [13].

Other occasional findings may be a combination of epithelioid CD68-positive histiocytes in the subcutaneous septa, multinucleated giant cells, osteoclast-like giant cells, foci of osteoid deposition, and/or calcified bone spicules [13]. Increased numbers of factor XIIIa positive dendritic cells or a coexpression of factor XIIIa and CD68 in the same cell have been observed as well. Vascularity is not typically prominent, although some cases of NSF show evidence of angiogenesis. Microthrombi and vasculitis have never been observed [13]. The fibrotic process may extend through the fascia and into the underlying skeletal muscle that can be swelling and hardened as well [13]. Patients suspected of NSF should be fully assessed by an experienced dermatologist.

How to minimize the risk of NSF

Step 1: Identify patients at risk

The first step should be to identify patients at risk for NSF, that is, those patients that suffer from severe (stages 4 and 5) chronic kidney disease, i.e., GFR below 30 mL/min/1.73 m^2, independently of their age, race or gender or acute kidney injury [14]. The risk of NSF development in patients with GFR between 30 and 44 mL/min/1.73 m^2 (stage 3b) is much smaller, but the American College of Radiology Subcommittee on MR Safety recommends to manage this group of patients as those with stage 4 or 5 chronic kidney disease, since eGFR determinations may fluctuate from one day to the next [14]. Therefore, it is important to identify patients with GFR <45 mL/min/1.73 m^2.

The level of GFR should be estimated from prediction equations that take into account the serum creatinine concentration and some or all of the following variables: age, gender, race, and body size [14]. Many experts (including the American College of Radiology Subcommittee on MR Safety) have recommended that an estimated GFR be obtained within six weeks of anticipated GBCA injection in patients who might have reduced renal function. It has been suggested that this would include any patient with a history of renal disease (including a solitary kidney, renal transplant, or renal neoplasm), anyone over the age of 60 years, and with a history of hypertension or diabetes mellitus [14].

The most widely used equations for adult patients are the Modification of Diet in Renal Disease (MDRD) study equation [15] and the Cockcroft-Gault formula [16]. Even if both equations provide a marked improvement over serum creatinine alone [17], the MDRD Study equation may perform better than the Cockroft-Gault formula, but the data are very limited [18-20]. Both prediction equations assume that the amount of creatinine produced by the patient is equal to the amount being removed by the kidneys. Therefore, both equations are not suitable if renal function is in an unstable condition—that is, in patients with acute renal failure or on dialysis. Results may also deviate from true values in patients with exceptional dietary intake (e.g., vegetarian diet, high protein diet, creatine supplements), extremes of body composition (e.g., very lean, obese, paraplegia), or severe liver disease. Among children, the Schwartz formula provides a clinically useful estimate of GFR [21].

Step 2: Assess risk-benefit of contrast-enhanced MRI in patients at risk

A patient at risk of NSF should receive a GBCA only when a risk–benefit assessment for that particular patient indicates that the benefit of doing so clearly outweighs the potential risk(s). The risk-benefit evaluation should be made by the radiologist in conjunction with the referring physician(s) and should be properly a prospectively documented. History of previous exposures to GBCAs or other factors that are thought to act as possible co-triggers of the disease, such as metabolic acidosis, vascular surgery, thrombotic events, etc. should be taken into account during the risk–benefit assessment of each individual patient.

Patients, or parents or guardians in case of minors, should be properly informed of the benefits, risks, and diagnostic alternatives, based on all the information available at that time, and provide their consent in writing.

Step 3: Perform any unenhanced MR sequence that may be helpful before injecting the contrast agent

In the United States, the Food and Drug Administration has requested the prescribing information of all GBCAs to be revised by adding a black boxed warning, according to which the use of GBCAs in risk patients should be avoided, unless the diagnostic information is essential and not available with non-contrast enhanced MRI. Therefore, the MR exam should be properly monitored. All unenhanced MR sequences that may be helpful to make a diagnosis should be performed, and the images evaluated by an experienced radiologist, in order to ensure that the administration of a GBCA is still deemed necessary.

Step 4: Do not expose risk patients to high doses of GBCAs

If the use of a GBCA is still deemed necessary, use the lowest dose needed to reliably provide the diagnostic information being clinically sought. According to boxed warning required by the FDA, the recommended doses should never be exceeded and dosing should not be repeated.

Which agent should be used?

In the USA, as in Europe and Japan, some GBCAs (gadodiamide, Omniscan; gadopentetate dimeglumine, Magnevist; gadoversetamide, OptiMARK) are specifically contraindicated for use in patients at risk of NSF [22]. The American College of Radiology recommends to never use these agents in patients with GFR <45 mL/min and in patients with known or suspected acute kidney injury, regardless of calculated GFR values [14]. Features of acute kidney injury consist of rapid (over hours to days) and usually reversible decrease in kidney function, commonly in the setting of surgery, severe infection, injury, or drug-induced kidney toxicity [22].

The other approved agents (Ablavar, gadofosveset trisodium; Eovist, gadoxetate disodium; MultiHance, gadobenate dimeglumine; ProHance, gadoteridol) should be used in patients at risk of NSF only if the diagnostic information is essential and not available with non-contrast enhanced MRI or other imaging modalities.

What to do after the MRI exam?

The usefulness of hemodialysis in the prevention of NSF is unknown. However, to enhance and speed up the GBCA elimination, many experts recommend that consideration be given to the performance of several dialysis sessions following GBCA administration in patients with end-stage renal disease on chronic dialysis, with use of prolonged dialysis times and increased flow rates and volumes to assist in the process of GBCA clearance [14]. Peritoneal dialysis provides much less potential NSF risk reduction compared to hemodialysis and should not be considered protective [14].

Patients at risk of NSF should be followed up at least for one year after a contrast-enhanced MR exam, to promptly identify any symptom or sign suggestive of NSF and confirm or rule out a diagnosis of NSF. Should a new diagnosis of NSF be made, it is recommended that all the regulatory authorities in the United States, Canada, Europe, Asia and other countries be properly notified.

[*Special thanks to Alberto Spinazzi, M.D., Senior Vice President, Group Regulatory and Medical Affairs, Bracco Diagnostics, Inc.]

REFERENCES

(1) Cowper SE, et al. Scleromyxoedema-like cutaneous disease in renal-dialysis patients. *Lancet* 2000, 356:1000–1001

(2) Cowper SE, Boyer PJ. Nephrogenic systemic fibrosis: an update. *Curr Rheumatol Rep* 2006, 8:151–157.

(3) DeHoratius D, Cowper SE. Nephrogenic systemic fibrosis: an emerging threat among renal patients. *Semin Dial* 2006; 19: 191–194.

(4) Introcaso CE, et al. Nephrogenic fibrosing dermopathy/ nephrogenic systemic fibrosis: a case series of nine patients and review of the literature. *Int J Dermatol* 2007, 46: 447–452.

(5) Mendoza FA, et al. Description of 12 cases of nephrogenic fibrosing dermopathy and review of the literature. *Semin Arthritis Rheum* 2006; 35: 238-249.

(6) Gibson SE, et al. Multiorgan involvement in nephrogenic fibrosing dermopathy; an autopsy case and review of the literature. *Arch Path Lab Med* 2006;130 : 209-212

(7) Keyrouz S, Rudnicki SA. Neuromuscular Involvement in nephrogenic systemic fibrosis. *J Clin Neuromusc Dis* 2007;9:297–302

(8) Ting WW, et al. Nephrogenic fibrosing dermopathy with systemic involvement. *Arch Dermatol* 2003; 139:903–9.

(9) Knopp EA, Cowper SE. Nephrogenic Systemic Fibrosis: Early Recognition and Treatment. *Semin Dial* 2008: DOI: 10.1111/j.1525-139X.2007.00399.x

(10) Cowper SE: Nephrogenic fibrosing dermopathy: the first 6 years. *Curr Opin Rheumatol* 15:785–790, 2003

(11) Cowper SE, et al. Nephrogenic fibrosing dermopathy. *Amer J Dermatopathol* 2001, 23:383–393

(12) Bucala R. Circulating fibrocytes: cellular basis for NSF. *J Am Coll Radiol* 2008;5:36-39

(13) Cowper SE, et al., Clinical and histological findings in nephrogenic systemic fibrosis, *Eur J Radiol* (2008), DOI:10.1016/j.ejrad.2008.01.016

(14) ACR Manual on Contrast Media - Version 7, 2010; Chapter 11. Available at http://www.acr.org/secondarymainmenucategories/quality_safety/contrast_m anual.aspx. Accessed on November 4, 2010

(15) Levey AS, et al. A more accurate method to estimate glomerular filtration rate from serum creatinine: a new prediction equation. Modification of Diet in Renal Disease Study Group. *Ann Intern Med* 1999;130:461–470

(16) Cockcroft DW, Gault MH. Prediction of creatinine clearance from serum creatinine. *Nephron* 1976;16:31–41

(17) Levey AS, et al. National Kidney Foundation. National Kidney Foundation practice guidelines for chronic kidney disease: evaluation, classification, and stratification. *Ann Intern Med* 2003; 139:137–147 [Erratum in *Ann Intern Med* 2003; 139:605]

(18) Stevens LA, et al. Impact of creatinine calibration on performance of GFR estimating equations in a pooled individual patient database. *Am J Kidney Dis* 2007; 50:21–35

(19) Levey AS, et al. Chronic Kidney Disease Epidemiology Collaboration. Expressing the Modification of Diet in Renal Disease Study equation for estimating glomerular filtration rate with standardized serum creatinine values. *Clin Chem* 2007; 53:766–772

(20) Levey AS, et al. Chronic Kidney Disease Epidemiology Collaboration. Using standardized serum creatinine values in the modification of diet in renal disease study equation for estimating glomerular filtration rate. *Ann Intern Med* 2006; 145:247–254

(21) Schwartz GJ, et al. A simple estimate of glomerular filtration rate in children derived from body length and plasma creatinine. *Pediatrics* 1976; 58:259–263

(22) http://www.fda.gov/Drugs/DrugSafety/ucm223966.htm - Accessed on November 4, 2010

MRI Contrast Agents and NSF: Websites and Links to Obtain Current Information*

American College of Radiology
www.acr.org
www.acr.org/SecondaryMainMenuCategories/quality_safety/contrast_manual.aspx
www.acr.org/SecondaryMainMenuCategories/quality_safety/contrast_manual/Nephrogenic
SystemicFibrosis.aspx

The International Center for Nephrogenic Fibrosing Dermopathy Research (ICNFDR)
www.icnfdr.org/

International Society for Magnetic Resonance in Medicine
www.ismrm.org/
www.ismrm.org/special/FDA.htm

United States Food and Drug Administration
www.fda.gov/cder/drug/infopage/gcca/qa_20061222.htm
www.fda.gov/cder/drug/advisory/gadolinium_agents.htm
www.fda.gov/bbs/topics/NEWS/2007/NEW01638.html
www.fda.gov/cder/drug/infopage/gcca/qa_200705.htm
www.fda.gov/cder/drug/infopage/gcca/default.htm
www.fda.gov/cder/drug/advisory/gadolinium_agents_20061222.htm
www.fda.gov/Drugs/DrugSafety/ucm223966.htm

[*For additional information, please refer to the following comprehensive review Shellock FG, Spinazzi A. MRI Safety Update: 2008, Part 1, MRI contrast agents and nephrogenic systemic fibrosis. American Journal of Roentgenology 2008;191:1-11. This article is available as a free downloadable PDF file at http://www.ajronline.org/]

Pregnant Patients and MR Procedures*

Magnetic resonance (MR) imaging has been used to evaluate obstetrical, placental, and fetal abnormalities in pregnant patients for more than 25 years. MR imaging is recognized as a beneficial diagnostic tool and is utilized to assess a wide range of diseases and conditions that affect the pregnant patient as well as the fetus.

Initially, there were substantial technical problems with the use of MR imaging primarily due to image degradation from fetal motion. However, several technological improvements, including the development of high-performance gradient systems and rapid pulse sequences, have provided major advances especially useful for imaging the pregnant patient and the fetus. Thus, MR imaging examinations for obstetrical and fetal applications may now be accomplished routinely in the clinical setting.

PREGNANCY AND MR SAFETY

The use of diagnostic imaging is often required in pregnant patients. Thus, it is not surprising, that the question of whether or not a patient should undergo an MR examination during pregnancy will often arise. Safety issues include possible bioeffects of the static magnetic field of the MR system, risks associated with exposure to the gradient magnetic fields, the potential adverse effects of radiofrequency (RF) energy, and possible adverse effects related to the combination of these three electromagnetic fields.

MR environment-related risks are difficult to assess for pregnant patients due to the number of possible permutations of the various factors that are present in this setting (e.g., differences in field strengths, pulse sequences, exposure times, etc.). This becomes even more complicated since new hardware and software is developed for MR systems on an on-going basis.

There have been a number of laboratory and clinical investigations conducted to determine the effects of using MR imaging during pregnancy. Most of the laboratory studies showed no evidence of injury or harm to the fetus, while a few studies reported adverse outcomes for laboratory animals. However, whether or not these findings can be extrapolated to human subjects is debatable.

By comparison, there have been relatively few studies performed in pregnant human subjects exposed to MR imaging or the MR environment. Each investigation reported no adverse outcomes for the subjects. For example, Baker et al. (1994) reported no demonstrable increase in disease, disability, or hearing loss in 20 children examined *in utero* using echo-planar MRI for suspected fetal compromise. Myers et al. (1998) reported no significant reduction in fetal growth vs. matched controls in 74 volunteer subjects exposed *in utero* to echo-planar MRI performed at 0.5-Tesla. A survey of reproductive health among 280 pregnant MR healthcare professionals performed by Kanal et al. (1993) showed no substantial increase in common adverse reproductive outcomes.

There has been on-going concern that acoustic noise associated with MRI may impact the fetus. Reeves et al. (2010) conducted an investigation to establish whether fetal exposure to the operating noise of 1.5-T MR imaging causes cochlear injury and subsequent hearing loss in neonates. The findings in this study provide some evidence that exposure of the fetus to 1.5-T MR imaging during the second and third trimesters is not associated with an increased risk of substantial neonatal hearing impairment.

With regard to the publications to date, there are discrepancies with respect to the experimental findings of the effects of electromagnetic fields used for MR procedures and the pertinent safety aspects of pregnancy. These discrepancies may be explained by a variety of factors, including the differences in the scientific methodology used, the type of organism examined, and the variance in exposure duration, as well as the conditions of the exposure to the electromagnetic fields. Additional investigations are warranted before the risks associated with exposure to MR procedures can be absolutely known and properly characterized.

GUIDELINES FOR THE USE OF MR PROCEDURES IN PREGNANT PATIENTS

As stated in the Policies, Guidelines, and Recommendations for MR Imaging Safety and Patient Management issued by the Safety Committee of the Society for Magnetic Resonance Imaging in 1991, "MR imaging may be used in pregnant women if other nonionizing forms of diagnostic imaging are inadequate or if the examination provides important information that would otherwise require exposure to ionizing radiation (e.g., fluoroscopy, CT, etc.). Pregnant patients should be informed that, to date, there has been no indication that the use of clinical MR imaging during pregnancy has produced deleterious effects." This policy has been adopted by the American College of Radiology and is considered to be the "standard of care" with respect to the use of MR procedures in pregnant patients. Importantly, this information applies to MR systems operating up to and including 3-Tesla.

Thus, MR procedures may be used in pregnant patients to address important clinical problems or to manage potential complications for the patient or fetus. The overall decision to utilize an MR procedure in a pregnant patient involves answering a series of important questions that will address risk:benefit including, the following:

- Is sonography satisfactory for diagnosis?
- Is the MR procedure appropriate to address the clinical question?
- Is obstetrical intervention prior to the MR procedure a possibility? That is, is termination of pregnancy a consideration? Is early delivery a consideration?

With regard to the use of MR procedures in pregnant patients, this diagnostic technique should not be withheld for the following cases:

- Patients with active brain or spine signs and symptoms requiring imaging.
- Patients with cancer requiring imaging.
- Patients with chest, abdomen, and pelvic signs and symptoms of active disease when sonography is non-diagnostic.
- In specific cases of suspected fetal anomaly or complex fetal disorder.

[*Portions of the content on this topic were excerpted with permission from Colletti P M. Magnetic Resonance Procedures and Pregnancy, In: Magnetic Resonance Procedures: Health Effects and Safety, FG Shellock, Editor, CRC Press, Boca Raton, FL, 2001. Reviewed and updated 2012.]

REFERENCES

Abdelazim IA, et al. Complementary roles of prenatal sonography and magnetic resonance imaging in diagnosis of fetal renal anomalies. Aust N Z J Obstet Gynaecol. 2010;50:237-41.

Beddy P, et al. Magnetic resonance imaging for the evaluation of acute abdominal pain in pregnancy. Semin Ultrasound CT MR. 2010;31:433-41.

Baker, P.N., et al, A three-year follow-up of children imaged *in utero* with echo-planar magnetic resonance. Am J Obstet Gynecol 170, 32-33, 1994.

Benson, R.C., Colletti, P.M., Platt, L.D., et al, MR imaging of fetal anomalies. Am. J. Roentgenol., 156, 1205, 1991.

Brown, C.E.L., and Weinreb, J.C., Magnetic resonance imaging appearance of growth retardation in a twin pregnancy. Obstet. Gynecol. 71, 987, 1988.

Carnes, K.I., and Magin, R.L., Effects of in utero exposure to 4.7 T MR imaging conditions on fetal growth and testicular development in the mouse. Magn. Reson. Imaging, 14, 263, 1996.

Carswell, H., Fast MRI of fetus yields considerable anatomic detail. Diag. Imaging, Nov, 11-12, 1988.

Chen MM, Coakley FV, et al. Guidelines for computed tomography and magnetic resonance imaging use during pregnancy and lactation. Obstet Gynecol. 2008;112 (2 Pt 1):333-40.

Colletti PM. Computer-assisted imaging of the fetus with magnetic resonance imaging. Comput. Med. Imaging Graph., 20, 491, 1996.

Colletti PM, Platt LD. When to use MRI in obstetrics. Diag. Imaging, 11, 84, 1989.

Colletti, P.M., and Sylvestre, P.B., Magnetic resonance imaging in pregnancy. MRI Clin. N. Am., 2, 291, 1994.

De Wilde JP, et al. A review of the current use of magnetic resonance imaging in pregnancy and safety implications for the fetus. Prog Biophys Mol Biol. 2005;87:335-353.

Dinh DH, et al. The use of magnetic resonance imaging for the diagnosis of fetal intracranial anomalies. Child Nerv. Syst., 6, 212, 1990.

Dunn, R.S., and Weiner, S.N., Antenatal diagnosis of sacrococcygeal teratoma facilitated by combined use of Doppler sonography and MR imaging. Am. J. Roentgenol., 156,1115, 1991.

Fitamorris-Glass, R., Mattrey, R.F., Cantrell, C.J., Magnetic resonance imaging as an adjunct to ultrasound in oligohydramnio. J Ultrasound Med. 8,159, 1989.

Fraser, R., Magnetic resonance imaging of the fetus. Initial experience [letter]. Gynecol. Obstet. Invest., 29, 255, 1990.

Garcia-Bournissen F, Shrim A, Koren G. Safety of gadolinium during pregnancy. Can Fam Physician. 2006 Mar;52:309-10.

Gardens AS, Weindling AM, Griffiths RD, et al, Fast-scan magnetic resonance imaging of fetal anomalies. Br J Obstet Gynecol 98,1217-1222, 1991

Hand JW, et al. Prediction of specific absorption rate in mother and fetus associated with MRI examinations during pregnancy. Magn Reson Med. 2006;55:883-893.

Hand JW, et al. Numerical study of RF exposure and the resulting temperature rise in the foetus during a magnetic resonance procedure. Phys Med Biol. 2010;55:913-30.

Hill MC, et al. Prenatal diagnosis of fetal anomalies using ultrasound and MRI. Radiol Clin North Am 26,287-307, 1988

Horvath L, Seeds JW. Temporary arrest of fetal movement with pancuronium bromide to enable antenatal magnetic resonance imaging of holosencephaly. Am. J. Roentgenol., 6,418-420, 1989

Heinrichs WL, et al.Midgestational exposure of pregnant BALB/c mice to magnetic resonance imaging conditions. Magn Reson Imaging, 6,305, 1988.

Huisman TA. Fetal magnetic resonance imaging. Semin Roentgenol. 2008;43:314-36.

International Commission on Non-Ionizing Radiation Protection Statement, Medical magnetic resonance procedures: protection of patients. Health Physics 2004;87:197-216.

Jackson HA, Panigrahy A. Fetal magnetic resonance imaging: the basics. Pediatr Ann. 2008;37:388-93.

Junkermann H. Indications and contraindications for contrast-enhanced MRI and CT during pregnancy. Radiologe. 2007;47:774-7.

Kanal E, Barkovich AJ, Bell C, et al. ACR guidance document for safe MR practices: 2007. AJR Am J Roentgenol. 2007;188:1447-1474.

Kanal E, Gillen J, Evans J, Savitz D, Shellock FG. Survey of reproductive health among female MR workers. Radiology 1993;187:395-399.

Kanal E, Shellock FG, Sonnenblick D. MRI clinical site safety: Phase I results and preliminary data. Magn. Reson. Imaging 7[Suppl] 1, 106, 1988.

Kay, H.H., Herfkens, R.J., and Kay, B.K., Effect of magnetic resonance imaging on Xenopus laevis embryogenesis. Magn. Reson. Imaging, 6, 501-6, 1988.

Kikuchi S, et al. Temperature elevation in the fetus from electromagnetic exposure during magnetic resonance imaging. Phys Med Biol. 2010;55:2411-26.

Kok RD, et al. Absence of harmful effects of magnetic resonance exposure at 1.5 T in utero during the third trimester of pregnancy: a follow-up study. Magn Reson Imaging. 2004;22:851-4.

Lee JW, et al. Genotoxic effects of 3 T magnetic resonance imaging in cultured human lymphocytes. Bioelectromagnetics. 2011;32:535-42.

Lenke RR, et al. Use of pancuronium bromide to inhibit fetal movement during magnetic resonance imaging. J. Reprod. Med. 34,315-317, 1989

Leithner K, et al. Psychological reactions in women undergoing fetal magnetic resonance imaging. Obstet Gynecol. 2008;111(2 Pt 1):396-402.

Levine D. Obstetric MRI. J Magn Reson Imaging 2006;24:1-15

Malko JA, et al. Search for influence of 1.5 T magnetic field on growth of yeast cells. Bioelectromagnetics, 15, 495, 1987.

Mansfield P, Stehling MK, Ordidge RJ, et al. Study of internal structure of the human fetus in utero at 0.5-T. Br J Radiol 13,314-318, 1990

Masselli G, et al. Acute abdominal and pelvic pain in pregnancy: MR imaging as a valuable adjunct to ultrasound? Abdom Imaging 2011;36:596-603.

McCarthy SM, et al. Uterine neoplasms: MR imaging. Radiology, 170, 125, 1989.

McRobbie, D., and Foster, M.A., Pulsed magnetic field exposure during pregnancy and implications for NMR foetal imaging. A study with mice. Magn. Reson. Imaging, 3, 231, 1985.

Myers C, et al. Failure to detect intrauterine growth restriction following in utero exposure to MRI. Br J Radiol, 71, 549, 1998.

Murakami J, et al. Fetal developmet of mice following intrauterine exposure to a static magnetic field of 6.3-T. Magn. Reson. Imaging, 10, 433, 1992.

Nara VR, et al., Effects of a 1.5T static magnetic field on spermatogenesis and embryogenesis in mice. Invest. Radiology 31, 586, 1996.

Oto A. MR imaging evaluation of acute abdominal pain during pregnancy. Magn Reson Imaging Clin N Am. 2006;14:489-501.

Reeves MJ, et al. Neonatal cochlear function: measurement after exposure to acoustic noise during in utero MR imaging. Radiology. 2010;257:802-809.

Ruckhäberle E, et al. In vivo intrauterine sound pressure and temperature measurements during magnetic resonance imaging (1.5 T) in pregnant ewes. Fetal Diagn Ther. 2008;24:203-10.

Shellock FG, Crues JV. MR procedures: biologic effects, safety, and patient care. Radiology, 2004;232:635-652.

Shellock FG, Kanal E. Policies, guidelines, and recommendations for MR imaging safety and patient management. J. Magn. Reson. Imaging, 1, 97, 1991.

Shellock, F.G., and Kanal, E. Magnetic resonance procedures and pregnancy. In, Magnetic Resonance Bioeffects, Safety, and Patient Management. Second Edition, Lippincott-Ravin, Philadelphia, New York, 1996, Chapter 4, pp. 49.

Smith FW, Kent C, et al. Nuclear magnetic resonance imaging – a new look at the fetus. Br J Gynaecol 92,1024-1033, 1985

Smith FW, Sutherland HW. Magnetic resonance imaging: The use of the inversion recovery sequence to display fetal morphology. Br J Radiol 61,338-341, 1988.

Stark, DD, et al. Pelvimetry by magnetic resonance imaging. Am. J. Roentgenol., 144, 947, 1985.

Tesky, G.C., et al. Survivability and long-term stress reactivity levels following repeated exposure to nuclear magnetic resonance imaging procedures in rats. Physiol. Chem. Phys. Med. NMR, 19, 43, 1987.

Tyndall, D.A., MRI effects on the teratogenicity of x-irradiation in the C57BL/6J mouse. Magn. Reson. Imaging, 8, 423, 1990.

Tyndall, R.J., and Sulik, K.K., Effects of magnetic resonance imaging on eye development in the C57BL/6J mouse. Teratology, 43, 263, 1991.

Tyndall, D.A., MRI effects on craniofacial size and crown-rump length in C57BL/6J mice in 1.5 T fields. Oral Surg. Oral Med. Oral Pathol. 76, 655, 1993.

Yip YP, et al. Effects of MR exposure at 1.5 T on early embryonic development of the chick. J. Magn. Reson. Imaging, 4, 742, 1994.

Yip YP, et al. Effects of MR exposure on axonal outgrowth in the sympathetic nervous system of the chick. J. Magn. Reson. Imaging, 4, 457, 1995.

Yip YP, et al. Effects of MR exposure on cell proliferation and migration of chick motor neurons. J. Magn. Reson. Imaging, 4,799, 1994.

Vadeyar SH, et al. Effect of fetal magnetic resonance imaging on fetal heart rate patterns. Am. J. Obstet. Gynecol., 182, 666, 2000.

Webb JA, et al. Members of Contrast Media Safety Committee of European Society of Urogenital Radiology (ESUR). The use of iodinated and gadolinium contrast media during pregnancy and lactation. Eur Radiol. 2005;15:1234-40.

Weinreb JC, et al.. Pelvic masses in pregnant patients, MR and US imaging. Radiology, 159, 717, 1986.

Weinreb JC, et al. Magnetic resonance imaging in obstetric diagnosis. Radiology 154,157-161, 1985.

Wenstrom KD, et al. Magnetic resonance imaging of fetuses with intracranial defects. Obstet Gynecol., 77,529-532, 1991.

Wieseler KM, et al. Imaging in pregnant patients: examination appropriateness. Radiographics. 2010;30:1215-29.

Wilcox A, et al. Incidence of early loss of pregnancy. New Engl. J. Med., 319,189-194, 1988.

Williamson, RA, et al. Magnetic resonance imaging of anomalous fetuses. Obstet Gynecol 71,952, 1988.

Pregnant Technologists and Other Healthcare Workers in the MR Environment

Due to the concern with regard to pregnant technologists and other healthcare workers in the MR environment, a survey of reproductive health among female MR system operators was conducted by Kanal et al. (1993). Questionnaires were sent to female MR technologists and nurses at the majority of the MRI facilities in the United States. The questionnaire addressed menstrual and reproductive experiences as well as work activities. This study attempted to account for known potential confounding variables (e.g., age, smoking, alcohol use, etc.) for this type of data.

Of the 1,915 completed questionnaires analyzed, there were 1,421 pregnancies: 280 occurred while working as an MR employee (technologist or nurse), 894 while employed at another job, 54 as a student, and 193 as a homemaker. Five categories were analyzed that included spontaneous abortion rate, pre-term delivery (less than 39 weeks), low birth weight (less than 5.5 pounds), infertility (taking more than eleven months to conceive), and gender of the offspring.

The data indicated that there were no statistically significant alterations in the five areas studied for MR healthcare professionals relative to the same group studied when they were employed elsewhere, prior to becoming MR healthcare employees. Additionally, adjustment for maternal age, smoking, and alcohol use failed to markedly change any of the associations. Menstrual regularity, menstrual cycle, and related topics were also examined in this study. These included inquiries regarding the number of days of menstrual bleeding, the heaviness of the bleeding, and the time between menstrual cycles.

Admittedly, this is a difficult area to objectively examine because it depends on both subjective memory and the memory of the respondent for a given topic. Subjective memory is often inadequate. Nevertheless, the data suggested that there were no clear correlations between MR workers and specific modifications of the menstrual cycle.

The data from this extensive epidemiological investigation were reassuring insofar as that there did not appear to be deleterious effects from exposure to the static magnetic field of the MR system. Therefore, a policy is recommended that permits pregnant technologists and healthcare workers to perform MR procedures, as well as to enter the MR system room, and attend to the patient during pregnancy, regardless of the trimester. Importantly, technologists and healthcare workers should not remain within the MR system room or bore of the magnet during the actual operation of the scanner.

This later recommendation is especially important for those healthcare workers involved in patient management or interventional MR-guided examinations and procedures, since it may be necessary for them to be directly exposed to the MR system's electromagnetic fields at levels similar to those used for patients. These recommendations are not based on indications of adverse effects, but rather, from a conservative point of view and the feeling that there are insufficient data pertaining to the effects of the other electromagnetic fields of the MR system to support or allow unnecessary exposures.

REFERENCES

Evans JA, Savitz DA, Kanal E, Gillen J. Infertility and pregnancy outcome among magnetic resonance imaging workers. J Occu Med 1993;12:1191-1195.

International Commission on Non-Ionizing Radiation Protection (ICNIRP) Statement, Medical magnetic resonance procedures: protection of patients. Health Physics 2004;87:197-216.

Kanal E, Gillen J, Evans J, Savitz D, Shellock FG. Survey of reproductive health among female MR workers. Radiology 1993;187:395-399.

Shellock FG. Magnetic Resonance Procedures: Health Effects and Safety. CRC Press, LLC, Boca Raton, FL, 2001.

Shellock FG, Kanal E. Policies, guidelines, and recommendations for MR imaging safety and patient management. J Magn Reson Imaging 1991;1: 97-101.

Prevention of Missile Effect Accidents

The "missile effect" refers to the capability of the fringe field of an MR system to attract a ferromagnetic object, drawing it rapidly into the scanner by considerable force. The missile effect can pose a significant risk to the patient inside the MR system and/or anyone in the path of the projectile. Furthermore, considerable damage to the MR system may result due to the impact of ferromagnetic object. Therefore, a strict policy must be established by the MRI facility to detect metallic objects prior to allowing individuals or patients to enter the MR environment. In addition, to guard against accidents from projectiles, the immediate area around the MR system should be clearly demarcated, labeled with appropriate danger signs, and secured by trained staff aware of proper MR safety procedures.

For patients preparing to undergo MR examinations, all metallic or other potentially problematic personal belongings and devices (i.e., hearing aids, analog watches, beepers, cell phones, jewelry, etc.) must be removed as well as clothing items that have metallic fasteners or other metallic components (e.g., clothing with metallic threads). One of the most effective means of preventing a ferromagnetic object from a patient inadvertently becoming a missile and to ensure that no inappropriate objects enter the MR environment is to require the patient to wear a gown or scrubs without pockets for the MR examination.

Non-ambulatory patients must only be allowed to enter the area of the MR system using a nonferromagnetic wheelchair or nonferromagnetic gurney. Wheelchairs and gurneys should also be inspected for the presence of a ferromagnetic oxygen tank, IV pole, sand bag (which may have metal shot), or other similar problematic component or accessory before allowing the patient into the MR setting. Fortunately, there are many commercially-available, specially-designed devices that are appropriate for use to transport and support patients in the MR environment.

Any individual accompanying the patient must be required to remove all metallic objects or other problematic items before entering the MR area and should undergo a careful and thorough screening procedure. All hospital and outside personnel that may need to enter the MR environment periodically or in response to an emergency (e.g., custodial staff, maintenance workers, housekeeping staff, bioengineers, nurses, security officers, fire fighters, etc.) should also undergo MRI screening and educated about the potential hazards associated with the MR system. These individuals should, likewise, be instructed to remove inappropriate objects before entering the MR environment.

Many serious incidents have occurred when individuals who were unaware of the potentially dangerous aspects of the MR system entered the MR environment with items such as steel oxygen tanks, wheel chairs, scissors, hand guns, monitors, and other similar objects.

In 2001, the first fatal accident occurred that illustrated the importance of careful attention to preventing ferromagnetic objects from entering the MR environment. In this widely publicized incident, a young patient suffered a blow to the head from a ferromagnetic oxygen tank that became a projectile in the presence of a 1.5-Tesla MR system.

While MR safety guidelines and procedures are well known, accidents related to the missile effect continue to occur. Guidelines for preventing these hazards are presented in **Table 1**.

Table 1. Guidelines for preventing hazards related to missile effects.*

1) Appoint an MRI safety officer or other appropriately trained person to be responsible for ensuring that proper procedures are in effect, enforced, and updated to ensure safety in the MR environment.

2) Establish and routinely review safety policies and procedures and assess the level of compliance by all staff members.

3) Provide all MR staff, along with other personnel who may need to enter the MR environment (e.g., transport personnel, security officers, housekeeping staff, maintenance workers, fire department personnel, etc.) with formal training on MR safety. This should be done especially for new employees and repeated on a regular basis (i.e., yearly).

4) Emphasize to all personnel that the MR system's powerful static magnetic field is always "on" and treat the MR environment, accordingly.

5) Don't allow equipment and devices containing ferromagnetic components into the MR environment, unless they have been tested and labeled "MR-safe" or "MR-conditional".

6) Adhere to the restrictions provided by suppliers regarding the use of MR-safe and/or MR-conditional equipment and devices in the MR environment.

7) Maintain a list of MR-safe and MR-conditional equipment, including restrictions for use. This list should be kept and updated in every MRI facility by the MR safety officer (refer to **www.MRIsafety.com** for comprehensive information).

8) Bring a non-ambulatory patient into the MR environment using a nonmagnetic wheelchair or gurney. Ensure that no oxygen tanks, IV poles, sandbags with metal shot, or other ferromagnetic objects are concealed under blankets or sheets or stowed away on the transport equipment.

9) Carefully screen all individuals and patients entering the MR environment to identify magnetic objects in their bodies (e.g., implants, bullets, shrapnel, etc.), on their bodies (e.g., hair pins, brassieres, buttons, zippers, jewelry, clothing with metallic threads), or attached to their bodies (e.g., body piercing jewelry, body modification implants, halo vests, cervical fixation devices, external fixation systems, prosthetic appliances). Ferromagnetic objects on or attached to the bodies of patients, family members, or staff members should be removed, if feasible, before the individuals enter the MR environment. Additional attention must also be given to items that are made from conducting metals, as these may pose hazards under certain conditions.

10) Have patients wear hospital gowns or scrubs without pockets and metallic fasteners for MR procedures. Clothing that contains metallic objects or threads that may pose a hazard in the MR environment.

[*Adapted and published permission from ECRI Report, 2001 and Shellock FG, 2001; updated 2007. Reviewed and updated 2012.]

REFERENCES

Chaljub G, et al. Projectile cylinder accidents resulting from the presence of ferromagnetic nitrous oxide or oxygen tanks in the MR suite. American Journal of Roentgenology 2001;177:27-30.

Colletti PM. Size "H" oxygen cylinder: accidental MR projectile at 1.5-Tesla. Journal of Magnetic Resonance Imaging 2004;19:141-143.

ECRI. Patient Death Illustrates the Importance of Adhering to Safety Precautions in Magnetic Resonance Environments. ECRI, Plymouth Meeting, PA, Aug. 6, 2001.

Kanal E, Barkovich AJ, Bell C, et al. ACR guidance document for safe MR practices: 2007. AJR Am J Roentgenol. 2007;188:1447-1474.

International Commission on Non-Ionizing Radiation Protection (ICNIRP) Statement, Medical magnetic resonance procedures: protection of patients. Health Physics 2004;87:197-216.

Joint Commission on Accreditation of Healthcare Organizations, USA. Preventing accidents and injuries in the MRI suite. Sentinel Event Alert. 2008 Feb 14; 1-3.

Shellock FG. Magnetic Resonance Procedures: Health Effects and Safety. CRC Press, LLC, Boca Raton, FL, 2001.

Signs to Help Control Access to the MR Environment

To guard against accidents and injuries to patients and other individuals as well as damage to magnetic resonance (MR) systems, the general and immediate areas associated with the scanner (also referred to as the MR environment) must have supervised and controlled access. Supervised and controlled access involves having MR safety-trained personnel present at all times during the operation of the facility to ensure that no unaccompanied or unauthorized individuals are allowed to enter the MR environment. MR safety-trained personnel must be responsible for performing comprehensive screening of patients and other individuals before allowing them to enter the MR system room. The area should be secured and/or controlled by appropriate means when MR safety-trained personnel are not present.

Importantly, it is necessary to educate and train individuals who need to enter the MR environment on a regular basis, those working on an intermittent basis, or responding to an emergency including custodial workers, transporters, security personnel, firefighters, nurses, anesthesiologists, and paramedics regarding the potential hazards related to the powerful magnetic field of the MR system. Unfortunately, even with proper MR safety procedures in place, many individuals and patients have inadvertently "wandered" unattended into the MR setting, and these situations have resulted in problematic or serious consequences.

As a means of helping to control access to the MR environment, the area must be clearly demarcated and labeled with prominently displayed signs to make individuals and patients aware of the risks associated with the MR system. Access to the MR environment must also be monitored and controlled on a continuous basis.

Signs with appropriate content and information were designed to promote a safe MR environment. According to the U.S. Food and Drug Administration document entitled, Guidance for the Submission Of Premarket Notifications for Magnetic Resonance Diagnostic Devices (issued November 14, 1998), Attachment B, states: "The controlled access area should be labeled "Danger - High Magnetic Field" at all entries." Also, this FDA document indicates, "Operators should be warned by appropriate signs about the presence of magnetic fields and their force and torque on magnetic materials, and that loose ferrous objects should be excluded."

"DANGER" Sign

In consideration of the above, the sign used for the MRI environment states: **DANGER!** Additionally, to inform everyone about the powerful static magnetic field associated with the MR system, especially individuals unacquainted with MR technology, the following information is prominently shown on this sign:

RESTRICTED ACCESS
STRONG MAGNETIC FIELD
THIS MAGNET IS ALWAYS ON!

With respect to the information for implants and devices, in addition to cardiac pacemakers, implantable cardioverter defibrillators (ICDs) are potentially hazardous for patients and individuals in the MR environment. Therefore, this information is included on the sign used for the MR environment. The peer-reviewed literature has reported that many types of metallic implants are acceptable for patients undergoing MR procedures, while others are not. As such, this information is clarified on the current sign, with individuals and patients informed to consult MRI professionals if there are questions regarding this matter, as follows:

"Persons with certain metallic, electronic, magnetic, or mechanically-activated implants, devices, or objects may not enter this area. Serious injury may result. <u>Do not enter</u> this area if you have any question regarding an implant, device, or object. Consult the MRI Technologist or Radiologist."

Finally, the sign also states:

"Objects made from ferrous materials must not be taken into this area. Serious injury or property damage may result. Electronic objects such as hearing aids, cell phones, and beepers may also be damaged."

Many individuals fail to realize that the MR system's static magnetic field is always on. In fact, investigations of accidents that involved relatively large ferromagnetic objects like oxygen cylinders, chairs, IV poles, and wheelchairs revealed that the offending personnel thought that the powerful magnetic field was activated *only* during the MR procedure. Therefore, a smaller sign or decal is particularly useful to emphasize the potentially hazardous nature of the MR environment, which states:

DANGER! THIS MAGNET IS ALWAYS ON!

Sign Placement. The strategic placement of signs in and around the MR environment is crucial to ensure that all individuals and patients see them before entering this area. In general, a sign should be placed on the door or entrance to MR system room and near or on the doorframe to be viewed by individuals and patients, especially if the door to the MR system room is open.

[*To obtain the afore-mentioned signs designed to help control access to the MR environment, please visit www.Magmedix.com]

REFERENCES

U. S. Department Of Health and Human Services, Center for Devices and Radiological Health Food and Drug Administration, the document entitled, Guidance for the, Submission Of Premarket Notifications for Magnetic Resonance Diagnostic Devices, Issued November 14, 1998.

Spatial Gradient Magnetic Field: How This Information is Applied to Labeling of Medical Implants and Devices*

*[*Excerpted with permission from, Regarding the Value Reported for the Term "Spatial Gradient Magnetic Field" and How This Information Is Applied to Labeling of Medical Implants and Devices*, Shellock FG, Kanal E, Gilk, TB. American Journal of Roentgenology, 2011;196:142-145. To obtain the original article including the illustrations, please visit www.IMRSER.org.]*

Differences in interpretations of testing and reporting criteria, methodologies, and perhaps even concerns about manufacturer legal liability have created a contemporary environment in which questions and confusion abound in the magnetic resonance imaging (MRI) industry. Of particular concern regarding the management of patients with implants and devices in the MRI environment is the disparities in the way that the spatial gradient magnetic field information is presented.

The intensity of the static magnetic field around an MR system varies with respect to the distance from the scanner. This so-called "fringe-field" of the MR system creates a "spatial gradient magnetic field". By definition, the spatial gradient magnetic field is a magnetic field that varies in intensity over distance. The spatial gradient magnetic field should not be confused with the time-varying, gradient magnetic fields produced by the gradient coils that are used during the imaging process for spatial encoding of the MRI signals.

The spatial gradient of the magnetic field produces an attractive displacement (or translational) force on ferromagnetic objects placed into the static magnetic field of the MR system (1-4). Importantly, the MRI-specific labeling that is used for medical implants and devices typically provides information for the "highest spatial gradient magnetic field" at which the medical device was tested and that is allowed for the object to be exposed to in order to ensure the safety of the patient relative to the device's translational attraction (1-6). The assessment of translational attraction (or displacement force) is just one aspect of implant testing that is performed when evaluating a medical device (1-5).

In most cases, the Food and Drug Administration (FDA) accepts the determination of translational attraction for a medical device that is conducted according to the procedure described by the American Society for Testing and Materials (ASTM) International Designation. F 2052, Standard test method for measurement of magnetically induced displacement force on passive implants in the magnetic resonance environment. Using this technique, a test apparatus with a protractor (also called the "fixture") is placed in an MR system with a horizontal magnetic field at the point of the highest "accessible" spatial gradient magnetic field (6). In general, the highest spatial gradient magnetic field used to assess translational attraction for a medical device is located off-axis, at a side-wall and near the opening of the bore of the scanner (1, 3). [Alternatively, the medical device is assessed for translational attraction at the point where the highest deflection angle occurs in association with the particular MR system used for the assessment.] The angular "deflection" of the device from the vertical is measured and the translational attraction is calculated (6).

Notably the placement of the test fixture (apparatus with the protractor) in the MR system is at a position where it can be utilized properly (i.e., securely positioned) for the test procedure. This is almost always a worst-case position of greatest attractive force that the patient with the device will "pass through" when entering the bore of the MR system for an examination.

With regard to the translational attraction measurement for a medical device, if the deflection angle is less than 45-degrees, and the magnetic force is in the horizontal direction, the deflection force is less than the gravitational force associated with the device's weight and it is assumed that any risk imposed by the application of the magnetically-induced deflection force is no greater than any risk imposed by normal daily activity in the Earth's gravitational field (4, 6). However, even if a device exceeds 45-degrees of deflection, it may still be acceptable for a patient undergoing an MRI examination if sufficient counter-forces are present (e.g., from sutures, scarring, tissue in-growth, etc.) that prevent it from being moved or dislodged (3).

There is confusion about the term "spatial gradient magnetic field" (or "highest spatial gradient" or "magnetic spatial gradient") and how this parameter is reported for a given MR system relative to this term's use in the labeling of a medical device. [Note: The term "spatial gradient magnetic field" may also be misunderstood because some MRI professionals see the term "gradient" and presume that it refers to the "time-varying or gradient magnetic fields" (dB/dt) used for spatial location in association with MR imaging (2).] The term "spatial gradient magnetic field" refers to the rate at which the static magnetic field strength changes over space or distance per unit length. This parameter is indicated as dB/dx, using the units of Tesla/meter or gauss/centimeter.

According to test reports and resulting labeling for many implants tested at 3-Tesla, the highest "accessible" spatial gradient magnetic field of 720-gauss/cm was determined using highly involved methodology for the 3-Tesla MR system used for the measurements of translational attraction. (Researchers and MRI professionals, however, must typically rely on the magnitude and location of the spatial gradient magnetic field as it is provided by the MR system manufacturer.) To test the device, the apparatus with the protractor was placed at that position (720-gauss/cm) to measure the deflection angle. This information (i.e., the value for the highest spatial gradient magnetic field) is reported in the labeling for the device. Thus, the MRI-specific labeling would then state that the acceptable static magnetic field information for a given implant would be, as follows (2):

"-3-Tesla or less
-Highest spatial gradient magnetic field of 720-gauss/cm or less"

To date, the Food and Drug Administration has approved MRI-specific labeling for more than three thousand medical devices according to the above-described process, especially with regard to how the displacement force is determined [i.e., by following the procedure described in the ASTM document (6)] and with respect to how the findings are presented in the labeling (i.e., reporting the value for the highest spatial gradient magnetic field that was used for the determination of the deflection angle for the medical device, which was based on where the apparatus with the protractor was positioned). Furthermore, the ASTM document that addresses the measurement of translational attraction for a medical device clearly states to report "10.1.7….the magnitude of the spatial gradient of the magnetic field, at the test location." That is why this particular spatial gradient magnetic field value has been used in the FDA-approved MRI labeling for thousands of medical devices. Of note is that the reported results describe the MR system variables under which the implant or device was tested and do not necessarily represent the safety threshold for translational forces.

Recently, MR system manufacturers have provided data to MRI professionals pertaining to the "spatial gradient magnetic field" values for a given scanner, including information for the highest spatial gradient magnetic field. Presumably, this was done in an effort to help address the case when a patient presents with a medical device that has labeling stating the "highest spatial gradient magnetic field" value permitted for that implant and that parameter is unknown for a specific MR system. The format, values, locations for measurement and presentation of these reported MR system values have varied, and even conflicted between and within the MR system vendors that have provided these data.

Considerable confusion has inadvertently arisen as a result of these recently reported spatial gradient magnetic field values. The reason for this misunderstanding is simple: The location, and, therefore, the values, of the highest spatial gradient magnetic field measured and reported by the MR system manufacturers is not the same as that which is utilized for the location at which the implant/device displacement force testing was performed. To elaborate, the location of measurement of the highest spatial gradient magnetic field that is used when evaluating the displacement force for a medical implant or device (i.e., the place in the MR system where the apparatus with the protractor is positioned; which is generally off-axis, near the opening of the bore of the scanner) is not necessarily the same as the location where the MR system manufacturer measures the scanner's highest spatial gradient magnetic field.

The MR system manufacturer may have performed the measurement with the covers or shroud removed from the MR system, and/or without the patient table present. This permits access to stronger static magnetic fields and spatial gradient magnetic fields and, thus, can result in a greater measured value for the "highest spatial gradient magnetic field" as it is reported by the manufacturer. This region and, therefore, the measured value, however, is not one that can be reached by a patient with an implant and, thus, it does not represent a reasonable assessment of risk exposure for that situation.

We recognize that the values reported for the regions not normally accessible to patients may have significance or relevance for MR system manufacturers and their manufacturing and/or service employees. Nevertheless, from the point of view of clinical patient care, these "patient inaccessible regions" and the spatial gradient magnetic field values reported for them are of no particular benefit. Indeed, reporting these values seems to have resulted in confusion.

Furthermore, making decisions regarding the patients with implants or devices based on these higher spatial gradient magnetic field values measured in patient inaccessible regions might inadvertently lead to canceling requested and needed clinical MRI examinations for patients with devices tested and cleared to the patient accessible region's translational forces – but not to those higher values reported at patient inaccessible regions.

Clinical personnel responsible for assessing the labeling that states the "MR conditional" aspects of an implant or device, rated as acceptable to a value of 720 gauss/cm, when their MR system by the specifications provided by the MR system manufacturer is identified as having a maximum value 200 gauss/cm higher (e.g., 900 gauss/cm), may refuse to scan the patient with the implant on that MR system which, ironically, is equivalent to the scanner used to demonstrate safety relative to translational attraction for the implant!

While the value for the highest spatial gradient magnetic field that the MR system manufacturer reports for a given scanner does not have direct relevance to a patient with a medical device, if the MR system manufacturer provides measurements that are obtained in radial increments from that position, these values may be useful for managing patients with medical implants and devices, if the position used to perform the deflection angle test on the device was known.

In consideration of the discrepancy between the MR system manufacturer's reported value for the highest spatial gradient magnetic field for a given scanner and the highest "accessible" spatial magnetic gradient value used for medical device testing that has led to confusion and frustration when MRI professionals must consider how to manage patients presented with MRI labeling information, we strongly recommend that standardization is necessary. Notably, it would be helpful and appropriate for all MR system manufacturers to report the greatest static magnetic field strength as well as the highest spatial gradient magnetic field values in regions that are readily accessible by patients and/or healthcare professionals working around an "intact" (i.e., with the covers or shroud not removed) MR system.

In order to accomplish such a task, the FDA needs to understand the nature of the present problems related to the MRI specific labeling for implants and devices, develop an appropriate strategy to address this matter, and implement a solution in a timely manner.

Clinical Implications. For today, a recognition that the spatial gradient magnetic field values provided by the MR system manufacturers may differ (i.e., typically the values are higher) from those at which the implant might have undergone testing for translational attraction is the first step towards understanding the important issues presented in this *Editorial Commentary*. Hopefully, this information will enable an appropriate determination of the risk-benefit for the management of patients with implants.

If the deflection angle information for the implant can be obtained from the device manufacturer, and the deflection angle value was somewhat trivial (e.g., 15-degrees or lower) for the specific MR system to be used for the examination, it would be reasonable to expect that a minor variation in the highest spatial gradient magnetic field value reported by the MR system manufacturer (i.e., compared to that reported in the labeling for the device) would not produce a clinically significant difference in the safety outcome. Of course, an entirely different conclusion might be reached if the translational attraction testing documented a significant deflection angle for the implant.

Conclusions. There are *two different positions* where the highest spatial gradient magnetic field may be measured and reported. One, the highest "patient accessible" spatial gradient magnetic field, which pertains to that used for the deflection angle test for a medical implant or device and through which a patient with an implant or device may pass. The other, the scanner's highest spatial gradient magnetic field, as reported in the specifications for the magnet of a given scanner, that reports the region of greatest dB/dx regardless of its accessibility to patients or healthcare providers. The values measured by the MR system manufacturers are inherently higher than those reported and used in the labeling of medical devices are of dubious clinical value, and should be replaced, or at the very least supplemented, with the greatest dB/dx values reachable or accessible by patients and healthcare professionals.

REFERENCES

(1) American Society for Testing and Materials (ASTM) International Designation: F 2503. Standard Practice for Marking Medical Devices and Other Items for Safety in the Magnetic Resonance Environment. West Conshohocken, PA.

(2) Shellock FG, Woods TO, Crues JV. MRI Labeling Information for Implants and Devices: Explanation of Terminology. Radiology 2009;253:26-30.

(3) Shellock FG. Reference Manual for Magnetic Resonance Safety Implants and Devices: 2011 Edition. Biomedical Research Publishing Group, Los Angeles, CA, 2011.

(4) Woods TO. Standards for medical devices in MRI: present and future. Journal of Magnetic Resonance Imaging 2007;26:1186-1189.

(5) www.MRIsafety.com

(6) American Society for Testing and Materials (ASTM) International Designation. F 2052. Standard test method for measurement of magnetically induced displacement force on passive implants in the magnetic resonance environment. West Conshohocken, PA.

Tattoos, Permanent Cosmetics, and Eye Makeup

Traditional (i.e., decorative) and cosmetic tattoo procedures have been performed for thousands of years. Cosmetic tattoos or "permanent cosmetics" are used to reshape, recolor, recreate, or modify eye shadow, eyeliner, eyebrows, lips, beauty marks, and cheek blush. Additionally, permanent cosmetics are used aesthetically to enhance nipple-areola reconstruction procedures and for other applications.

Unfortunately, there is confusion regarding the overall safety aspects of permanent cosmetics. For example, based on a few reports of symptoms localized to the tattooed area during MR imaging, radiologists have refused to perform examinations on individuals with permanent cosmetics, particularly tattooed eyeliner. This undue and unwarranted concern for possible adverse events prevents patients with cosmetic tattoos access to an important diagnostic imaging technique.

While it is well-known that permanent cosmetics and decorative tattoos may cause artifacts and may be associated with relatively minor, short-term cutaneous reactions, the exact frequency and severity of soft tissue reactions or other problems related to MR imaging, while unknown, is considered to be quite low.

In 2002, Tope and Shellock conducted a study to determine the frequency and severity of adverse events associated with MR imaging in a population of subjects with permanent cosmetics. A questionnaire was distributed to clients of cosmetic tattoo technicians. This survey asked subjects for demographic data, information about their tattoos, and for their experiences during MR imaging procedures. Results from 1,032 surveys were tabulated. One hundred thirty-five (13.1%) study subjects underwent MR imaging after having permanent cosmetics applied. Only two individuals (1.5%) experienced problems associated with MR imaging. One subject reported a sensation of "slight tingling" and the other reported a "burning" sensation. Both incidents were transient and did not prevent the MR procedures from being performed. Based on these findings and additional information in the peer-reviewed literature, it appears that MR imaging may be performed in patients with permanent cosmetics without serious soft tissue reactions or adverse events.

Therefore, the presence of permanent cosmetics should not prevent a patient from undergoing MR imaging.

Before undergoing an MR procedure, the patient should be asked if he or she has ever had a permanent coloring technique (i.e., tattooing) applied to the body. This includes cosmetic applications such as eyeliner, lip-liner, lip coloring, as well as decorative designs. This question is necessary because of the associated imaging artifacts and, more importantly, because a small number of patients (fewer than 10 documented cases) have experienced transient skin irritation, cutaneous swelling, or heating sensations at the site of the permanent colorings in association with MR procedures (review of Medical Device Reports, 1985 to 2011).

Interestingly, decorative tattoos tend to cause worse problems (including first- and second-degree burns) for patients undergoing MR imaging compared to those that have been reported for cosmetic tattoos. With regard to decorative tattoos, a letter to the editor described a second-degree burn that occurred on the skin of the deltoid from a decorative tattoo. The authors suggested that "the heating could have come either from oscillations of the gradients or, more likely from the RF-induced electrical currents". However, the exact mechanisms responsible for complications or adverse events in the various cases that have occurred related to decorative tattoos is unknown.

Additionally, Kreidstein et al. reported that a patient experienced a sudden burning pain at the site of a decorative tattoo while undergoing MR imaging of the lumbar spine using a 1.5-Tesla MR system. Swelling and erythema was resolved within 12 hours, without evidence of permanent sequelae. The tattoo pigment used in this case was ferromagnetic, which possibly explained the symptoms experienced by the patient. Surprisingly, in order to permit the MRI examination, an excision of the tattooed skin was performed.

The authors of this report stated, "Theoretically, the application of a pressure dressing of the tattoo may prevent any tissue distortion due to ferromagnetic pull". (However, this relatively benign procedure was not attempted for this patient.) The authors also indicated that, "In some cases, removal of the tattoo may be the most practical means of allowing MRI".

Kanal and Shellock (1998) commented on this report in a letter to the editor, suggesting that the response to this situation was "rather aggressive". Clearly the trauma, expense, and morbidity associated with excision of a tattoo far exceed those that may be associated with ferromagnetic tattoo interactions. A firmly applied pressure bandage may be used if there is concern related to "movement" of the ferromagnetic particles in the tattoo pigment. Additionally, direct application of a cold compress to the site of a tattoo would likely mitigate any heating sensation that may occur in association with MR imaging.

Artifacts. Imaging artifacts associated with permanent cosmetics and certain types of eye makeup have been reported. These artifacts are predominantly associated with the presence of pigments that use iron oxide or other type of metal and occur in the immediate area of the applied pigment or material. As such, tattoo- and makeup-related MR imaging artifacts should not prevent a diagnostically adequate MR imaging procedure from being performed, especially in consideration that careful selection of imaging parameters may minimize artifacts related to metallic materials.

The only possible exception to this is if the anatomy of interest is in the *exact* same position of where the tattoo was applied using a metal-based pigment. For example, Weiss et al. reported that heavy metal particles used in the pigment base of mascara and eyeliner tattoos have a paramagnetic effect that causes alteration of the local magnetic field in adjacent tissues. Changes in the MR signal pattern may result in distortion of the globes. In some cases, the artifact and distortion may mimic actual ocular disease, such as a ciliary body melanoma or cyst.

GUIDELINES AND RECOMMENDATIONS

In consideration of the available literature and experience pertaining to MR procedures and patients with permanent cosmetics and tattoos, guidelines to manage these individuals include, the following:

1) The screening form used for patients should include a question to identify the presence of permanent cosmetics or decorative tattoos.
2) Before undergoing an MR procedure, the patient should be asked if he or she had a permanent coloring technique (i.e., tattooing) applied to any part of the body. This includes cosmetic applications such as eyeliner, lip-liner, lip coloring, as well as decorative designs.
3) The patient should be informed of the potential risks associated with the site of the tattoo.
4) The patient should be advised to immediately inform the MRI technologist regarding any unusual sensation felt at the site of the tattoo in association with the MR procedure.
5) The patient should be closely monitored using visual and auditory means throughout the operation of the MR system to ensure safety. In the event that the patient reports a problem, the MR examination

must be stopped immediately and an investigation conducted to ensure patient safety.

6) As a precautionary measure, a cold compress (e.g., wet washcloth) may be applied to the tattoo site during the MR procedure.

In addition to the above, information and recommendations have been provided for patients by the United States Food and Drug Administration, Center for Food Safety and Applied Nutrition, Office of Cosmetics and Colors Fact Sheet, as follows: "... the risks of avoiding an MRI when your doctor has recommended one are likely to be much greater than the risks of complications from an interaction between the MRI and tattoo or permanent makeup. Instead of avoiding an MRI, individuals who have tattoos or permanent makeup should inform the radiologist or technician of this fact in order to take appropriate precautions, avoid complications, and assure the best results."

REFERENCES

Becker H. The use of intradermal tattoo to enhance the final result of nipple-areola reconstruction. Plast Reconstr Surg 1986;77:673.

Carr JJ. Danger in performing MR imaging on women who have tattooed eyeliner or similar types of permanent cosmetic injections. AJR Am J Roentgenol 1995;165:1546-1547.

DeBoer S, et al. Body piercing/tattooing and trauma diagnostic imaging: medical myths vs realities. J Trauma Nurs. 2007;14:35-8.

Gomey M. Tattoo pigments, patient clothing, and magnetic resonance imaging. Risk Management Bulletin #12748-8/95, The Doctors' Company, Napa, CA. August, 1995.

Halder RM, et al. Micropigmentation for the treatment of vitiligo. J Dermatol Surg Oncol 1989;15:1092-1098.

Jackson JG, Acker H. Permanent eyeliner and MR imaging. (letter) AJR Am J Roentgenol 1987;149:1080.

Kanal E, Barkovich AJ, et al. ACR guidance document for safe MR practices: 2007. AJR Am J Roentgenol. 2007;188:1447-1474.

Kanal E, Shellock FG. MRI interaction with tattoo pigments. (letter) Plast Reconstr Surg 1998;101:1150-1151.

Klitscher D, et al. MRT-induced burns in tattooed patients. Case report of a traumatic surgery patient. Unfallchirurg 2005;108:410-414.

Kreidstein ML, et al. MRI interaction with tattoo pigments: case report, pathophysiology, and management. Plast Reconstr Surg 1997;99:1717-1720.

Laumann AE, Derick AJ. Tattoos and body piercings in the United States: a national data set. J Am Acad Dermatol. 2006;55:413-21.

Lund A, et al. Tattooing of eyelids: magnetic resonance imaging artifacts. Ophthalmic Surg 1986;17:550-553.

Morishita Y, et al. Influence of mechanical effect due to MRI-magnet on tattoo seal and eye makeup. Nippon Hoshasen Gijutsu Gakkai Zasshi. 2008;64:587-90.

Offret H, et al. Permanent cosmetics and magnetic resonance imaging. J Fr Ophtalmol. 2009;32:131.e1-3.

Sacco D, et al. Artifacts caused by cosmetics in MR imaging of the head. Am J Roentgenol 1987;148:1001-1004.

Shellock FG. Magnetic Resonance Procedures: Health Effects and Safety, CRC Press, LLC, Boca Raton, FL, 2001.

Tattoos. FDA Medical Bulletin 1994;24:8.

Tope WD, Shellock FG. Magnetic resonance imaging and permanent cosmetics (tattoos): survey of complications and adverse events. J Magn Reson Imaging 2002;15:180-184.

Vahlensieck M. Tattoo-related cutaneous inflammation (burn grade I) in a mid-field MR scanner. (letter) Eur Radiol 2000;10:97.

Wagle WA, Smith M. Tattoo-induced skin burn during MR imaging. (letter) Am J Roentgenol 2000: 174:1795.

Weiss RA, et al. Mascara and eye-lining tattoos: MRI artifacts. Ann Ophthalmology 1989;21:129-131.

Terminology for Implants and Devices

MRI Labeling Information for Implants and Devices: Explanation of Terminology*

Summary Statement. This Editorial presents the recommendations from the Food and Drug Administration for MR safety terminology and labeling for medical devices and provides an explanation of how this information is applied.

The magnetic resonance (MR) environment may pose risks or problems to patients with certain implants and other medical devices primarily due to factors that include electromagnetic field interactions, MRI-related heating, and the creation of artifacts (1-5). In addition, for electrically-activated implants and other medical devices, there are concerns that the MR system may affect the operation of the medical device and/or to induce currents in the device (1-3, 5). With the growing use of MRI in the 1990s, the Food and Drug Administration (FDA) recognized the need for standardized tests to address MRI safety issues for implants and other medical devices (4, 6). Thus, over the years, test methods have been developed by various organizations including the American Society for Testing and Materials (ASTM) International (formerly the American Society for Testing and Materials), with an ongoing commitment to ensure patient safety in the MR environment (7-10).

The FDA is responsible for reviewing the MR terminology and labeling that manufacturers provide to their devices. The MR terminology, as it pertains to performing MR examinations in patients with implants and other medical devices, has continued to evolve to keep pace with advances in MRI technology (4, 6, 11). Unfortunately, members of the MRI community frequently do not always understand the terms that are used and are often confused by the conditions that are specified in "MR Conditional" labeling. This lack of understanding may result in patients with implants being exposed to potentially hazardous MRI conditions or in inappropriately preventing them from undergoing needed MRI examinations. Importantly, there is now new labeling terminology, which is associated with expanded labeling information. Therefore, the goal of this <u>Editorial</u> is to present background information about the terms used for MRI labeling of implants and other medical devices, to define the current terms, and to illustrate the use of the new labeling by providing a sample label with a detailed explanation of how the terminology is used.

Prior Terminology

In 1997, the FDA's Center for Devices and Radiological Health (CDRH) first proposed terms to be used to label MRI information for medical devices, which was presented in the draft document, "A Primer on Medical Device Interactions with Magnetic Resonance Imaging Systems (6). These terms were defined, as follows (6):

MR Safe: This term indicates that the device, when used in the MR environment, has been demonstrated to present no additional risk to the patient, but may affect the quality of the diagnostic information.

MR Compatible: This term indicates that the device, when used in the MR environment, is MR Safe and has been demonstrated to neither significantly affect the quality of the diagnostic information nor have its operations affected by the MR device."

This document further stated that, "The use of the terms, "MR Compatible" and "MR Safe" without specification of the MR environment in which the device was tested should be avoided since interpretation of these claims may vary and are difficult to substantiate rigorously. Statements such as "intended for use in the MR environment" or similar claims along with appropriate qualifying information are preferred (i.e. test conditions should be specifically stated)(6)." Here, the term "MR environment" encompasses the static, gradient (time-varying), and RF electromagnetic fields that may impact an implant or device.

Using this terminology, MRI testing of an implant or device for "MR safety" involved *in vitro* assessments of static magnetic field interactions, MRI-related heating, and, in some cases, induced electrical currents (i.e., from gradient magnetic fields), while "MR compatibility" testing required all of these as well as characterization of artifacts. In addition, it may have been necessary to evaluate the effect of various MRI conditions on the functional or operational aspects of an implant or device (2, 3, 4, 6, 7-10).

Revised Terminology

In time, it became apparent that the terms, "MR Safe" and "MR Compatible" were confusing and often used interchangeably or incorrectly (2-4, 11, 12). In particular, the terms were sometimes used without including the list of conditions for which the device had been demonstrated to be safe, in some cases inappropriately giving the impression that the device is "safe" or "compatible" in all MR environments. Therefore, in an effort to develop more appropriate terminology and, more importantly, because the misuse of these terms could result in serious accidents for patients and others in the MR environment, the MR Task Group of ASTM International Committee F04 on Medical and Surgical Materials and Devices developed standard ASTM F2503 which includes a new set of MR labeling terms with associated icons (4). The new terms defined in ASTM F2503 (released in August 2005) and currently recognized by the FDA are (11, 13), as follows:

MR Safe - an item that poses no known hazards in all MRI environments. Using the terminology, "MR Safe" items are non-conducting, non-metallic, and non-magnetic items such as a plastic Petri dish. An item may be determined to be MR Safe by providing a scientifically based rationale rather than test data.

MR Conditional - an item that has been demonstrated to pose no known hazards in a specified MR environment with specified conditions of use. "Field" conditions that define the MR environment include static magnetic field strength, spatial gradient, dB/dt (time rate of change of the magnetic field), radio frequency (RF) fields, and specific absorption rate (SAR). Additional conditions, including specific configurations of the item (e.g., the routing of leads used for a neurostimulation system), may be required.

For MR Conditional items, the item labeling includes results of testing sufficient to characterize the behavior of the item in the MR environment. In particular, testing for items that may be placed in the MR environment should address magnetically induced displacement force and torque, and RF heating. Other possible safety issues include but are not limited to, thermal injury, induced currents/voltages, electromagnetic compatibility, neurostimulation, acoustic noise, interaction among devices, and the safe functioning of the item and the safe operation of the MR system. Any parameter that affects the safety of the item should be listed and any condition that is known to produce an unsafe condition must be described.

MR Unsafe - an item that is known to pose hazards in all MRI environments. MR Unsafe items include magnetic items such as a pair of ferromagnetic scissors.

Associated Icons. In addition to the terms, MR Safe, MR Conditional, and MR Unsafe, the ASTM International MR marking standard introduced corresponding icons, consistent with international standards for colors and shapes of safety signs (13). These icons are intended for use on items that may be brought into or near the MR environment as well as in product labeling for implants and other medical devices. The icons may be reproduced in color or in black and white, however, the use of color is encouraged because of the added visibility (13).

The "MR Safe" icon consists of the letters 'MR' in green in a white square with a green border, or the letters 'MR' in white within a green square. The "MR Conditional" icon consists of the letters 'MR' in black inside a yellow triangle with a black border. The "MR Unsafe" icon consists of the letters 'MR' in black on a white field inside a red circle with a diagonal red band. Importantly, for "MR Conditional" items, the item's labeling must include the parameters and results used for testing that are sufficient to characterize the behavior of the item in the MRI environment (13).

Further details and a comprehensive discussion of the labeling applied to passive implants are presented in the recent FDA document, "Guidance for Industry and FDA Staff - Establishing Safety and Compatibility of Passive Implants in the Magnetic Resonance (MR) Environment" (11).

Use of Terminology: Reasons for Confusion

Because of the variety of MR systems and MR conditions in clinical use today (e.g., ranging from 0.2- to 9.4-Tesla), the current terminology is intended help elucidate labeling matters for medical devices and other items that may be used in the MR environment to ensure the safe use of MRI technology. However, it should be noted that this updated terminology has not been applied *retrospectively* to the many implants and devices that previously received FDA approved labeling using the terms "MR Safe" or "MR Compatible" (in general, this applies to those objects tested prior to the release of the ASTM International standard for labeling, around August 2005).

Therefore, this important point must be understood to avoid undue confusion regarding the matter of the labeling that has been applied to previously tested implants (i.e., labeled as "MR safe" or "MR Compatible") versus those that have recently undergone MRI testing (i.e., now labeled as "MR Conditional")(2, 3).

The labeling for medical devices that were **appropriately** labeled using the historical definitions for MR Safe or MR Compatible, **including the list of conditions** for which the device has been determined to be safe or compatible, is still accurate. Indeed, part of the confusion that exists on this matter is due to the use coexistence of the newer terminology with the prior labeling terminology.

In order to eliminate this ongoing confusion, in 2005 FDA recognized the new set of terms in ASTM F2503 and asks manufacturers to use them for all new products. When manufacturers make a submission to FDA for an existing device, FDA requests the manufacturers of these previously approved devices update their labeling to use the new MR safety terminology. Labeling information for implants and other medical devices has been compiled and is available in published and on-line formats (2, 14). Specific testing and labeling for active implants (e.g., those involving electronics) is currently being developed by an ISO (International Standards Organization) – IEC (International Electrotechnical Commission) joint working group.

MR Conditional Labeling Information: Explanation of the Content

In addition to the frequent problems associated with understanding the MRI labeling, the actual content of the label is often misunderstood with respect to the conditions indicated for a given implant that is labeled "MR Conditional". Therefore, the following is an example of "MR Conditional" labeling for an implant, *Example Implant*, along with an explanation of the content, provided for each aspect of the label (1-4, 11, 13) (**Table 1**):

MRI Information

Non-clinical testing has demonstrated the Example Implant is MR Conditional. It can be scanned safely under the following conditions:

-Static magnetic field of 3-Tesla

This is the static magnetic field for which the implant gave acceptable test results, generally the largest static magnetic field used for testing the implant. In some cases the labeling will state, "Static magnetic field of 3-Tesla or less" or "Static magnetic field of 3-Tesla, *only*" or *"static magnetic field of 1.5-Tesla or 3-Tesla."* Therefore, carefully reading and implementing this portion of the labeling for the implant is advised in order to avoid possible injuries to patients.

-Spatial gradient magnetic field of 720-Gauss/cm or less.

This is a frequently misinterpreted parameter because the MRI user sees the term "gradient field" and presumes that it refers to the time-varying or gradient fields used during MR imaging. However, the term, "**spatial** gradient magnetic field" for medical device labeling relates to the rate at which the static magnetic field strength changes over space per unit length (thus, indicated as dB/dx or, in this case, as 720-Gauss/cm for this example). Notably, the point of the highest spatial magnetic gradient is the position where translational attraction (i.e., determined using the deflection angle method) is typically assessed for an implant or device, according to ASTM F2052 - 06e1. The MR system manufacturer is able to provide spatial gradient magnetic field information for a particular MR system or it may determined using a Gauss meter.

-Maximum MR system reported, whole body averaged specific absorption rate (SAR) of 2-W/kg for 15-minutes of scanning.

Confusion commonly exists with respect to this stated parameter insofar as the term "scanning" is presumed to apply to the entire MRI procedure when, in fact, it applies to only each particular pulse *sequence* that is used and, of course, multiple sequences are utilized when performing the MRI examination. Therefore, to adequately safeguard the patient, the whole body averaged SAR for each scan sequence must be maintained at or below 2-W/kg for each scan sequence.

-In non-clinical testing, the Example Implant produced a temperature rise of less than 2.0°C at a maximum MR system reported, whole body averaged specific absorption rate (SAR) of 2- W/kg for 15 minutes of MR scanning in a (static magnetic field strength _____) (model _____) (MR system manufacturer _____) (software version _____) MR scanner.

The labeling for the implant has additional information with respect to the temperature rise that is associated with certain MRI parameters, that is based on the findings obtained in the MRI-related heating test. Therefore, as seen in this example, the expected "worst case" temperature rise is 2.0 degrees C or less during MRI performed at a whole body averaged SAR of 2-W/kg for 15-min., using a particular MR system type (i.e., with the make, model, and software of the scanner indicated). The MR system reported, whole body averaged SAR of 2-W/kg is the level specified in the ASTM F2182 - 02a and is the level commonly reported in device labeling, although higher or lower SAR levels may also be indicated. (It should be noted that, in this labeling section, certain labels for implants and other medical devices may state that this information applies to the use of a particular type of transmit RF coil that should be used, such as a transmit body or transmit head RF coil.)

Image Artifact
MR image quality may be compromised if the area of interest is in the same area or relatively close to the position of the device. Therefore, it may be necessary to optimize MR imaging parameters for the presence of this implant.

This is a common statement for many different implants and devices. Since the size of the artifact for an implant or device may impact the diagnostic use of MR imaging, information is typically provided in the label that characterizes the size and shape of the artifacts associated with certain pulse sequences (e.g., T1-weighted spin echo and gradient echo), according to ASTM F2119 - 07 or an equivalent method. For devices with a lumen (e.g., stent), the labeling may indicate whether the lumen is obscured by the size of the artifact.

The FDA also recommends that the patient register the conditions under which their MR Conditional implant can be scanned safely with the MedicAlert Foundation or other equivalent organization, and so the device labeling may include contact information for MedicAlert (11).

Table 1. Example of MRI labeling information for a medical implant or device.

MRI Information

Non-clinical testing has demonstrated the <u>Example Implant</u> is MR Conditional. It can be scanned safely under the following conditions:

- Static magnetic field of 3-Tesla.
- Spatial gradient magnetic field of 720-Gauss/cm or less.
- Maximum MR system reported, whole body averaged specific absorption rate (SAR) of 2-W/kg for 15-minutes of scanning.
- In non-clinical testing, the <u>Example Implant</u> produced a temperature rise of less than 2.0°C at a maximum MR system reported, whole body averaged specific absorption rate (SAR) of 2- W/kg for 15 minutes of MR scanning in a (static magnetic field strength _____) (model _____) (MR system manufacturer _____) (software version _____) MR scanner.

Image Artifact

MR image quality may be compromised if the area of interest is in the same area or relatively close to the position of the device. Therefore, it may be necessary to optimize MR imaging parameters for the presence of this implant.

Summary and Conclusions

This Editorial presents current FDA recommendations for MR safety terminology and labeling for implants and other medical devices and provides an explanation of how this information may be applied. Notably, the specific content of the MR labeling may take other forms (especially for electrically active implants and devices) as the format continues to be refined by the FDA in an ongoing effort to properly communicate this information to ensure patient safety.

REFERENCES

(1) Shellock FG, Crues JV. MR procedures: biologic effects, safety, and patient care. Radiology, 2004; 232:635-652.

(2) Shellock FG. Reference Manual for Magnetic Resonance Safety Implants and Device: 2009 Edition. Biomedical Research Publishing Group, Los Angeles, CA, 2009.

(3) Shellock FG, Spinazzi A. MRI Safety Update: 2008, Part 2, Screening patients for MRI. American Journal of Roentgenology 2008;191:12-21.

(4) Woods TO. Standards for medical devices in MRI: present and future. J Magn Reson Imaging. 2007; 26:1186-9.

(5) Levine GN, Gomes AS, Arai AE, Bluemke DA, Flamm SD, Kanal E, Manning WJ, Martin ET, Smith JM, Wilke N, Shellock FG. Safety of magnetic resonance imaging in patients with cardiovascular devices: an American Heart Association Scientific Statement from the Committee on Diagnostic and Interventional Cardiac Catheterization. Circulation 2007; 116:2878-2891.

(6) United States Food and Drug Administration, Center for Devices and Radiological Health, A Primer on Medical Device Interactions with Magnetic Resonance Imaging Systems. http://www.fda.gov/cdrh/ode/primerf6.html, 1997.

(7) American Society for Testing and Materials (ASTM) International, Designation: ASTM F2052 - 06e1, Standard Test Method for Measurement of Magnetically Induced Displacement Force on Medical Devices in the Magnetic Resonance Environment. ASTM International, West Conshohocken, PA.

(8) American Society for Testing and Materials (ASTM) International, Designation: ASTM F2213-06, Standard Test Method for Measurement of Magnetically Induced Torque on Medical Devices in the Magnetic Resonance Environment. ASTM International, West Conshohocken, PA.

(9) American Society for Testing and Materials (ASTM) International, Designation: ASTM F2119 – 07, Standard Test Method for Evaluation of MR Image Artifacts from Passive Implants. ASTM International, West Conshohocken, PA.

(10) American Society for Testing and Materials (ASTM) International, Designation: ASTM F2182 - 02a, Standard Test Method for Measurement of Radio Frequency Induced Heating Near Passive Implants During Magnetic Resonance Imaging. ASTM International, West Conshohocken, PA.

(11) Guidance for Industry and FDA Staff - Establishing Safety and Compatibility of Passive Implants in the Magnetic Resonance (MR) Environment. Document issued on: August 21, 2008; http://www.fda.gov/cdrh/osel/guidance/1685.html

(12) Shellock FG, Crues JV. Commentary: MR safety and the American College of Radiology White Paper. American Journal of Roentgenology 2002; 178:1349-1352.

(13) American Society for Testing and Materials (ASTM) International, Designation: F2503-08, Standard Practice for Marking Medical Devices and Other Items for Safety in the Magnetic Resonance Environment. ASTM International, West Conshohocken, PA.

(14) http://www.mrisafety.com/ accessed June, 2009.

[*Portions of this content were excerpted with permission from Shellock FG, Woods TO, Crues JV. MRI Labeling Information for Implants and Devices: Explanation of Terminology. Radiology 2009;253:26-30. The full-length article may be downloaded from www.IMRSER.org]

SECTION II

MR Procedures and Implants, Devices, and Materials

General Information

Magnetic resonance (MR) procedures may be contraindicated for patients primarily because of risks associated with movement or dislodgment of a ferromagnetic biomedical implant, material, or device. There are other possible hazards and problems related to the presence of a metallic object that include induction of currents (e.g., in materials that are conductors), excessive heating, changes in the operational aspects of the device, and the difficulty in interpretation or the misinterpretation of an imaging artifact as an abnormality.

Induced Electrical Currents. The potential for MR procedures to injure patients by inducing electrical currents in conductive materials or devices such as gating leads, indwelling catheters with metallic components (e.g., thermodilution catheters), guide wires, pacemaker leads, neurostimulation system leads, disconnected or broken surface coils, external fixation devices, cervical fixation devices, cochlear implants, infusion pumps, or improperly used physiologic monitors has been previously reported. Recommendations have been presented to protect patients from injuries related to induced currents that may develop during MR procedures.

Heating. Temperature increases produced in association with MR procedures have been studied using *ex vivo* techniques to evaluate various metallic implants, devices, and objects with a variety of sizes, shapes, and metallic compositions. In general, reports have indicated that only minor temperature changes occur in association with MR procedures involving relatively small metallic objects that are "passive" implants (i.e., those that are not electronically-activated), including implants such as aneurysm clips, hemostatic clips, prosthetic heart valves, vascular access ports, and similar devices. Therefore, heat generated during an MR procedure involving a patient with a "small" metallic "passive" implant does not appear to be a substantial hazard. In fact, to date, there has been no report of a patient being seriously injured as a result of excessive heat that developed in a relatively small passive metallic implant or device.

However, MRI-related heating is potentially problematic for implants that have an elongated shape or those that form a conducting loop of a certain diameter. For example, substantial heating can occur under some MR conditions for objects that form resonant conducting loops or for elongated implants (e.g., leads, wires, etc.) that form resonant antennae.

Artifacts. The type and extent of artifacts caused by the presence of metallic implants, materials, and devices have been described and tend to be easily recognized on MR images. Artifacts and image distortion associated with metallic objects are predominantly caused by a disruption of the local magnetic field that perturbs the relationship between position and frequency. Additionally, artifacts associated with metallic objects may be caused by gradient switching due to the generation of eddy currents.

The relative amount of artifact seen on an MR image is dependent on the magnetic susceptibility, quantity, shape, orientation, and position of the object in the body as well as the technique used for imaging (i.e., the specific pulse sequence parameters) and the image processing method. An artifact caused by the presence of a metallic object in a patient during MR imaging is seen typically as a signal void or loss and may include a local or regional distortion of the image. In some cases, there may be areas of high signal intensity seen along the edge of a signal void or when there is an abrupt change in the shape (e.g., the tip of a biopsy needle).

Magnetic Field Interactions. Numerous studies have assessed magnetic field interactions for implants and othe items by measuring translational attraction, torque or other interactions associated with the static magnetic fields of MR systems. These investigations demonstrated that, for certain implants, MR procedures may be performed safely in patients with metallic objects that are nonferromagnetic or "weakly" ferromagnetic (i.e., only minimally attracted by the magnetic field in relation to its *in vivo* application), such that the associated magnetic field interactions are insufficient to move or dislodge them, *in situ*. Furthermore, the "intended *in vivo* use" of the implant or device must be taken into consideration, because this can impact whether or not a given object is safe for a patient undergoing an MR procedure. Notably, sufficient counter-forces may exist to retain even a ferromagnetic implant, *in situ*.

In general, each implant or other item (particularly those made from unknown materials) should be evaluated using *ex vivo* techniques before allowing an individual or patient with the object to enter the MR environment and/or before performing the MR procedure. By following this guideline, the magnetic susceptibility for an object may be determined so that a competent decision can be made concerning possible risks associated with exposure to the MR system. Because movement or dislodgment of an implanted metallic object in a patient undergoing an MR procedure is the primary mechanism responsible for an injury, this aspect of testing is considered to be of utmost importance and should involve the use of an MR system operating at an appropriate static magnetic field strength. As previously mentioned, it may also be necessary to assess MRI-related heating for the implant or device.

Various factors influence the risk of performing an MR procedure in a patient with a metallic object including the strength of the static magnetic field, the magnetic susceptibility of the object, the mass of the object, the geometry of the object, the location and orientation of the object *in situ*, the presence of retentive mechanisms (i.e., fibrotic tissue, sutures, etc.) and the length of time the object has been implanted. These factors should be carefully considered before subjecting a patient or individual with a ferromagnetic object to an MR procedure or allowing entrance to the MR environment. This is particularly important if the object is located in a potentially dangerous area of the body such as a vital neural, vascular, of soft tissue structure where movement or dislodgment could injure the patient.

Furthermore, in certain cases, there is a possibility of changing the operational or functional aspects of the implant or device as a result of exposure to the electromagnetic fields of the MR system. Therefore, this important aspect must be evaluated using comprehensive testing techniques to verify that specific MR conditions will not impact the operation of the device.

Patients with certain implants or devices that have relatively strong ferromagnetic qualities may be safely scanned using MR procedures because the objects are held in place by sufficient retentive forces that prevent them from being moved or dislodged with reference to the "intended *in vivo* use" of an implant or device. For example, there is an interference screw (i.e., the Perfix Interference Screw) used for reconstruction of the anterior cruciate ligament that is highly ferromagnetic. However, once this implant is screwed into the patient's bone, this prevents it from being moved, even if the patient is exposed to a 1.5-Tesla MR system. Other implants that exhibit substantial ferromagnetic qualities may likewise be safe for patients undergoing MR procedures under highly specific conditions as a result of the presence of counter-forces that prevent movement of these objects.

MR systems with very low (0.2-Tesla or less) or very high (9.4-Tesla) static magnetic fields are currently used for clinical and research applications. Considering that most metallic objects evaluated for magnetic field interactions were assessed at 1.5-Tesla, an appropriate variance or modification of the information provided regarding the safety of performing an MR procedure in a patient with a metallic object may exist when an MR system with a lower or higher static magnetic field strength is used. That is, it may be acceptable to adjust safety recommendations depending on the static magnetic field strength and other aspects of a given MR system. Obviously, performing an MR procedure using a 0.2-Tesla MR system has different risk implications for a patient with a ferromagnetic object compared with using a 9.4-Tesla MR system.

Information Pertaining to Implants, Materials, Devices and Objects. The information contained in this textbook is a compilation of the current data available relative to the assessment of magnetic field interactions, MRI-related heating, and other tests conducted on implants, materials, and devices and is based primarily on published reports in the peer-reviewed literature. This compilation also includes unpublished data acquired from *ex vivo* testing performed on implants and devices using standardized or well-accepted techniques. Furthermore, MRI-related information obtained from manufacturers (e.g., the *Product Insert* or *Instructions for Use* information) is provided for various implants and devices.

Although every attempt was made to provide comprehensive and accurate information, there are many other implants, materials, devices, and objects that remain to be evaluated with regard to the MR environment. In addition, new or updated information may exist for a given implant, especially those that are electronically-activated, since the procedures used to assess these devices continues to evolve. Therefore, to ensure the safety of an individual or patient in the MR environment or undergoing an MR procedure, MR healthcare professionals should follow the guideline whereby MR examinations should only be performed in a patient with a metallic object that has been previously tested and demonstrated to be safe. A similar guideline should be followed with regard to whether or not to allow an individual with an implant or device to enter the MR environment. Finally, for electronically-activated implants, the most current safety guidelines must be obtained and followed. Therefore, the MR healthcare professional is advised to confirm the latest MRI labeling information with the respective manufacturer prior to performing an MRI examination on the patient.

Terminology Applied to Implants and Devices

To ensure proper understanding of the terminology applied to implants and devices, please review the following section in this textbook:

- **Terminology for Implants and Devices**

REFERENCES

American Society for Testing and Materials (ASTM) International, Designation: F2503. Standard Practice for Marking Medical Devices and Other Items for Safety in the Magnetic Resonance Environment. ASTM International, West Conshohocken, PA.

American Society for Testing and Materials (ASTM) International, Designation: F 2052. Standard test method for measurement of magnetically induced displacement force on passive implants in the magnetic resonance environment. ASTM International, West Conshohocken, PA.

Arena L, Morehouse HT, Safir J. MR imaging artifacts that simulate disease: how to recognize and eliminate them. Radiographics 1995;15:1373-1394.

Calcagnini G, et al. In vitro investigation of pacemaker lead heating induced by magnetic resonance imaging: role of implant geometry. J Magn Reson Imaging. 2008;28:879-86.

Davis PL, et al. Potential hazards in NMR imaging: heating effects of changing magnetic fields and RF fields on small metallic implants. AJR Am J Roentgenol 1981;137:857-860.

Dempsey MF, Condon B, Hadley DM. Investigation of the factors responsible for burns during MRI. J Magn Reson Imaging 2001;13:627-631.

Diaz F, Tweardy L, Shellock FG. Cervical fixation devices: MRI issues at 3-Tesla. Spine 2010;35:411-5.

Graf H, Steidle G, Martirosian P, Lauer UA, Schick F. Metal artifacts caused by gradient switching. Magnetic Resonance in Medicine 2005;54:231-234.

Hargreaves BA, et al. Metal-induced artifacts in MRI. AJR Am J Roentgenol. 2011;197:547-55.

Kanal E, Barkovich AJ, et al. ACR guidance document for safe MR practices: 2007. AJR Am J Roentgenol. 2007;188:1447-1474.

Kainz W. MR heating tests of MR critical implants. J Magn Reson Imaging. 2007;26:450-1.

Knott PT, et al. A comparison of magnetic and radiographic imaging artifact after using three types of metal rods: stainless steel, titanium, and vitallium. Spine J. 2010;10:789-94.

Koch KM, et al. Magnetic resonance imaging near metal implants. J Magn Reson Imaging. 2010;32:773-87.

Levine GN, Gomes AS, Arai AE, Bluemke DA, Flamm SD, Kanal E, Manning WJ, Martin ET, Smith JM, Wilke N, Shellock FG. Safety of magnetic resonance imaging in patients with cardiovascular devices: an American Heart Association scientific statement from the Committee on Diagnostic and Interventional Cardiac Catheterization. Circulation 2007;116:2878-2891.

Masaki F, et al. Iatrogenic second-degree burn caused by a catheter encased tubular braid of stainless steel during MRI. Burns. 2007;33:1077-9.

Mattei E, et al. Temperature and SAR measurement errors in the evaluation of metallic linear structures heating during MRI using fluoroptic probes. Phys Med Biol. 2007;52:1633-46.

Muranaka H, et al. Evaluation of RF heating due to various implants during MR procedure. Magn Reson Med Sci. 2011;10:11-9.

Neufeld E, et al. Measurement, simulation and uncertainty assessment of implant heating during MRI. Phys Med Biol. 2009;54:4151-69.

Nordbeck P, et al. Spatial distribution of RF-induced E-fields and implant heating in MRI. Magn Reson Med. 2008;60:312-9.

Nordbeck P, et al. Measuring RF-induced currents inside implants: Impact of device configuration on MRI safety of cardiac pacemaker leads. Magn Reson Med. 2009;61:570-8.

Nordbeck P, et al. Impact of imaging landmark on the risk of MRI-related heating near implanted medical devices like cardiac pacemaker leads. Magn Reson Med. 2011;65:44-50.

Nyenhuis JA, et al. Heating near implanted medical devices by the MRI RF-magnetic field. IEEE Trans Magn 1999;35:4133-4135.

Nyenhuis JA, Park SM, Kamondetdacha R, Amjad A, Shellock FG, Rezai A. MRI and implanted medical devices: basic interactions with an emphasis on heating. IEEE Transactions on Device and Materials Reliability 2005;5:467-478.

Rezai AR, Baker K, Tkach J, Phillips M, Hrdlicka G, Sharan A, Nyenhuis J, Ruggieri P, Henderson J, Shellock FG. Is magnetic resonance imaging safe for patients with neurostimulation systems used for deep brain stimulation (DBS)? Neurosurgery 2005;57:1056-1062.

Roguin A, et al. Magnetic resonance imaging in individuals with cardiovascular implantable electronic devices. Europace. 2008;10:336-46.

Schenck JF. Chapter 1, Health Effects and Safety of Static Magnetic Fields. In: Magnetic Resonance Procedures: Health Effects and Safety. CRC Press, LLC, Boca Raton, FL, 2001; pp. 1-31.

Shellock FG. Magnetic Resonance Procedures: Health Effects and Safety. CRC Press, LLC, Boca Raton, FL, 2001.

Shellock FG. Guest Editorial. Comments on MRI heating tests of critical implants. Journal of Magnetic Resonance Imaging 2007;26:1182-1185.

Shellock FG. Excessive temperature increases in pacemaker leads at 3-T MR imaging with a transmit-received head coil. Radiology 2009;251:948-949.

Shellock FG. Biomedical implants and devices: assessment of magnetic field interactions with a 3.0-Tesla MR system. J Magn Reson Imaging 2002;16:721-732.

Shellock FG. MR safety update 2002: Implants and devices. J Magn Reson Imaging 2002;16:485-496.

Shellock FG. Surgical instruments for interventional MRI procedures: assessment of MR safety. J Magn Reson Imaging 2001;13:152-157.

Shellock FG, Crues JV. High-field strength MR imaging and metallic biomedical implants: an *ex vivo* evaluation of deflection forces. AJR Am J Roentgenol 1988;151:389-392.

Shellock FG, Crues JV. MR procedures: biologic effects, safety, and patient care. Radiology, 2004;232:635-652.

Shellock FG, Kanal E, Gilk T. Regarding the value reported for the term "spatial gradient magnetic field" and how this information is applied to labeling of medical implants and devices. American Journal of Roentgenology, 2011;196:142-145..

Shellock FG, Kanal E. Magnetic Resonance: Bioeffects, Safety, and Patient Management. Second Edition, Lippincott-Raven Press, New York, 1996.

Shellock FG, et al. MRI and orthopedic implants used for anterior cruciate ligament reconstruction: assessment of ferromagnetism and artifacts. J Magn Reson Imaging 1992;2:225-228.

Shellock FG, Spinazzi A. MRI Safety Update: 2008, Part 2, Screening patients for MRI. American Journal of Roentgenology 2008;191:12-21.

Shellock FG, et al. Aneurysm clips: evaluation of magnetic field interactions and translational attraction using "long-bore" and "short-bore" 3.0-Tesla MR systems. Am J Neuroradiology 2003;24:463-471.

Shellock FG, Tkach JA, Ruggieri PM, Masaryk TJ. Cardiac pacemakers, ICDs, and loop recorder: Evaluation of translational attraction using conventional ("long-bore") and "short-bore" 1.5- and 3.0-Tesla MR systems. Journal of Cardiovascular Magnetic Resonance 2003;5:387-397.

Shellock FG, Woods TO, Crues JV. MRI Labeling information for implants and devices: explanation of terminology. Radiology 2009;253:26-30.

Shinbane J, Colletti P, Shellock FG. MR in patients with pacemakers and ICDs: Defining the Issues. Journal of Cardiovascular Magnetic Resonance 2007;9:5-13.

Smith CD, et al. Interactions of MRI magnetic fields with elongated medical implants. J Appl Physics 2000; 87:6188-6190.

Smith CD, et al. Chapter 16. Health effects of induced electrical currents: Implications for implants. In: Magnetic resonance: Health Effects and Safety, FG Shellock, Editor, CRC Press, Boca Raton, FL, 2001; pp. 393-413.

Stradiotti P, et al. Metal-related artifacts in instrumented spine. Techniques for reducing artifacts in CT and MRI: state of the art. Eur Spine J. 2009;18 Suppl 1:102-8.

Woods TO. Guidance for Industry and FDA Staff - Establishing Safety and Compatibility of Passive Implants in the Magnetic Resonance (MR) Environment. 2008; http://www.fda.gov/cdrh/osel/guidance/1685.html

Woods TO. Standards for medical devices in MRI: present and future. J Magn Reson Imaging. 2007;26:1186-9.

Yang CW, Liu L, et al. Magnetic resonance imaging of artificial lumbar disks: safety and metal artifacts. Chin Med J (Engl). 2009;20;122:911-6.

Zanchi MG, et al. An optically coupled system for quantitative monitoring of MRI-induced RF currents into long conductors. IEEE Trans Med Imag. 2010;29:169-78.

3-Tesla MR Safety Information for Implants and Devices

Because previous investigations performed to evaluate MR safety issues for implants and devices used mostly scanners with static magnetic fields of 1.5-Tesla or less, it is crucial to perform *ex vivo* testing at 3-Tesla to determine possible risks for these objects with respect to magnetic field interactions and heating. Importantly, a metallic object that displayed "weakly" ferromagnetic qualities at 1.5-Tesla may exhibit substantial magnetic field interactions at 3-Tesla.

Furthermore, for elongated devices or those that form a loop of a certain diameter, the effects of MRI-related heating may be substantially different. Evidence from an *ex vivo* study conducted by Shellock et al. (2005) reported that significantly *less* MRI-related heating occurred at 3-Tesla/128-MHz (MR system reported, whole body averaged SAR, 3-W/kg) versus 1.5-Tesla/64-MHz (MR system reported, whole body averaged SAR, 1.4-W/kg) for a pacemaker lead not connected to a pulse generator (same lead length, positioning, etc.). This phenomenon, whereby less heating was observed at 3-Tesla/128-MHz vs. 1.5-Tesla/64-MHz, has also been observed for external fixation devices, Foley catheters with temperature sensors, neurostimulation systems, relatively long peripheral vascular stents, and other objects (Unpublished Observations, F.G. Shellock, 2011). Therefore, it is crucial to conduct *ex vivo* testing to assess magnetic field interactions and, for certain devices, MRI-related heating to identify potentially hazardous objects prior to subjecting individuals to the MR environment or patients to an MR examination at 3-Tesla.

Magnetic Field Interactions at 3-Tesla. From a magnetic field interaction consideration, translational attraction and/or torque may cause movement or dislodgment of a ferromagnetic implant resulting in an uncomfortable sensation or injury. Translational attraction is dependent on the strength of the static magnetic field, the spatial gradient magnetic field, the mass of the object, the shape of the object, and its magnetic susceptibility. The effects of translational attraction on external and implanted ferromagnetic objects are predominantly responsible for serious hazards in the immediate area of the MR system. That is, as one moves closer to the MR system or is moved into the scanner for an examination. An evaluation of torque is also important for a metallic object, especially if it has an elongated configuration. Qualitative and quantitative techniques have been used to determine magnetic field-related torque for implants and devices.

From a practical consideration, in addition to the findings for translational attraction and torque, the "intended *in vivo* use" of the implant or device must be considered as well as mechanisms that may provide retention of the object *in situ* (e.g., implants or devices held in place by sutures, granulation or ingrowth of tissue, fixation devices, or by other means) with regard to potential risks for the metallic object (for further information on this topic, please refer to the prior section in this textbook, **General Information**).

Long-Bore vs. Short-Bore 3-Tesla MR Systems. Different magnet designs exist for commercially available 3-Tesla MR systems, including configurations that are conventional "long-bore" scanners and "short-bore" systems. Because of physical differences in the position and magnitude of the highest spatial gradient magnetic fields for different magnets, measurements of deflection angles for implants using long-bore vs. short-bore MR systems can produce substantially different results for deflection angle measurements (i.e., translational attraction), as reported by Shellock et al. Studies conducted using 3-Tesla MR systems indicated that, in general, there were significantly ($p<0.01$) higher deflection angles measured for implants using short-bore vs. the long-bore MR systems. The differences in deflection angle measurements for the metallic objects were related to differences in the highest spatial gradient magnetic fields for short-bore vs. long-bore scanners.

The safety implications are primarily for magnetic field-related translational attraction with respect to short-bore vs. long-bore 3-Tesla MR systems. For example, the deflection angle measured for an implant on a short-bore can be substantially higher (and thus, potentially unsafe from a magnetic field interaction consideration) compared to the deflection angle measured on a long-bore MR system. Therefore, safety information for measurements of magnetic field interactions for metallic objects must be considered with regard to the specific type of MR system used for the evaluation or, more accurately, with respect to the level of the highest spatial gradient magnetic field that was used for the test.

Heating of Implants and Devices at 3-Tesla. *Ex vivo* testing has been used to evaluate MRI-related heating for various metallic implants, materials, devices, and objects of a variety of sizes, shapes, and metallic compositions. In general, reports have indicated that only minor temperature changes occur in association with MR procedures involving metallic objects that are relatively small passive implants (e.g., those that are not electronically-activated). Therefore, heat generated during an MR procedure performed at 3-Tesla on a patient with a relatively small, passive metallic implant does not appear to be a substantial hazard.

However, because excessive heating and burns have occurred in implants and devices that have elongated configurations or that form conducting loops of certain diameter, patients with these objects should not undergo MR procedures at 3-Tesla until *ex vivo* heating assessments are performed to determine the relative risks. *Ex vivo* investigations have demonstrated that excessive heating may occur for certain implants related to MRI performed at 3-Tesla under certain operating conditions.

REFERENCES

American Society for Testing and Materials (ASTM) International Designation: F 2052. Standard test method for measurement of magnetically induced displacement force on passive implants in the magnetic resonance environment. West Conshohocken, PA..

Bottomley PA, Kumar A, et al. Designing passive MRI-safe implantable conducting leads with electrodes. Med Phys 2010;37:3828-43.

Davis P L, et al. Potential hazards in NMR imaging: heating effects of changing magnetic fields and RF fields on small metallic implants. AJR Am J Roentgenol 1981;137:857-860.

Dempsey MF, Condon B, Hadley DM. Investigation of the factors responsible for burns during MRI. J Magn Reson Imaging 2001;13:627-631.

Diaz F, Tweardy L, Shellock FG. Cervical fixation devices: MRI issues at 3-Tesla. Spine 2010;35:411-5.

Edwards M-B, et al. Mechanical testing of human cardiac tissue: some implications for MRI safety. J Cardiovasc Magn Resonance 2005;7:835-840.

Gimbel JR. Magnetic resonance imaging of implantable cardiac rhythm devices at 3-Tesla. Pacing Clin Electrophysiol. 2008;31:795-801.

Hennemeyer CT, et al. In vitro evaluation of platinum Guglielmi detachable coils at 3-T with a porcine model: safety issues and artifacts. Radiology 2001;219:732-737.

Kakizawa Y, et al. Cerebral aneurysm clips in the 3-tesla magnetic field. Laboratory investigation. J Neurosurg. 2010;113:859-69.

Martin AD, et al. Safety evaluation of titanium middle ear prostheses at 3-Tesla. Otolaryngol Head Neck Surg 2005;132:537-42.

Medtronic Heart Valves, Medtronic, Inc., Minneapolis, MN, Permission to publish 3-Tesla MR testing information for Medtronic Heart Valves provided by Kathryn M. Bayer, Senior Technical Consultant, Medtronic Heart Valves, Technical Service.

Nyehnuis JA, et al. Heating near implanted medical devices by the MRI RF-magnetic field. IEEE Trans Magn 1999;35:4133-4135.

Schenck JF. Chapter 1, Health Effects and Safety of Static Magnetic Fields. In: Magnetic Resonance Procedures: Health Effects and Safety. CRC Press, LLC, Boca Raton, FL, 2001; pp. 1-31.

Shellock FG. Radiofrequency-induced heating during MR procedures: A review. J Magn Reson Imaging 2000;12:30-36.

Shellock FG. MR safety update 2002: Implants and devices. J Magn Reson Imaging 2002;16:485-496.

Shellock FG. Biomedical implants and devices: assessment of magnetic field interactions with a 3.0-Tesla MR system. J Magn Reson Imaging 2002;16:721-732.

Shellock FG. Begnaud J, Inman DM. VNS Therapy System: *In vitro* evaluation of MRI-related heating and function at 1.5- and 3-Tesla. Neuromodulation 2006;9:204-213.

Shellock FG. Forder J. Drug eluting coronary stent: *In vitro* evaluation of magnetic resonance safety at 3-Tesla. Journal of Cardiovascular Magnetic Resonance 2005;7:415-419.

Shellock FG, Woods TO, Crues JV. MRI labeling information for implants and devices: Explanation of terminology. Radiology 2009;253:26-30.

Shellock FG, Kanal E, Gilk T. Regarding the value reported for the term "spatial gradient magnetic field" and how this information is applied to labeling of medical implants and devices. American Journal of Roentgenology 2011;196:142-145.

Shellock FG, Gounis M, Wakhloo A. Detachable coil for cerebral aneurysms: *In vitro* evaluation of magnet field interactions, heating, and artifacts at 3-Tesla. American Journal of Neuroradiology 2005;26:363-366.

Shellock FG, Habibi R, Knebel J. Programmable CSF shunt valve: *In vitro* assessment of MRI safety at 3-Tesla. American Journal of Neuroradiology 2006;27:661-665.

Shellock FG, Wilson SF, Mauge CP. Magnetically programmable shunt valve: MRI at 3-Tesla. Magnetic Resonance Imaging 2007;25:1116-21.

Shellock FG, et al. Cardiac pacemakers, ICDs, and loop recorder: Evaluation of translational attraction using conventional ("long-bore") and "short-bore" 1.5- and 3.0-Tesla MR systems. Journal of Cardiovascular Magnetic Resonance 2003;5:387-397.

Shellock FG, et al. Aneurysm clips: evaluation of magnetic field interactions and translational attraction using "long-bore" and "short-bore" 3.0-Tesla MR systems. American Journal of Neuroradiology 2003;24:463-471.

Shellock FG, Valencerina S. Septal repair implants: evaluation of MRI safety at 3-Tesla. Magnetic Resonance Imaging 2005;23:1021-1025.

Shellock FG, Valencerina S, Fischer L. MRI-related heating of pacemaker at 1.5- and 3-Tesla: Evaluation with and without pulse generator attached to leads. Circulation 2005;112;Supplement II:561.

Shellock FG. Valencerina S. In vitro evaluation of MR imaging issues at 3-T for aneurysm clips made from MP35N: Findings and information applied to 155 additional aneurysm clips. AJNR Am J Neuroradiol. 2010;31:615-619

Smith CD, et al. Interactions of MRI magnetic fields with elongated medical implants. J Appl Physics 2000;87:6188-6190.

Smith CD, et al. Chapter 16. Health effects of induced electrical currents: Implications for implants. In: Magnetic resonance: health effects and safety, FG Shellock, Editor, CRC Press, Boca Raton, FL, 2001; pp. 393-413.

Sommer T, et al. High field MR imaging: magnetic field interactions of aneurysm clips, coronary artery stents and iliac artery stents with a 3.0 Tesla MR system. Rofo Fortschr Geb Rontgenstr Neuen Bildgeb Verfahr 2004;176:731-8.

Woods TO. Standards for medical devices in MRI: present and future. J Magn Reson Imaging. 2007;26:1186-9.

Woods TO. Guidance for Industry and FDA Staff - Establishing Safety and Compatibility of Passive Implants in the Magnetic Resonance (MR) Environment. Document issued on: August 21, 2008; http://www.fda.gov/cdrh/osel/guidance/1685.html

AccuRx Constant Flow Implantable Pump and DuraCath Intraspinal Catheter

AccuRx Constant Flow Implantable Pump. The AccuRx Constant Flow Implantable Pump (Advanced Neuromodulation Systems, Plano, TX) is an implantable device that stores and dispenses medication at a constant factory-set flow rate to a specific site. The pumps are available in a range of flow rates to allow physicians to tailor therapy to the needs of the patient.

The AccuRx Constant Flow Implantable Pump consists of a single sealed chamber formed between a rigid titanium shell and a polymeric diaphragm. The chamber holds the drug to be infused. The diaphragm exerts pressure on the medication causing it to flow out of the chamber through a series of filters and a flow restrictor, and then out the catheter (see DuraCath Intraspinal Catheter information below) to the delivery site. The AccuRx Constant Flow Implantable Pump is refilled through a raised refill port in the center of the titanium shell. Refilling the pump expands the diaphragm outward and starts the pump on the next cycle of drug infusion.

DuraCath Intraspinal Catheter. The DuraCath Intraspinal Catheter (Advanced Neuromodulation Systems, Plano, TX) is designed for long-term intraspinal (epidural or intrathecal) implantation. The trimmable, flexible, elastic radiopaque catheter incorporates insertion depth markings and a removable guide wire to facilitate implantation. This catheter has a closed tip and multiple side-exit channels to facilitate dispersion of the drug to reduce the probability of catheter tip complications. There are one- and two-piece versions of the DuraCath Intraspinal Catheter to suite a variety of clinical needs. The DuraCath Intraspinal Catheter is made from silicone and has a small connector made from 316L stainless steel.

MAGNETIC RESONANCE IMAGING (MRI) INFORMATION

Exposure of the AccuRx Constant Flow Implantable Pump and DuraCath Intraspinal Catheter to magnetic resonance imaging (MRI) fields of 1.5-Tesla has demonstrated no impact on pump or catheter performance and a limited effect on the quality of the diagnostic information. Testing performed on the AccuRx Constant Flow Implantable Pump and DuraCath Intraspinal Catheter has established the following with regard to MRI safety and diagnostic issues:

Static Magnetic Field. Testing demonstrated that a 1.5-Tesla magnetic resonance environment produced no measurable magnetic field interactions (i.e., translational attraction and torque) for the AccuRx Constant Flow Implantable Pump and DuraCath Intraspinal Catheter.

Heating During MRI. Testing demonstrated that little heating occurred for the AccuRx Constant Flow Implantable Pump in association with MR imaging conducted using an excessive amount of RF energy (i.e., a whole-body averaged specific absorption rate of 1.5 W/kg). Furthermore, heating was considered to be physiologically inconsequential and will not pose an additional risk to the patient undergoing an MR procedure under the conditions used for the evaluation. In the unlikely event that the patient experiences warmth near the pump, the MR procedure should be stopped immediately.

Peripheral Nerve Stimulation. The presence of the AccuRx Constant Flow Implantable Pump may cause a one-fold increase (doubling) of the induced gradient current in tissues near the device. This increase in the induced gradient current is similar to that already present elsewhere in the body (e.g., at bone-tissue interfaces) and, as such, will not cause nerve stimulation. In the unlikely event that the patient reports stimulation during the scan, the MR procedure should be stopped immediately.

REFERENCE

AccuRX Constant Flow Implantable Pumps, Technical Manual, Advanced Neuromodulation Systems, Inc., Plano, TX.

ActiFlo Indwelling Bowel Catheter System

The ActiFlo Indwelling Bowel Catheter System (also known as the Zassi Bowel Management System, Hollister, Libertyville, IL) is intended for diversion of fecal matter to minimize external contact with the patient's skin, to facilitate the collection of fecal matter for patients requiring stool management, to provide access for colonic irrigation and to administer enema or medications. This system consists the catheter, the collection bag, and the irrigation bag. The ActiFlo Indwelling Bowel Catheter System allows stool to drain directly from the rectum into a closed or drainable collection bag.

MRI Information

The ActiFlo Indwelling Bowel Catheter System was determined to be MR conditional:

Non-clinical testing demonstrated that this product is MR Conditional according to the following conditions:

-Static magnetic field of 3-Tesla or less
-Highest spatial gradient magnetic field of 720-Gauss/cm or less

Important note: A metallic spring used for this device is located outside of the patient's body during the intended *in vivo* use of this product. Therefore, the only possible MRI-related issue pertains to magnetic field interactions. Heating and artifacts are of no concern. As such, the assessment of magnetic field interactions for this product specifically involved evaluations of translational attraction and torque in relation to exposure to a 3-Tesla MR system, *only.* Evaluations of MRI-related heating and artifacts were not conducted and are unnecessary.

REFERENCE

http://www.hollister.co.za/us/

ActiPatch

ActiPatch (BioElectronics, Frederick, MD) is a medical, drug-free device that delivers pulsed electromagnetic frequency therapies to accelerate healing of soft tissue injuries. The ActiPatch has an embedded battery-operated microchip that delivers continuous pulsed therapy to reduce pain and swelling.

MRI and the ActiPatch

The ActiPatch must be removed prior to performing an MRI procedure to prevent possible damage to this device and the potential risk of excessive heating.

REFERENCE

http://www.bielcorp.com

Alsius Intravascular Temperature Management

Alsius Corporation (a Zoll Corporation, Chelmsford, MA) products are designed for placement in the central venous system. Via a proprietary, "closed loop" internal cooling circuit, the catheter cools or warms the patient's blood as it circulates past the catheter. The catheters (Cool Line, Icy, and Fortius) are attached to the CoolGard 3000 Thermal Regulation System. This is an electronic cooling system that regulates the cooling performance of the catheter via remote sensing of the patient's temperature. Alsius catheters are also designed to facilitate critical care management with features similar to those found in conventional central venous catheters.

CoolGard 3000. All Alsius heat exchange catheters connect to the CoolGard 3000 Thermal Regulation System, which achieves and maintains a target temperature input by the user. It remotely senses changes in patient core temperature and automatically adjusts the temperature of the circulating saline within the catheter (0-42 degrees C), providing consistent maintenance of temperature.

Cool Line Catheter. The Cool Line Catheter is inserted into the subclavian or jugular vein and resides in the superior vena cava. The Cool Line Catheter combines temperature control and central venous catheter capabilities.

Icy Catheter. The Icy catheter is inserted into the femoral vein and resides in the inferior vena cava.

Fortius Catheter. The Fortius catheter is inserted percutaneously into the femoral vein residing in the inferior vena cava, just below the heart. The Fortius catheter provides maximum heat exchange power with minimum time to target temperature.

MRI Information

The following models of Alsius Heat Exchange catheters have been determined to be MR-safe:

1) Cool Line
2) Icy
3) Fortius

Magnetic resonance imaging (MRI) procedures must be performed according to the following guidelines:

Through non-clinical testing, these catheters were shown to be MR safe* at a field strength of 1.5 Tesla or less and a maximum whole body averaged specific absorption rate (SAR) of 2.0 W/kg for 20 minutes of MRI. MRI at 1.5-Tesla (highest spatial gradient magnetic field, 2.4 Tesla/meter) or less may be performed immediately following the insertion of the one of these catheters.

MR image quality may be compromised if the area of interest is in the exact same area or relatively close to the position of these catheters. Therefore, it may be necessary to optimize the MRI parameters for the presence of these metallic devices.

IMPORTANT NOTE: The Alsius CoolGard 3000 system is NOT MRI Safe NOR Compatible NOR Intended for Use in an MRI environment. The Catheter should be disconnected from the System prior to moving the patient to the MRI facility.

[*Note the use of the term "MR Safe". These products underwent testing and labeling prior to the implementation of the current terminology. For further explanation, please refer to the section in this textbook, entitled: **Terminology for Implants and Devices.**]

REFERENCES

http://www.alsius.com
http://www.zoll.com

Ambulatory Infusion Systems

Ambulatory Infusion Systems (Smiths Medical) are designed to help healthcare providers administer medications accurately, monitor patient's response to therapy, stimulate early clinical assessment and facilitate patient recovery. These devices include, the following:

CADD – 1 Ambulatory Infusion Pump
CADD – Legacy 1 Ambulatory Infusion Pump
CADD – Legacy Ambulatory Infusion Pump
CADD – Legacy PCA Ambulatory Infusion Pump
CADD – Legacy PLUS Ambulatory Infusion Pump
CADD – Micro Ambulatory Infusion Pump
CADD – MS 3 Ambulatory Infusion Pump
CADD – PCA Ambulatory Infusion Pump
CADD – PLUS Ambulatory Infusion Pump
CADD – Prizm PCS Ambulatory Infusion Pump
CADD – Prizm PCS II Ambulatory Infusion Pump
CADD – Prizm VIP Ambulatory Infusion Pump
CADD – Solis Ambulatory Infusion Pump
CADD – TPN Ambulatory Infusion Pump

MRI Information
Regarding the pump used for each device, the Operator's Manual states: "Magnetic fields produced by magnetic resonance imaging (MRI) equipment may adversely affect the operation of the pump. Remove the pump from the patient during MRI procedures and keep it at a safe distance from magnetic energy."

REFERENCE

http://www.smiths-medical.com/

Aneurysm Clips

The surgical management of intracranial aneurysms and arteriovenous malformations (AVMs) by the application of aneurysm clips is a well-established procedure. The presence of an aneurysm clip in a patient referred for an MR procedure represents a situation that requires the utmost consideration because of the associated risks.

Certain types of intracranial aneurysm clips (e.g., those made from martensitic stainless steels such as 17-7PH or 405 stainless steel) are a contraindication to the use of MR procedures because excessive, magnetically induced forces can displace these implants and cause serious injury or death. By comparison, aneurysm clips classified as "nonferromagnetic" or "weakly ferromagnetic" (e.g., those made from Phynox, Elgiloy, austentitic stainless steels, titanium alloy, or commercially pure titanium) are acceptable for patients undergoing MR examinations. Additional information on performing MR procedures in patients with aneurysm clips is provided in the section entitled, **Extremity MR System.**

[For the sake of discussion, the term "weakly magnetic" refers to metal that may demonstrate some extremely low ferromagnetic qualities using highly sensitive measurements techniques (e.g., vibrating sample magnetometer, superconducting quantum interference device or SQUID magnetometer, etc.) and as such, may not be technically referred to as being "nonmagnetic." All metals possess some degree of magnetism, such that no metal is entirely "nonmagnetic".]

MR procedures have been used to evaluate patients with certain types of aneurysm clips. Becker et al., using MR systems that ranged from 0.35 to 0.6-Tesla, studied three patients with nonferromagnetic aneurysm clips (one patient, Yasargil, 316 LVM stainless steel; two patients, Vari-Angle McFadden, MP35N; 316 LVM) and one patient with a ferromagnetic aneurysm clip (Heifetz aneurysm clip) without incident. Dujovny et al. similarly reported no adverse effects in patients with nonferromagnetic aneurysm clips that underwent procedures using 1.5-Tesla MR systems.

Pride et al. performed a study in patients with nonferromagnetic aneurysm clips that underwent MR imaging. There were no adverse outcomes for the patients, confirming that MR procedures can be performed safely in patients with nonferromagnetic clips. Brothers et al.

also demonstrated that MR imaging at 1.5-Tesla can be performed safely in patients with nonmagnetic aneurysm clips. This report was particularly important because, according to Brothers et al., MR imaging was found to be better than CT in the postoperative assessment of aneurysm patients, especially with regard to showing small zones of ischemia.

To date, only one ferromagnetic aneurysm clip-related fatality has been reported in the peer-reviewed literature. According to this report, the patient became symptomatic at a distance of approximately 1.2-meters from the bore of the MR system, suggesting that translational attraction of the aneurysm clip was likely responsible for dislodgment of this implant.

This incident was the result of erroneous information pertaining to the type of aneurysm clip that was present in the patient. That is, the clip was thought to be a nonmagnetic Yasargil aneurysm clip (Aesculap Inc., Central Valley, PA) and turned out to be a magnetic Vari-Angle clip (Codman & Shurtleff, Randolf, MA).

There has never been a report of an injury to a patient or individual in the MR environment related to the presence of an aneurysm clip made from a nonmagnetic or "weakly" magnetic material. In fact, there have been cases in which patients with ferromagnetic aneurysm clips (based on the extent of the artifact seen during MR imaging or other information) have undergone MR procedures without sustaining injuries (Personal communications, D. Kroker, 1995; E. Kanal, 1996; A. Osborne, 2002).

In these cases, the aneurysm clips were exposed to magnetic-induced translational attraction and torque associated with MR systems operating at 1.5-Tesla or less. Although these cases do not prove safety, they do demonstrate the difficulty of predicting the outcome for patients with ferromagnetic aneurysm clips that undergo MR procedures. Variables to consider include the size, shape (especially the length of the blade), mass, and material of the aneurysm clip.

There is controversy regarding the amount of ferromagnetism that needs to be present in an aneurysm clip to constitute a hazard for a patient in the MR environment. Consequently, this issue has not only created problems for MR healthcare professionals but for manufacturers of aneurysm clips, as well.

For example, MR healthcare professionals performing tests on aneurysm clips similar to the method described in the report by Kanal et al. (1996) identified the presence of magnetic field interactions and returned several clips made from Phynox to the manufacturer (Personal Communication, Aesculap, Inc., South San Francisco, CA, 1997). However, the testing method used by Kanal et al. (1996) was admittedly crude and developed to primarily obtain rapid, qualitative screening data for large numbers of aneurysm clips to determine if quantitative assessments were necessary. Importantly, the test technique used by Kanal et al. (1996) may be problematic and yield spurious results, especially if the aneurysm clip has a shape or configuration that is somewhat "unstable" (Unpublished Observations, F.G. Shellock, 1997). For example, aneurysm clips with blades that are bayonet, curved, or angled shapes are less stable on a piece of plate glass (i.e., using the testing method described by Kanal et al.) when placed in certain orientations compared with aneurysm clips with straight blades.

A variety of more appropriate testing techniques have been developed and utilized over the years to evaluate the relative amount of ferromagnetism present for implants and devices prior to allowing patients with these objects to enter the MR environment. In 2002, the American Society for Testing and Materials (ASTM) provided recommendations for testing passive implants that involves the use of the deflection angle test, originally described by New et al., to assess translational attraction. Additionally, the U.S. Food and Drug Administration recommends that an evaluation of torque should be performed on aneurysm clips. Thus, procedures such as the deflection angle test and some form of evaluation of torque (qualitative or quantitative) are the most appropriate means of determining which specific aneurysm clip may present a hazard to a patient or individual in the MR environment.

Aneurysm Clips and MRI Procedures: Guidelines. In consideration of the knowledge pertaining to aneurysm clips, the following guidelines are recommended with regard to performing an MR procedure in a patient or before allowing an individual with an aneurysm clip into the MR environment:

1) Specific information (i.e., manufacturer, type or model, material, lot and serial numbers) about the aneurysm clip must be known, especially with respect to the material used to make the aneurysm clip, so that only patients or individuals with nonferromagnetic or weakly ferromagnetic clips are allowed into the MR environment. The manufacturer provides this information in the labeling of the aneurysm clip. The implanting surgeon is responsible for properly recording and communicating this information in the patient's or individual's records.

2) An aneurysm clip that is in its original package and made from Phynox, Elgiloy, MP35N, titanium alloy, commercially pure titanium or other material known to be nonferromagnetic or weakly

ferromagnetic does not need to be evaluated for ferromagnetism. Aneurysm clips made from nonferrromagnetic or "weakly" ferromagnetic materials in original packages do not require testing of ferromagnetism because the manufacturers ensure the pertinent MR safety or conditional aspects of these clips and, therefore, are responsible for the accuracy of the labeling.

3) If the aneurysm clip is not in its original package and/or properly labeled, it should undergo testing for magnetic field interactions following appropriate testing procedures to determine if it is safe.

4) The radiologist and implanting surgeon are responsible for evaluating the information pertaining to the aneurysm clip, verifying its accuracy, obtaining written documentation, and deciding to perform the MR procedure after considering the risk vs. benefit aspects for a given patient.

5) Consideration must be give to the static magnetic field strength that is to be used for the MRI procedure and the strength of the static magnetic field used to test magnetic field interactions for the aneurysm clip in question.

MRI at 3-Tesla and Aneurysm Clips. Many aneurysm clips have been tested for magnetic field interactions in association with 3-Tesla MR systems (refer to **The List** for information for aneurysm clips tested at 3-Tesla). Findings for these specific implants indicated that they either exhibited no magnetic field interactions or relatively minor or "weak" magnetic field interactions. Accordingly, these particular aneurysm clips are considered acceptable for patients undergoing MR procedures using MR systems operating at 3-Tesla or less.

Yasargil Aneurysm Clips (Information dated 11/11/09 - Aesculap Inc., Center Valley, PA)

Aesculap currently markets two lines of YASARGIL aneurysm clips, one from a cobalt-chrome alloy ("Phynox") and one from a titanium alloy. Phynox clips have been available since 1983 and have catalog numbers that begin with "FE". Titanium clips have been available since 1997 and have catalog numbers that begin with "FT". All "FE" and "FT" model YASARGIL aneurysm clips are non-ferromagnetic and may be safely exposed to MRI. Both implant materials have been tested and proven MR-safe as per ASTM-2052-02 up to 3.0 Tesla*.

Prior to 1985, Aesculap distributed various models of aneurysm clips manufactured from stainless steel. These aneurysm clips were identified with the letters "FD" and have not been proven safe under exposure to MRI. For this reason, **Aesculap does not recommend the use of MRI**

on a patient implanted with a YASARGIL aneurysm clip identified with the letters "FD".

For additional information, please refer to the following three scientific publications:

1) Dujovny, M., et. al. (1985). *Aneurysm clip motion during magnetic resonance imaging: in vivo experimental study with metallurgical factor analysis, Journal of Neurosurgery,. 17(4), 543-548.*

2) *Shellock, F.G, Kanal, E.,. (1998). Aneurysm clips: evaluation of MR imaging artifacts at 1.5. Radiology, 209(2), 563-566.*

3) Romner, B., et. al. (1989). *Magnetic resonance imaging and aneurysm clips, Journal of Neurosurgery, 70(3), 426-431.*

*These Aesculap devices were cleared by FDA as "MR-Safe" per ASTM 2052-02. Due to a change in definition within this standard (F 2503 2005-08), these devices are now termed as "MR Conditional" by ASTM. The FDA has not mandated a revision to our labeling because the device material and performance have not changed.

Aneurysm Clips, Codman & Shurtleff, Inc., a Johnson & Johnson Company, Raynham, MA

Recently, three different MP35N aneurysm clips (Codman Slim-Line Aneurysm Clip, Straight, Blade length 25-mm; Codman Slim-Line Aneurysm Clip Graft, 5-mm Diameter X 5-mm width; Codman Slim-Line Aneurysm Clip, Reinforcing 30-degree angle, 6-mm X 18-mm; Codman & Shurtleff, Inc., a Johnson & Johnson Company, Raynham, MA) underwent MRI testing that represented the largest mass for 155 additional clips made from MP35N. The clips were evaluated at 3-Tesla for magnetic field interactions, heating, and artifacts. Each aneurysm clip showed relatively minor magnetic field interactions that will not cause movement *in situ*. Heating was not excessive (highest temperature change, < 1.8°C). Artifacts may create issues if the area of interest is in the same area or close to the aneurysm clip. The results of this investigation demonstrated that it would be acceptable (i.e., "MR conditional" using current terminology) for patients with these aneurysm clips to undergo MRI at 3-Tesla or less. Notably, in consideration of the sizes of the clips that underwent testing, these findings pertain to 155 additional aneurysm clips made from the same material including, the following:

Codman Slim-Line Aneurysm Clip
Codman AVM Micro Clip
Codman Slim-Line Aneurysm Clip Graft
Codman Slim-Line Mini Aneurysm Clip
Codman Slim-Line Temporary Vessel Aneurysm Clip

The following information is the MRI labeling for these aneurysm clips approved by the Food and Drug Administration:

Magnetic Resonance Imaging Information

Non-clinical testing of representative configurations of **Codman Slim-Line Aneurysm, Mini, Micro and Graft Clips** (Codman Slim-Line Clips) up to 25-mm in blade length has demonstrated that they are **MR Conditional.** A patient with one such clip up to 25-mm in blade length (i.e., Codman Slim-Line Aneurysm, Mini, Micro and Graft Clips (Codman Slim-Line Clips) can be scanned safely, immediately after placement under the following conditions.

3.0 Tesla Systems:

- Static magnetic field of 3.0 Tesla.
- Spatial gradient magnetic field of 720 Gauss/cm or less.
- Maximum MR system reported, whole-body-averaged specific absorption rate (SAR) of 3.0 W/kg for 15 minutes of scanning (i.e., per pulse sequence).

MRI Related Heating

MRI related heating was assessed for the representative configurations of the Codman clips (up to 25-mm in blade length) following guidelines provided in ASTM F2182. A maximum temperature change equal to or less than 1.8 ° C was observed during testing (parameters listed below).

Parameters:

- Maximum MR system-reported, whole-body-averaged SAR of 3.0 W/kg (associated calorimetry measured whole body averaged value of 2.8 W/kg).
- 15-minute duration MR scanning (i.e., per pulse sequence).
- 3 Tesla MR System (EXCITE MR Scanner, Software G3 .0-052B, General Electric Healthcare, Milwaukee, WI) using a transmit/receive RF body coil.

Artifact Information

Artifacts were assessed for representative clip configurations using T1-weighted spin echo (T1-SE) and gradient echo (GRE) pulse sequences following methods similar to the guidelines provided in ASTM F2119-07. The 25-mm blade-length aneurysm clip imaged using a GRE pulse sequence produced an artifact that extended approximately 5-cm from the clip in the parallel (long-axis) imaging plane. The void size corresponding to this artifact was approximately 1251-mm^2. MR image quality may be compromised if the area of interest is in the exact location or within a few centimeters of the Codman Slim-Line Clip. In general, the GRE pulse sequence produced larger artifacts than the T1-SE sequence for each clip. However, MRI artifacts can be minimized by careful selection of pulse sequence parameters.

MRI at 8.0-Tesla and Aneurysm Clips. *Ex vivo* testing has been conducted to identify potentially hazardous implants and devices using an 8-Tesla MR system. The first investigation of this type was conducted by Kangarlu and Shellock.

Twenty-six different aneurysm clips were tested for magnetic field interactions using previously-described techniques. These implants were specifically selected for this investigation because they represent various types of clips used for temporary or permanent treatment of aneurysms or arteriovenous malformations. Additionally, these aneurysm clips were reported to be safe for patients undergoing MR procedures using MR systems with static magnetic field strengths of 1.5-Tesla or less.

According to the results, six aneurysm clips (i.e., type, model, blade length) made from stainless steel alloy (Perneczky) and Phynox (Yasargil, Models FE 748 and FE 750) displayed deflection angles above 45 degrees (i.e., referring to the guideline stated by the American Society for Testing and Materials, ASTM) and relatively high qualitative torque values. These findings indicated that these specific aneurysm clips may be unsafe for individuals or patients in an 8.0-Tesla or higher MR environment.

Aneurysm clips made from commercially pure titanium (Spetzler), Elgiloy (Sugita), titanium alloy (Yasargil, Model FE 750T), and MP35N (Sundt) displayed deflection angles less than 45 degrees (i.e., referring to the ASTM guideline) and qualitative torque values that were relatively minor. Accordingly, these aneurysm clips are considered to be acceptable for patients or individuals exposed to an 8.0-Tesla MR system.

As previously indicated, at 1.5-Tesla, aneurysm clips that are considered to be acceptable for patients or others in the MR environment include those made from commercially pure titanium, titanium alloy, Elgiloy, Phynox, and austentic stainless steel. By comparison, findings from the 8.0-Tesla study indicated that deflection angles for the aneurysm clips made from commercially pure titanium and titanium alloy ranged from 5 to 6 degrees, suggesting that these aneurysm clips would be safe for patients or individuals in the 8.0-Tesla MR environment. However, deflection angles for aneurysm clips made from Elgiloy ranged from 36 to 42 degrees, such that further consideration must be given to the specific type of Elgiloy clip that is present. For example, an Elgiloy clip that has a greater mass (e.g., due to a longer blade length) than those tested in this study may exceed a deflection angle of 45 degrees (i.e., referring to the ASTM guideline of 45 degrees or less being acceptable for translational attraction) in association with an 8.0-Tesla MR system.

Depending on the actual dimensions and mass, an aneurysm clip made from Elgiloy may or may not be acceptable for a patient or individual in the 8.0-Tesla MR environment. Notably, the results of this investigation are specific to the types of intracranial aneurysm clips that underwent testing (i.e., with regard model, shape, size, blade length, material, etc.) as well as the spatial gradient magnetic field associated with the 8.0-Tesla MR system.

Effects of Long-Term and Multiple Exposures to the MR System. MR testing procedures used for aneurysm clips, if performed routinely prior to implantation, would result in the reintroduction of aneurysm clips into strong magnetic fields several times prior to use in the patient. Furthermore, there are patients with implanted aneurysm clips previously designated as "MR-safe" or "MR-conditional" that have undergone repeated exposures to strong magnetic fields during follow-up MR examinations.

A concern has emerged that a potential alteration in the magnetic properties of pre-or post-implanted aneurysm clips may occur due to long-term or multiple exposures to strong magnetic fields. Long-term or multiple exposures to strong magnetic fields (such as those associated with MR imaging systems) have been suggested to grossly "magnetize" aneurysm clips, even if they are made from nonferromagnetic or weakly ferromagnetic materials. This theoretical problem could present a substantial hazard to an individual in the MR environment. Therefore, an *in vitro* investigation was conducted by Kanal and Shellock to study intracranial aneurysm clips prior to and following long-term and multiple exposures to 1.5-Tesla MR systems. This was done to quantify possible alterations in the magnetic properties of these aneurysm clips.

Aneurysm clips made from Elgiloy, Phynox, titanium alloy, commercially pure titanium, and austenitic stainless steel were tested in association with long-term and multiple exposures to 1.5-Tesla MR systems. The findings indicated a lack of response to the magnetic field exposure conditions that were used, such that long-term or multiple exposures to 1.5-Tesla MR systems should not result in significant changes in their magnetic properties.

Artifacts Associated with Aneurysm Clips. An additional problem related to aneurysm clips is that artifacts produced by these metallic implants may substantially detract from the diagnostic aspects of MR procedures. MR imaging, MR angiography, and functional MRI are frequently used to evaluate the brain or cerebral vasculature of patients with aneurysm clips. For example, to reduce morbidity and mortality after subarachnoid hemorrhage, it is imperative to assess the results of the surgical treatment of cerebral aneurysms.

The extent of the artifact produced by an aneurysm clip will have a direct effect on the diagnostic aspects of the MR procedure. Therefore, an investigation was conducted to characterize artifacts associated with aneurysm clips made from nonferromagnetic or weakly ferromagnetic materials. Five different aneurysm clips made from five different materials were evaluated in this investigation, as follows:

1) Yasargil, Phynox (Aesculap, Inc., Central Valley, PA),
2) Yasargil, titanium alloy (Aesculap, Inc., Central Valley, PA),
3) Sugita, Elgiloy (Mizuho American, Inc., Beverly, MA),
4) Spetzler Titanium Aneurysm Clip, commercially pure titanium (Elekta Instruments, Inc., Atlanta, GA), and
5) Perneczky, cobalt alloy (Zepplin Chirurgishe Instrumente, Pullach, Germany).

These aneurysm clips were selected for testing because they are made from nonferromagnetic or weakly ferromagnetic materials. These aneurysm clips were previously reported to be acceptable for patients in the 1.5-Tesla MR environment and, as such, are often found in patients referred for MR procedures.

Artifact testing revealed that the size of the signal voids were directly related to the type of material (i.e., the magnetic susceptibility) used to make the particular clip. Arranged in decreasing order of artifact size, the materials responsible for the artifacts associated with the aneurysm clips were, as follows: Elgiloy (Sugita), cobalt alloy (Perneczky), Phynox (Yasargil), titanium alloy (Yasargil), and commercially pure titanium (Spetzler). These results have implications when one considers the various critical factors that are responsible for the decision to use a particular type of aneurysm clip (e.g., size, shape, closing force, biocompatibility, corrosion resistance, material-related effects on diagnostic imaging examinations, etc.).

An aneurysm clip that causes a relatively large artifact is less desirable because it can impact the diagnostic capabilities of the MR procedure if the area of interest is in the immediate location of where the aneurysm clip was implanted. Fortunately, aneurysm clips exist that are made from materials (i.e., commercially pure titanium and titanium alloy) that created minimal artifacts.

Burtscher et al. conducted additional artifact research with the intent of determining the extent to which titanium aneurysm clips could improve the quality of MR imaging compared to stainless steel aneurysm clips and to assess whether the artifacts could be reduced by controlling MR imaging parameters. The results indicated that the use of titanium aneurysm clips reduced MR artifacts by approximately 60% compared to stainless steel aneurysm clips. MR imaging artifacts were further reduced by using spin echo pulse sequences with high bandwidths or, if necessary, gradient echo pulse sequences with a low echo times (TE).

REFERENCES

American Society for Testing and Materials (ASTM) Designation: F 2052. Standard test method for measurement of magnetically induced displacement force on passive implants in the magnetic resonance environment. ASTM, West Conshohocken, PA.

Becker RL, Norfray JF, Teitelbaum GP, et al. MR imaging in patients with intracranial aneurysm clips. Am J Roentgenol 1988;9:885-889.

Brothers MF, et al. MR imaging after surgery for vertebrobasilar aneurysm. Am J Neuroradiol 1990;11:149-161.

Brown MA, Carden JA, Coleman RE, et al. Magnetic field effects on surgical ligation clips. Magn Reson Imaging 1987;5:443-453.

Burtscher IM, et al. Aneurysm clip MR artifacts. Titanium versus stainless steel and influence of imaging parameters. Acta Radiology 1998;39:70-76.

Dujovny M, et al. Aneurysm clip motion during magnetic resonance imaging: *in vivo* experimental study with metallurgical factor analysis. Neurosurgery 1985;17:543-548.

FDA stresses the need for caution during MR scanning of patients with aneurysm clips. In: Medical Devices Bulletin, Center for Devices and Radiological Health. March, 1993;11:1-2.

Johnson GC. Need for caution during MR imaging of patients with aneurysm clips [Letter]. Radiology 1993;188:287.

Kakizawa Y, et al. Cerebral aneurysm clips in the 3-tesla magnetic field. Laboratory investigation. J Neurosurg. 2010;113:859-69.

Kanal E, Barkovich AJ, Bell C, et al. ACR guidance document for safe MR practices: 2007. AJR Am J Roentgenol. 2007;188:1447-1474.

Kanal E, Shellock FG. MR imaging of patients with intracranial aneurysm clips. Radiology 1993;187:612-614.

Kanal E, Shellock FG. Aneurysm clips: effects of long-term and multiple exposures to a 1.5-Tesla MR system. Radiology 1999;210:563-565.

Kanal E, Shellock FG, Lewin JS. Aneurysm clip testing for ferromagnetic properties: clip variability issues. Radiology 1996;200:576-578.

Kangarlu A, Shellock FG. Aneurysm clips: evaluation of magnetic field interactions with an 8.0-T MR system. J Magn Reson Imaging 2000;12:107-111.

Klucznik RP, et al. Placement of a ferromagnetic intracerebral aneurysm clip in a magnetic field with a fatal outcome. Radiology 1993;187:855-856.

Lauer UA, et al. Radio frequency versus susceptibility effects of small conductive implants-a systematic MRI study on aneurysm clips at 1.5 and 3 T. Magn Reson Imaging 2005;23:563-9.

New PFJ, et al. Potential hazards and artifacts of ferromagnetic and nonferromagnetic surgical and dental materials and devices in nuclear magnetic resonance imaging. Radiology 1983;147:139-148.

Olsrud J, et al. Magnetic resonance imaging artifacts caused by aneurysm clips and shunt valves: dependence on field strength (1.5 and 3 T) and imaging parameters. J Magn Reson Imaging 2005;22:433-7.

Pride GL, et al. Safety of MR scanning in patients with nonferromagnetic aneurysm clips. J Magn Reson Imaging 2000;12:198-200.

Shellock FG. Magnetic Resonance Procedures: Health Effects and Safety. CRC Press, LLC, Boca Raton, FL, 2001.

Shellock FG. Biomedical implants and devices: assessment of magnetic field interactions with a 3.0-Tesla MR system. J Magn Reson Imaging 2002;16:721-732.

Shellock FG, et al. Aneurysm clips: evaluation of magnetic field interactions and translational attraction using "long-bore" and "short-bore" 3.0-Tesla MR systems. American Journal of Neuroradiology 2003;24:463-471.

Shellock FG, Crues JV. High-field strength MR imaging and metallic biomedical implants: an *ex vivo* evaluation of deflection forces. Am J Roentgenol 1988;151:389-392.

Shellock FG, Crues JV. Aneurysm clips: Assessment of magnetic field interaction associated with a 0.2-T extremity MR system. Radiology 1998;208:407-409.

Shellock FG, Kanal E. Aneurysm clips: Evaluation of MR imaging artifacts at 1.5-Tesla. Radiology 1998;209:563-566.

Shellock FG, Kanal E. Magnetic Resonance: Bioeffects, Safety, and Patient Management. Second Edition, Lippincott-Raven Press, New York, 1996.

Shellock FG, Kanal E. Yasargil aneurysm clips: evaluation of interactions with a 1.5-Tesla MR system. Radiology 1998;207:587-591.

Shellock FG, Shellock VJ. MR-compatibility evaluation of the Spetzler titanium aneurysm clip. Radiology 1998;206:838-841.

Shellock FG. Valencerina S. In vitro evaluation of MR imaging issues at 3-T for aneurysm clips made from MP35N: Findings and information applied to 155 additional aneurysm clips. AJNR Am J Neuroradiol. 2010;31:615-619

Baha, Bone Conduction Implant

What is Baha?

The Baha System (Cochlear Americas, Englewood, Colorado) utilizes the body's natural ability to conduct sound. Bone, like air, conducts sound vibrations. For people with hearing loss, this provides another pathway to perceive sound.

Typical hearing aids rely on air conduction and a functioning middle ear. In cases where the middle ear function may be blocked, damaged or occluded, the Baha system may be a better option as it bypasses the middle ear altogether. Instead, sound is sent around the damaged or problematic area, naturally stimulating the cochlea through bone conduction. Once the cochlea receives these sound vibrations, the organ 'hears' in the same manner as through air conduction; the sound is converted into neural signals and is transferred to the brain, allowing a Baha recipient to perceive sound.

How does it work?

We receive sound in two ways, by air conduction via the ear canal, eardrum, and ossicles, and by bone conduction. Bone conduction transmits sound directly though the bones in the jaw and skull, bypassing the outer and middle ear.

In most cases, those with a hearing loss will be fitted with traditional air conduction devices. Typically, these hearing aids are placed inside the ear canal or behind the ear. However, some people are unable to benefit from this type of device.

The Baha system, which is based on bone conduction, utilizes a titanium implant, which is placed in the skull bone behind the ear. An abutment connects the sound processor with the implant in the bone. This creates direct (percutaneous) bone conduction. In contrast, traditional bone conductors connect indirectly to the bone through unbroken skin (transcutaneous) and work by exerting pressure against the skull.

Direct bone conduction, provided by Baha, gives improved access to sound when compared to traditional bone conductors since sound is not weakened when passing through the skin. This unique hearing treatment is the only system of its kind cleared by the U.S. Food and Drug Administration (FDA) to treat hearing loss.

One reason the Baha system works so well is due to its simple design. The Baha system combines a sound processor with an abutment and a small titanium implant. The implant is placed behind the non-functioning ear. Surgery is minor, and Baha recipients report a wide range of advantages over other hearing devices.

MRI INFORMATION

Can I wear the sound processor if I have to undergo an MRI?

The sound processor should be removed prior to undergoing an MRI, but the titanium implant will not pose any risk. Cochlear (Cochlear Americas, Englewood, Colorado) provides wearers with MRI and security check information card.

MRI (Magnetic Resonance Imaging)
If you are to undergo an MRI (Magnetic Resonance Imaging), remove the sound processor prior to the procedure. The implant and abutment remain in place.

[MR healthcare professionals are advised to contact the respective manufacturer in order to obtain the latest safety information to ensure patient safety relative to the use of an MR procedure.]

REFERENCES

http://www.cochlearamericas.com/

http://products.cochlearamericas.com/baha

http://products.cochlearamericas.com/support/baha/mri-other-medical-questions

Biopsy Needles, Markers, and Devices

Magnetic resonance (MR) imaging has been used to guide tissue biopsy and apply markers for many years. These specialized procedures require tools that are acceptable for use with MR systems. Many commercially available biopsy needles, markers, and devices (i.e., guidewires, stylets, marking wires, marking clips, biopsy guns, etc.) have undergone MRI evaluations with respect to safety issues and artifacts. The results indicated that most of the commercially available tools are not useful for MR-guided biopsy procedures due to the presence of excessive ferromagnetism and the associated artifacts that may limit or obscure the area of interest. Fortunately, several needles, markers, and devices have been developed using materials with low magnetic susceptibility specifically for utilization in MR-guided procedures.

Although most of the biopsy guns tested for magnetic field interactions and artifacts were found to be ferromagnetic, since these are not used in the immediate area of the target tissue, artifacts associated with these devices are unlikely to affect the resulting images during MR-guided biopsy procedures. Nevertheless, the presence of ferromagnetism may preclude the optimal use of most biopsy guns in the MR environment, especially at 3-Tesla. Currently, there are several commercially available biopsy devices, including vacuum-assisted systems, that have been developed specifically for use in MR-guided procedures.

REFERENCES

Causer PA, Piron CA, Jong RA, et al. MR imaging-guided breast localization system with medial or lateral access. Radiology. 2006;240:369-79.

Chen X, et al. MRI-guided breast biopsy: clinical experience with 14-gauge stainless steel core biopsy needle. AJR Am J Roentgenol. 2004;182:1075-80.

Daniel BL, et al. An MRI-compatible semiautomated vacuum-assisted breast biopsy system: initial feasibility study. J Magn Reson Imaging. 2005;21:637-44.

Hall WA, Galicich W, Bergman T, Truwit CL. 3-Tesla intraoperative MR imaging for neurosurgery. J Neurooncol. 2006;77:297-303.

Lehman CD, et al. MR imaging-guided breast biopsy using a coaxial technique with a 14-gauge stainless steel core biopsy needle and a titanium sheath. AJR Am J Roentgenol. 2003;181:183-5.

Lewin JS, et al. Needle localization in MR-guided biopsy and aspiration: Effect of field strength, sequence design, and magnetic field orientation. AJR Am J Roentgenol 1996;166:1337-1341.

Lufkin R, Layfield L. Coaxial needle system of MR- and CT-guided aspiration cytology. J Computer Assist Tomogr 1989;13:1105-1107.

Lufkin R, Teresi L, Hanafee W. New needle for MR-guided aspiration cytology of the head and neck. AJR Am J Roentgenol 1987;149:380-382.

Moscatel M, Shellock FG, Morisoli S. Biopsy needles and devices: assessment of ferromagnetism and artifacts during exposure to a 1.5-Tesla MR system. J Magn Reson Imaging 1995;5:369-372.

Shellock FG. Magnetic Resonance Procedures: Health Effects and Safety. CRC Press, LLC, Boca Raton, FL, 2001.

Shellock FG, Kanal E. Magnetic Resonance: Bioeffects, Safety, and Patient Management. Second Edition, Lippincott-Raven Press, New York, 1996.

Shellock FG, Shellock VJ. Additional information pertaining to the MR-compatibility of biopsy needles and devices. J Magn Reson Imaging 1996;6:411.

Shellock FG, Shellock VJ. Metallic marking clips used after stereotactic breast biopsy: *ex vivo* testing of ferromagnetism, heating, and artifacts associated with MRI. AJR Am J Roentgenol 1999;172:1417-1419.

Thomas C, Wojtczyk H, et al. Carbon fibre and nitinol needles for MRI-guided interventions: First in vitro and in vivo application. Eur J Radiol. 2010 [Epub ahead of print]

Veltman J, Boetes C, Wobbes T, Blickman JG, Barentsz JO. Magnetic resonance-guided biopsies and localizations of the breast: initial experiences using an open breast coil and compatible intervention device. Invest Radiol. 2005;40:379-84.

Zangos S, Herzog C, Eichler K, et al. MR-compatible assistance system for punction in a high-field system: device and feasibility of transgluteal biopsies of the prostate gland. Eur Radiol. 2007;17:1118-24.

Bone Fusion Stimulator/Spinal Fusion Stimulator

The implantable bone fusion or spinal fusion stimulator (EBI, LLC, Biomet, Inc.) is designed for use as an adjunct therapy to a spinal fusion procedure. The implantable spinal fusion stimulator consists of a direct current generator with a lithium iodine battery and solid-state electronics encased in a titanium shell, partially-coated with platinum that acts as an anode. The generator is implanted beneath the skin and muscle near the vertebral column and provides the full-rated current for approximately 24 to 26 weeks. The use of this electronic implant provides a faster consolidation of the bone grafts, leading to higher fusion rates and improved surgical outcomes, along with a reduced need for orthopedic instrumentation.

Studies using relatively high electromagnetic fields under specific experimental conditions and modeling scenarios for the lumbar/torso area (i.e., 1.5-Tesla MR system, excessive exposures to RF fields, excessive exposures to gradient magnetic fields, etc.) demonstrated that the implantable spinal fusion stimulator will not present a hazard to a patient undergoing MR imaging with respect to movement, heating, or induced electrical fields during the use of conventional MR techniques associated with 1.5-Tesla/64-MHz.

Additionally, there was no evidence of malfunction of the implantable spinal fusion stimulator based on *in vitro* and *in vivo* experimental findings. These studies addressed the use of conventional pulse sequences and parameters with an acknowledgement that other imaging parameters will have different implications and consequences for the patient with an implantable spinal fusion stimulator.

To date, MR examinations have been performed in many patients (conceivably, using MR imaging conditions that involved a wide-variety of imaging parameters and conditions) with implantable spinal fusion stimulators with no reports of substantial adverse events (based on a review of data obtained through the Freedom of Information Act and Unpublished Observations, Simon BJ, EBI, LLC, Parsippany, NJ).

In a clinical study, there were no reports of immediate or delayed (minimum of one month follow up) adverse events from patients with implantable spinal fusion stimulators who underwent MR imaging at 1.5-Tesla. Each patient was visually inspected following the MRI study and there was no evidence of excessive heating.

One patient indicated a sensation of "warming" felt at the site of the stimulator, however, this feeling was described as minor and the MR examination was completed without further indication of unusual sensations or problems. Of further note is that there were no reports of excessive heating or neuromuscular stimulation in association with the presence of implantable spinal fusion stimulators in patients that underwent MR procedures.

Chou et al. conducted an investigation of the effect of heating of the implantable spinal fusion stimulator associated with MR imaging. This work was performed using a human phantom during MR procedures involving whole body averaged specific absorption rates of approximately 1.0-W/kg. Fluoroptic thermometry probes were placed at various positions on and near the cathodes, leads, and the stimulator for each experiment to record temperature changes.

The phantom used by Chou et al. did not include the effects of blood flow, which obviously would help dissipate heating that may occur during MR imaging and, therefore, it further represents an excessive RF exposure condition. With the implantable spinal fusion stimulator in place and the leads intact, the maximum temperature rise after 25 minutes of scanning occurred at the center of the stimulator and was less than 2 degrees C.

The temperature rise at the cathodes was less than 1 degree C. When the stimulator was removed, the maximum temperature rise was less than 1.5 degrees C, recorded at the tip of the electrode with insignificant temperature changes occurring at the cathode. These temperature changes are within physiologically acceptable ranges for the tissues where the implantable spinal fusion stimulator is implanted, especially considering that the temperatures for muscle and subcutaneous tissues are at levels that are known to be several degrees below the normal core temperature of 37 degrees C.

Chou et al. also investigated heating of the tips of broken leads of the implantable spinal fusion stimulator (this device was the same as that which underwent testing in the present study). Temperature changes occurred in localized regions that were within a few millimeters of the cut ends of the leads, with maximum temperature increases that ranged from 11 to 14 degrees C.

If these levels of temperatures occurred during MR imaging, the amount of possible tissue damage would be comparable in characteristics and clinical significance to a small electrosurgical lesion and would likely occur in the scar tissue that typically forms around the implanted leads. Additionally, the potential for tissue damage is only theoretical and a brief temperature elevation around a broken lead over an approximated volume of 2- to 3-mm radius may not be clinically worse than the scar tissue that forms over the leads during implantation. Fortunately, broken leads are rare, occurring in approximately 10 out of the 70,000 devices implanted over the last ten years (Personal Communication, Simon BJ, EBI, LLC, Parsippany, NJ).

Based on findings from the various investigations that have been conducted, RF energy-induced heating during MR imaging does not appear to present a major problem for a patient with the implantable spinal fusion stimulator, as long as there is no broken lead. Accordingly, the integrity of the leads should be assessed using a radiograph prior to the MR procedure.

MRI Safety Information - SpF-XL IIb
SpF-XL IIb Model

Safety information for the use of Magnetic Resonance Imaging (MRI) procedures (i.e., imaging, angiography, functional imaging, spectroscopy, etc.) pertains to shielded MRI systems with static magnetic fields of 1.5 Tesla or less (maximum spatial gradient 450 gauss/cm), gradient magnetic fields of 20 Tesla/second or less, and a maximum whole body averaged Specific Absorption Rate (SAR) of 1.1 W/kg for 25 minutes of imaging. The effects of MRI procedures using MR systems and conditions above these levels have not been determined.

The **SpF** devices have been determined to be MR safe, thereby (when used in the MRI environment) there is no additional risk to the patient, but may affect image quality. MRI procedures must only be performed according to the following guidelines:

- Plain films (radiographs) must be obtained to assess the site of the implanted **SpF** prior to the MRI examination to verify that there are no broken leads present.
- If this cannot be reliably determined, then the potential risks and benefits to the patient requiring the MRI examination must be

carefully assessed in consideration of the possibility of excessive heating to develop in the leads.

- The patient must be continuously observed during the MRI procedure and instructed to report any unusual sensations including any feelings of warming, burning, or neuromuscular excitation or stimulation.
- If these occur, the MRI procedure must be discontinued.

Static Magnetic Field of MR Systems

A patient with a **SpF** may safely undergo an MRI procedure using a shielded MR system with a static magnetic field of 1.5 Tesla or less (maximum spatial gradient 450 gauss/cm)

Gradient Magnetic Fields of MR Systems

Pulse sequences (e.g., echo planar imaging techniques or other rapid imaging pulse sequences), gradient coils or other techniques, and procedures that exceed a gradient magnetic field of 20 Tesla/second must not be used for MRI procedures. The use of unconventional or non-standard MRI techniques must be avoided. Standard or conventional pulse sequences (e.g., spin echo, fast spin echo, gradient echo, etc.) may be used for MRI examinations.

Radio Frequency (RF) Fields of MR Systems

MRI procedures must not exceed exposures to RF fields greater than a whole body averaged specific absorption rate (SAR) of 1.1 W/kg for 25 minutes of imaging. The use of unconventional or non-standard MRI techniques must be avoided.

MRI Artifacts

Artifacts for the **SpF** have been characterized using a 1.5 Tesla MR system (maximum spatial gradient 450 gauss/cm) and various pulse sequences. Based on this information, implantation of the **SpF** (i.e., with reference to the center of the device) a distance of at least 5 to 8 cm from the imaging area of interest is likely to maintain the diagnostic quality of the MRI examination. Artifact size is dependent on the type of pulse sequence used for imaging (e.g., larger for gradient echo pulse sequences and smaller for fast spin echo pulse sequences), the direction of the frequency encoding direction (larger if the frequency encoding direction is perpendicular to the device and smaller if it is parallel to the device), and the size of the field of view. Positional errors and artifacts on MR images may be larger for MR systems with static magnetic field strengths greater than 1.5 Tesla or smaller for MR systems with lower static magnetic fields strengths using the same imaging parameters.

Implant the **SpF** as far as possible from the spinal canal and bone graft is desirable since this will decrease the possibility that artifacts will affect this area of interest on MRI examinations. The use of fast spin echo pulse sequences will minimize the amount of artifact associated with the presence of the **SpF** compared to the use of other imaging techniques.

Nerve Excitation

The cathodes of the implantable spinal fusion stimulator must be positioned a minimum of 1 cm from nerve roots to reduce the possibility of nerve excitation during a MRI procedure.

Torque

To minimize the possibility of magnetically induced torque during MR imaging, the stimulator should be oriented with its broad face (36 mm x 23 mm plane) parallel to the body and to the static field lines inside the bore.

MRI Safety Information - SpF PLUS-Mini
SpF PLUS-Mini 60μA/W and 60μA/M

Safety information for the use of Magnetic Resonance Imaging (MRI) procedures (i.e., imaging, angiography, functional imaging, spectroscopy, etc.) pertains to shielded MRI systems with static magnetic fields of 1.5 Tesla or less (maximum spatial gradient magnetic field of 250 gauss/cm), gradient magnetic fields of 20 Tesla/second or less, and a maximum whole body averaged Specific Absorption Rate (SAR) of 1.1 W/kg for 25 minutes of imaging. The effects of MRI procedures using MR systems and conditions above these levels have not been determined.

The **SpF** devices have been determined to be MR safe, thereby (when used in the MRI environment) there is no additional risk to the patient, but may affect image quality. MRI procedures must only be performed according to the following guidelines:

- Plain films (radiographs) must be obtained to assess the site of the implanted **SpF** prior to the MRI examination to verify that there are no broken leads present.
- If this cannot be reliably determined, then the potential risks and benefits to the patient requiring the MRI examination must be carefully assessed in consideration of the possibility of excessive heating to develop in the leads.

- The patient must be continuously observed during the MRI procedure and instructed to report any unusual sensations including any feelings of warming, burning, or neuromuscular excitation or stimulation.
- If these occur, the MRI procedure must be discontinued.

Static Magnetic Field of MR Systems

A patient with a **SpF** may safely undergo an MRI procedure using a shielded MR system with a static magnetic field of 1.5 Tesla or less (maximum spatial gradient magnetic field of 250 gauss/cm)

Gradient Magnetic Fields of MR Systems

Pulse sequences (e.g., echo planar imaging techniques or other rapid imaging pulse sequences), gradient coils or other techniques, and procedures that exceed a gradient magnetic field of 20 Tesla/second must not be used for MRI procedures. The use of unconventional or non-standard MRI techniques must be avoided. Standard or conventional pulse sequences (e.g., spin echo, fast spin echo, gradient echo, etc.) may be used for MRI examinations.

Radio Frequency (RF) Fields of MR Systems

MRI procedures must not exceed exposures to RF fields greater than a whole body averaged specific absorption rate (SAR) of 1.1 W/kg for 25 minutes of imaging. The use of unconventional or non-standard MRI techniques must be avoided.

MRI Artifacts

Artifacts for the **SpF** have been characterized using a 1.5 Tesla MR system (maximum spatial gradient 250 gauss/cm) and various pulse sequences. Based on this information, implantation of the **SpF** (i.e., with reference to the center of the device) a distance of at least 5 to 8 cm from the imaging area of interest is likely to maintain the diagnostic quality of the MRI examination. Artifact size is dependent on the type of pulse sequence used for imaging (e.g., larger for gradient echo pulse sequences and smaller for fast spin echo pulse sequences), the direction of the frequency encoding direction (larger if the frequency encoding direction is perpendicular to the device and smaller if it is parallel to the device), and the size of the field of view. Positional errors and artifacts on MR images may be larger for MR systems with static magnetic field strengths greater than 1.5 Tesla or smaller for MR systems with lower static magnetic fields strengths using the same imaging parameters.

Implant the **SpF** as far as possible from the spinal canal and bone graft is desirable since this will decrease the possibility that artifacts will affect this area of interest on MRI examinations. The use of fast spin echo pulse sequences will minimize the amount of artifact associated with the presence of the **SpF** compared to the use of other imaging techniques.

Nerve Excitation

The cathodes of the implantable spinal fusion stimulator must be positioned a minimum of 1 cm from nerve roots to reduce the possibility of nerve excitation during a MRI procedure.

Torque

To minimize the possibility of magnetically induced torque during MR imaging, the stimulator should be oriented with its broad face (39 mm x 27 mm plane) parallel to the body and to the static field lines inside the bore.

[MR healthcare professionals are advised to contact the respective manufacturer in order to obtain the latest safety information to ensure patient safety relative to the use of an MR procedure.]

REFERENCES

http://www.biomet.com

Chou C-K, McDougall JA, Chan KW. RF heating of implanted spinal fusion stimulator during magnetic resonance imaging. IEEE Trans Biomed Engineering 1997;44:357-373.

Shellock FG. Magnetic Resonance Procedures: Health Effects and Safety. CRC Press, LLC, Boca Raton, FL, 2001.

Shellock FG, Hatfield M, Simon BJ, Block S, Wamboldt J, Starewicz PM, Punchard WFB. Implantable spinal fusion stimulator: assessment of MRI safety. J Magn Reson Imaging 2000;12:214-223.

Bravo pH Monitoring System

Indications for Use. The Bravo pH Monitoring System with Accessories (Medtronic, Inc., Minneapolis, MN and Given Imaging) is intended for measurement of gastroesophageal pH and monitoring gastric reflux. The pH probe (capsule) can be delivered and placed endoscopically or with standard manometric procedures. The pH Software Analysis Program is intended to record, store, view and analyze gastroesophageal pH data.

Warnings and Precautions. Potential complications associated with gastrointestinal endoscopy include but are not limited to: perforation, hemorrhage, aspiration, fever, infection, hypertension, respiratory arrest, cardiac arrhythmia or arrest. Potential complications associated with nasal intubation include but are not limited to: sore throat, trauma to nasopharynx or bloody nose. Complications associated with the Bravo System include premature detachment of the capsule, failure of the capsule to slough off in a timely period, or discomfort associated with the capsule requiring endoscopic removal.

The Bravo pH Capsule with Delivery System is a single use, disposable device. Reuse or any other misuse of a Bravo pH Capsule with Delivery System will result in an increased potential for damage to the device and ancillary equipment.

Prior to use, all equipment for the procedure should be examined carefully to verify proper function.

MRI Information
Patients are restricted from undergoing an MRI study within 30 days of the Bravo procedure.

[MR healthcare professionals are advised to contact the respective manufacturer in order to obtain the latest safety information to ensure patient safety relative to the use of an MR procedure.]

REFERENCE

http://www.givenimaging.com
http://www.medtronic.com

Breast Tissue Expanders and Implants

Adjustable breast tissue expanders and mammary implants are utilized for breast reconstruction following mastectomy, for the correction of breast and chest-wall deformities and underdevelopment, for tissue defect procedures, and for cosmetic augmentation. These devices are typically equipped with either an integral injection site or a remote injection dome that is utilized to accept a needle for placement of saline for expansion of the prosthesis intra-operatively and/or postoperatively.

There are many different types of breast tissue expanders. For example, the Becker and the Siltex prostheses provide a choice of a standard injection dome or a micro-injection dome. The Radovan expander is indicated for temporary implantation only. The injection port for this device contains 316L stainless steel to guard against piercing the injection port by the needle used to fill the implant.

Notably, there are various breast tissue expanders that have *magnetic* ports to allow for a more accurate detection of the injection site. These devices are substantially attracted to the static magnetic fields of MR systems and, therefore, may be uncomfortable, injurious, or contraindicated for patients undergoing MR procedures. One such device is the Contour Profile Tissue Expander (Mentor, Santa Barbara, CA), which contains a magnetic injection dome and is considered to be unsafe for an MR examination.

Breast tissue expanders with magnetic ports produce relatively large artifacts on MR images and, as such, assessment of the breast using MR imaging is problematic. Importantly, there may be a situation during which a patient is referred for MR imaging for the determination of breast cancer or a breast implant rupture, such that the presence of the metallic artifact could obscure the precise location of the abnormality. In view of this possibility, it is recommended that a patient with a breast tissue expander that has a metallic component be identified prior to MRI so that the radiologist is aware of the potential problems related to the generation of artifacts as well as a possible injury.

McGhan Medical Breast Tissue Expanders and MRI Issues. McGhan Medical Breast Tissue Expanders are intended for temporary subcutaneous implantation to develop surgical flaps and additional tissue coverage (Product Information documents, McGhan Medical/INAMED Aesthetics; Allergan, Inc.). These breast tissue expanders are constructed from silicone elastomer and consist of an expansion envelope with a textured surface, and a MAGNA-SITE integrated injection site. The expanders are available in a wide range of styles and sizes to meet diverse surgical needs. Specific styles include: Style 133 FV with MAGNA-SITE injection site, Style 133 LV with MAGNA-SITE injection site, Style 133 MV with MAGNA-SITE injection site, and Style 133 V with MAGNA-SITE injection site.

The MAGNA-SITE injection site and MAGNA-FINDER external locating device contain rare-earth, permanent magnets for an accurate injection system. When the MAGNA-FINDER is passed over the surface of the tissue being expanded, its rare-earth, permanent magnet indicates the location of the MAGNA-SITE injection site.

The Product Information documents for these breast tissue expanders states: "DO NOT use MAGNA-SITE expanders in patients who already have implanted devices that would be affected by a magnetic field (e.g., pacemakers, drug infusion devices, artificial sensing devices). DO NOT perform diagnostic testing with Magnetic Resonance Imaging (MRI) in patients with MAGNA-SITE expanders in place."

Furthermore, in the Warnings section of the Product Information document, the following is indicated: "Diagnostic testing with Magnetic Resonance Imaging (MRI) is contraindicated in patients with MAGNA-SITE expanders in place. The MRI equipment could cause movement of the MAGNA-SITE breast tissue expander, and result in not only patient discomfort, but also expander displacement, requiring revision surgery. In addition, the MAGNA-SITE magnet could interfere with MRI detection capabilities."

Therefore, MR procedures are deemed unsafe for patients with these specific breast tissue expanders.

Zegzula et al. presented a case of bilateral tissue expander infusion port dislodgment associated with an MRI examination. The report involved a 56-year-old woman that underwent bilateral mastectomy and immediate reconstruction with McGhan BIOSPAN tissue expanders. As noted, these implants contain the "MAGNA-SITE" components. Several weeks postoperatively the patient underwent MR imaging of her spine. Subsequently, the infusion ports could not be located with the finder magnet (used to re-fill the tissue expander). A chest radiograph was obtained that demonstrated bilateral dislodgment of the infusion ports.

Surgical removal and replacement of the tissue expanders were required. This incident emphasizes that all patients undergoing tissue expansion with implants that contain magnetic ports should be thoroughly warned about the potential hazards of MR imaging and managed appropriately.

In another incident involving a tissue expander, Duffy and May reported a case of a woman who developed a burning sensation at the site of the tissue expander during an MR procedure. The sensation resolved rapidly once the scan was discontinued. The implications of the symptoms in this case are unclear. Nevertheless, a patient with a tissue expander that requires an MR procedure should be alerted to the possibility of localized symptoms in the region of the implant during scanning.

REFERENCES

Duffy FJ Jr, May JW Jr. Tissue expanders and magnetic resonance imaging: the "hot" breast implant. Ann Plast Surg 1995;5:647-9.

Fagan LL, Shellock FG, Brenner RJ, Rothman B. Ex vivo evaluation of ferromagnetism, heating, and artifacts of breast tissue expanders exposed to a 1.5-T MR system. J Magn Reson Imaging 1995;5:614-616.

Liang MD, Narayanan K, Kanal E. Magnetic ports in tissue expanders: a caution for MRI. Magn Reson Imaging 1989;7:541-542.

Product Information, Style 133 Family of Breast Tissue Expanders with Magna-Site Injection Sites, McGhan Medical/INAMED Aesthetics, Santa Barbara, CA.

Product Information, Directions for Use, Style 133V Series Tissue Expander Matrix, With Magna-Site Injection Sites, Allergan, Inc.

Shellock FG, Kanal E. Magnetic Resonance: Bioeffects, Safety, and Patient Management. Second Edition, Lippincott-Raven Press, New York, 1996.

Zegzula HD, Lee WP. Infusion port dislodgment of bilateral breast tissue expanders after MRI. Ann Plast Surg 2001;46:46-8.

Cardiac Pacemakers and Implantable Cardioverter Defibrillators

Cardiac pacemakers and implantable cardioverter defibrillators (ICDs) are crucial implanted devices for patients with heart conditions and serve to maintain quality of life and substantially reduce morbidity. Expanded indications for cardiac pacemakers and ICDs (e.g., heart failure, obstructive sleep apnea, and other conditions) emphasize that an increasing number of patients will be treated with these devices. Currently, these cardiovascular implants are considered a relative contraindication for patients referred for MR procedures. Additionally, individuals with cardiac pacemakers and ICDs should be prevented from entering the MR environment because of potential risks.

MR conditional cardiac pacing systems are now available for patients referred for MR examinations and a comprehensive review of this topic has recently been presented in the Journal of Cardiovascular Magnetic Resonance (JCMR) by Shinbane, Colletti, and Shellock (Magnetic resonance imaging in patients with cardiac pacemakers: Era of MR conditional design. Journal of Cardiovascular Magnetic Resonance 2011;197:W457-9).

For additional information on the topic of cardiac pacing systems and MRI, please refer to the following sections, including the sections that refer to "MR Conditional" cardiac pacing systems: **Cardiac Pacemaker: Accent MRI Pacemaker System, Cardiac Pacemaker: Advisa DR MRI SureScan Pacing System, Cardiac Pacemaker: Ensura DR MRI SureScan Pacing System, Cardiac Pacemaker: EnRhythm MRI SureScan Pacing System, Cardiac Pacemaker: Revo MRI SureScan Pacing System, Cardiac Pacemakers: ProMRI Pacing Systems, and Extremity MR System**.

Cardiac pacemakers and ICDs have been suggested to present potential problems to patients undergoing MR procedures from various mechanisms, including:

1) Movement and/or vibration of the pulse generator or lead(s)

2) Temporary or permanent modification of the function (i.e., damage) of the device
3) Inappropriate sensing, triggering, or activation of the device
4) Excessive heating of the leads
5) Induced currents in the leads
6) Electromagnetic interference

The effects of the MR environment and MR procedures on the functional and operational aspects of cardiac pacemakers and ICDs vary, depending on several factors including the type of device, how the device is programmed, the static magnetic field strength of the MR system, and the imaging conditions used for the procedure (i.e., the anatomic region imaged relative to the transmit RF coil, type of transmit RF coil used, the pulse sequence, amount of radiofrequency energy used, etc.). Notably, most of the data concerning the deleterious effects of MR imaging on cardiac pacemakers involved the use of older versions (i.e., pre-1996) of these devices.

More recently, many compelling reports have been published concerning "modern-day" pacemakers (i.e. devices with decreased ferromagnetic components and more sophisticated circuitry) that indicate that certain patients may undergo MR examinations without harmful effects by following specific guidelines to minimize or prevent risks. Thus, there is evidence that it may be possible to perform MR procedures safely in patients with cardiovascular devices under highly controlled conditions (see below). Alternatively, as previously mentioned, MR conditional cardiac pacing systems now exist that were specifically designed to provide a high margin of safety for patients referred for MR procedures.

Implantable cardioverter defibrillators (ICDs) are medical devices designed to automatically detect and treat episodes of ventricular fibrillation, ventricular tachycardias, bradycardia, and other conditions. When a problem is identified, the device can deliver defibrillation, cardioversion, antitachycardia pacing, bradycardia pacing, or other therapy.

In general, exposure to an MR system or to an MR procedure has similar effects on an ICD as those previously described for a cardiac pacemaker. However, there are several unique aspects of ICDs that impact the possible safe performance of MR procedures in patients with these devices. Therefore, patients and individuals with these cardiac devices are generally not allowed to enter the MR environment. In addition, since ICDs have electrodes placed in the myocardium, patients are typically not permitted to undergo MR examinations because of the inherent risks related to the presence of these conductive materials.

Similar to cardiac pacemakers, it is anticipated that, in lieu of developing a truly acceptable ICD for the MR environment, safety criteria may be determined for "modern-day" ICDs that entail using specialized programming, monitoring procedures, and MR conditions to allow patients to undergo MR examinations safely. Several recent studies have described patients with ICDs examined by MR imaging without serious problems with the caveat that ICDs, in fact, tend to be more problematic than pacemakers relative to the use of MR examinations. Notably, potential problems remain even for "modern" cardiac pacemakers and ICDs as indicated by reports by Gimbel (2009) and Mollerus et al. (2009), such that extreme caution must be exercised when scanning patients with these devices.

Growing Evidence for Performing MR Procedures in Nonpacemaker Dependent Patients

Harmful effects related to performing MRI procedures in patients with cardiac pacemakers have been documented. In virtually every case involving a fatality, the patient apparently entered the MR environment without the staff knowing a cardiac pacemaker was present. Importantly, these deaths were poorly characterized, no electrocardiographic data were available for review, it was unknown whether these patients were pacemaker dependent, and the actual causes or mechanisms of death were not confirmed or otherwise verified. By comparison, no irreversible harm has been reported when patients with cardiac pacemakers were carefully monitored during MR procedures and/or the devices underwent reprogramming prior to the scans.

Regardless of the known hazards of subjecting a patient with a cardiac pacemaker to the MR environment, numerous patients (1,000+) have now undergone MR imaging during purposeful, monitored procedures performed in order to conduct necessary diagnostic examinations. These patients were safely and successfully imaged using MR systems operating at static magnetic fields ranging from 0.2- to 3-Tesla without serious adverse events.

In consideration of the above, there is increasing evidence from *in vitro*, laboratory, and clinical studies that strict restrictions prohibiting MR procedures in patients with "modern" cardiac pacemakers and ICDs may be modified. Similar to performing MR procedures in patients with other electronically-activated devices (e.g., bone fusion stimulators, cochlear implants, neurostimulation systems, programmable injusion pumps, etc.), scanning patients with cardiac pacemakers and ICDs involves following highly specific procedures to ensure patient safety.

Interestingly, a study by Gimbel (2008) reported scanning patients with cardiac pacemakers at 3-Tesla with no restrictions placed on pacemaker dependency, region scanned, device type, or manufacturer. This somewhat limited experience suggested that patients may undergo carefully tailored 3-Tesla MRI scans when pre-MRI reprogramming of the device occurs in conjunction with extensive monitoring, supervision, and follow-up.

Proposed Guidelines for Performing MRI in Nonpacemaker Dependent Patients

Guidelines have been presented by Martin et al. (2004), Roquin et al. (2004), Loewy et al. (2004), the American College of Radiology (2007) and the American College of Cardiology/American Heart Association (2007) with regard to performing MR procedures in nonpacemaker dependent patients. These guidelines include, the following:

- Establish a risk-benefit ratio for the patient
- Obtain written and verbal informed consent
- Pretest pacemaker functions using appropriate equipment outside of the MR environment
- A cardiologist/electrophysiologist should decide whether it is necessary to program the pacemaker prior to the MR examination
- A cardiologist/electrophysiologist with Advanced Cardiac Life Support (ACLS) training must be in attendance for the entire MRI examination
- The patient should be monitored continuously during the MR procedure using proper procedures and technology (e.g., blood pressure, pulse rate, oxygen saturation, and ECG)
- Appropriate personnel, a crash cart, and defibrillator must be available throughout the procedure to address an adverse event
- Maintain visual and voice contact throughout the procedure with the patient
- Instruct the patient to alert the MR system operator of any unusual sensations or problems so that, if necessary, the MR system operator can immediately terminate the procedure
- After the MRI examination, a cardiologist/electrophysiologist should interrogate the pacemaker to confirm that the function is consistent with the pre-MR procedure state

MRI at 1.5 and 3-Tesla and Cardiac Pacemakers and ICDs: Magnetic Field Interactions

As previously discussed, one important safety aspect of the MR environment on cardiac pacemakers and ICDs is related to magnetic field interactions. Component parts of pacemakers and ICDs, such as batteries, reed-switches, or transformer core materials may contain ferromagnetic materials. Therefore, substantial magnetic field interactions may exist, causing these implants to move or be uncomfortable for patients or individuals. Therefore, as an important part of evaluating pacemakers and ICDs, tests for magnetic field interactions have been conducted using MR systems operating at static magnetic field strengths ranging from 0.2-Tesla (i.e., the dedicated-extremity MR system) to 3-Tesla.

Luechinger et al. investigated magnetic field interactions for thirty-one cardiac pacemakers and thirteen ICDs in association with exposure to a 1.5-Tesla MR system (Gyroscan ACS NT, Philips Medical Systems, Best, The Netherlands). The investigators reported that "newer" cardiac pacemakers had relatively low magnetic force values compared to older devices. With regard to ICDs, with the exception of one newer model (GEM II, 7273 ICD, Medtronic, Inc., Minneapolis, MN), all ICDs showed relatively high magnetic field interactions. Luechinger et al. concluded that modern-day pacemakers present no safety risk with respect to magnetic field interactions at 1.5-Tesla, while ICDs could pose problems due to strong magnet-related mechanical forces.

The use of 3-Tesla MR systems for brain, musculoskeletal, body, cardiovascular, and other applications has become routine in many clinical settings.. Because previous investigations performed to determine MR safety for pacemakers and ICDs used MR systems with static magnetic fields of 1.5-Tesla or less, it is crucial to perform *ex vivo* testing at 3-Tesla to characterize magnetic field-related safety for these implants, with full appreciation that additional safety issues exist for these devices, as described-above.

A critical aspect of determining magnetic field interactions for metallic implants involves the measurement of translational attraction. Translational attraction is assessed for metallic implants using the standardized deflection angle test recommended by the American Society for Testing and Materials (ASTM) International. According to ASTM International guidelines, the deflection angle for an implant or device is generally measured at the point of the "highest spatial gradient" for the specific MR system used for testing. Notably, the deflection angle test is commonly performed as an integral part of safety testing for metallic implants and devices.

Various types of magnets exist for commercially available 1.5- and 3-Tesla MR systems, including magnet configurations that are used for conventional "long-bore" scanners and newer "short-bore" systems. Because of physical differences in the position and magnitude of the highest spatial gradient for different magnets, measurements of deflection angles for implants using long-bore vs. short-bore MR systems can produce substantially different results for magnetic field-related translational attraction, as reported by Shellock et al.

The implications are primarily for magnetic field-related translational attraction with regard to long-bore vs. short-bore 3-Tesla MR systems (with short-bore scanners producing greater translational attraction for a given implant). Therefore, a study was conducted on fourteen different cardiac pacemakers and four ICDs to evaluate translational attraction for these devices in association with long-bore and short-bore 1.5- and 3-Tesla MR systems. Deflection angles were measured based on guidelines from the ASTM International.

In general, deflection angles for the cardiovascular implants that underwent evaluation were significantly ($p<0.01$) higher on 1.5- and 3-Tesla short-bore scanners compared to long-bore MR systems. For the 1.5-Tesla MR systems, three cardiac pacemakers (Cosmos, Model 283-01 Pacemaker, Intermedics, Inc., Freeport, TX; Nova Model 281-01 Pacemaker, Intermedics, Inc., Freeport, TX; Res-Q ACE, Model 101-01 Pacemaker; Intermedics, Inc., Freeport, TX) exhibited deflection angles greater than 45 degrees (i.e., exceeding the recommended ASTM International criteria) on both long-bore and short-bore 1.5-Tesla MR systems. The findings indicated that these devices are potentially problematic for patients from a magnetic field interaction consideration.

With regard to the 3-Tesla MR systems, seven implants exhibited deflection angles greater than 45 degrees on the long-bore 3-Tesla scanner, while 13 exhibited deflection angles greater than 45 degrees on the short-bore 3-T MR system (refer to **The List** for information on the cardiac pacemakers and ICDs that underwent testing). Importantly, the findings for magnetic field-related translational attraction were substantially different comparing the long-bore (i.e., lower values) and short-bore (i.e., higher values) MR systems.

As stated, other factors exist that may impact MRI issues for these cardiac pacemakers and ICDs. Therefore, regardless of the fact that magnetic field interactions may not present a risk for some of the cardiovascular implants that have been tested, these potentially hazardous mechanisms must also be considered carefully for these devices.

[MR healthcare professionals are advised to contact the respective manufacturer in order to obtain the latest safety information to ensure patient safety relative to the use of an MR procedure.]

REFERENCES

Achenbach S, et al. Effects of magnetic resonance imaging on cardiac pacemakers and electrodes. Am Heart J 1997;134:467-473.

Alagona P, et al. Nuclear magnetic resonance imaging in a patient with a DDD pacemaker. Pacing Clin Electrophysiol 1989;12:619 (letter).

American Society for Testing and Materials (ASTM) Designation: F 2052. Standard test method for measurement of magnetically induced displacement force on passive implants in the magnetic resonance environment. West Conshohocken, PA.

Anfinsen OG, et al. Implantable cardioverter defibrillator dysfunction during and after magnetic resonance imaging. Pacing Clin Electrophysiol 2002;25:1400-1402.

Baikoussis NG, et al. Safety of magnetic resonance imaging in patients with implanted cardiac prostheses and metallic cardiovascular electronic devices. Ann Thorac Surg. 2011;91:2006-11.

Bailey SM, et al. Magnetic resonance imaging (MRI) of the brain in pacemaker dependent patients. Pacing and Clinical Electrophysiology 2005;2:S128.

Baser K, et al. High ventricular lead impedance of a DDD pacemaker after cranial magnetic resonance imaging. Pacing Clin Electrophysiol. 2011 Feb 8 [Epub ahead of print]

Bhachu DS, Kanal E. Implantable pulse generators (pacemakers) and electrodes: safety in the magnetic resonance imaging scanner environment. J Magn Reson Imaging 2000; 12:201-204.

Boilson BA, et al. Safety of magnetic resonance imaging in patients with permanent pacemakers: a collaborative clinical approach. J Interv Card Electrophysiol. 2011 Sep 21. [Epub ahead of print]

Bonnet CA, Elson JJ, Fogoros RN. Accidental deactivation of the automatic implantable cardioverter defibrillator. Am Heart J 1990;3:696-697.

Buendía F, et al. Nuclear magnetic resonance imaging in patients with cardiac pacing devices. Rev Esp Cardiol. 2010;63:735-9.

Buendía F, et al. Cardiac magnetic resonance imaging at 1.5 T in patients with cardiac rhythm devices. Europace. 2011;13:533-8.

Burke PT, et al. A protocol for patients with cardiovascular implantable devices undergoing magnetic resonance imaging (MRI): should defibrillation threshold testing be performed post-(MRI). J Interv Card Electrophysiol. 2010;28:59-66.

Calcagnini G, et al. In vitro investigation of pacemaker lead heating induced by magnetic resonance imaging: role of implant geometry. J Magn Reson Imaging. 2008;28:879-86.

Colletti PM, Shinbane JS, Shellock FG. "MR-conditional" pacemakers: The radiologist's role in multidisciplinary management. AJR Am J Roentgenol. 2011;197:W457-9.

Del Ojo JL, et al. Is magnetic resonance imaging safe in cardiac pacemaker recipients? Pacing Clin Electrophysiol 2005;28:274-8.

Duru F, et al. Pacing in magnetic resonance imaging environment: clinical and technical considerations on compatibility. Eur Heart J 2001;22:113-124.

Duru F, Luechinger R, Candinas R. MR imaging in patients with cardiac pacemakers. Radiology 2001;219:856-858.

Erlebacher JA, Cahill PT, Pannizzo F, Knowles RJR. Effect of magnetic resonance imaging on DDD pacemakers. Am J Cardio 1986;57:437-440.

Faris OP, Shein M. Food and Drug Administration perspective: Magnetic resonance imaging of pacemaker and implantable cardioverter-defibrillator patients. Circulation 2006;114:1232-1233.

Fetter J, Aram G, Holmes DR, Gray JE, Hayes DL. The effects of nuclear magnetic resonance imagers on external and implantable pulse generators. Pacing Clin Electrophysiol 1984;7:720-727.

Fiek M, et al. Complete loss of ICD programmability after magnetic resonance imaging. Pacing Clin Electrophysiol 2004;27:1002-4.

Fontaine JM, et al. Rapid ventricular pacing in a pacemaker patient undergoing magnetic resonance imaging. Pacing Clin Electrophysiol 1998;21:1336-1339.

Forleo GB, et al. Safety and efficacy of a new magnetic resonance imaging-compatible pacing system: early results of a prospective comparison with conventional dual-chamber implant outcomes. Heart Rhythm. 2010;7:750-4

Garcia-Bolao I, Albaladejo V, et al. Magnetic resonance imaging in a patient with a dual chamber pacemaker. Acta Cardiol 1998;53:33-35.

Gimbel JR. Unexpected asystole during 3T magnetic resonance imaging of a pacemaker dependent patient with a 'modern' pacemaker. Europace. 2009;11:1241-2.

Gimbel JR. Unexpected pacing inhibition upon exposure to the 3T static magnetic field prior to imaging acquisition: what is the mechanism? Heart Rhythm. 2011;8:944-5.

Gimbel JR. Letter to the Editor. Pacing Clin Electrophysiol 2003;26:1.

Gimbel JR. Magnetic resonance imaging of implantable cardiac rhythm devices at 3-Tesla. Pacing Clin Electrophysiol. 2008;31:795-801.

Gimbel JR. The safety of MRI scanning of pacemakers and ICDs: what are the critical elements of safe scanning? Ask me again at 10,000. Europace. 2010;12:915-7.

Gimbel JR, et al. Safe performance of magnetic resonance imaging on five patients with permanent cardiac pacemakers. Pacing Clin Electrophysiol 1996;19:913-919.

Gimbel JR, et al. Outcome of magnetic resonance imaging (MRI) in selected patients with implantable cardioverter defibrillators (ICDs). Pacing Clin Electrophysiol 2005;28:270-3.

Goldsher D, et al. Magnetic resonance imaging for patients with permanent pacemakers: initial clinical experience. Isr Med Assoc J 2006;8:91-94.

Goldsher D, et al. Successful cervical MR scan in a patient several hours after pacemaker implantation. Pacing Clin Electrophysiol. 2009;32:1355-6.

Halshtok O, et al. Pacemakers and magnetic resonance imaging: no longer an absolute contraindication when scanned correctly. Isr Med Assoc J. 2010;12:391-5.

Harden SP. MRI conditional pacemakers: the start of a new era. Br J Radiol. 2011;84:773-4.

Hayes DL, et al. Effect of 1.5 Tesla nuclear magnetic resonance imaging scanner on implanted permanent pacemakers. J Am Coll Cardiol 1987;10:782-786.

Heatlie G, Pennell DJ. Cardiovascular magnetic resonance at 0.5-T in five patients with permanent pacemakers. J Cardiovasc Magn Reson. 2007;9:15-9.

Holmes DJ, et al. The effects of magnetic resonance imaging on implantable pulse generators. Pacing Clin Electrophysiol 1986;9:360-370.

http://www.medtronic.com/mrisurescan

Inbar S, Larson J, et al. Case report: nuclear magnetic resonance imaging in a patient with a pacemaker. Am J Med Sci 1993;3:174-175.

Irnich W, Irnich B, et al. Do we need pacemakers resistant to magnetic resonance imaging? Europace. 2005;7:353-65.

International Commission on Non-Ionizing Radiation Protection (ICNIRP) Statement, Medical magnetic resonance procedures: protection of patients. Health Physics 2004;87:197-216.

Junttila MJ, et al. Safety of serial MRI in patients with implantable cardioverter defibrillators. Heart. 2011 Aug 26 [Epub ahead of print]

Kanal E, Barkovich AJ, et al. ACR guidance document for safe MR practices: 2007. AJR Am J Roentgenol. 2007;188:1447-1474.

Langman DA, Finn JP, Ennis D. Abandoned pacemaker leads are a potential risk for patients undergoing MRI. Pacing Clin Electrophysiol 2011;34:1051-3.

Langman DA, et al. Pacemaker lead tip heating in abandoned and pacemaker-attached leads at 1.5 Tesla MRI. J Magn Reson Imaging. 2011;33:426-31.

Lauck G, et al. Effects of nuclear magnetic resonance imaging on cardiac pacemakers. Pacing Clin Electrophysiol 1995;18:1549-55.

Levine PA. Industry Viewpoint: St. Jude Medical: Pacemakers, ICDs and MRI. Pacing and Clinical Electrophysiology 2005;28:266.

Levine GN, Gomes AS, Arai AE, Bluemke DA, Flamm SD, Kanal E, Manning WJ, Martin ET, Smith JM, Wilke N, Shellock FG. Safety of magnetic resonance imaging in patients with cardiovascular devices: an American Heart Association scientific statement from the Committee on Diagnostic and Interventional Cardiac Catheterization. Circulation 2007;116:2878-2891.

Loewy J, Loewy A, Kendall EJ. Reconsideration of pacemakers and MR imaging. Radiographics 2004;24:1257-1268.

Luechinger RC. Safety Aspects of Cardiac Pacemakers in Magnetic Resonance Imaging. Swiss Institute of Technology, Zurich, Dissertation, 2002

Luechinger RC, et al. Pacemaker reed-switch behavior in 0.5, 1.5, and 3.0 Tesla magnetic resonance units: Are reed switches always closed in strong magnetic fields? Pacing Clin Electrophysiol 2002;25:1419-1423.

Luechinger RC, et al. Force and torque effects of a 1.5 Tesla MRI scanner on cardiac pacemakers and ICDs. Pacing Clin Electrophysiol 2001;24:199-205.

Luechinger R, et al. *In vivo* heating of pacemaker leads during magnetic resonance imaging. Eur Heart J 2005;26:376-83.

Martin TE, Coman JA, Shellock FG, Pulling C, Fair R, Jenkins K. Magnetic resonance imaging and cardiac pacemaker safety at 1.5-Tesla. Journal of the American College of Cardiology 2004;43:1315-1324.

Mattei E, et al. Role of the lead structure in MRI-induced heating: In vitro measurements on 30 commercial pacemaker/defibrillator leads. Magn Reson Med. 2011 Jul 11. [Epub ahead of print]

Mollerus M, et al. Ectopy in patients with permanent pacemakers and implantable cardioverter-defibrillators undergoing an MRI scan. Pacing Clin Electrophysiol. 2009;32:772-8.

Mollerus M, et al. Magnetic resonance imaging of pacemakers and implantable cardioverter-defibrillators without specific absorption rate restrictions. Europace. 2010;12:947-51.

Naehle CP, et al. Evaluation of cumulative effects of MR imaging on pacemaker systems at 1.5 Tesla. Pacing Clin Electrophysiol. 2009;32:1526-35.

Naehle CP, et al. Safety of brain 3-T MR imaging with transmit-receive head coil in patients with cardiac pacemakers: pilot prospective study with 51 examinations. Radiology. 2008;249:991-1001.

Naehle CP, et al. Magnetic resonance imaging at 1.5-T in patients with implantable cardioverter-defibrillators. J Am Coll Cardiol. 2009;54:549-55.

Naehle CP, et al. Safety, feasibility, and diagnostic value of cardiac magnetic resonance imaging in patients with cardiac pacemakers and implantable cardioverters/defibrillators at 1.5 T. Am Heart J. 2011;161:1096-105.

Nazarian S, Halperin HR. How to perform magnetic resonance imaging on patients with implantable cardiac arrhythmia devices. Heart Rhythm. 2009;6:138-43.

Nazarian S, et al. Clinical utility and safety of a protocol for noncardiac and cardiac magnetic resonance imaging of patients with permanent pacemakers and implantable-cardioverter defibrillators at 1.5 Tesla. Circulation 2006;114:1277-1284.

Nazarian S, et al. A prospective evaluation of a protocol for magnetic resonance imaging of patients with implanted cardiac devices. Ann Intern Med 2011;155:7 415-424

Nordbeck P, et al. Measuring RF-induced currents inside implants: Impact of device configuration on MRI safety of cardiac pacemaker leads. Magn Reson Med. 2009;61:570-8.

Nordbeck P, et al. Impact of imaging landmark on the risk of MRI-related heating near implanted medical devices like cardiac pacemaker leads. Magn Reson Med. 2011;65:44-50.

Pfeil A, et al. Compatibility of temporary pacemaker myocardial pacing leads with magnetic resonance imaging: an ex vivo tissue study. Int J Cardiovasc Imaging. 2011 Feb 24 [Epub ahead of print]

Pavlicek W, Geisinger M, et al. The effects of nuclear magnetic resonance on patients with cardiac pacemakers. Radiology 1983;147:149-153.

Pulver AF,et al. Safety and imaging quality of MRI in pediatric and adult congenital heart disease patients with pacemakers. Pacing Clin Electrophysiol. 2009;32:450-6.

Quarta G, et al. Cardiovascular magnetic resonance in cardiac sarcoidosis with MR conditional pacemaker in situ. J Cardiovasc Magn Reson. 2011;13:26.

Raj V, et al. MRI and cardiac pacing devices - beware the rules are changing. Br J Radiol. 2011;84:857-9.

Roguin A, et al. Magnetic resonance imaging in individuals with cardiovascular implantable electronic devices. Europace. 2008;10:336-46.

Roguin A, et al. Cardiac magnetic resonance imaging in a patient with implantable cardioverter-defibrillator. Pacing Clin Electrophysiol 2005;28:336-8.

Roguin A, et al. Modern pacemaker and implantable cardioverter-defibrillator systems can be MRI-safe. Circulation 2004;110:475-482.

Sasaki T, et al. Quantitative assessment of artifacts on cardiac magnetic resonance imaging of patients with pacemakers and implantable cardioverter defibrillators. Circ Cardiovasc Imaging. 2011 Sep 23. [Epub ahead of print]

Schmiedel A, et al. Magnetic resonance imaging of the brain in patients with cardiac pacemakers. In-vitro- and in-vivo-evaluation at 1.5 Tesla. Rofo 2005;177:731-44.

Shellock FG. Guest Editorial. Comments on MRI heating tests of critical implants. Journal of Magnetic Resonance Imaging 2007;26:1182-1185.

Shellock FG. Excessive temperature increases in pacemaker leads at 3-T MR imaging with a transmit-received head coil. Radiology 2009;251:948-949.

Shellock FG. Cardiac pacemakers: growing evidence for MRI safety. Signals, No. 48, Issue 1, pp. 14-15, 2004.

Shellock FG, Magnetic Resonance Procedures: Health Effects, Safety, and Patient Management CRC Press, LLC, Boca Raton, FL, 2001.

Shellock FG, Crues JV. MR procedures: biologic effects, safety, and patient care. Radiology 2004;232:635-652.

Shellock FG, Fieno DS, et al. Cardiac pacemaker: *in vitro* assessment of MR safety at 1.5-Tesla. American Heart Journal 2006;151:436-443.

Shellock FG, Fischer L, Fieno DS. Cardiac pacemakers and implantable cardioverter defibrillators: in *vitro* evaluation of MRI safety at 1.5-Tesla. Journal of Cardiovascular Magnetic Resonance 2007;9:21-31.

Shellock FG, et al. Cardiac pacemakers and implantable cardiac defibrillators are unaffected by operation of an extremity MR system. AJR Am J Roentgenol 1999;72:165-170.

Shellock FG, Tkach JA, Ruggieri PM, Masaryk TJ. Cardiac pacemakers, ICDs, and loop recorder: Evaluation of translational attraction using conventional ("long-bore") and "short-bore" 1.5- and 3.0-Tesla MR systems. Journal of Cardiovascular Magnetic Resonance 2003;5:387-397.

Shellock FG, Valencerina S, Fischer L. MRI-related heating of pacemaker at 1.5- and 3-Tesla: Evaluation with and without pulse generator attached to leads. Circulation 112;Supplement II:561, 2005.

Shinbane J, Colletti P, Shellock FG. MR in patients with pacemakers and ICDs: Defining the issues. Journal of Cardiovascular Magnetic Resonance 2007;9:5-13.

Shibane J, Colletti P, Shellock FG. MRI in patients with cardiac pacemakers and other biomedical devices: Engineering the future. Journal of the American College of Cardiology Imaging 201;13:63. [Epub ahead of print]

Shibane J, Colletti P, Shellock FG. Magnetic resonance imaging in patients with cardiac pacemakers: Era of "MR conditional" designs. Journal of Cardiovascular Magnetic Resonance 2011;197:W457-9.

Sommer T, Vahlhaus C, et al. MR imaging and cardiac pacemakers: in vitro evaluation and in vivo studies in 51 patients at 0.5 T. Radiology 2000;215:869-879.

Sommer T, et al. Strategy for safe performance of extrathoracic magnetic resonance imaging at 1.5 Tesla in the presence of cardiac pacemakers in non-pacemaker-dependent patients: a prospective study with 115 examinations. Circulation 2006;114:1285-92

Strach K, et al. Low-field magnetic resonance imaging: increased safety for pacemaker patients? Europace. 2010;12:952-60.

Sutton R, Kanal E, Wilkoff BL, et al. Safety of magnetic resonance imaging of patients with a new Medtronic EnRhythm MRI SureScan pacing system: clinical study design. Trials. 2008;9:68.

Tandri H, et al. Determinants of gradient field-induced current in a pacemaker lead system in a magnetic resonance imaging environment. Heart Rhythm. 2008;5:462-8

Ubee SS, et al. Implications of pacemakers and implantable cardioverter defibrillators in urological practice. J Urol. 2011;186:1198-205

Vahlhaus C, et al. interference with cardiac pacemakers by magnetic resonance imaging: Are there irreversible changes at 0.5 Tesla? Pacing Clin Electrophysiol 2001;24(Pt. I):489-95.

Weishaupt D, et al. Pacemakers and magnetic resonance imaging: Current status and survey in Switzerland. Swiss Med Wkly. 2011;141:w13147.

Wollmann C, et al. Safe performance of magnetic resonance imaging on a patient with an ICD. Pacing Clin Electrophysiol 2005;28:339-42.

Wilkoff BL, et al. Magnetic resonance imaging in patients with a pacemaker system designed for the magnetic resonance environment. Heart Rhythm. 2011;8:65-73.

Wilkoff BL, et al. EnRhythm MRI SureScan Pacing System Study Investigators. Magnetic resonance imaging in patients with a pacemaker system designed for the magnetic resonance environment. Heart Rhythm. 2011;8:65-73.

Zikria JF, et al. MRI of patients with cardiac pacemakers: a review of the medical literature. AJR Am J Roentgenol. 2011;196:390-401.

Zimmermann BH, Faul DD. Artifacts and hazards in NMR imaging due to metal implants and cardiac pacemakers. Diagn Imaging Clin Med 1984;53:53-56.

Cardiac Pacemaker: Accent MRI Pacemaker System

The **Accent MRI** and **Accent ST MRI Cardiac Pacemaker Systems** (Models PM1224, PM2224, PM1226, PM2226, PM1124, PM2124) (St. Jude Medical, Inc., St. Paul, MN) have been designed and tested for performance of a full-body MRI scan, using a 1.5 T (Tesla) field-strength MRI scanner. The St. Jude Medical MR Conditional Cardiac Pacemaker System must be used in conjunction with the Tendril MRI Pacing Lead or other MRI lead from St. Jude Medical. The system must be used in accordance with MR Conditional labeling requirements.

For specific information, please visit www.SJMprofessional.com/MRI

SJM MRI Activator Handheld Device

An optional, easy-to-use handheld device (SJM MRI Activator device) can be used to enable and disable pre-approved MRI settings in the Accent MRI pacemaker pre- and post-MRI scan. The pre-approved settings can be pre-programmed by the physician at any follow-up visit. The Accent MRI pacemaker and Tendril MRI lead are currently CE marked. At the present time, these products are not approved for use in the United States (11/2011).

MRI Conditions for Use

- Patients implanted with the St. Jude Medical MR Conditional pacing system can be scanned under the following conditions:
- Horizontal closed-bore clinical scanner working in the Normal Operating Mode or First Level Controlled Operating Mode, whole body specific absorption rate (SAR) less than or equal to 4.0 W/kg and head SAR less than or equal to 3.2 W/kg
- Static magnetic field strength of 1.5 Tesla (T) only
- Maximum gradient slew rate of 200 T/m/s per axis
- Use of local transmit-only coils or local transmit and receive coils placed directly over the pacing system has not been studied and such use is contraindicated.
- All spectroscopy and imaging for atoms other than hydrogen are contraindicated.
- A patient with an implanted St. Jude Medical MR Conditional Pacing System must not be positioned on his or her side within

the MRI system bore. This position is contraindicated for an MRI scan.

- Patients with a St. Jude Medical MR Conditional Pacing System implanted in sites other than the left and right pectoral region are contraindicated for an MRI scan.

Patient Monitoring

Proper patient monitoring must be provided during the MRI scan. This includes continuous monitoring of the patient's hemodynamic function. Since the MRI environment may interfere with the patient monitoring system, it is recommended that more than one of the following systems be used: electrocardiography, pulse oximetry, noninvasive blood pressure measurements. If the patient's hemodynamic function is compromised during the MRI scan, discontinue the MRI scan and take the proper measures to restore the patient's hemodynamic function. Verbal communication with the patient during the MRI scan is recommended.

Additional MRI conditions exist over and above those indicated here.

Please see the _MRI Procedure Information_ document for additional details before performing an MRI scan.

For more information please visit http://www.SJMprofessional.com/MRI

[MR healthcare professionals are advised to contact the respective manufacturer in order to obtain the latest safety information to ensure patient safety relative to the use of an MR procedure.]

REFERENCE

www.SJMprofessional.com/MRI

Cardiac Pacemaker: Advisa DR MRI SureScan Pacing System

A cardiac pacemaker has been developed that permits MRI procedures to be performed in patients by following specific labeling requirements (http://www.medtronic.com/mrisurescan). The Advisa MRI SureScan Pacing System (Medtronic, Inc., Minneapolis, MN; was designed to minimize the potential interactions with the electromagnetic fields used for MR systems.

Note: The Advisa MRI SureScan Pacing System is also now available but not in the United States.

Comprehensive labeling information must be reviewed and adhered to ensure patient safety and includes, but is not limited to:

MRI conditions for use

Non-clinical testing has demonstrated that the SureScan pacing system is safe for use in the MRI environment when used according to the instructions in this manual.

The SureScan pacing system can be scanned in patients under the following conditions:

-Cylindrical bore magnet, clinical MRI systems with a static magnetic field of 1.5 T (tesla) must be used.

-Gradient systems with maximum gradient slew rate performance per axis of ≤ 200 T/m/s must be used.

-Whole body averaged specific absorption rate (SAR) as reported by the MRI equipment must be ≤ 2.0 W/kg; head SAR as reported by the MRI equipment must be < 3.2 W/kg.

-Patients and their implanted systems must be screened per the contraindications:

-Patients with previously implanted (active or abandoned) medical devices, leads, lead extenders, or lead adaptors are contraindicated for an MRI scan.

-Patients with broken or intermittent leads are contraindicated for an MRI scan.

-Patients with a SureScan pacing system that has been implanted for less than 6 weeks are contraindicated for an MRI scan.

-Patients with a SureScan pacing system implanted in sites other than the left and right pectoral region are contraindicated for an MRI scan.

-Patients who do not have a complete SureScan pacing system, which includes a SureScan device and both atrial and ventricular SureScan leads, are contraindicated for an MRI scan.

-Patients with pacing capture threshold values of > 2.0 V at a pulse width of 0.4 ms are contraindicated for an MRI scan.

Note: Patients experiencing atrial fibrillation may be scanned if all other pre-MRI scan requirements are satisfied.

-Patients whose device will be programmed to an asynchronous pacing mode when MRI SureScan is on, and who have diaphragmatic stimulation at a pacing output of 5.0 V and at a pulse width of 1.0 ms are contraindicated for an MRI scan.

-Patients with a lead impedance value of < 200 ohms or > 1500 ohms are contraindicated for an MRI scan.

-A patient with an implanted SureScan pacing system must not be positioned on his or her side within the MRI bore. This position, called the lateral decubitus position, is contraindicated for all MRI scans.

-Use of local transmit-only coils or local transmit and receive coils placed directly over the pacing system has not been studied and such use is contraindicated

-Continuous patient monitoring must be provided:

Preparation for patient rescue –
Keep an external defibrillator available during the MRI scan.

Patient monitoring –
During the MRI scan, the patient's hemodynamic function must be continuously monitored using at least one of the following monitoring systems:
-electrocardiography

-pulse oximetry-
-noninvasive blood pressure measurements

Note: If the patient's hemodynamic function is compromised during the MRI scan, discontinue the MRI scan and take the proper measures to restore the patient's hemodynamic function.

The patient must be positioned according to the contraindications:

-A patient with an implanted SureScan pacing system must not be positioned on his or her side within the MRI bore. This position, called the lateral decubitus position, is contraindicated for all MRI scans.

-Use of local transmit-only coils or local transmit and receive coils placed directly over the pacing system has not been studied and such use is contraindicated.

-There are no patient positioning restrictions relative to the MRI isocenter landmark when using the body coil.

-There are no patient positioning restrictions relative to the use of any receive-only coils.

-The implanted system must consist solely of a SureScan device and SureScan leads. Any other combination may result in a hazard to the patient during MRI scans.

The Advisa MRI SureScan Pacing System is commercially available in Europe but is not currently available for sale in the United States.

[MR healthcare professionals are advised to contact the respective manufacturer in order to obtain the latest safety information to ensure patient safety relative to the use of an MR procedure.

REFERENCES

http://www.medtronic.com/mrisurescan

Instructions for Use, SURESCAN MRI procedural information for Advisa MRI SureScan A3DR01, CapSureFix MRI 5086MRI, Medtronic, Inc., Minneapolis, MN

Sutton R, Kanal E, Wilkoff BL, et al. Safety of magnetic resonance imaging of patients with a new Medtronic EnRhythm MRI SureScan pacing system: clinical study design. Trials. 2008;2;9:68.

Cardiac Pacemaker: Ensura DR MRI SureScan Pacing System

A cardiac pacemaker has been developed that permits MRI procedures to be performed in patients by following specific labeling requirements (http://www.medtronic.com/mrisurescan). The Ensura MRI SureScan Pacing System (Medtronic, Inc., Minneapolis, MN; was designed to minimize the potential interactions with the electromagnetic fields used for MR systems.

Note: The Ensura MRI SureScan Pacing System is also now available but not in the United States.

Comprehensive labeling information must be reviewed and adhered to ensure patient safety and includes, but is not limited to:

MRI conditions for use:

Non-clinical testing has demonstrated that the SureScan pacing system is safe for use in the MRI environment when used according to the instructions in this manual.

-The SureScan pacing system can be scanned in patients under the following conditions:

-Cylindrical bore magnet, clinical MRI systems with a static magnetic field of 1.5 T (tesla) must be used.

-Gradient systems with maximum gradient slew rate performance per axis of ≤ 200 T/m/s must be used.

-Whole body averaged specific absorption rate (SAR) as reported by the MRI equipment must be ≤ 2.0 W/kg; head SAR as reported by the MRI equipment must be < 3.2 W/kg.

-Patients and their implanted systems must be screened per the contraindications:

-Patients with previously implanted (active or abandoned) medical devices, leads, lead extenders, or lead adaptors are contraindicated for an MRI scan.

-Patients with broken or intermittent leads are contraindicated for an MRI scan.

-Patients with a SureScan pacing system that has been implanted for less than 6 weeks are contraindicated for an MRI scan.

-Patients with a SureScan pacing system implanted in sites other than the left and right pectoral region are contraindicated for an MRI scan.

-Patients who do not have a complete SureScan pacing system, which includes a SureScan device and both atrial and ventricular SureScan leads, are contraindicated for an MRI scan.

-Patients with pacing capture threshold values of > 2.0 V at a pulse width of 0.4 ms are contraindicated for an MRI scan.

Note: Patients experiencing atrial fibrillation may be scanned if all other pre-MRI scan requirements are satisfied.

-Patients whose device will be programmed to an asynchronous pacing mode when MRI SureScan is on, and who have diaphragmatic stimulation at a pacing output of 5.0 V and at a pulse width of 1.0 ms are contraindicated for an MRI scan.

-Patients with a lead impedance value of < 200 ohms or > 1500 ohms are contraindicated for an MRI scan.

-A patient with an implanted SureScan pacing system must not be positioned on his or her side within the MRI bore. This position, called the lateral decubitus position, is contraindicated for all MRI scans.

-Use of local transmit-only coils or local transmit and receive coils placed directly over the pacing system has not been studied and such use is contraindicated

Continuous patient monitoring must be provided:

Preparation for patient rescue – Keep an external defibrillator available during the MRI scan.

Patient monitoring – During the MRI scan, the patient's hemodynamic function must be continuously monitored using at least one of the following monitoring systems:

-electrocardiography

-pulse oximetry

-noninvasive blood pressure measurements

Note: If the patient's hemodynamic function is compromised during the MRI scan, discontinue the MRI scan and take the proper measures to restore the patient's hemodynamic function.

The patient must be positioned according to the contraindications:

-A patient with an implanted SureScan pacing system must not be positioned on his or her side within the MRI bore. This position, called the lateral decubitus position, is contraindicated for all MRI scans.

-Use of local transmit-only coils or local transmit and receive coils placed directly over the pacing system has not been studied and such use is contraindicated.

-There are no patient positioning restrictions relative to the MRI isocenter landmark when using the body coil.

-There are no patient positioning restrictions relative to the use of any receive-only coils.

-The implanted system must consist solely of a SureScan device and SureScan leads. Any other combination may result in a hazard to the patient during MRI scans.

The Ensura MRI SureScan Pacing System is commercially available in Europe but is not currently available for sale in the United States

[MR healthcare professionals are advised to contact the respective manufacturer in order to obtain the latest safety information to ensure patient safety relative to the use of an MR procedure.]

REFERENCE

http://www.medtronic.com/mrisurescan

Cardiac Pacemaker: EnRhythm MRI SureScan Pacing System

A cardiac pacemaker has been developed that permits MRI procedures to be performed in patients by following specific labeling requirements (http://www.medtronic.com/mrisurescan). The EnRhythm MRI SureScan Pacing System (Medtronic, Inc., Minneapolis, MN; was designed to minimize the potential interactions with the electromagnetic fields used for MR systems.

Note: the EnRhythm MRI SureScan Pacing System is also now available but not in the United States.

Comprehensive labeling information must be reviewed and adhered to ensure patient safety and includes, but is not limited to:

MRI conditions for use

-Non-clinical testing has demonstrated that the SureScan pacing system is safe for use in the MRI environment when used according to the instructions in this manual.

-The SureScan pacing system can be scanned in patients under the following conditions:

-Cylindrical bore magnet, clinical MRI systems with a static magnetic field of 1.5 T (tesla) must be used.

-Gradient systems with maximum gradient slew rate performance per axis of ≤ 200 T/m/s must be used.

-Whole body averaged specific absorption rate (SAR) as reported by the MRI equipment must be ≤ 2.0 W/kg; head SAR as reported by the MRI equipment must be < 3.2 W/kg.

-Patients and their implanted systems must be screened per the contraindications:

-Patients with previously implanted (active or abandoned) medical devices, leads, lead extenders, or lead adaptors are contraindicated for an MRI scan.

-Patients with broken or intermittent leads are contraindicated for an MRI scan.

-Patients with a SureScan pacing system that has been implanted for less than 6 weeks are contraindicated for an MRI scan.

-Patients with a SureScan pacing system implanted in sites other than the left and right pectoral region are contraindicated for an MRI scan.

-Patients who do not have a complete SureScan pacing system, which includes a SureScan device and both atrial and ventricular SureScan leads, are contraindicated for an MRI scan.

-Patients with pacing capture threshold values of > 2.0 V at a pulse width of 0.4 ms are contraindicated for an MRI scan.

Note: Patients experiencing atrial fibrillation may be scanned if all other pre-MRI scan requirements are satisfied.

-Patients whose device will be programmed to an asynchronous pacing mode when MRI SureScan is on, and who have diaphragmatic stimulation at a pacing output of 5.0 V and at a pulse width of 1.0 ms are contraindicated for an MRI scan.

-Patients with a lead impedance value of < 200 ohms or > 1500 ohms are contraindicated for an MRI scan.

-A patient with an implanted SureScan pacing system must not be positioned on his or her side within the MRI bore. This position, called the lateral decubitus position, is contraindicated for all MRI scans.

-Use of local transmit-only coils or local transmit and receive coils placed directly over the pacing system has not been studied and such use is contraindicated

Continuous patient monitoring must be provided:

-Preparation for patient rescue – Keep an external defibrillator available during the MRI scan.

-Patient monitoring – During the MRI scan, the patient's hemodynamic function must be continuously monitored using at least one of the following monitoring systems:

-electrocardiography
-pulse oximetry
-noninvasive blood pressure measurements

Note: –If the patient's hemodynamic function is compromised during the MRI scan, discontinue the MRI scan and take the proper measures to restore the patient's hemodynamic function.

The patient must be positioned according to the contraindications:

-A patient with an implanted SureScan pacing system must not be positioned on his or her side within the MRI bore. This position, called the lateral decubitus position, is contraindicated for all MRI scans.

-Use of local transmit-only coils or local transmit and receive coils placed directly over the pacing system has not been studied and such use is contraindicated.

-There are no patient positioning restrictions relative to the MRI isocenter landmark when using the body coil.

-There are no patient positioning restrictions relative to the use of any receive-only coils.

-The implanted system must consist solely of a SureScan device and SureScan leads. Any other combination may result in a hazard to the patient during MRI scans.

The EnRhythm MRI SureScan Pacing System is commercially available in Europe but is not currently available for sale in the United States. In the United States the device is limited by federal law to investigational use only.

[MR healthcare professionals are advised to contact the respective manufacturer in order to obtain the latest safety information to ensure patient safety relative to the use of an MR procedure.]

REFERENCE

http://www.medtronic.com/mrisurescan

Cardiac Pacing Systems: ProMRI Pacing Systems

ProMRI Pacing Systems (BIOTRONIK) provide patients access to MRI scanning and physicians more options in MR conditional single and dual chamber pacemaker systems.

For specific information, please visit
www.www.biotronik.com/en/de/28956

The ProMRI Pacing Systems are currently CE marked; These products are not approved for use in the United States (11/2011)

REFERENCE

www.biotronik.com/en/de/28956

Cardiac Pacemaker: Revo MRI SureScan Pacing System

A new cardiac pacemaker has been developed that permits MRI procedures to be performed in patients by following specific labeling requirements (http://www.medtronic.com/mrisurescan). The Revo MRI SureScan Pacing System (Medtronic, Inc., Minneapolis, MN; was designed to minimize the potential interactions with the electromagnetic fields used for MR systems.

Comprehensive labeling information must be reviewed and adhered to ensure patient safety and includes, but is not limited to:

MRI conditions for use

A complete SureScan pacing system including a Revo MRI SureScan IPG and two SureScan leads is required for use in the MRI environment. Any other combination may result in a hazard to the patient during an MRI scan. The SureScan feature must be programmed to 'On' prior to scanning a patient according to the specified conditions for use.

Clinical and pre-clinical testing has demonstrated that the SureScan pacing system is safe for use in the MRI environment when used according to the instructions in the Revo MRI SureScan Pacing System Technical Manual.

The SureScan pacing system can be scanned in patients under the following conditions:

(1) Horizontal, cylindrical bore magnet, clinical MRI systems with a static magnetic field of 1.5 Tesla (T) must be used.

(2) Gradient systems with maximum gradient slew rate performance per axis of less than or equal to 200 Teslas per meter per second (T/m/s) must be used.

(3) The scanner must be in Normal Operating Mode:

-Whole body averaged specific absorption rate (SAR) as reported by the MRI equipment must be equal to or less than or equal to 2.0 Watts per kilogram (W/kg)

-The head SAR must be less than 3.2 W/kg.

(4) The patient must be positioned within the bore such that the isocenter (center of the MRI bore) is superior to the C1 vertebra or inferior to the T12 vertebra.

(5) Proper patient monitoring must be provided during the MRI scan. The methods include visual and verbal contact with the patient, electrocardiography, and pulse oximetry (plethysmography).

(6) Patients and their implanted systems must be screened to meet the following requirements:

-no previously implanted (active or abandoned) medical devices, leads, lead extenders, or lead adaptors

-no broken leads or leads with intermittent electrical contact as confirmed by lead impedance history

-a SureScan pacing system that has been implanted for a minimum of 6 weeks

-a SureScan pacing system implanted the left or right pectoral region

-pacing capture threshold values of ≤ 2.0 volts (V) at a pulse width of 0.4 milliseconds (ms)

-a lead impedance value of ≥ 200 ohms or ≤ 1500 ohms

-no diaphragmatic stimulation at a pacing output of 5.0 V and at a pulse width of 1.0 ms in patients whose device will be programmed to an asynchronous pacing mode when MRI SureScan is on

(7) A health professional who has completed cardiology SureScan training must be present during the programming of the SureScan feature.

(8) A health professional who has completed radiology SureScan training must be present during the MRI scan.

(9) The implanted system must consist solely of a SureScan device and SureScan leads. Any other combination may result in a hazard to the patient during MRI scans.

[MR healthcare professionals are advised to contact the respective manufacturer in order to obtain the latest safety information to ensure patient safety relative to the use of an MR procedure.]

REFERENCE

http://www.medtronic.com/mrisurescan

Cardiovascular Catheters and Accessories

Cardiovascular catheters and accessories are indicated for use in the assessment and management of critically-ill or high-risk patients including those with acute heart failure, cardiogenic shock, severe hypovolemia, complex circulatory abnormalities, acute respiratory distress syndrome, pulmonary hypertension, certain types of arrhythmias and other serious conditions. In these cases, cardiovascular catheters are used to measure intravascular pressures, intracardiac pressures, cardiac output, and oxyhemoglobin saturation. Secondary indications include venous blood sampling and therapeutic infusion of solutions or medications. In addition, some cardiovascular catheters are designed for temporary cardiac pacing and intra-atrial or intraventricular electrocardiographic monitoring.

Because patients with cardiovascular catheters and associated accessories may require evaluation using MR procedures or these devices may be considered for use during MR-guided or interventional procedures, it is imperative that a thorough *ex vivo* assessment of MRI issues be conducted to ascertain the potential risks. For example, MR imaging, angiography, and spectroscopy procedures may play an important role in the diagnostic evaluation of these patients. Furthermore, the performance of certain MR-guided procedures may require the utilization of cardiovascular catheters and accessories to monitor patients during biopsies, interventions, or treatments.

There is at least one report of a cardiovascular catheter, the Swan-Ganz Triple Lumen Thermodilution Catheter, that "melted" in a patient undergoing MR imaging. This catheter has a wire made from a conductive material that was considered to be responsible for this problem. Thus, there are realistic concerns pertaining to the use of similar devices in patients undergoing MR examinations. Therefore, an investigation was performed using *ex vivo* testing techniques to evaluate various cardiovascular catheters and accessories with regard to magnetic field interactions, heating, and artifacts associated with MR imaging.

A total of fifteen different cardiovascular catheters and accessories (Abbott Laboratories, Morgan Hill, CA) were selected for evaluation because they represent a wide-variety of the styles and types of devices that are commonly-used in the critical care setting (i.e., the basic structures of these devices are comparable to those made by other manufacturers). Of these devices, the 3-Lumen CVP Catheter, CVP-PVC Catheter (used for central venous pressure monitoring, administration of fluids, and venous blood sampling; polyurethane and polyvinyl chloride, respectively), Thermoset-Iced and Thermoset-Room (used as accessories for determination of cardiac output using the thermodilution method; plastic), and Safe-set with In-Line Reservoir (used for in-line blood sampling; plastic) were determined to have no metallic components (Personal communications, Ann McGibbon, Abbott Laboratories, 1997). Thus, these devices were deemed safe for patients undergoing MR procedures and were not included in the overall *ex vivo* tests for MR issues. The remaining ten devices were evaluated for potential MRI issues.

Excessive heating of implants or devices made from conductive materials has been reported to be a hazard for patients who undergo MR procedures. This is particularly a problem for a device that is a certain length or in the form of a loop or coil of a certain diameter because current can be induced during MR imaging, resulting in a serious injury.

Additional physical factors responsible for this problem have not been well-characterized (i.e., possible gradient field effects, size of the loop associated with excessive heating, etc.). Therefore, the afore-mentioned study examining cardiovascular catheters and accessories did not attempt to investigate the effect of various "coiled" catheter shapes on the development of substantial heating during an MR procedure, especially since there are many factors in addition to the shape or configuration of the catheter with a conductive component that can influence the amount of heating that occurs.

The thermodilution Swan-Ganz catheter and other similar cardiovascular catheters have nonferromagnetic materials that include conductive wires. A report indicated that a portion of a Swan-Ganz thermodilution catheter that was outside the patient melted during MR imaging. It was postulated that the high-frequency electromagnetic fields induced heating of either the wires within the thermodilution catheter or the radiopaque material used in the construction of the catheter.

This incident suggests that patients with this catheter or similar device that has conductive wires or other component parts, could be potentially injured during an MR examination. Furthermore, heating of the wire or lead of a temporary pacemaker (e.g., the RV Pacing Lead) is of at least a theoretical concern for any similar wire in the area of the transmit RF coil. Cardiac pacemaker leads are typically intravascular for most of their length and heat transfer and dissipation from the leads into the blood may prevent dangerous levels of lead heating to be reached or maintained for the intravascular segments of the leads.

It is theoretically possible that sufficient RF power deposition and heating may be induced within the leads (i.e., those unconnected to a pulse generator) to result in local tissue injury or burn during an MR procedure. An *ex vivo* study conducted by Achenbach et al. substantiates this, whereby temperature increases of up to 63.1 degrees C were recorded at the tips of pacemaker electrodes during MR imaging performed in phantoms. An investigation conducted by Shellock et al. (2005) further demonstrated that excessive temperatures can occur for unconnected cardiac pacing leads.

A case report by Masaki et al. described an iatrogenic second-degree burn caused by a catheter (percutaneous transluminal coronary angioplasty or PTCA) encased by tubular, braided stainless steel. The presence of this PTCA catheter caused a superficial burn of the abdomen during an MRI procedure performed at 1.5-Tesla and further illustrates the potential risks associated with cardiovascular catheters that are made from conducting, metallic materials.

Because of possible deleterious and unpredictable effects, patients referred for MR procedures with cardiovascular catheters and accessories that have internally or externally-positioned conductive wires or similar components should not undergo MR procedures without a thorough assessment of risk:benefit because of the possible associated risks, unless findings from MR imaging tests demonstrate otherwise. Further support of this recommendation is based on the fact that inappropriate use of monitoring devices during MR procedures is often the cause of patient injuries. For example, burns have resulted in the MR environment in association with the use of devices that utilize conductive wires.

[MR healthcare professionals are advised to contact the respective manufacturer in order to obtain the latest safety information to ensure patient safety relative to the use of an MR procedure.]

REFERENCES

Achenbach S, Moshage W, Diem B, Bieberle T, Schibgilla V, Bachmann K. Effects of magnetic resonance imaging on cardiac pacemakers and electrodes. Am Heart J 1997;134:467-473

Dempsey MF, Condon B, Hadley DM. Investigation of the factors responsible for burns during MRI. J Magn Reson Imaging 2001;13:627-631.

ECRI, Health devices alert. A new MRI complication? May 27, 1988.

Masaki F, Shuhei Y, Riko K, Yohjiro M. Iatrogenic second-degree burn caused by a catheter encased tubular braid of stainless steel during MRI. Burns. 2007;33:1077-9.

Shellock FG. Magnetic Resonance Procedures: Health Effects and Safety. CRC Press, LLC, Boca Raton, FL, 2001.

Shellock FG, Kanal E. Magnetic Resonance: Bioeffects, Safety, and Patient Management. Second Edition, Lippincott-Raven Press, New York, 1996.

Shellock FG, Shellock VJ. Cardiovascular catheters and accessories: *Ex vivo* testing of ferromagnetism, heating, and artifacts associated with MRI. J Magn Reson Imaging 1998;8:1338-1342.

Shellock FG, Valencerina S, Fischer L. MRI-related heating of pacemaker at 1.5- and 3-Tesla: Evaluation with and without pulse generator attached to leads. Circulation 112;Supplement II:561, 2005.

Carotid Artery Vascular Clamps

A carotid artery vascular clamp is a medical device that is surgically placed around the carotid artery and used to temporarily block blood flow through the carotid artery in order to treat a brain (cerebral) aneurysm. To date, each carotid artery vascular clamp tested in association with a 1.5-Tesla MR system displayed positive magnetic field interactions. However, only the Poppen-Blaylock carotid artery vascular clamp is considered contraindicated for patients undergoing MR procedures due to the existence of substantial ferromagnetism. The other carotid artery clamps were considered safe for patients exposed to MR systems because they were deemed "weakly" ferromagnetic. With the exception of the Poppen-Blaylock clamp, patients with the other carotid artery vascular clamps that have been evaluated for magnetic field interactions have been imaged by MR systems with static magnetic fields up to 1.5-Tesla without experiencing discomfort or neurological sequelae.

REFERENCES

Shellock FG. Magnetic Resonance Procedures: Health Effects and Safety. CRC Press, LLC, Boca Raton, FL, 2001.

Shellock FG, Kanal E. Magnetic Resonance: Bioeffects, Safety, and Patient Management. Second Edition, Lippincott-Raven Press, New York, 1996.

Teitelbaum GP, Lin MCW, Watanabe AT, et al. Ferromagnetism and MR imaging: safety of carotid vascular clamps. AJNR Am J Neuroradiol 1990;11:267-272.

Celsius Control System or Temperature Modulation Therapy

The **Celsius Control System** (or **Temperature Modulation Therapy**) Philips Innercool Systems, Philips Healthcare) provides physicians with state-of-the-art, endovascular technology that can safely and rapidly lower the patient's body temperature, precisely maintain a chosen target temperature, and rewarm the patient to normothermic levels.

Medical research suggests there are a number of potential clinical applications for the Celsius Control System such as inducing mild hypothermia in surgery, stroke, and heart attack or for temperature control in surgical and critical care procedures.

The Celsius Control System consists of an endovascular catheter, console and proprietary disposables. The distal portion of the catheter incorporates a flexible Temperature Control Element (TCE) that is cooled or warmed with saline solution circulated in a closed-loop manner from the console. When placed in the inferior vena cava, the TCE exchanges thermal energy directly with the blood, resulting in cooling or warming of the downstream organs and body. The Celsius Control System does not infuse fluid into the patient, nor is blood circulated outside of the body.

Celsius Control System

The Celsius Control System consists of a disposable endovascular heat transfer catheter, administration cassette, and a console. The distal portion of the catheter (10.7 Fr. and 14 Fr.) has a flexible, metallic temperature control element (TCE) that is cooled or warmed by sterile saline circulated within it from the Celsius Control Console. The administration cassette connects the catheter to the console, maintaining the sterility of the saline conduit. The TCE does not expand inside the body so the outer diameter of the TCE will remain consistent throughout the entire cooling/warming procedure unlike balloon based cooling systems which expand to outer diameters of 24 Fr.-47 Fr. during use.

Accutrol Catheter

The Accutrol Catheter contains an integrated temperature sensor, which can accurately determine the patient's core body temperature <u>within</u>

0.1°C of pulmonary artery temperature. The proprietary, novel Accutrol software control algorithm provides automated body temperature control. The Accutrol system eliminates the need to place bladder or rectal probes, which can be slow to react to actual decreases in core body temperature, may be uncomfortable to the patient, and time-consuming to place. The Accutrol catheter is beneficial in the critical care environment where gradual rewarming may be warranted.

Standard catheter
The Standard catheter incorporates the same design features as the Accutrol catheter including performance attributes. However, an external core temperature feedback probe is required for operation

MAGNETIC RESONANCE IMAGING (MRI)

The Celsius Control Catheter is "MR Conditional" according to the American Society for Testing and Materials (ASTM) International, Designation: F2503. Standard Practice for Marking Medical Devices and Other Items for Safety in the Magnetic Resonance Environment. The Celsius Control Catheter demonstrates no known hazards when a "head-only" MRI procedure is performed according to the conditions stated in this labeling.

It is important to read and understand this document in its entirety before conducting a head-only MRI (magnetic resonance imaging) procedure on a patient with an indwelling Celsius Control Catheter. Failure to strictly adhere to these guidelines may result in serious injury to the patient. This information applies to the following INNERCOOL Therapies products:

Catalog No.
11-10-65-1 Celsius Control Standard Catheter 10.7 Fr.
11-14-65-1 Celsius Control Standard Catheter 14 Fr.
11-10-65-2 Celsius Control Accutrol Catheter 10.7 Fr.
11-14-65-2 Celsius Control Accutrol Catheter 14 Fr

Warnings
-Disconnect Celsius Control Catheter from the Celsius Control Console completely prior to entering the MRI environment. Failure to do so may result in serious injury to the patient. It is not possible to continue therapy with the system during an MRI procedure.

-This labeling information applies to "head-only" MRI procedures conducted using a 1.5- Tesla transmit/receive RF head coil or a transmit RF body/receive-only head coil, *ONLY*.

MRI examinations of other parts of the body is strictly prohibited with the Celsius Control Catheter *in situ*.

-Testing has not been performed using other MR systems operating at other static magnetic field strengths (i.e., 1.5-Tesla, <u>*only*</u>) and, therefore, other scanners should not be used to perform an MRI examination on a patient who has an indwelling Celsius Control Catheter.

-The Celsius Control Catheter must be properly positioned per the directions for use with the catheter introduced through the femoral vein of either the left or right groin of the patient and advanced into the IVC such that the catheter is parallel to the bore of the MR system. Do not perform the MRI examination with the Celsius Control Catheter placed in any other configuration. Failure to follow this guideline may result in serious injury to the patient.

-Using the transmit/receive RF head coil, do not exceed an MR system reported, whole body averaged specific absorption rate (SAR) greater than 0.4-W/Kg.

-Using the transmit RF body coil/receive-only head coil, do not exceed an MR system reported, whole body averaged SAR of greater than 3.5-W/Kg.

Overview

The Celsius Control Catheter has undergone extensive *in vitro* testing to demonstrate that, by following specific guidelines, it is safe to perform a head-only MRI procedure on a patient with this device in a 1.5-Tesla MR system, ONLY. Variability among MR systems, differences in how scanners estimate or calculate specific absorption rates (SAR) cannot be simulated comprehensively using *in vitro* techniques. This document outlines recommended guidelines and specific conditions under which the Celsius Control Catheter has been shown to pose minimal risk to a patient undergoing a head only MRI procedure. Deviation from these guidelines may increase the potential for serious harm to the patient. MRI conditions utilizing MR systems with higher or lower static magnetic fields have not been assessed for the Celsius Control Catheter and, as such, must be avoided to ensure patient safety. The user of this information assumes full responsibility for the consequences of conducting a MRI examination on a patient with an indwelling Celsius Control Catheter.

Magnetic Field Interactions

Translation Attraction and Torque. Magnetic materials contained within an implanted or indwelling device may experience translational or rotational forces when brought into the static magnetic field of a MRI system. The Celsius Control Catheter contains relatively minor magnetic materials. In vitro testing demonstrated that the Celsius Control Catheter is not substantially affected by translational attraction and torque related to exposure to a 1.5 Tesla MR system.

MRI-Related Heating
Under certain conditions, RF fields generated by MRI can induce substantial currents in metallic components contained within medical device products. This may rapidly produce significant heating of a device. Failure to follow the recommendations contained in this communication may result in the generation of thermal lesions and serious patient harm. In vitro testing demonstrated that the Celsius Control Catheter is not substantially affected by the RF fields related to exposure to a 1.5 Tesla MR system under the conditions used for testing.

MRI Artifacts
The presence of the Celsius Control Catheter will cause moderate artifacts on the MR image depending on the pulse sequence parameters used for MRI. However, the artifacts are confined to the position of the Celsius Control Catheter and, as such, will not affect the diagnostic use of MR imaging for head only MRI examinations.

Procedure
In addition to standard safety procedures for MRI, the following precautions must be followed specific to the Celsius Control Catheter:

1) Inform the patient of the potential risks of undergoing a MRI procedure with the Celsius Control Catheter.
2) Disconnect all cables and patient monitoring devices attached to the Celsius Control Catheter prior to transporting the patient into the MRI environment.
3) The MRI procedure must be performed using a 1.5-Tesla MR system, *only*.
4) MRI examinations must be performed to image the *head only.* Use only the following types of radio frequency (RF) coils for the MRI procedure:
   a) Transmit/receive RF head coil
   b) Transmit body RF coil/receive-only head coil.
5) Using the transmit/receive RF head coil, do not exceed an MR system reported SAR of 0.4-W/kg. Using the transmit RF body coil/receive-only RF head coil, do not exceed an MR system reported SAR of 3.5-W/kg.
6) It is important to place the Celsius Control Catheter in a specific geometry to minimize the potential for excessive heating during the MRI procedure. The Celsius Control Catheter must be properly positioned as per the directions for use with the catheter introduced

through the femoral vein of either the left or right groin of the patient and advanced into the IVC such that the catheter is parallel to the bore of the MR system (but not touching the bore of the MR system). Do not perform the MRI examination with the Celsius Control Catheter placed in any other configuration. Failure to follow this guideline may result in serious injury to the patient.

7) Ensure that the proper patient weight is used for the SAR calculations. Verify that the MRI system has appropriately calculated and updated the SAR value after all parameter changes have been made.

8) A knowledgeable MRI expert (e.g., MRI physicist, MRI-trained radiologist, etc.) must verify that all set-up steps and settings have been properly implemented and checked prior to performing the head only MRI procedure.

9) Verify that all proposed MRI examination parameters and conditions for the Celsius Control Catheter comply with the instructions described herein. If they do not comply, do not perform the head only MRI procedure.

10) Provide the patient with a means by which he/she can alert the MR system operator during the MRI procedure if any discomfort or unusual sensations should occur.

11) Monitor the patient continuously during the head only MRI examination and be prepared respond or to terminate the MRI procedure immediately in the event of a complaint.

12) Determine if the patient has any other implants or conditions that would prohibit or contraindicate a head only MRI examination. Do not conduct a head only MRI examination if any conditions or implanted devices that would prohibit or contraindicate a MRI are present.

[MR healthcare professionals are advised to contact the manufacturer to ensure that the latest safety information is obtained and carefully followed in order to ensure patient safety relative to the use of an MR procedure.]

REFERENCE

www.Philips.com/Innercool

http://www.healthcare.philips.com/main/products/temperature_modulation_thera
py/index.wpd

Cerebrospinal Fluid (CSF) Shunt Valves

Hydrocephalus is the accumulation of cerebrospinal fluid in the brain, resulting from increased production, or more commonly, pathway obstruction or decreased absorption of the fluid. Cerebrospinal fluid (CSF) shunts have been used for decades for the treatment of hydrocephalus. A CSF shunt involves establishing an accessory pathway for the movement of CSF to bypass an obstruction of the natural pathways.

The shunt is positioned to enable the CSF to be drained from the cerebral ventricles or sub-arachnoid spaces into another absorption site (e.g., the right atrium of the heart or the peritoneal cavity) through a system of small catheters. A regulatory device, such as a valve, may be inserted into the pathway of the catheters. In general, the valve keeps the CSF flowing away from the brain and moderates the pressure or flow rate. Some valves are fixed pressure valves (i.e., monopressure valves) and others have adjustable or programmable settings. The drainage system using catheters and valves enables the excess CSF within the brain to be evacuated and, thereby, the pressure within the cranium to be reduced.

There are many different types of CSF shunt valves and associated accessories used for treatment of hydrocephalus. In general, for shunt valves that utilize magnetic components, highly specific safety guidelines must be followed in order to perform MRI procedures safely in patients with these devices.

CODMAN CERTAS Programmable Valve, CSF Shunt Valve (Codman, a Johnson & Johnson Company)

Warnings

- The use of Magnetic Resonance (MR) systems operating at 3 Tesla or less will not damage the valve mechanism and testing shows that the valve is resistant to unintended changes in the setting. However, it is recommended that the clinician confirm the valve setting after a magnetic resonance imaging (MRI) procedure.

- The valve setting is adjusted with the application and manipulation of strong magnets. A change to the valve setting is unlikely to occur under normal circumstances. However, magnetic fields should not be placed in close proximity to the valve due to the possibility of an unintentional setting change.

- Read *MRI Information* before performing an MRI procedure on a patient implanted with the valve.

Magnetic Resonance Imaging (MRI) Information

The CODMAN CERTAS Therapy Management System (TMS) is considered "MR Unsafe" in accordance with the American Society for Testing and Materials (ASTM) Standard F2503-05. Do not use the TMS in the MR suite. The CODMAN CERTAS Programmable Valve contains small metallic parts that are insulated and isolated from patient tissue by nonmetallic, non-conducting materials. There is no metal in contact with the patient. Non-clinical testing has demonstrated that the CODMAN CERTAS Programmable Valve is considered "MR Conditional" in accordance with ASTM F2503-05 and it can be scanned safely under the following conditions and specific guidelines at any time after implantation:

Conditions
- Static magnetic field of 3 Tesla or less.
- Highest spatial gradient magnetic field of 720 Gauss/cm or less.
- The MR system can be operated in either of the following modes:

-**Normal Operating Mode** (i.e., mode of operation of the MR EQUIPMENT in which none of the outputs has a value that might cause physiological stress to PATIENTS) only with a maximum whole-body averaged specific absorption rate of 2.0-W/kg.

- **First Level Controlled Operating Mode** (i.e., mode of operation of the MR EQUIPMENT in which one or more outputs reach a value that might cause physiological stress to PATIENTS that needs to be controlled by MEDICAL SUPERVISION) with a whole-body-averaged specific absorption rate of 4.0 W/kg.

Specific Guidelines. It is recommended that the valve setting be verified after the MRI procedure (see *Post Implantation Adjustment Procedure* Steps 1 through 3 in the *Instructions for Use*).

MRI TESTING INFORMATION
Static Magnetic Field. Translational attraction and torque associated with a 3 Tesla or lower field strength MR system are at levels that are less than those related to gravity and will not pose an additional hazard or risk to the patient in an MRI environment at 3 Tesla or less.

MRI-Related Heating. In non-clinical testing, the valve produced a temperature rise of 1.8 degrees C at a maximum MR system reported whole-body-averaged specific absorption rate (SAR) of 3.0 W/kg as assessed by calorimetry for 15 minutes of MR scanning (per pulse sequence) in a 3 T EXCITE MR Scanner, HDx, Software 14X.M5, General Electric Healthcare, Milwaukee, WI, USA.

MRI Artifacts. Artifacts were assessed using T1-weighted spin echo (SE) and gradient echo (GRE) pulse sequences. The details of these pulse sequences and the corresponding artifact sizes are listed in Table 2 (please refer to *Instructions for Use*). MR image quality might be compromised if the area of interest is in the exact location or relatively close to the location of the CODMAN CERTAS Programmable Valve. However, MRI artifacts can be minimized by careful selection of pulse sequence parameters. **Note:** The maximum artifact size, as seen on the gradient echo pulse sequence, extends approximately15-mm relative to the size and shape of the valve.

Codman Hakim Precision Valve, CSF Shunt Valve

Description. The CODMAN HAKIM Precision Fixed Pressure Valve (CSF shunt valve, Codman, a Johnson & Johnson Company, Raynham, MA) offers five distinct and narrow bandwidths to assure the correct pressure setting for each individual case. It also uses the proven ball and cone technology to insure that each pressure range is correct within a + / - 10mm H2O variance. The CODMAN HAKIM Precision Fixed Pressure Valve is available in eight basic configurations, and each of these configurations can be purchased with a unitized distal catheter or as a valve only.

The Codman Hakim Precision CSF Shunt Valve (CSF shunt valve, Codman, a Johnson & Johnson Company, Raynham, MA) is "MR Conditional" according to ASTM F2503. The valve demonstrates no known hazards when an MRI is performed under the following conditions:

- MRI can be performed at any time after implantation
- Use an MR system with a static magnetic field of 3-T or less
- Use an MR System with a spatial gradient of 720 gauss/cm or less
- Limit the exposure to RF energy to a whole-body-averaged specific absorption rate (SAR) of 3 W/kg for 15 minutes (per pulse sequence)

MR image quality may be compromised if the area of interest is relatively close to the device. Distortion may be seen at the boundaries of the artifact. Therefore, optimization of the MR imaging parameters may be necessary.

CODMAN HAKIM Programmable Valves

Description. The CODMAN HAKIM Programmable Valve (CSF shunt valve, Codman, a Johnson & Johnson Company, Raynham, MA) includes a valve mechanism that incorporates a flat 316L stainless steel spring in which the calibration is accomplished by a combination between a pillar and a micro-adjustable telescoping fulcrum. The valve chassis is made of titanium. The ball and cone are manufactured from synthetic ruby. Intraventricular pressure is maintained at a constant level by the ball and cone valve seat design.

The pressure setting of the spring in the inlet valve unit is noninvasively adjusted by the use of an external programmer, which activates the stepper motor within the valve housing. The programmer transmits a codified magnetic signal to the motor allowing eighteen pressure settings, ranging from 30 mm to 200 mm H_2O (294 to 1960 Pa) in 10 mm (98 Pa) increments. These are operating pressures of the valve unit and have been determined with a flow rate of 15 to 25 ml H_2O per hour.

The valve is classified by its working pressure with a specified flow rate and not by the opening and closing pressures. The pressure that a valve sustains with a given flow is the parameter that reflects the working pressure of the valve once it is implanted. Before shipment, each valve is calibrated with special equipment: Duplication of these test procedures cannot be accomplished in the operating room.

Indications. The CODMAN HAKIM Programmable Valves are implantable devices that provide constant intraventricular pressure and drainage of CSF for the management of hydrocephalus.

Programmable Valve Configurations

- In-line with SIPHONGUARD Device
- In-line
- Right Angle with SIPHONGUARD Device
- Right Angle
- Cylindrical with Prechamber
- Cylindrical
- Micro with RICKHAM® Reservoir
- Micro

CODMAN HAKIM In-line and Right Angle Valves include a programmable valve with a low profile and flat bottom, and an in-line or right angle integral reservoir with or without SIPHONGUARD.

CODMAN HAKIM Cylindrical Valves include a programmable valve, a pumping chamber, and an outlet valve available with or without a prechamber.

CODMAN HAKIM Micro Valves include a programmable valve with or without an integral RICKHAM reservoir.

WARNINGS. Subjecting the valve to strong magnetic fields may change the setting of the valve.

- The use of Magnetic Resonance (MR) systems up to 3-Tesla will not damage the valve mechanism, but may change the setting of the valve. Confirm the valve setting after an MRI procedure.
- Common magnets greater than 80 gauss, such as household magnets, loudspeaker magnets, and language lab headphone magnets may affect the valve setting when placed close to the valve.
- Magnetic fields generated from microwaves, high-tension wires, electric motors, transformers, etc., do not affect the valve setting.

Read the *MRI Information* before performing an MRI procedure on a patient implanted with the programmable valve.

MRI Information

The CODMAN HAKIM Programmable Valve (CSF shunt valve, Codman, a Johnson & Johnson Company, Raynham, MA) is "MR Conditional" according to ASTM F 2503. The valve demonstrates no known hazards when an MRI is performed under the following conditions:

- MRI can be performed at any time after implantation
- Use an MR system with a static magnetic field of 3 T or less
- Use an MR System with a spatial gradient of 720 gauss/cm or less
- Limit the exposure to RF energy to a whole-body-averaged specific absorption rate (SAR) of 3 W/kg for 15 minutes
- Verify the valve setting after the MRI procedure (see *Programming the Valve*)

In non-clinical testing, the valve produced a temperature rise of 0.4-degrees C at a maximum whole-body-averaged specific absorption rate

(SAR) of 3-W/kg for 15 minutes of MR scanning in a 3-T Excite General Electric MR scanner.

MR image quality may be compromised if the area of interest is relatively close to the device. Distortion may be seen at the boundaries of the artifact. Therefore, optimization of the MR imaging parameters may be necessary.

The following table provides a comparison between the signal void and imaging pulse sequence at 3-Tesla:

Signal Void	Pulse Sequence	Imaging plane
1,590-mm^2	T1-weighted, spin echo	Parallel
1,022-mm^2	T1-weighted, spin echo	Perpendicular
2,439-mm^2	Gradient echo	Parallel
2,404-mm^2	Gradient echo	Perpendicular

Delta Shunt Assembly

The Delta Shunt Assembly (Medtronic Neurosurgery, Goleta, CA) combines the Delta valve with an integral, open-end, radiopaque peritoneal catheter. All Delta shunt assemblies incorporate the same product features as the Delta valves. These include injectable reservoir domes, occluders for selective flushing, and a completely non-metallic design. The valves are fabricated of dissimilar materials - polypropylene and silicone elastomer - reducing the chance of valve sticking and deformation. The normally closed Delta chamber mechanism minimizes over-drainage by utilizing the principles of hydrodynamic leverage. Because of the non-metallic design, the Delta shunt is safe for patients undergoing MRI procedures.

POLARIS Adjustable Pressure Valve

The POLARIS Adjustable Pressure Valve (Sophysa USA, Inc., Crown Point, IN) has magnets made of Samarium-Cobalt, which are specially treated to preserve permanent magnetization, even after repeated exposure to MRI at 3-Tesla. The principle of the POLARIS Adjustable Pressure Valve is based on the variation in pressure exerted on a ball by a semicircular spring at different points along its curvature. The flat semicircular calibrated spring determines an operating pressure. Because of the unique design of the POLARIS Adjustable Pressure Valve, it is considered to be acceptable for patients undergoing MRI procedures at 3-Tesla or less.

Although the magnetic self-locking system for the POLARIS Adjustable Pressure Valve is designed to be insensitive to magnetic fields associated with exposure to MRI, it is recommended that the following procedure be performed when a patient undergoes an MRI examination:

1) Confirm the position of the rotor before entering the MR system room, using the locating instrument and the reading/adjustment instrument.
2) Perform the MRI examination.
3) Check the position of the rotor (i.e., the setting) as soon as the patient leaves the MR system room.
4) If the position of the rotor has changed, reset it to its original position using the reading/adjustment instrument following the described procedure.

proGAV Programmable Valve

The programmable valve, proGAV (Aesculap, Inc., Center Valley, PA), has magnetic components used for the programming mechanism. This device underwent evaluation relative to the use of a 3-Tesla MR system (i.e., tested for magnetic field interactions, heating, artifacts, and functional alterations). In consideration of the results of these tests, in order to take proper precautions to ensure patient safety, the following guidelines are recommended for scanning a patient with this device:

1) A patient with the programmable valve, proGAV, may undergo MRI at 3-T or less immediately after implantation.
2) Prior to MRI, the programmable valve setting should be determined by appropriate personnel using proper equipment.
3) The exposure to RF energy should be limited to a whole body averaged SAR of 2.1-W/kg for 15-min. (i.e., per pulse sequence)
4) After MRI, the proGAV programmable valve setting should be determined and re-set, as needed.

Pulsar Valve

The Pulsar Valve (Sophysa USA, Inc., Costa Mesa, CA) for CSF drainage is a monopressure valve. Its principal is based on the play of a silicone membrane, calibrated in low, medium, or high pressure, ensuring a proximal regulation of CSF flow through the shunt system. The Pulsar Valve is safe for patients undergoing MRI procedures.

Sophy Mini Monopressure Valve

The Sophy Mini Monopressure Valve (Sophysa USA, Inc., Costa Mesa, CA) for CSF drainage has a ball-in-cone mechanism. This device is safe for patients undergoing MRI procedures.

Strata, Strata II, and Strata NSC Programmable CSF Shunt Valves

MRI Information

The Strata, Strata NSC, and Strata II Programmable CSF shunt valves (Medtronic Neurosurgery, Goleta, CA) are Magnetic Resonance Conditional (MR conditional) in accordance with ASTM F2503. MRI systems of up to 3.0-Tesla may be used any time after implantation and will not damage the Strata, Strata NSC, or Strata II valve mechanisms, but can change the performance level setting. The performance level setting should always be checked before and after MRI exposure. The results of the tests performed to assess magnetic field interactions, artifacts, and heating, indicated the presence of the valves evaluated should present no substantial risk to a patient undergoing an MRI procedure using the following conditions:

- Static magnetic field of 3.0 Tesla or less
- Spatial gradient magnetic field of 720 Gauss/cm or less
- Radio Frequency (RF) Fields with an average Specific Absorption Rate (SAR) of 3 W/kg for 15 minutes. Using the GE 3T Excite HD Magnetic Resonance Imaging System, the valve experienced a maximum temperature change of 0.4°C over a 15 minute exposure period. The table below provides maximum signal voids (artifact sizes) for standard imaging pulse sequences at 3 Tesla per ASTM F2119.

Signal Void	Pulse Sequence	Imaging plane
35.16-cm^2	T1-weighted, spin echo	Parallel
33.03-cm^2	T1-weighted, spin echo	Perpendicular
75.91-cm^2	Gradient echo	Parallel
66.55-cm^2	Gradient echo	Perpendicular

Adjustment Kits

Do **NOT** take the Adjustment Tool into an MRI facility as these magnets could potentially be a safety hazard to the patient and/or user. Proximity to MRI suite may impede the mechanism in the Indicator Tool due to the field strength of an MRI magnet. Move out of the vicinity prior to attempting to verify a valve setting.

SOPHY Adjustable Pressure Valve

The principle of the SOPHY Adjustable Pressure Valve (Sophysa USA, Inc., Costa Mesa, CA) resides in the variation in pressure exerted on a ball by a semi-circular spring at various points along its circumference. The spring is attached to a magnetic rotor whose position can be noninvasively altered using an adjustment magnet. A series of indentations allows a variety of positions to be selected, each position representing a different pressure setting. The valve's ball-in-cone mechanism maintains the selected pressure constant without significant drift.

Because a magnetic component is associated with this device, special MR safety precautions exist for scanning patients with the SOPHY Adjustable Pressure Valve, as follows:

- The pressure settings should always be checked in case of shock on the implantation site.
- Changing pressure settings must only be performed by a neurosurgeon.
- The patient must be advised that carrying his Patient Identification Card is important and necessary for the follow-up of the clinical conditions.
- Patients undergoing MRI exposure should be advised that they might feel a small yet harmless effect due to MRI.
- The pressure settings should always be checked before and after MRI exposure, or after strong magnetic field exposure.
- The patient must be advised that in the case of implantation on the skull vibrations due to CSF flow may be perceived.
- Patients with implanted valve systems must be kept under close observation for symptoms of shunt failure.

[MR healthcare professionals are advised to contact the respective manufacturer in order to obtain the latest safety information to ensure patient safety relative to the use of an MR procedure.]

REFERENCES

Akbar M, et al. Adjustable cerebrospinal fluid shunt valves in 3.0-Tesla MRI: a phantom study using explanted devices. Rofo. 2010;182:594-602.

Anderson RCE, et al. Adjustment and malfunction of a programmable valve after exposure to toy magnets. J Neurosurg (Pediatrics) 2004;101:222-225.

Codman, a Johnson and Johnson Company, http://www.codman.com

Fransen P. Transcutaneous pressure-adjustable valves and magnetic resonance imaging: an ex vivo examination of the Codman-Medos programmable valve and the Sophy adjustable pressure valve. Neurosurgery 1998;42:430.

Fransen P, Dooms G, Thauvoy C. Safety of the adjustable pressure ventricular valve in magnetic resonance imaging: problems and solutions. Neuroradiology 1992;34:508-509.

Inoue T, et al. Effect of 3-Tesla magnetic resonance imaging on various pressure programmable shunt valves. J Neurosurg 2005;103(2 Suppl):163-5.

Lindner D, et al. Effect of 3-T MRI on the function of shunt valves--evaluation of Paedi GAV, Dual Switch and proGAV. Eur J Radiol 2005;56:56-9.

Lollis SS, et al. Programmable CSF shunt valves: radiographic identification and interpretation. AJNR Am J Neuroradiol. 2010;31:1343-6.

Ludemann W, Rosahl SK, Kaminsky J, Samii M. Reliability of a new adjustable shunt device without the need for readjustment following 3-Tesla MRI. Childs Nerv Syst 2005;21:227-229.

Medtronic Neurosurgery, Goleta, CA; Cerebral Spinal Fluid Shunt Valves and Accessories, http://www.medtronic.com/neurosurgery/shunts.html

Miwa K, Kondo H, Sakai N. Pressure changes observed in Codman-Medos programmable valves following magnetic exposure and filliping. Childs Nerv Syst 2001;17:150-153.

Ortler M, et al. Transcutaneous pressure-adjustable valves and magnetic resonance imaging: an ex vivo examination of the Codman-Medos programmable valve and the Sophy adjustable pressure valve. Neurosurgery 1997;40:1050-1057.

Schneider T, et al. Electromagnetic field hazards involving adjustable shunt valves in hydrocephalus. J Neurosurg 2002;96:331-334.

Shellock FG. MR safety and Cerebral Spinal Fluid Shunt (CSF) Valves. Signals, No. 51, Issue 4, pp. 10, 2004.

Shellock FG, Bedwinek A, Oliver-Allen M, Wilson SF. Assessment of MRI issues for a 3-T "immune" programmable CSF shunt valve. AJR Am J Roentgenol. 2011;197:202-7.

Shellock FG, Habibi R, Knebel J. Programmable CSF shunt valve: *In vitro* assessment of MRI safety at 3-Tesla. American Journal of Neuroradiology, 2006;27:661-665.

Shellock FG, Wilson SF, Mauge CP. Magnetically-programmable shunt valve: MRI at 3-Tesla. Magnetic Resonance Imaging 2007;25:1116-21.

Sophysa USA, Inc., Cerebral Spinal Fluid Shunt Valves and Accessories, http://www.sophysa.com

Toma AK, et al. Adjustable shunt valve-induced magnetic resonance imaging artifact: a comparative study. J Neurosurg. 2010;113:74-8.

Watanabe A, et al. Overdrainage of cerebrospinal fluid caused by detachment of the pressure control cam in a programmable valve after 3-tesla magnetic resonance imaging. J Neurosurg. 2010;112:425-7.

Zemack G, Romner B. Seven years of clinical experience with the programmable Codman Hakim valve: a retrospective study of 583 patients. J Neurosurg 2000;92:941-8.

Cochlear Implants

Cochlear implants are electronically-activated devices. Consequently, an MR procedure may be contraindicated for a patient with this type of implant because of the possibility of injuring the patient and/or altering or damaging the function of the device. In general, individuals with cochlear implants should be prevented from entering the MR environment unless specific guidelines exist to ensure safety for these devices.

Investigations have been conducted to determine if there are situations and specific conditions for a patient with a cochlear implant to safely undergo an MR procedure. These studies have resulted in highly specific guidelines that must be followed in order to safely perform MR examinations in patients with certain cochlear implants. Notably, some cochlear implants require the use of a 0.2-Tesla or 0.3-Tesla MR system, *only,* as part of the guidelines. In other cases, the magnet associated with the cochlear implant may require removal prior to the MRI examination and the replacement following the scan. Additional MRI concerns include possible demagnetization of the internal magnet associated with the cochlear implant be exposure to the powerful static magnetic field of the MR system, as well as the substantial artifacts that exist if this magnet remains in place during an MRI examination. See specific information below.

HiRes 90K Implant and MRI (Advanced Bionics, Sylmar, CA)*

Information for MRI Healthcare Workers
The HiRes 90K implant, with the internal magnet removed, has been tested with 1.5-Tesla/64-MHz and 0.3-Tesla/12-MHz MRI systems. MRI is contraindicated except under the circumstances described below.

Do not allow patients with a HiRes 90K cochlear implant to be in the area of an MRI system unless the following conditions have been met:

- The internal magnet must be surgically removed and replaced with the Magnet Insert Dummy before the patient undergoes an MRI procedure.
- The external sound processor and headpiece are removed before entering a room where an MRI scanner is located.

- MRI parameters should be selected to ensure a Specific Absorption Rate (SAR) of less than 1.0 W/kg in the head region.
- Continuous verbal and visual monitoring of the patient should be performed throughout the MRI procedure.

Image shadowing may extend as far as 7-cm squared area from the implant, resulting in loss of diagnostic information in the implant vicinity. The extent of the shadowing may be minimized by adjusting the signal parameters.

For additional information regarding the use of MRI with the HiRes 90K implant, please contact Advanced Bionics Technical Support.

Information for Patients

What is Magnetic Resonance Imaging? Magnetic resonance imaging (MRI) is a technique for taking remarkably clear and detailed pictures of internal organs and tissues using radio waves and a strong magnetic field.

When might a person be referred for an MRI? MRI is a sensitive exam for brain tumors, strokes, and certain chronic disorders of the nervous system such as multiple sclerosis. In addition, MRI might be recommended as a means of documenting disease of the cardiovascular system, pituitary gland, eye or inner ear.

Is the cochlear implant safe with MRI? Only after the magnet has been removed. As referrals for MRI are increasing, it is comforting to know that your implant is safe with this imaging technique. But you must be sure to have the magnet removed first.

The United States Food and Drug Administration (FDA) cleared the HiResolution Bionic Ear System's HiRes 90K implant for Magnetic Resonance Imaging (MRI) at 0.3-Tesla and 1.5-Tesla with the internal magnet removed.

The magnetic and electrical properties of an MRI machine can potentially cause harm to a patient with a cochlear implant and damage the device. Therefore a patient with a cochlear implant should not be near an MRI machine, whether or not in use, unless the following conditions have been met:

- Internal magnet has been removed
- External processor and headpiece have been removed

A cochlear implant recipient should always consult with their implant surgeon before any imaging is performed, regardless of the imaging technique.

If an MRI is needed, what are the steps required to remove the magnet of the cochlear implant? Removing the magnet is a quick and easy procedure typically performed under local anesthesia. Your surgeon will shave a small area of hair directly over the implant. A small incision will be made exposing the implant. The magnet is gently removed and replaced with a sterilized insert. The incision is then closed. You may experience some swelling and slight discomfort following the procedure.

Will I be able to wear my processor after the magnet is removed? Once the incision has healed, you will be able to wear your processor. You should check with your implant center before resuming device use. Your audiologist will assist you in coupling the headpiece to the implant. Typically, a small hair clip is attached to hold the headpiece in place over the implant.

Can the magnet be replaced after an MRI? Yes, your surgeon can replace the magnet after an MRI is completed, provided that further MRI evaluations are not anticipated. Under local anesthesia, your surgeon will shave the hair over the implant and make a small incision. The sterilized insert is removed and replaced with a new sterilized magnet ordered from Advanced Bionics.

If necessary, can the HiResolution Bionic Ear System's HiRes 90K be implanted without the magnet? Yes, your surgeon can elect to remove the magnet from the HiRes 90K before the device is implanted. In this case, the surgeon will order the sterilized insert with the device and replace the magnet with the sterilized insert at the time of surgery.

What recommendations should be provided to the radiologist/technologist when an MRI is ordered for a cochlear implant recipient? Your implant center can provide the MRI technologist or radiologist with the HiResolution Bionic Ear System's HiRes 90K package insert. Further instructions are provided when the implant center orders the sterilized insert or replacement magnet from Advanced Bionics that can be forwarded to the MRI technologist as well.

Are other imaging techniques available? How is MRI different? There are many imaging techniques used today including x-rays, computed tomography (CT) scans, positron emission tomography (PET) scans, and ultrasound. MRI requires specialized equipment and expertise and allows evaluation of some body structures that may not be as visible with other imaging methods. Your medical team will discuss these options with you and determine which technique is optimal for your healthcare needs.

What do we need to do if we want to replace the magnet after the MRI? Provided additional MRIs are not anticipated, the center can order a sterilized "replacement magnet" CI-1412 from Advanced Bionics' Customer Service. The replacement magnet will come with a surgical insert title "MRI for HiRes 90k implant" which provides detailed surgical instructions.

The Insert Dummy and Replacement Magnets are ordered SEPARATELY.

Can we implant the HiRes 90K without the magnet to begin with? Yes, order the Insert Dummy with the device. The surgical insert titled "MRI for HiRes 90K implant" that accompanies the insert dummy includes detailed surgical instructions for removing the magnet prior to implantation.

What specific recommendations can we provide the MRI technologist? The HiRes 90K implant is FDA approved for PRI testing at 0.3-Tesla and 1.5-Tesla with the magnet removed. The external hardware must also be removed before the patient enters the MRI testing room/suite. The center can provide the technologist with the "MRI for HiRes 90K implant" surgical insert that accompanies the insert dummy or replacement magnet.

[*Information provided with permission from Advanced Bionics, Sylmar, CA]

[MR healthcare professionals are advised to contact the manufacturer to ensure that the latest safety information is obtained and carefully followed in order to ensure patient safety relative to the use of an MR procedure.]

PULSAR COCHLEAR IMPLANT, PULSARCI[100] COCHLEAR IMPLANT, MED-EL CORPORATION

The Pulsar Cochlear Implant, PULSARCI[100] Cochlear Implant, MED-EL Corporation, Durham, NC) has the following information stated with regard to using MR imaging in patients with this device:

MRI Safe - Without Magnet Removal

Many cochlear implant users will require an MRI (Magnetic Resonance Imaging) scan at some point in their lifetime, so MRI compatibility is an important consideration when selecting a cochlear implant. MED-EL is the only cochlear implant manufacturer to offer MRI safety without surgical removal of the internal magnet. At MED-EL, we recognize the importance of providing access to critical medical treatment, including MRI, without disruption to your life or your hearing.

PULSARCI[100] is MRI safe at 0.2-Tesla

- No need for surgery to remove and replace the internal magnet
- No incision or swelling to heal after an MRI scan
- No recovery time to affect implant use or performance
- No additional risk to the patient
- No significant impact on MRI image quality
- No limitations on daily activities following an MRI scan
- No risk of magnet displacement

[MR healthcare professionals are advised to contact the manufacturer to ensure that the latest safety information is obtained and carefully followed in order to ensure patient safety relative to the use of an MR procedure.]

MED-EL, CONCERT Cochlear Implant, MED-EL Corporation

Magnetic Resonance Imaging. MED-EL must be consulted prior to conducting a 0.2 Tesla (T) MRI examination on any patient having a MED-EL CONCERT Device (www.medel.com)

-Do not, under any circumstance, scan a MED-EL CONCERT patient with field strength greater than 0.2 T

-Scanning at 0.2-T, confirm that the patient is positioned with the magnetic field of the internal magnet in the same orientation as the magnetic field of the scanner. This is necessary to minimize torque on the internal magnet and induced voltage in the receiver.

-Note that there exist many types of 0.2 T MRI scanners. In some, the coil used for head imaging is attached to the MRI bed (i.e., the scanner table). Further counseling and recommendations will be provided to the cochlear implant professional and radiologist in the event of head imaging.

-Bilaterally implanted MED-EL CONCERT patients, straight orientation of the head is acceptable

[MR healthcare professionals are advised to contact the manufacturer to ensure that the latest safety information is obtained and carefully followed in order to ensure patient safety relative to the use of an MR procedure.]

Nucleus 24 Series, Cochlear Implant (Cochlear Corporation)

Magnetic Resonance Imaging (MRI)

The Nucleus 24 cochlear implant and some Nucleus 22 cochlear implants have a removable magnet and specific design characteristics to enable it to withstand MRI up to 1.5 tesla, but not higher.

For patients with a Nucleus 22 cochlear implant without a removable magnet, MRI is contraindicated.

The Nucleus 24 cochlear implant has a removable magnet and specific design characteristics to enable it to withstand MRI up to 1.5 Tesla static field, a 64 MHz RF pulsed field, and pulsed gradient fields up to 20 Tesla/ sec. If the cochlear implant's magnet is in place, it must be removed surgically before the patient undergoes a MRI procedure.

Magnetic Resonance Imaging (MRI) is contraindicated except under the circumstances described below. Patients with a cochlear implant should not enter a room where a MRI scanner is located except under the following special circumstances. The patient must remove the speech processor and headset before entering a room where a MRI scanner is located.

If the implant's magnet is still in place, the implant may move, causing pain and/or tissue damage if the recipient is exposed to MRI. Once the magnet is surgically removed, the metal in the cochlear implant will affect the quality of the MRI, but no damage to the implant will occur. Image shadowing may extend as far as 6-cm from the implant, thereby resulting in loss of diagnostic information in the vicinity of the implant.

The MRI static field exerts a small force on the implant, even without the magnet. Without the magnet, the maximum force is less than the normal weight of the implant. This may be perceptible during the MRI procedure but is not harmful.

If there is doubt that the patient has a cochlear implant with a removable magnet, the physician should use an x-ray to check the radiopaque lettering on the implant. There are three platinum letters printed on each implant. If the middle letter is a "C", "H", "J", "L", "P", "T", "2", "5" or "7" the implant has a removable magnet. Once the magnet has been removed, MRI can be performed.

Removing the Magnet
(when the patient needs a single MRI)

If an implant user develops a condition likely to require a single MRI examination, the magnet must be surgically removed. Surgery is usually performed under local anesthetic in a minor procedure room. A local injection of lidoocaine with 1:100,000 or 1:200,000 Epinephrine is used. The area over the magnet is shaved and the area is prepared for the incision. A curved incision is made posterior to the implant. The surgeon cuts through any fibrous growth around the implant to expose the magnet.

If a retaining suture runs across the magnet, the surgeon may bend the suture to expose the magnet. A dry sterile dressing is applied over the wound and the patient is taken for MRI examination. The recess may remain empty, with sterility maintained for a period of up to four hours. After the examination, a sterile magnet is replaced and the wound closed. A sterile dressing is applied overnight.

Magnet Removal
(when it is anticipated that the patient will need repeated MRIs in the future)

If it is anticipated that a patient will need repeated MRIs in the future, the surgeon may elect to remove the magnet on a more long-term basis. If it is known prior to implantation that the patient will need repeated MRIs in the future, the surgeon may elect to remove the magnet from the implant prior to implantation.

In these cases, the magnet may be removed and replaced with a non-magnetic titanium plug. The plug prevents the growth of fibrous tissue into the recess, which could make the future placement of a magnet difficult.

If the device has not yet been implanted, the magnet should be removed under sterile conditions. The cochlear implant is removed from its sterile packaging and placed on a flat stable surface with the magnet's star symbol facing upward. The protective tubing should not be removed from the electrode array until implantation. Using an elevator, the lip of the silicone recess may be gently lifted in order to shell the magnet out of the recess. When removing the magnet, the pressure applied to the antenna of the implant should be minimized. If the device is already implanted, a similar method should be used to shell out the magnet while leaving the device in-situ. The sterile non-magnetic plug may then be inserted into the recess.

Replacing the Magnet

The magnet is replaced when there is no further need for MRI examinations. After exposure of the magnet recess, an elevator may be used to lift the lip of the recess and position the magnet. A sterile magnet should be inserted with the star symbol (denoting polarity) facing up. The wound is closed and a sterile dressing is applied.

Note to MR Healthcare Professionals: Different MRI guidelines exist for different countries. As such, use the appropriate information for your country. Visit www.Cochlear.com to obtain the proper information.

[MR healthcare professionals are advised to contact the respective manufacturer in order to obtain the latest safety information to ensure patient safety relative to the use of an MR procedure.]

REFERENCES

Chou H-K, et al. Absence of radiofrequency heating from auditory implants during magnetic resonance imaging. Bioelectromagnetics 1995;16:307-316.

Deneuve S, Loundon N, et al. Cochlear implant magnet displacement during magnetic resonance imaging. Otol Neurotol. 2008;29:789-190.

Gubbels SP, McMenomey SO. Safety study of the Cochlear Nucleus 24 device with internal magnet in the 1.5 Tesla magnetic resonance imaging scanner. Laryngoscope. 2006;116:865-71.

Heller JW, et al. Evaluation of MRI compatibility of the modified nucleus multi-channel auditory brainstem and cochlear implants. Am J Otol 1996;17:724-729.

http://www.Cochlear.com

http://www.MEDEL.com

Majdani O, Rau TS, Gotz F, et al. Artifacts caused by cochlear implants with non-removable magnets in 3T MRI: phantom and cadaveric studies. Eur Arch Otorhinolaryngol. 2009;266:1885-90

Majdani O, et al. Demagnetization of cochlear implants and temperature changes in 3.0T MRI environment. Otolaryngol Head Neck Surg. 2008;139:833-9.

Ouayoun M, et al. Nuclear magnetic resonance and cochlear implant. Ann Otolaryngol Chir Cervicofac 1997;114:65-70.

Shellock FG. Magnetic Resonance Procedures: Health Effects and Safety. CRC Press, LLC, Boca Raton, FL, 2001.

Teissl C, Kremser C, Hochmair ES, Hochmair-Desoyer IJ. Cochlear implants: *in vitro* investigation of electromagnetic interference at MR imaging-compatibility and safety aspects. Radiology 1998;208:700-708.

Teissl C, Kremser C, Hochmair ES, Hochmair-Desoyer IJ. Magnetic resonance imaging and cochlear implants: compatibility and safety aspects. J Magn Reson Imaging 1999;9:26-38.

Coils, Stents, Filters, and Grafts

Coils, stents, filters and vascular grafts have been evaluated relative to the use of MR systems. Several of these demonstrated magnetic field interactions. Fortunately, the devices that exhibited positive magnetic field interactions typically become incorporated securely in tissue within six weeks after implantation due to ingrowth and other mechanisms. Therefore, for most coils, filters, stents and grafts that have been tested, it is unlikely that these implants would become moved or dislodged as a result of exposure to MR systems operating at 1.5-Tesla or less. Additionally, many of these items have been evaluated at 3-Tesla (see below). MRI-related heating may also be of concern for certain configurations or shapes for coils, stents, filters, and vascular grafts.

Many of these implants are made from nonferromagnetic materials, such as the LGM IVC filter (Vena Tech) used for caval interruption and the Wallstent biliary endoprosthesis [Schneider (USA), Inc.] used for treatment of biliary obstruction. As such, these implants are acceptable for patients undergoing MR procedures relative to the use of the particular field strength utilized in the *ex vivo* testing (for specific information, see **The List**). Notably, it is unnecessary to wait after surgery to perform an MR procedure in a patient with a "passive" metallic implant that is made from a nonmagnetic material (see **Guidelines for the Management of the Post-Operative Patient Referred for a Magnetic Resonance Procedure**). In fact, there are reports in the peer-reviewed literature that describe placement of vascular stents or other similar devices using MR-guidance at 1.5-Tesla and 3-Tesla.

Patients with the specific coils, stents, filters and vascular grafts indicated in **The List** have had procedures using MR systems operating at static magnetic field strengths of 3-Tesla or less without reported injuries or other problems. Despite the past track record of safety, MRI facilities should never have a "general" policy to scan patients with these implants if the acceptable MRI conditions are unknown or if there is no specific MRI labeling available. One of the reasons for this is that new coils, stents, filters, and vascular grafts are developed on an ongoing basis. Additionally, to date, not all such devices have undergone comprehensive MRI testing, including with respect to the 3-Tesla MRI environment.

A study by Taal et al. supports the fact that not all stents are safe for patients undergoing MR procedures. This investigation was performed to evaluate potential problems for four different types of stents: the Ultraflex (titanium alloy), the covered Wallstent (Nitinol), the Gianturco stent (Cook), and the modified Gianturco stent (Song) - the last two are made from stainless steel. Taal et al. reported "an appreciable attraction force and torque" found for both types of Gianturco stents. Taal et al. stated, "the Gianturco (Cook) stent pulled toward the head with a force of 7 g…however, it is uncertain whether this is a potential risk for dislodgment." In consideration of these results, the investigators advised, "…specific information on the type of stent is necessary before a magnetic resonance imaging examination is planned."

Zenith Flex AAA Endovascular Graft (MRI information and labeling includes the Zenith AAA Spiral Z Iliac Leg Graft)

Recently, the MRI labeling information was revised for the Zenith Flex AAA Endovascular Graft (Cook Incorporated) which was previously labeled as a contraindicated implant. As such, this illustrates the need to remain informed and up to date with regard to MRI information for implants and devices, since the information may change. The revised MRI information applies to the following Zenith devices:

- Zenith AAA Endovascular Grafts (main body and iliac legs)
- Zenith Flex AAA Endovascular Grafts (main body, iliac legs and main body extensions)
- Zenith AAA Endovascular Graft Ancillary Components (main body extensions, iliac leg extensions, converters, occluders and iliac plugs)
- Zenith Renu AAA Ancillary Grafts (main body extension and converter configurations)
- Zenith TX2 TAA Endovascular Grafts (proximal components, proximal-tapered components, distal components, proximal extensions and distal extensions)

The current MRI labeling information for the Zenith Flex AAA Endovascular Graft (Cook Incorporated) is, as follows (excerpted from the IFU):

MRI Information

Non-clinical testing has demonstrated that the Zenith AAA Endovascular Graft is MR Conditional. It can be scanned safely under the following conditions:

Static Magnetic Field

Static magnetic field of 3.0 Tesla or less.

Spatial magnetic gradient field of 720 Gauss/cm

MRI-Related Heating, 1.5 Tesla Systems

Maximum whole body averaged specific absorption rate (SAR) of 2W/kg for 15 minutes of scanning (i.e., per pulse sequence). In non-clinical testing, the Zenith AAA Endovascular Graft produced a temperature rise of less than or equal to 1.4 degrees C at a maximum MR system reported, whole body averaged specific absorption rate (SAR) of 2.8 W/kg, as assessed by calorimetry for 15 minutes of MR scanning (i.e., per pulse sequence) in a 1.5 Tesla Magnetom, Siemens Medical Magnetom, Numaris/4 Software, Version Syngo MR 2002B DHHS MR Scanner. The maximum MR system reported, whole body averaged specific absorption rate (SAR) was 2.8 W/kg, which corresponds to a calorimetry measured value of 1.5 W/kg.

MRI-Related Heating, 3.0 Tesla Systems

Maximum whole body averaged specific absorption rate (SAR) of 2 W/kg for 15 minutes of scanning (i.e., per pulse sequence). In non-clinical testing, the Zenith AAA Endovascular Graft produced a temperature rise of less than or equal to 1.9 degrees C at a maximum MR system reported, whole body averaged specific absorption rate (SAR) of 3.0 W/kg, as assessed by calorimetry for 15 minutes of MR scanning in a 3.0 Tesla Excite, GE Electric Healthcare, G3.0-052B Software, MR Scanner. The maximum MR system reported, whole body averaged specific absorption rate (SAR) was 3.0 W/kg, which corresponds to a calorimetry measured value of 2.8 W/kg.

Artifacts

The image artifact extends throughout the anatomical region containing the device, obscuring the view of immediately adjacent anatomical structures within approximately 20 cm of the device, as well as the entire device and its lumen, when scanned in nonclinical testing using the sequence: Fast spin echo, in a 3.0 Tesla, Excite, GE Electric Healthcare, with G3.0-052B software, MR system with body radiofrequency coil.

For all scanners, the image artifact dissipates as the distance from the device to the area of interest increases. MR scans of the head and neck and lower extremities may be obtained without image artifacts. Image artifacts may be present in scans of the abdominal region and upper extremities, depending on the distance from the device to the area of interest.

Clinical information is available for seventeen patients who received MRI scans after stent-graft implantation. There have been no reported adverse events or device problems in any of these patients as a result of having received an MRI. Additionally, there have been approximately 100,000 Zenith AAA Endovascular Grafts distributed world wide, in which there have been no reported adverse events or device problems as a result of MRI.

MRI at 3-Tesla and Coils, Stents, Filters and Vascular Grafts. Different coils, stents, filters and vascular grafts have been evaluated at 3-Tesla. Of these implants, two displayed magnetic field interactions that exceeded the American Society for Testing and Materials (ASTM) International guideline for safety (i.e., the deflection angles were greater than 45 degrees). However, similar to other comparable implants, tissue ingrowth and other mechanims are sufficient to prevent them from posing a substantial risk to a patient or individual in the 3-Tesla MR environment. Thus, these issues warrant further consideration.

MRI at 3-Tesla: Bare Metal and Drug Eluting Coronary Stents. Patients with coronary artery disease are often treated by percutaneous transluminal coronary angioplasty (PTCA). Re-narrowing at the angioplasty site, or restenosis, occurs in as many as 50% of patients following PTCA. Therefore, after coronary artery intervention, either a bare metal or drug eluting stent may be placed in an effort to prevent restenosis.

MRI information has been obtained for many bare metal and drug eluting coronary artery stents, which have been reported to be acceptable for patients undergoing MR procedures at 3-Tesla or less (i.e., based on assessments of magnetic field interactions and MRI-related heating). Of note is that, for most of these coronary artery stents, patients with these implants may undergo MRI procedures immediately after placement. Please refer to **The List** for specific information.

REFERENCES

Ahmed S, Shellock FG. Magnetic resonance imaging safety: implications for cardiovascular patients. Journal of Cardiovascular Magnetic Resonance 2001;3:171-181.

Bueker A, et al. Real-time MR fluoroscopy for MR-guided iliac artery stent placement. J Magn Reson Imaging 2000;12:616-622.

Girard MJ, et al. Wallstent metallic biliary endoprosthesis: MR imaging characteristics. Radiology 1992;184:874-876.

Green SR, Gianchandani YB. Wireless magnetoelastic monitoring of biliary stents. Journal of Microelectromechanical Systems. 2009;18:64-78.

http://www.cookmedical.com/ai/productMri.do

http://www.cookmedical.com/di/productMri.do

http://www.cookmedical.com/ai/resourceJsp.do?mediaId=1581&id=5230&label=
MRI_Compatibility&file=zenithMRIfaq.jsp

Hennemeyer CT, Wicklow K, Feinberg DA, Derdeyn CP. In vitro evaluation of
platinum Guglielmi detachable coils at 3-T with a porcine model: safety
issues and artifacts. Radiology 2001;219:732-737.

Hiramoto JS, Reilly LM, Schneider DB, et al. Long-term outcome and
reintervention after endovascular abdominal aortic aneurysm repair using the
Zenith stent graft. J Vasc Surg. 2007;45:461-452

Hiramoto JS, et al. The effect of magnetic resonance imaging on stainless-steel Z-
stent-based abdominal aortic prosthesis. J Vasc Surg. 2007;45:472-474

Hug J, et al. Coronary arterial stents: safety and artifacts during MR imaging.
Radiology 2000;216:781-787.

Kaya MG, et al. Long-term clinical effects of magnetic resonance imaging in
patients with coronary artery stent implantation. Coron Artery Dis. 2009;
20:138-42.

Kiproff PM, et al. Magnetic resonance characteristics of the LGM vena cava
filter: technical note. Cardiovasc Intervent Radiol 1991;14:254-255.

Leibman CE, Messersmith RN, Levin DN, et al. MR imaging of inferior vena
caval filter: safety and artifacts. AJR Am J Roentgenol 1988;150:1174-1176.

Manke C, Nitz WR, Djavidani B, et al. MR imaging-guided stent placement in
iliac arterial stenoses: A feasibility study. Radiology 2001;219:527-534.

Marshall MW, Teitelbaum GP, Kim HS, et al. Ferromagnetism and magnetic
resonance artifacts of platinum embolization microcoils. Cardiovasc
Intervent Radiol 1991;14:163-166.

Nehra A, Moran CJ, Cross DT, Derdeyn CP. MR safety and imaging of
Neuroform Stents at 3-T. Am J Neuroradiol 2004;25:1476-1478.

Patel M, Albert TSE, Kandzari DE, et al. Acute myocardial infarction: safety of
cardiac MR imaging after percutaneous revascularization with stents.
Radiology 2006;674-680.

Porto I, Selvanayagam J, Ashar V, Neubauer S, Banning AP. Safety of magnetic
resonance imaging one to three days after bare metal and drug-eluting stent
implantation. Am J Cardiol 2005;96:366-8.

Rutledge JM, Vick GW, Mullins CE, Grifka RG. Safety of magnetic resonance
immediately following Palmaz stent implant: a report of three cases.
Catheter Cardiovasc Interv 2001;53:519-523.

Shellock FG. MR Safety at 3-Tesla: Bare Metal and Drug Eluting Coronary
Artery Stents. Signals No. 53, Issue 2, pp. 26-27, 2005.

Shellock FG. Biomedical implants and devices: assessment of magnetic field
interactions with a 3.0-Tesla MR system. J Magn Reson Imaging
2002;16:721-732.

Shellock FG. Magnetic Resonance Procedures: Health Effects and Safety. CRC
Press, LLC, Boca Raton, FL, 2001.

Shellock FG, Detrick MS, Brant-Zawadski M. MR-compatibility of the Guglielmi detachable coils. Radiology 1997;203:568-570.

Shellock FG. Forder J. Drug eluting coronary stent: *In vitro* evaluation of magnetic resonance safety at 3-Tesla. Journal of Cardiovascular Magnetic Resonance 2005;7:415-419.

Shellock FG, Gounis M, Wakhloo A. Detachable coil for cerebral aneurysms: *In vitro* evaluation of magnet field interactions, heating, and artifacts at 3-Tesla. American Journal of Neuroradiology 2005;26:363-366.

Shellock FG, Morisoli S, Kanal E. MR procedures and biomedical implants, materials, and devices: 1993 update. Radiology 1993;189:587-599.

Shellock FG, Shellock VJ. Stents: Evaluation of MRI safety. Am J Roentgenol 1999;173:543-546.

Sommer T, et al. High field MR imaging: magnetic field interactions of aneurysm clips, coronary artery stents and iliac artery stents with a 3.0 Tesla MR system. Rofo Fortschr Geb Rontgenstr Neuen Bildgeb Verfahr 2004;176:731-8.

Spuentrup E, et al. Magnetic resonance-guided coronary artery stent placement in a swine model. Circulation 2002;105:874-879.

Taal BG, Muller SH, Boot H, Koop W. Potential risks and artifacts of magnetic resonance imaging of self-expandable esophageal stents. Gastrointestinal Endoscopy 1997;46;424-429.

Teitelbaum GP, Bradley WG, Klein BD. MR imaging artifacts, ferromagnetism, and magnetic torque of intravascular filters, stents, and coils. Radiology 1988;166:657-664.

Teitelbaum GP, Lin MCW, Watanabe AT, et al. Ferromagnetism and MR imaging: safety of cartoid vascular clamps. AJNR Am J Neuroradiol 1990;11:267-272.

Teitelbaum GP, Ortega HV, Vinitski S, et al. Low artifact intravascular devices: MR imaging evaluation. Radiology 1988;168:713-719.

Teitelbaum GP, Raney M, Carvlin MJ, et al. Evaluation of ferromagnetism and magnetic resonance imaging artifacts of the Strecker tantalum vascular stent. Cardiovasc Intervent Radiol 1989;12:125-127.

Watanabe AT, Teitelbaum GP, Gomes AS, et al. MR imaging of the bird's nest filter. Radiology 1990;177:578-579.

Cranial Flap Fixation Clamps and Similar Devices

After performing a craniotomy, bone flaps are typically fixed with wire, suture material, or small plates and screws. Problems related to cranial bone flap fixation after craniotomy are more common with the trend for performing smaller craniotomies that are frequently utilized for minimally invasive surgical procedures. The use of small plates and screws for fixation of cranial bone flaps has improved the overall attachment process and end result. However, this technique requires a considerable amount of time and expense compared to using wire and suture techniques.

Because of the various problems with bone flap fixation, a special metallic implant system, named the Craniofix (Aesculap, Inc., Central Valley, PA) was developed for fixation of cranial bone flaps after craniotomy. MR tests conducted to assess magnetic field interaction, heating, and artifacts indicated that the clamps used for the cranial bone flap fixation system present no risk to the patient in the MR environment of MR systems operating at 1.5-Tesla or less. Furthermore, the quality of the diagnostic MR images was acceptable, particularly for the use of conventional spin echo or fast spin echo pulse sequences. Other similar devices used for these applications have been evaluated for MRI issues.

MRI at 3-Tesla and Cranial Fixation Implants and Devices. Several different cranial or burr hole fixation implants and devices made from titanium or titanium alloy have been tested at 3-Tesla. These were found to be acceptable for patients undergoing MR procedures.

CranioFix Titanium Clamps (Information dated 11/11/09 - Aesculap Inc., Center Valley, PA) are indicated for the fixation of cranial bone flaps after a craniotomy. They are manufactured from a titanium alloy (Ti_6Al_4V) which is non-ferromagnetic and may be safely exposed to MRI. All CranioFix Titanium Clamps (FF099T, FF100T, FF101T, FF490T, FF491T, and FF492T) have been tested and proven acceptable for MRI procedures up to and including 3-Tesla.

For additional information, please refer to the following publications:

(1) Shellock, F.G. (2010). Reference manual for MR safety, implants, and devices. Los Angeles: Biomedical Research Publishing Group, 2011.

(2) Shellock, F.G. (2002). Biomedical implants and devices: Assessment of magnetic field interactions with a 3.0 Tesla MR system. JMRI, 16, 721-732

*These Aesculap devices were cleared by the FDA as "MR-Safe" per ASTM-2052-02. Due to a change in definition within this standard, F 2503, these devices are now termed as "MR Conditional" according to the new terminology. The FDA has not mandated a revision to the labeling because the device material and performance have not changed.

REFERENCES

Shellock FG. Biomedical implants and devices: assessment of magnetic field interactions with a 3.0-Tesla MR system. J Magn Reson Imaging 2002;16:721-732.

Shellock FG. Magnetic Resonance Procedures: Health Effects and Safety. CRC Press, LLC, Boca Raton, FL, 2001.

Shellock FG, Shellock VJ. Evaluation of cranial flap fixation clamps for compatibility with MR imaging. Radiology 1998;207:822-825.

Shellock FG, Woods TO, Crues JV. MRI labeling information for implants and devices: Explanation of terminology. Radiology 2009;253:26-30.

Dental Implants, Devices, and Materials

Many of the dental implants, devices, materials, and objects evaluated for ferromagnetic qualities exhibited measurable deflection forces (e.g., brace bands, brace wires, etc.) but only the ones with magnetically-activated components appear to present potential problems for patients during MR procedures (also, see **Magnetically-Activated Implants and Devices**). The issues that exist for magnetically-activated dental implants include possible demagnetization of the magnetic components and the substantial artifacts that these magnets produce on MR imaging.

In general, most dental implants, devices, and materials made from ferromagnetic materials tend to be held in place with sufficient counter-forces to prevent them from causing problems related to movement or dislodgment in association with MR systems operating 3-Tesla or less.

REFERENCES

Blankenstein FH, et al. Signal loss in magnetic resonance imaging caused by intraoral anchored dental magnetic materials. Rofo. 2006;178:787-93.

Gegauff A, Laurell KA, Thavendrarajah A, et al. A potential MRI hazard: forces on dental magnet keepers. J Oral Rehabil 1990;17:403-410.

Hubalkova H, La Serna P, Linetskiy I, Dostalova T. Dental alloys and magnetic resonance imaging. Int Dent J. 2006;56:135-41.

Lissac MI, Metrop D, Brugigrad, et al. Dental materials and magnetic resonance imaging. Invest Radiol 1991;26:40-45.

New PFJ, Rosen BR, Brady TJ, et al. Potential hazards and artifacts of ferromagnetic and nonferromagnetic surgical and dental materials and devices in nuclear magnetic resonance imaging. Radiology 1983;147:139-148.

Shellock FG. *Ex vivo* assessment of deflection forces and artifacts associated with high-field strength MRI of "mini-magnet" dental prostheses. Magn Reson Imaging 1989;7 (Suppl 1):38.

Shellock FG. Magnetic Resonance Procedures: Health Effects and Safety. CRC Press, LLC, Boca Raton, FL, 2001.

Shellock FG, Crues JV. High-field strength MR imaging and metallic biomedical implants: an *ex vivo* evaluation of deflection forces. Am J Roentgenol 1988;151:389-392.

Diaphragms

A contraceptive diaphragm may have a metallic ring that maintains it in position during use. Thus, certain contraceptive diaphragms with metallic components may display positive magnetic field interactions in association with exposure to MR systems and, because of the metallic parts, substantial artifacts may be found. MR examinations have been performed in patients with these devices without complaints or adverse sensations related to movement. Furthermore, there is no danger of heating for a contraceptive diaphragm during an MR procedure under conditions currently recommended by the United States Food and Drug Administration. Therefore, the presence of a contraceptive diaphragm is not a contraindication for a patient undergoing an MR examination using an MR system operating at 3-Tesla or less. Regardless of the afore-mentioned information, it is best to remove a contraceptive diaphragm prior to an MRI examination.

REFERENCES

Shellock FG. Magnetic Resonance Procedures: Health Effects and Safety. CRC Press, LLC, Boca Raton, FL, 2001.

Shellock FG, Kanal E. Magnetic Resonance: Bioeffects, Safety, and Patient Management. Second Edition, Lippincott-Raven Press, New York, 1996.

Dressings Containing Silver and MRI Procedures

Clarification: Antimicrobial Dressings Containing Silver Aren't Necessarily Hazardous during MR Scans*

[*ECRI Institute. Antimicrobial dressings containing silver may cause pain and burns during MR scans [Hazard Report and clarification]. Health Devices 2007 Jul;36(7):232-3 and 2008 Feb; 37(2):60-2. Copyright 2007, 2008 ECRI Institute. Content reprinted with permission.]

In our July 2007 issue, we published a Hazard Report titled "Antimicrobial Dressings Containing Silver May Cause Pain and Burns during MR Scans" in which we reported on a patient who suffered pain during a magnetic resonance (MR) scan. The patient was wearing dressings containing silver, which acts as an antimicrobial agent. We discussed the possibility that the silver in the dressings might have been heated by the radio-frequency (RF) energy that is present during any MR scan.

Our report on this incident has given some readers the impression that patients wearing dressings containing silver should never undergo MR scans. That is not the case. We are publishing this update to further explain the issue and clarify our recommendations. In particular, we want to make the following points clear:

First, the fact that a patient is wearing silver-containing dressings should not keep the patient from having an MR examination.

Second, the reason that some silver-containing dressings are contraindicated by the dressing manufacturer for use during MR scans is because they could produce artifacts and distortions in the MR image, not because of any risk they might pose to the patient (although such risk cannot be conclusively ruled out).

Third, the exact cause of the patient's pain in the reported incident was never determined; the silver-containing dressings are only one of the possible causes.

DISCUSSION

Our position on silver-containing dressings in MR scans. We believe that the presence of antimicrobial dressings containing silver should not disqualify a patient from undergoing an MR scan. We do advise, whenever feasible, that such dressings be removed before a scan and that the wound be washed with water to remove as many traces of silver as possible. The reason for doing so is to minimize any detrimental effects the silver might have on the quality of the image. If it isn't feasible to remove the dressings, we believe the scan should still be carried out.

However, clinicians should be aware that there may be a risk, albeit remote, that the silver in the dressing— some of which will have been absorbed into the wound and its exudate—could become heated by the RF energy present during the scan (see Possible Causes of Pain, below). As in any MR procedure, the patient should be monitored closely, and any report of unusual pain or heating should be promptly addressed, as described in our Recommendations.

Note that the dressings are only likely to be a concern if the dressed area will be included in the scanned area. If, for example, a head scan is being performed and there are silver-containing dressings on the patient's foot, there is probably no reason the dressings need to be disturbed.

Possible causes of pain.

In the reported incident, the patient was an amputee whose stump was being scanned. The stump had been covered with silver-containing dressings. During the MR acquisition, the patient experienced significant pain, and the scan was aborted.

A week later, the study was continued, after the dressing had been removed and the wound lightly washed with water at the advice of the dressing manufacturer. However, the patient still experienced significant pain, and the reporting hospital noted that the amputation stump retained a silvery sheen despite the washing. It was suspected that the MR energy had interacted with the silver. But no further testing was undertaken to verify that suspicion.

Silver is not ferromagnetic, so the patient's pain could not have been caused by any magnetic effects of the MR field on the silver. As discussed above, though, MR scans create RF energy, which can induce electrical currents within electrical conductors. These currents can cause heating and lead to patient burns. This has been previously reported by Wagle and Smith (2000) and Franiel et al. (2006). However, empirical testing with implants and devices shows that excessive heating only occurs for those that have an elongated shape forming a closed loop of a certain diameter (Dempsey and Condon 2001). In the case that we reported, it is conceivable that the silver formed a large conducting loop around the wound; but the large amount of silver that would be needed makes this unlikely. Also, although the patient felt a burning sensation, there were no visible signs of a burn. So the evidence is far from conclusive.

RECOMMENDATIONS

Until further empirical testing is done to establish the required conditions, if any, necessary to produce a heating effect, the following revised recommendations should be followed:

1) Alert MR healthcare workers that some silver-containing antimicrobial dressings are contraindicated for MR exams in order to avoid artifacts. Therefore, if contraindicated dressings are close to the region being scanned or within the transmit RF coil, they should be removed if possible. However, a patient wearing such a dressing should not be prevented from having an MR procedure.

2) In some cases, it may be possible to reapply the same dressing to the patient after the scan. Whether this can be done depends in part on the amount of exudates on the dressing. The decision to reapply a dressing must be made by qualified staff.

3) As with any MR procedure, the patient should be carefully monitored and instructed to immediately report any unusual pain or heating. All such cases should be investigated immediately. If it is not possible to determine the cause of the pain and alleviate the problem (e.g., by applying a cold compress), then the procedure should be abandoned.

4) Report any similar occurrences of patient pain or burns to the dressing manufacturer and to ECRI Institute. Full details of the procedure should be recorded, including the field strength, coil used, and scan parameters.

REFERENCES

Dempsey MF, Condon B. Thermal injuries associated with MRI. Clin Radiol. 2001 Jun;56:457-65

Franiel T, Schmidt S, Klingebiel R. First-degree burns on MRI due to nonferrous tattoos. AJR Am J Roentgenol. 2006;187(5):W556

Tope WD, Shellock FG. Magnetic resonance imaging and permanent cosmetics (tattoos): survey of complications and adverse events. J Magn Reson Imaging. 2002;15:180-4.

Wagle WA, Smith M. Tattoo-induced skin burn during MR imaging. AJR Am J Roentgenol. 2000;174:1795.

Wagner M, Lanfermann H, Zanella F. MR-induced burn-reaction in a female patient with "permanent make-up" Rofo. 2006;178:728-30.

Yuh WT, Fisher DJ, Shields RK, Ehrhardt JC, Shellock FG. Phantom limb pain induced in amputee by strong magnetic fields. J Magn Reson Imaging. 1992;2:221-3.

Dressings Containing Silver and MRI Procedures: Aquacel AG

Aquacel Ag (ConvaTec, Skillman, New Jersey) is a dressing that contains ionic silver, which combines the antibacterial action of silver with a barrier dressing that utilizes Hydrofiber technology (E.R. Squibb & Sons, LLC, New Brunswick, NJ) to absorb large amounts of wound exudate without requiring frequent dressing changes.

Nyenhuis and Duan (2009) evaluated MRI issues for this dressing at 1.5- and 3-Tesla. Based on the findings, the Aquacel Ag wound dressing impregnated with ionic silver was reported to be "MR safe" (i.e., an item that poses no known hazards in all MRI environments), particularly since it exhibited magnetic and electric properties similar to human tissues. Therefore, an Aquacel Ag dressing may be left in place in a patient undergoing an MRI procedure at 3-Tesla or less.

REFERENCE

Nyenhuis J, Duan L. An evaluation of MRI safety and compatibility of a silver-impregnated antimicrobial wound dressing. J Am Coll Radiol. 2009;6:500-5.

Shellock FG, Woods TO, Crues JV. MRI labeling information for implants and devices: Explanation of terminology. Radiology 2009;253:26-30.

ECG Electrodes

To ensure patient safety and proper recording of the electrocardiogram during an MRI procedure, it is strongly recommended to only use electrocardiograph (ECG) electrodes tested specifically with regard to the MRI environment and recommended by the monitor's manufacturer. Tests should include an evaluation of magnetic field interactions, MRI-related heating, and characterization of artifacts.

Various ECG electrodes have been specially developed for use during MRI examinations to protect the patient from potentially hazardous conditions and to minimize MRI-related artifacts. **The List** provides a compilation of ECG electrodes that have been evaluated for MRI issues using MR systems operating with static magnetic fields up to 1.5-Tesla. Some have been assessed at 3-Tesla, as well. Importantly, these electrodes should be used according to the guidelines provided by the manufacturers of the ECG monitoring devices.

In general, for patients undergoing MRI procedures, ECG electrodes should be removed if they are not connected to acceptable monitoring equipment and/or needed for the examination.

REFERENCES

Shellock FG. MRI and ECG electrodes. Signals, No. 29, Issue 1, pp. 10-14, 1999.

Shellock FG. Magnetic Resonance Procedures: Health Effects and Safety. CRC Press, LLC, Boca Raton, FL, 2001.

EmpowerMR Contrast Injection System

The **EmpowerMR Contrast Injection System** is uniquely designed for seamless integration within the magnetic resonance imaging (MRI) setting. This device has the following features:

-Virtually eliminates RF transients in the scanner room

-MR conditional up to 7-Tesla

-The compact, rotating head adapts to workflow and the environment

The EmpowerMR Injector Head, which is MR Conditional, can be positioned on either the right or left side of the MR scanner, on either side of the patient gantry. The controls on the Injector Head should be outward facing to the clinician to ensure that the patient can be observed concurrently with the injector controls.

There is no minimum distance requirement within these locations to the exterior of the MR scanner, within these prescribed locations for static magnetic field strengths up to 7-Tesla.

Two system configurations are possible. The only difference between the two system configurations is the location of the Hydraulic Controller. In one configuration, the Hydraulic Controller is located in the Equipment Room and in the other it is located in the Control Room.

The Equipment Room is the preferred location due to the noise of the Hydraulic Controller. As a general rule, the hydraulic controller must be located beyond the ten gauss level.

Additional MRI information may be obtained at www.acist.com/radiology/empower_mr.asp or by contacting Bracco Diagnostics, Inc.

Epidural Pump, ambIT Epidural Pump

ambIT Epidural Pump, Model 22028

The ambIT Trialing Drug Infusion Pump/ambIT external epidural pump (Medtronic, Inc.,   Sorensen Medical, Inc.) is used to infuse medication and/or fluids into patients primarily for pain management. Routes of delivery are generally intravenous, epidural and/or regional.

MRI Information
Warnings
Safety hazards such as under infusion may be associated with external radio frequency interference (RFI) or electromagnetic radiation. Typical equipment which may generate such radiation include x-ray machines, MRI equipment, and any other non-shielded electrical equipment.

REFERENCE

http://www.medtronic.com

Essure Device

The Essure Device (Conceptus Incorported, Mountain View, CA) is a metallic implant developed for permanent female contraception. The presence of this implant is intended to alter the function and architecture of the fallopian tube, resulting in permanent contraception. The Essure Device is composed of 316L stainless steel, platinum, iridium, nickel-titanium alloy, silver solder, and polyethylene terephthalate (PET) fibers.

The MRI assessment of this device involved testing for magnetic field interactions (1.5-Tesla), heating, induced electrical currents, and artifacts using previously described techniques. There were no magnetic field interactions, the highest temperature changes were $\leq +0.6°C$, and the induced electrical currents were minimal. Furthermore, artifacts should not create a substantial problem for diagnostic MR imaging unless the area of interest is in the exact same position as where this implant is located. Thus, the findings indicated that it is acceptable for a patient with the Essure Device to undergo an MR procedure at 1.5-Tesla or less.

MRI at 3-Tesla and the Essure Device. The Essure Device has been evaluated (i.e., tested for magnetic field interactions and MRI-related heating) at 3-Tesla and found to be acceptable for patients undergoing MR procedures.

REFERENCES

Shellock FG. Biomedical implants and devices: assessment of magnetic field interactions with a 3.0-Tesla MR system. J Magn Reson Imaging 2002;16:721-732.

Shellock FG. New metallic implant used for permanent female contraception: evaluation of MR safety. Am J Roentgenol 2002;178:1513-1516.

External Fixation Devices

Most orthopedic implants and materials do not pose substantial problems for patients undergoing MR procedures. However, because of the length of the implant and/or the formation of a conductive loop, MR examinations may be hazardous for certain orthopedic implants, including external fixation systems.

External fixation systems comprise specially designed frames, clamps, rods, rod-to-rod couplings, pins, posts, fasteners, wire fixations, fixation bolts, washers, nuts, hinges, sockets, connecting bars, screws and other components used in orthopedic and reconstructive surgery. Indications for external fixation systems are varied and include the following treatment applications:

- Open and closed fracture fixation;
- Pseudoarthroses of long bones (both congenital and acquired);
- Limb lengthening by metaphyseal or epiphyseal distraction;
- Correction of bony or soft tissue defects; and
- Correction of bony or soft tissue deformities.

The assessment of MRI issues for external fixation systems is especially challenging because of the myriad of possible components (many of which are made from conductive materials) and configurations used for these devices. The primary concern is MRI-related heating which is dependent on the particular aspects (e.g., the lengths of the component parts) of the external fixation system. Importantly, the MRI conditions (strength of the static magnetic field, RF field, RF transmit coil, pulse sequence, body part imaged, position of the fixation device relative to the transmit RF coil, etc.) directly impact the safety aspects of scanning patients with external fixation systems.

For example, Luechinger et al. used MRI to study "large orthopedic external fixation clamps and related components". Forces induced by a 3-Tesla MR scanner were compiled for newly designed nonmagnetic clamps and older clamps that contained ferromagnetic components. Heating trials were performed in 1.5- and 3-Tesla MR systems for two assembled external fixation frames. Forces acting on the newly designed clamps were more than a factor of two lower as the gravitational force on the devices whereas, magnetic forces on the older devices showed over

10 times the force induced by earth acceleration of gravity. No torque effects could be found for the newly designed clamps.

Furthermore, the investigators recorded temperatures at the tips of Schanz screws in the 1.5-Tesla MR system and reported a rise of 0.7 degrees C for a pelvic frame and of 2.1 degrees C for a diamond knee bridge frame when normalized to a specific absorption rate (SAR) of 2 W/kg. The normalized temperature increases at 3-Tesla MR system were 0.9 degrees C for the pelvic frame and 1.1 degrees C for the knee bridge frame. Large external fixation frames assembled with the newly designed clamps (390 Series Clamps), carbon fiber reinforced rods, and implant quality 316L stainless steel Schanz screws met acceptable safety guidelines when tested at 3-Tesla. Notably, this information pertains to the specific configuration of the fixation devices that underwent testing, relative to the MRI conditions that were used.

To ensure patient safety, guidelines for external fixation devices must be applied on a case-by-case and configuration-by-configuration basis. Therefore, MR healthcare professionals are referred to product labeling approved by the U.S. Food and Drug Administration for a given external fixation system. Importantly, this information may only apply to a particular configuration for the external fixation device.

Vibration Associated With MR Procedures. Graf et al. reported that considerable torque may act on metallic implants or instruments due to eddy-current induction in associated with MR imaging. Larger implants (such as fixation devices) made from conducting materials are especially affected. Gradient switching was shown to produce fast alternating torque. Significant vibrations at off-center positions of the metal parts may explain why some patients with metallic implants may report feeling sensations of "heating" during MR examinations.

[MR healthcare professionals are advised to contact the respective manufacturer in order to obtain the latest safety information to ensure patient safety relative to the use of an MR procedure.]

REFERENCE

Graf H, Lauer UA, Schick F. Eddy-current induction in extended metallic parts as a source of considerable torsional moment. Journal of Magnetic Resonance Imaging 2006;23:585-590.

Luechinger R, Boesiger P, Disegi JA. Safety evaluation of large external fixation clamps and frames in a magnetic resonance environment. J Biomed Mater Res B Appl Biomater. 2007;82:17-22.

Shellock FG. External Fixation Devices and MRI Safety. Signals, No. 56, Issue 1, pp. 15, 2006.

Foley Catheters With and Without Temperature Sensors

Most Foley catheters utilized to drain the bladder have no or few metallic components. Accordingly, these devices tend to be acceptable for patients undergoing MR procedures. However, certain Foley catheters have sensors to measure the temperature of the urine in the bladder, which is an appropriate means of determining "deep" body or core temperature. This type of Foley catheter typically has a thermistor or thermocouple located on or near the tip of the device and a wire that runs the length of the catheter to a connector that plugs into a temperature monitor. Sometimes an additional external cable is also used, which may or may not be removable. A Foley catheter with a temperature sensor should never be connected to an external cable and/or the temperature monitor because this equipment has not been shown to be safe for patients undergoing MR examinations.

Several Foley catheters with temperature sensors have been evaluated for MRI issues by determining magnetic field interactions, heating, and artifacts. In general, the findings indicated that it would be acceptable to perform MR procedures in patients with certain Foley catheters with temperature sensors as long as specific recommendations and conditions are followed.

Similar to other devices with conductive components, the position of the wire and/or cable associated with the Foley catheter with a temperature sensor has an important effect on the amount of heating that develops during an MR procedure. Therefore, to prevent excessive heating associated with an MR examination, a Foley catheter with a temperature sensor must be positioned in a straight configuration (without a loop) down the center of the MR system and away from transmit RF coil or inside of the bore of the scanner. The metal connector, cable, or wire, must not touch the patient. Additional recommendations for the specific Foley catheters with temperature sensors that have undergone MRI testing include, the following:

1) If the Foley catheter with a temperature sensor has a removable connector cable or extension, it should be disconnected prior to the MR procedure.

2) Remove all electrically conductive material from the bore of the MR system that is not required for the procedure (i.e., unused surface coils, cables, etc.).

3) Keep electrically conductive material that must remain in the bore of the MR system from directly contacting the patient by placing insulation or space between the conductive material and the patient.

4) Position the Foley catheter with a temperature sensor in a straight configuration down the center of the MR system table to prevent cross points, coils, and loops.

5) Ensure that the connector, cable, or wire does not touch the patient.

6) MR imaging should be performed using MR systems shown to be acceptable and safe for patients (e.g., operating at a specific static magnetic field and frequency, 1.5-Tesla/64-MHz, or other tested field strength/frequency level) and all pertinent safety guidelines must be followed.

7) Follow the **Instructions for Use** for a given Foley catheter with a temperature sensor with regard to the MR system reported, whole body averaged specific absorption rate (SAR).

8) Monitor the patient continuously using a verbal means (e.g., intercom).

9) If the patient reports any unusual sensation, discontinue the MR procedure immediately.

10) Notably, MRI procedures should not be performed in patients that are unable to communicate (e.g., sedated, anesthetized, etc.).

Specific labeling instructions for a given Foley catheter with temperature sensor must be carefully followed. Importantly, not all Foley catheters with temperature sensors are acceptable for patients undergoing MR procedures.

An example of specific instructions for a Foley catheter with temperature sensor that has MRI labeling approved by the Food and Drug Administration is, as follows:

Foley Catheter with Temperature Sensor, Bardex Latex-Free Temperature-Sensing 400-Series Foley Catheter (C. R. Bard, Inc., Covington, GA)

MRI Safety Instructions

Warning: This product should never be connected to the temperature monitor or connected to a cable during an MRI procedure. Failure to follow this guideline may result in serious injury to the patient. Refer to *Instructions for Use.* It is important to closely follow these specific conditions that have been determined to permit the examination to be conducted safely. Any deviation may result in a serious injury to the patient.

Non-clinical testing demonstrated that these Foley catheters with temperature sensors are MR Conditional. A patient with one of these devices can be scanned safely, immediately after placement under the following conditions:

- Static magnetic field of 3-Tesla or less with regard to magnetic field interactions.
- Spatial gradient magnetic field of 720-Gauss/cm or less with regard to magnetic field interactions.
- Maximum MR system reported, whole-body-averaged specific absorption rate (SAR) of 3.5-W/kg at 1.5-Tesla or 3-W/kg at 3-Tesla for 15 minutes of scanning (i.e., per pulse sequence).

Importantly, the MRI procedure should be performed using an MR system operating at a static magnetic field strength of 1.5-Tesla or 3-Tesla, ONLY. The safe use of an MR system operating at lower or higher static magnetic field strength for a patient with a Foley catheter with temperature sensor has not been determined.

Special Instructions: The position of the wire of the Foley Catheter with Temperature Sensor has an important effect on the amount of heating that may develop during an MRI procedure. Accordingly, the Foley catheter with temperature sensor must be positioned in a straight configuration down the center of the patient table (i.e., down the center of the MR system without any loop) to prevent possible excessive heating associated with an MRI procedure.

Additional safety instructions include the following:

1) The Foley catheter with temperature sensor should not be connected to the temperature monitoring equipment during the MRI procedure.

2) If the Foley catheter with temperature sensor has a removable catheter connector cable, it should be disconnected prior to the MRI procedure.

3) Remove all electrically conductive material from the bore of the MR system that is not required for the procedure (i.e., unused surface coils, cables, etc.).

4) Keep electrically conductive material that must remain in the bore of the MR system from directly contacting the patient by placing thermal and/or electrical insulation (including air) between the conductive material and the patient.

5) Position the Foley catheter with a temperature sensor in a straight configuration down the center of the patient table to prevent cross points and conductive coils or loops.

6) The wire and connector of the Foley catheter with temperature sensor should not be in contact with the patient during the MRI procedure. Position the device, accordingly.

7) MR imaging should be performed using an MR system with static magnetic strength of 1.5-Tesla or 3-Tesla, ONLY.

8) At 1.5-Tesla, the MR system reported whole body averaged SAR should not exceed 3.5- W/kg for 15-min. of scanning (i.e., per pulse sequence).

9) At 3-Tesla, the MR system reported whole body averaged SAR should not exceed 3-W/kg for 15-min of scanning (i.e., per pulse sequence).

DeRoyal Foley Catheter With Temperature Sensor, MR Conditional at 3-Tesla, Only (DeRoyal, www.deroyal.com)

The DeRoyal Foley Catheter With Temperature Sensor, 18-Fr, REF 81-080718 was determined to be MR-conditional according to the terminology specified in the American Society for Testing and Materials (ASTM) International, Designation: F2503.

Non-clinical testing demonstrated that the DeRoyal Foley Catheter With Temperature Sensor, 18-Fr, REF 81-080718 is MR Conditional. A patient with this device can be scanned safely, immediately after placement under the following conditions:

Static Magnetic Field

-Static magnetic field of 3-Tesla or less

-Maximum spatial gradient magnetic field of 720-Gauss/cm or less

MRI-Related Heating

In non-clinical testing, the DeRoyal Foley Catheter With Temperature Sensor, 18-Fr, REF 81-080718 produced the following temperature rise during MRI performed for 15-min of scanning (i.e., per pulse sequence) in the 3-Tesla (3-Tesla/128-MHz, Excite, HDx, Software 14X.M5, General Electric Healthcare, Milwaukee, WI) MR system: *Highest temperature change*   +4.2 degrees C

Therefore, the MRI-related heating experiments for the DeRoyal Foley Catheter With Temperature Sensor, 18-Fr, REF 81-080718 at 3-Tesla using a transmit/receive RF body coil at an MR system reported whole body averaged SAR of 2.9-W/kg (i.e., associated with a calorimetry measured whole body averaged value of 2.7-W/kg) indicated that the greatest amount of heating that occurred in association with these specific conditions was equal to or less than +4.2 degrees C.

Artifact Information

MR image quality may be compromised if the area of interest is in the exact same area or relatively close to the position of the DeRoyal Foley Catheter With Temperature Sensor, 18-Fr, REF 81-080718. Therefore, optimization of MR imaging parameters to compensate for the presence of this device may be necessary.

Pulse Sequence	T1-SE	T1-SE	GRE	GRE
Signal Void Size	1,956-mm^2	159-mm^2	3,262-mm^2	763-mm^2
Plane Orientation	Parallel	Perpendicular	Parallel	Perpendicular

Important Note: *This labeling information pertains to MRI conditions at 3-Tesla ONLY (no other MR system field strength/frequency, higher or lower).*

Additional MRI Information: Importantly, the MRI procedure should be performed using an MR system operating at a static magnetic field strength of 3-Tesla, ONLY. The safe use of an MR system operating at lower or higher field strength for a patient with a DeRoyal Foley Catheter With Temperature Sensor, 18-Fr, REF 81-080718 has not been determined.

Special Instructions: The position of the wire and connector of the DeRoyal Foley Catheter With Temperature Sensor, 18-Fr, REF 81-080718 has an important effect on the amount of heating that may develop during an MRI procedure. Accordingly, the DeRoyal Foley Catheter With Temperature Sensor, 18-Fr, REF 81-080718 must be positioned in a straight configuration down the center of the patient table (i.e., down the center of the MR system without any loop) to prevent possible excessive heating associated with an MRI procedure. The wire and connector must not touch the patient.

Additional instructions include the following:

1) The DeRoyal Foley Catheter With Temperature Sensor, 18-Fr, REF 81-080718 should not be connected to the temperature monitoring equipment during the MRI procedure.

2) If the DeRoyal Foley Catheter With Temperature Sensor, 18-Fr, REF 81-080718 has a removable catheter connector cable, it should be disconnected prior to the MRI procedure.

3) Remove all electrically conductive material from the bore of the MR system that is not required for the procedure (i.e., unused surface coils, cables, etc.).

4) Keep electrically conductive material that must remain in the bore of the MR system from directly contacting the patient by placing thermal and/or electrical insulation (including air) between the conductive material and the patient.

5) Position the Foley catheter with a temperature sensor in a straight configuration down the center of the patient table to prevent cross points and conductive coils or loops.

6) The wire and connector of the DeRoyal Foley Catheter With Temperature Sensor, 18-Fr, REF 81-080718 should not be in contact with the patient during the MRI procedure. Position the device, accordingly.

7) MR imaging should be performed using an MR system with static magnetic strength of 3-Tesla, ONLY.

8) At 3-Tesla, the MR system reported whole body averaged SAR should not exceed 2.9-W/kg for 15-min of scanning (per pulse sequence).

In addition to the above, the **Guidelines to Prevent Excessive Heating and Burns Associated with Magnetic Resonance Procedures** should be considered and implemented, as needed.

[MR healthcare professionals are advised to contact the respective manufacturer in order to obtain the latest safety information to ensure patient safety relative to the use of an MR procedure.]

REFERENCES

Dempsey MF, Condon B, Hadley DM. Investigation of the factors responsible for burns during MRI. J Magn Reson Imaging 2001;13:627-631.

http://www.bardmedical.com/

Shellock FG. Magnetic Resonance Procedures: Health Effects and Safety. CRC Press, LLC, Boca Raton, FL, 2001.

Shellock FG, Kanal E. Magnetic Resonance: Bioeffects, Safety, and Patient Management. Second Edition, Lippincott-Raven Press, New York, 1996.

FREEHAND Implantable Functional Neurostimulator System (FNS)

The FREEHAND Implantable Functional Neurostimulator System (FNS)(NeuroControl, Cleveland, OH) is a radiofrequency (RF) powered motor control neuroprosthesis that consists of both implanted and external components. It utilizes low levels of electrical current to stimulate the peripheral nerves that innervate muscles in the forearm and hand providing functional hand grasp patterns. The NeuroControl FREEHAND System is intended to improve a patient's ability to grasp, hold, and release objects. It is indicated for use in patients who:

- are tetraplegic due to C5 or C6 level spinal cord injury (ASIA Classification)
- have adequate functional range of motion of the upper extremity
- have intact lower motor neuron innervation of the forearm and hand musculature and
- are skeletally mature

PRECAUTIONS

- **MRI**: Testing of the FREEHAND System in a 1.5-Tesla scanner exposed to a whole body averaged Specific Absorption Rate (SAR) of 1.1 W/kg for a 30 minute duration resulted in localized temperature rises no more than 2.7 degrees C in a gelled saline filled phantom (without blood flow) and translational force less than that of a 3-gram mass and torque of 0.063 N-cm (significantly less than produced by the weight of the device). A patient with a FREEHAND System may undergo an MR procedure using a shielded or unshielded MR system with a static magnetic field of 1.5-Tesla <u>only</u>. The implantable components may obscure the view of other nearby anatomic structures. Artifact size is dependent on a variety of factors including the type of pulse sequence used for imaging (e.g. larger for gradient echo pulse sequences and smaller for spin echo and fast spin echo pulse sequences), the direction of the frequency encoding, and the size of the field of view used for imaging. The use of non-standard scanning modes to minimize image artifact or improve visibility should be applied with caution and with the Specific Absorption Rate (SAR) not to exceed an average of 1.1 W/kg and gradient magnetic fields no greater than 20 Tesla/sec. The use of Transmit Coils other than the scanner's Body Coil or a Head Coil is prohibited. Testing of the function of each electrode should be conducted prior to MRI scanning to ensure that no leads are broken. Do not expose patients to MRI if any lead is broken or if integrity cannot be established as excessive heating may result in a broken lead. The external components of the FREEHAND System must be removed prior to MRI scanning. Patients must be continuously observed during the MR procedure and instructed to report any unusual sensations (e.g., warming, burning, or neuromuscular stimulation). Scanning must be discontinued immediately if any unusual sensation occurs. Contact NeuroControl Corporation for additional information.

Important Note: Only the pertinent MRI information is shown above, however, there is substantial labeling for the FREEHAND System that must be carefully reviewed prior to conducting MRI examination on a patient with this device. Additional *Warnings*, *Precautions*, and *Contraindications* are stated in the **Product Insert** and **Instructions for Use** for this product.

[Excerpted with permission from the Package Insert, FREEHAND System, NeuroControl Corporation, Cleveland, OH]

[MR healthcare professionals are advised to contact the respective manufacturer in order to obtain the latest safety information to ensure patient safety relative to the use of an MR procedure.]

Glaucoma Drainage Implants (Shunt Tubes)

A glaucoma drainage implant or device, also known as a shunt tube, is implanted to maintain an artificial drainage pathway to control intraocular pressure for patients with glaucoma. Intraocular pressure is lowered when aqueous humor flows from inside the eye through the tube into the space between the plate that rests on the scleral surface and surrounding fibrous capsule. The implantation of a glaucoma drainage device is used to treat glaucoma that is refractory to medical and standard surgical therapy. These are usually cases where standard drainage procedures have been unsuccessful or have a poor prognosis including failed trabeculectomy, juvenile glaucoma, neovascular glaucoma and glaucoma secondary to uveitis, traumatic glaucoma, cataract with glaucoma and high risk cases of primary glaucoma.

Importantly, for certain glaucoma drainage implants, radiographic findings may suggest the diagnosis of an orbital foreign body if the ophthalmic history is unknown, as reported by Ceballos and Parrish (2002). In this case report, a patient was denied an MRI examination for fear of dislodging an apparent "metallic foreign body." In fact, the patient had a Baerveldt glaucoma drainage implant that was mistakenly identified as an orbital metallic object based on its radiographic characteristics (i.e., due to the presence of barium-impregnated silicone).

At least one glaucoma drainage implant, the Ex-PRESS miniature glaucoma shunt (Optonol Ltd., Neve Ilan, Israel) is made from 316L stainless steel which, according to De Feo et al., may affect MRI examinations of the optic nerve. Geffen et al. reported that the Ex-PRESS glaucoma shunt is acceptable for patients undergoing MRI at 3-Tesla or less.

Many other glaucoma drainage implants are made from nonmetallic materials and are safe for patients undergoing MRI procedures. Commonly used devices that do not contain metal include, the following:

- Baerveldt glaucoma drainage implant (Pharmacia Co., Kalamazoo, MI)
- Krupin-Denver eye valve to disc implant (E. Benson Hood Laboratories, Pembroke, MA)

- Ahmed glaucoma valve (New World Medical, Rancho Cucamonga, CA)
- Molteno drainage device (Molteno Ophthalmic Ltd., Dunedin, New Zealand)
- Joseph valve (Valve Implants Limited, Hertford, England)

REFERENCES

Ceballos EM, Parrish RK. Plain film imaging of Baerveldt glaucoma drainage implants. American Journal of Neuroradiology 2002;23;935-937.

Dahan E, Carmichael TR. Implantation of a miniature glaucoma device under a scleral flap. J Glaucoma 2005;14:98-102.

De Feo F, Roccatagliata L, Bonzano L, et al. Magnetic resonance imaging in patients implanted with Ex-PRESS stainless steel glaucoma drainage microdevice. Am J Ophthalmol. 2009;147:907-11.

Geffen N, Trope GE, et al. Is the Ex-PRESS Glaucoma Shunt Magnetic Resonance Imaging Safe? J Glaucoma. 2010;19:116-8

Hong CH, Arosemena A, Zurakowski D, Ayyala RS. Glaucoma drainage devices: a systematic literature review and current controversies. Surv Ophthalmol 2005;50:48-60.

Jeon TY, Kim HJ, Kim ST, Chung TY, Kee C. MR imaging features of giant reservoir formation in the orbit: an unusual complication of Ahmed glaucoma valve implantation. AJNR Am J Neuroradiol. 2007;28:1565-1566.

Seibold LK, Rorrer RA, Kahook MY. MRI of the Ex-PRESS stainless steel glaucoma drainage device. Br J Ophthalmol. 2011;95:251-4.

Sidoti PA, Baerveldt G. Glaucoma drainage implants. Curr Opin Ophthalmol 1994;5:85-98.

Traverso CE, De Feo F, Messas-Kaplan A, Denis P, Levartovsky S, Sellem E, Badalà F, Zagorski Z, Bron A, Belkin M. Long term effect on IOP of a stainless steel glaucoma drainage implant (Ex-PRESS) in combined surgery with phacoemulsification. British Journal of Ophthalmology 2005;89:425-429.

Guidewires

Advances in interventional MR procedures have resulted in the need for guidewires that are acceptable for endovascular therapy, drainage procedures, and other similar applications. Conventional guidewires are made from stainless steel or Nitinol, materials known to be conductive. Accordingly, radiofrequency fields used for MR procedures may induce substantial currents in guidewires, leading to excessive temperature increases and potential injuries.

Liu et al. studied the theoretical and experimental aspects of the RF heating resonance phenomenon of an endovascular guidewire. A Nitinol-based guidewire (Terumo, Tokyo, Japan) was inserted into a vessel phantom and imaged using 1.5-T and 0.2-T MR systems with continuous temperature monitoring at the guidewire tip. The guidwire was deployed in the phantom in a "straight" manner. Heating effects due to different experimental conditions were examined. A model was developed for the resonant current and the associated electric field produced by the guidewire acting as an antenna. Temperature increases of up to 17 degrees C were measured while imaging the guidewire at an off-center position in the 1.5-Tesla MR system. Power absorption produced by the resonating wire decreased as the repetition time was increased. No temperature rise was measured during MRI performed using the 0.2-Tesla MR system. Thus, considering the potential utility of low-field, open MR systems for MR-guided endovascular interventions, it is important to be aware of the safety of such applications for metallic guidewires and the potential hazards associated with using a guidewire with MR systems operating at higher static magnetic field strengths, including 3-Tesla.

An investigation conducted by Konings et al. examined the radiofrequency (RF) heating of an endovascular guidewire frequently used in interventional MR procedures. A Terumo guidewire was partly immersed in an oblong saline bath to simulate an endovascular intervention. The temperature rise of the guidewire tip during MR imaging was measured using a Luxtron fluoroptic thermometry system. Starting from a baseline level of 26 degrees C, the tip of the guidewire reached temperatures up to 74 degrees C after 30 seconds of scanning using a 1.5-Tesla MR system. Touching the guidewire produced a skin burn.

The excessive heating of a linear conductor, like the guidewire that underwent evaluation, was explained by the resonating RF waves. According to Konings et al., the capricious dependencies of this resonance phenomenon have potentially severe consequences for safety guidelines of interventional MR procedures involving guidewires.

Recent advances in guidewire designs reported by Kocaturk et al. and Kramer et al. have yielded guidewires that appear to be more acceptable for interventional MRI procedures with respect to both safety and visualization aspects.

REFERENCES

Buecker A. Safety of MRI-guided vascular interventions. Minim Invasive Ther Allied Technol. 2006;15:65-70.

Johnston T, et al. Intraoperative MRI: safety. Neurosurg Clin N Am. 2009;20:147-53.

Kocaturk O, et al. Whole shaft visibility and mechanical performance for active MR catheters using copper-nitinol braided polymer tubes. J Cardiovasc Magn Reson. 2009;11:29.

Konings MK, Bartels LW, Smits HJ, Bakker CJ. Heating around intravascular guidewires by resonating RF waves. J Magn Reson Imaging 2000;12:79-85.

Kramer NA, et al. Preclinical evaluation of a novel fiber compound MR guidewire in vivo. Invest Radiol. 2009;44:390-7.

Lin C-Y, Farahani K, Lu DSK, Shellock FG. Safety of MRI-guided endovascular guidewire applications. Proceedings of the International Society of Magnetic Resonance Imaging, 1999;7:1015.

Shellock FG. Magnetic Resonance Procedures: Health Effects and Safety. CRC Press, LLC, Boca Raton, FL, 2001.

Shellock FG. Radiofrequency-induced heating during MR procedures: A review. Journal of Magnetic Resonance Imaging. 2000;12: 30-36.

van den Bosch MR, et al. New method to monitor RF safety in MRI-guided interventions based on RF induced image artefacts. Med Phys. 2010;37:814-21.

Halo Vests and Cervical Fixation Devices

Halo vests and cervical fixation devices are typically constructed from a combination of metallic components and other materials. Although some commercially available halo vests and cervical fixation devices are composed entirely of nonferromagnetic metals, there may be hazards due to excessive MRI-related heating that can be generated because of the conductive nature of the metallic parts. Additionally, there is a potential for the patient's tissue to be involved in part of a current loop, such that excessive heating and burns may occur. The currents generated within a "ring" or conductive loop is of additional concern because eddy current induction can cause image degradation. Adjusting the phase encoding direction of the pulse sequence so that it is parallel to the axis of the halo ring may reduce artifacts associated with eddy currents.

Serious injuries have occurred in patients with halo vests and cervical fixation devices that have undergone MR procedures. For example, Kim et al. (2003) described a case of a patient that underwent MRI at 1.5-Tesla wearing a titanium-based halo vest system (the name, model and manufacturer of this device were not provided). After the MR procedure, substantial burns were evident on the scalp of the right two posterior skull pins. According to the report, "the stoic patient had clearly perceived significant burning pain during MR imaging, but did not notify the technicians."

Fortunately, several halo vests and cervical fixation devices have been designed to specifically be acceptable for patients undergoing MR procedures at 1.5-Tesla and 3-Tesla (see **The List**).

Vibration Effects. A study was conducted to evaluate the possible heating of halo vests and cervical fixation devices during MR imaging performed at 1.5-Tesla MR system using a variety of pulse sequences. The data indicated that no substantial heating was detected for the specific devices tested. Of interest is that there appeared to be subtle, rapid motions of the halo ring associated with a magnetization transfer contrast (MTC) pulse sequence, as shown by recordings obtained using a motion sensitive, laser-Doppler flow monitor.

Apparently, the imaging parameters used for the MTC pulse sequence and other MR imaging techniques can produce sufficient vibration of the "halo" ring to create the sensation of heating. Accordingly, patients may interpret rapid movements or vibrations as a "heating" sensation. This is likely to occur when the vibration frequency is at a level that stimulates nerve receptors located in the subcutaneous region, which detect sensations of pain and temperature changes.

The aforementioned is a hypothesis based on the available experimental data and requires further investigation to substantiate this theory. However, additional support for this premise is provided in a report by Hartwell and Shellock (1997). In this case, a halo ring and vest (removed from a patient who complained of severe "burning" in a front skull pin during MR imaging) was evaluated for heating and other potential problems associated with MR imaging. This work was performed in conjunction with the neurosurgeon who applied the device to the patient. The halo ring and vest were connected similar to the manner used on the patient. A fluid-filled Plexiglas phantom was placed within the vest. The device was then placed in a 1.5-Tesla MR system and imaging was performed using the same parameters that were associated with the "burning" sensation experienced by the patient. The neurosurgeon remained inside of the MR system to visually observe the cervical fixation device and to maintain physical contact (i.e., touching the skull pins and other components of the cervical fixation device) during the MR procedure.

No perceivable temperature change was noted for the metallic components during MR imaging. However, the components (e.g., halo ring, vertical supports, vest bolts, etc.) vibrated substantially during MR imaging. Furthermore, when the skull pins were held firmly during the scan, there was a "drilling" sensation, which could be interpreted as a "burning" effect. Nevertheless, the skull pins remained cool to the touch throughout the MR procedure. Recent work conducted at 3-Tesla likewise supports the fact that substantial vibration can occur in cervical fixation devices (Unpublished observations, F.G. Shellock, 2009).

Graf et al. reported that torque acting on metallic implants or instruments due to eddy-current induction in associated with MR imaging can be considerable. Larger implants (such as fixation devices) made from well-conducting materials are especially affected. Gradient switching was shown to produce fast alternating torque. Significant vibrations at off-center positions of the metal parts may explain why some patients with metallic implants sometimes report feeling heating sensations during MR examinations.

In consideration of the above, it is inadvisable to permit patients with certain cervical fixation devices to undergo MR procedures using an MTC pulse sequence until this problem can be further characterized to avoid unwanted patient responses, regardless of the lack of safety concern related to excessive heating. Other comparable pulse sequences should likewise be avoided when performing MR imaging of patients with cervical fixation devices until the precise cause of this problem is determined and fully characterized. Importantly, all Instructions for Use (IFU) and patient application information provided by halo vest and cervical fixation device manufacturers should be carefully followed.

MRI at 3-Tesla and Cervical Fixation Devices. To date, several cervical fixation devices have undergone MRI testing at 3-Tesla. MRI information for these devices are, as follows:

'LiL Angel Pediatric Halo System with Jerome Halo Vest and Resolve Glass-composite Halo Ring and Resolve Ceramic-tipped Skull Pins

'LiL Angel Pediatric Halo System with Resolve Halo Vest and Resolve Glass-composite Halo Ring and Resolve Ceramic-tipped Skull Pins

Resolve Halo System with Jerome Halo Vest and Resolve Glass-composite Halo Ring and Resolve Ceramic-tipped Skull Pins

Resolve Halo System with Resolve Halo Vest and Resolve Glass-composite Halo Ring and Resolve Ceramic-tipped Skull Pins (Each product above is from OSSUR Reykjavik, Iceland and OSSUR AMERICAS, Aliso Viejo, CA)

Non-clinical testing has demonstrated that each product indicated above used as a cervical fixation or cervical traction device or system is *MR Conditional*. A patient with this system may undergo MRI safely under the following conditions:

- Static magnetic field of 3-Tesla or less
- Maximum spatial gradient magnetic field of 720 Gauss/cm or less
- Maximum MR system reported, specific absorption rate (SAR) of 3.0 W/kg for 15 minutes of scanning (i.e., per pulse sequence)

In non-clinical testing, this system produced maximum temperature changes of 0.6 degrees C or less at a maximum MR system reported, specific absorption rate (SAR) of 3.0 W/kg for 15 minutes of MRI using a 3-Tesla MR system (Excite, Software G3.0-052B, General Electric

Healthcare, Milwaukee, WI). MR image quality may be compromised if the area of interest is in the exact same area or relatively close to the position of the Skull Pins. Therefore, it may be necessary to optimize MR imaging parameters for the presence of these metallic objects.

Important Note: All of the materials used for the above products included metals with very low magnetic susceptibility (e.g., commercially pure titanium, Titanium alloy, Aluminum, etc.) or are nonmetallic and nonconductors. Accordingly, little or no substantial magnetic field interactions are present for these products in association with the 3-Tesla MR system.

PMT Halo System with Carbon Graphite Open Back Ring and Titanium Skull Pin (PMT Corporation, Chanhassen, MN)

Non-clinical testing has demonstrated that the PMT Halo System with Carbon Graphite Open Back Ring and Titanium Skull Pins used as a cervical fixation or cervical traction device or system is *MR Conditional*. A patient with this system may undergo MRI safely under the following conditions:

- Static magnetic field of 3-Tesla and 1.5-Tesla only.
- Maximum spatial gradient magnetic field of 720 Gauss/cm or less
- Maximum MR system reported, specific absorption rate (SAR) of 3.0 W/kg for 15 minutes of scanning (i.e., per pulse sequence)

In non-clinical testing, this system produced maximum temperature changes of 0.5 degrees C or less at a maximum MR system reported, specific absorption rate (SAR) of 3.0 W/kg for 15 minutes of MRI using a 3-Tesla MR system (Excite, Software G3.0-052B, General Electric Healthcare, Milwaukee, WI). MR image quality may be compromised if the area of interest is in the exact same area or relatively close to the position of the Titanium Skull Pins. Therefore, it may be necessary to optimize MR imaging parameters for the presence of these metallic objects.

Important Note: All of the materials used for the above products included metals with very low magnetic susceptibility (e.g., commercially pure titanium, Titanium alloy, Aluminum, etc.) or are nonmetallic and nonconductors. Accordingly, little or no substantial magnetic field interactions are present for these products in association with the 3-Tesla MR system.

Bremer Halo Crown System with Bremer Air Flo Vest and Titanium Skull Pins (DePuy Spine Inc., Raynham, MA)

Non-clinical testing has demonstrated that the Bremer Halo Crown System with Bremer Air Flo Vest and Titanium Skull Pins used as a cervical fixation or cervical traction device or system is *MR Conditional*. A patient with this system may undergo MRI safely under the following conditions:

- Static magnetic field of 3-Tesla or less
- Maximum spatial gradient magnetic field of 720 Gauss/cm or less
- Maximum MR system reported, specific absorption rate (SAR) of 3.0 W/kg for 15 minutes of scanning (i.e., per pulse sequence)

In non-clinical testing, this system produced maximum temperature changes of 0.6 degrees C or less at a maximum MR system reported, specific absorption rate (SAR) of 3.0 W/kg for 15 minutes of MRI using a 3-Tesla MR system (Excite, Software G3.0-052B, General Electric Healthcare, Milwaukee, WI). MR -image quality may be compromised if the area of interest is in the exact same area or relatively close to the position of the Titanium Skull Pins. Therefore, it may be necessary to optimize MR imaging parameters for the presence of these metallic objects.

Important Note: All of the materials used for the above products included metals with very low magnetic susceptibility (e.g., commercially pure titanium, Titanium alloy, Aluminum, etc.) or are nonmetallic and nonconductors. Accordingly, little or no substantial magnetic field interactions are present for these products in association with the 3-Tesla MR system.

Bremer 3D Halo Crown System with Bremer Air Flo Vest and Titanium Skull Pins (DePuy Spine Inc., Raynham, MA)
Non-clinical testing has demonstrated that the Bremer 3D Halo Crown System with Bremer Air Flo Vest and Titanium Skull Pins used as a cervical fixation or cervical traction device or system is *MR Conditional*. A patient with this system may undergo MRI safely under the following conditions:

- Static magnetic field of 3-Tesla or less
- Maximum spatial gradient magnetic field of 720 Gauss/cm or less
- Maximum MR system reported, specific absorption rate (SAR) of 3.0 W/kg for 15 minutes of scanning (i.e., per pulse sequence)

In non-clinical testing, this system produced maximum temperature changes of 0.6 degrees C or less at a maximum MR system reported, specific absorption rate (SAR) of 3.0 W/kg for 15 minutes of MRI using a 3-Tesla MR system (Excite, General Electric). MR image quality may be compromised if the area of interest is in the exact same area or relatively close to the position of the Titanium Skull Pins. Therefore, it may be necessary to optimize MR imaging parameters for the presence of these metallic objects.

Important Note: All of the materials used for the above products included metals with very low magnetic susceptibility (e.g., commercially pure titanium, Titanium alloy, Aluminum, etc.) or are nonmetallic and nonconductors. Accordingly, little or no substantial magnetic field interactions are present for these products in association with the 3-Tesla MR system.

[MR healthcare professionals are advised to contact the respective manufacturer in order to obtain the latest safety information to ensure patient safety relative to the use of an MR procedure.]

REFERENCES

Ballock RT, et al. The quality of magnetic resonance imaging, as affected by the composition of the halo orthosis. J Bone Joint Surg 1989;71-A:431-434.

Clayman DA, et al. Compatibility of cervical spine braces with MR imaging. A study of nine nonferrous devices. AJNR Am J Neuroradiol 1990;11:385-390.

Diaz F, Tweardy L, Shellock FG. Cervical fixation devices: MRI issues at 3-Tesla. Spine 2010;35:411-5.

Graf H, et al. Eddy-current induction in extended metallic parts as a source of considerable torsional moment. Journal of Magnetic Resonance Imaging 2006;23:585-590.

Hartwell CG, Shellock FG. MRI of cervical fixation devices: Sensation of heating caused by vibration of metallic components. J Magn Reson Imaging 1997;7:771.

Hua J, Fox RA. Magnetic resonance imaging of patients wearing a surgical traction halo. J Magn Reson Imaging 1996;:1:264-267.

Kim LJ, et al. Scalp burns from halo pins following magnetic resonance imaging. Case Report. Journal of Neurosurgery 2003:99:186.

Malko JA, Hoffman JC, Jarrett PJ. Eddy-current-induced artifacts caused by an "MR-compatible" halo device. Radiology 1989;173:563-564.

Shellock FG. MR imaging and cervical fixation devices: assessment of ferromagnetism, heating, and artifacts. Magn Reson Imaging 1996;14:1093-1098.

Shellock FG, Slimp G. Halo vest for cervical spine fixation during MR imaging. AJR Am J Roentgenol 1990;154:631-632.

Hearing Aids and Other Hearing Systems

External hearing aids are included in the category of electronically-activated devices that may be found in patients referred for MR procedures. Exposure to the magnetic fields used for MR examinations can damage these devices. Therefore, a patient or other individual with an external hearing aid must not enter the MR system room. Fortunately, most external hearing aids can be readily identified and removed from the patient or individual to prevent damage associated with the MRI environment.

Other hearing devices may have external components as well as pieces that are surgically implanted. Hearing devices with external and internal components may be especially problematic for patients and individuals in relative to the use of MR procedures. Accordingly, patients and individuals with these particular hearing devices may not be allowed into the MR environment because of the risk of damage to the components. The manufacturers of these devices should be contacted for current MRI information.

(For information on other hearing systems, refer to the sections: **Baha, Bone Conduction Implant**, **Cochlear Implants**, and **InSound XT Series and Lyric Hearing Device**).

[MR healthcare professionals are advised to contact the respective manufacturer in order to obtain the latest safety information to ensure patient safety relative to the use of an MR procedure.]

REFERENCES

Shellock FG. Magnetic Resonance Procedures: Health Effects and Safety. CRC Press, LLC, Boca Raton, FL, 2001.

Shellock FG, Kanal E. Magnetic Resonance: Bioeffects, Safety, and Patient Management. Second Edition, Lippincott-Raven Press, New York, 1996.

Heart Valve Prostheses and Annuloplasty Rings

Many heart valve prostheses and annuloplasty rings have been evaluated for MR issues, especially with regard to the presence of magnetic field interactions associated with exposure to MR systems operating at field strengths of as high as 4.7-Tesla. Of these, the majority displayed measurable yet relatively minor magnetic field interactions. That is, because the attractive forces exerted on the heart valve prostheses and annuloplasty rings were minimal compared to the force exerted by the beating heart (i.e., approximately 7.2-N), to date, an MR procedure is not considered to be hazardous for a patient that has any heart valve prosthesis or annuloplasty ring tested relative to the field strength of the magnet (i.e., MR system) used for the evaluation. Importantly, this recommendation includes the Starr-Edwards Model Pre-6000 heart valve prosthesis previously suggested to be a potential risk for a patient undergoing an MR examination.

With respect to the clinical use of MR procedures, there has been no report of a patient incident or injury related to the presence of a heart valve prosthesis or annuloplasty ring. However, it should be noted that not all heart valve prostheses have been evaluated and at least one prototype (to date, not commercially available) exists that has magnetic components.

A study by Edwards et al. examined the effects of aging on cardiac tissue strength and its ability to withstand forces associated with a 4.7-T magnet. The goal of this research was to determine the forces required to cause partial or total detachment of a heart valve prosthesis in patients with age-related degenerative diseases exposed to MRI. Edwards et al. concluded that specific age-related degenerative cardiac diseases stiffen and strengthen tissue, resulting in significant forces required to pull a suture through valve annulus tissue. Importantly, these forces are substantially greater than those magnetically-induced at 4.7-T. Therefore, patients with degenerative valvular diseases are unlikely to be at risk during exposure to static magnetic fields less than or equal to 4.7-T.

Heart Valve Prostheses and the Lenz Effect. Condon and Hadley reported the theoretical possibility of a previously unconsidered electromagnetic interaction with heart valves that contain metallic disks or leaflets. Basically, any metal (i.e., not just ferromagnetic material) moving through a magnetic field will develop another magnetic field that opposes the primary magnetic field. This phenomenon is referred to as the "Lenz effect". In theory, "resistive pressure" may develop with the potential to inhibit both the opening and closing aspects of the mechanical heart valve prosthesis. The Lenz effect is proportional to the strength of the static magnetic field. Accordingly, there may be problems for patients with heart valves that have metal leaflets undergoing MR procedures using MR systems operating at static magnetic fields greater than 1.5-Tesla. However, this phenomenon has not been observed in association with MR examinations.

MRI at 3-Tesla and Heart Valve Prostheses and Annuloplasty Rings. Findings obtained at 3-Tesla for various heart valve prostheses and annuloplasty rings that underwent testing indicated that certain implants exhibit relatively minor magnetic field interactions. Similar to heart valve prostheses and annuloplasty rings tested at 1.5-Tesla, because the attractive forces exerted on these implants are deemed minimal compared to the force exerted by the beating heart, MR procedures at 3-Tesla are not considered to be hazardous for patients or individuals that have these devices. To date, for the heart valves and annuloplasty rings that have been tested, MRI-related heating does not reach substantial levels.

REFERENCES

Ahmed S, Shellock FG. Magnetic resonance imaging safety: implications for cardiovascular patients. Journal of Cardiovascular Magnetic Resonance 2001;3:171-181.

Condon B, Hadley DM. Potential MR hazard to patients with metallic heart valves: the Lenz effect. Journal of Magnetic Resonance Imaging 2000;12:171-176.

Edwards, M-B, Taylor KM, Shellock FG. Prosthetic heart valves: evaluation of magnetic field interactions, heating, and artifacts at 1.5-Tesla. Journal of Magnetic Resonance Imaging. 2000;12:363-369.

Edwards MB, Draper ER, Hand JW, Taylor KM, Young IR. Mechanical testing of human cardiac tissue: some implications for MRI safety. J Cardiovasc Magn Reson. 2005;7:835-40

Frank H, Buxbaum P, Huber L, et al. *In vitro* behavior of mechanical heart valves in 1.5-T superconducting magnet. Eur J Radiol 1992;2:555-558.

Hassler M, Le Bas JF, Wolf JE, et al. Effects of magnetic fields used in MRI on 15 prosthetic heart valves. J Radiol 1986;67:661-666.

Levine GN, Gomes AS, Arai AE, Bluemke DA, Flamm SD, Kanal E, Manning WJ, Martin ET, Smith JM, Wilke N, Shellock FG. Safety of magnetic resonance imaging in patients with cardiovascular devices: an American Heart Association scientific statement from the Committee on Diagnostic and Interventional Cardiac Catheterization. Circulation 2007;116:2878-2891.

Medtronic Heart Valves, Medtronic, Inc., Minneapolis, MN, Permission to publish 3-Tesla MR testing information for Medtronic Heart Valves provided by Kathryn M. Bayer, Senior Technical Consultant, Medtronic Heart Valves, Technical Service.

Pruefer D, et al. In vitro investigation of prosthetic heart valves in magnetic resonance imaging: evaluation of potential hazards. J Heart Valve Disease 2001;10:410-414.

Randall PA, et al. Magnetic resonance imaging of prosthetic cardiac valves *in vitro* and *in vivo*. Am J Cardiol 1988;62:973-976.

Shellock FG. Magnetic Resonance Procedures: Health Effects and Safety. CRC Press, LLC, Boca Raton, FL, 2001.

Shellock FG. Biomedical implants and devices: assessment of magnetic field interactions with a 3.0-Tesla MR system. J Magn Reson Imaging 2002;16:721-732.

Shellock FG. Prosthetic heart valves and annuloplasty rings: assessment of magnetic field interactions, heating, and artifacts at 1.5-Tesla. Journal of Cardiovascular Magnetic Resonance 2001;3:159-169.

Shellock FG, Morisoli SM. *Ex vivo* evaluation of ferromagnetism, heating, and artifacts for heart valve prostheses exposed to a 1.5-Tesla MR system. J Magn Reson Imaging 1994;4:756-758.

Shellock FG, Shellock VJ. MRI Safety of cardiovascular implants: evaluation of ferromagnetism, heating, and artifacts. Radiology 2000;214:P19H.

Soulen RL. Magnetic resonance imaging of prosthetic heart valves [Letter]. Radiology 1986;158:279.

Soulen RL, Budinger TF, Higgins CB. Magnetic resonance imaging of prosthetic heart valves. Radiology 1985;154:705-707.

Hemostatic Clips, Other Clips, Fasteners, and Staples

Various hemostatic vascular clips, other types of clips, fasteners, and staples evaluated for magnetic field interactions were not attracted by static magnetic fields of MR systems operating at 3-Tesla or less. These implants were made from nonferromagnetic materials such as tantalum, commercially pure titanium, and nonferromagnetic forms of stainless steel. Additionally, some forms of ligating, hemostatic, or other types of clips are made from biodegradable materials. Therefore, patients that have the implants made from nonmagnetic or "weakly" magnetic materials listed in **The List** are not at risk for injury during MR procedures. Importantly, for the devices that have been tested to date, there has been no report of an injury to a patient in association with a hemostatic vascular clip, other type of clip, fastener, or staple associated with the MR environment. Patients with nonferromagnetic versions of these implants may undergo MR procedures immediately after they are placed.

Vascular grafts frequently have clips or fasteners applied that may present problems for MR imaging because of the associated artifacts. Weishaupt et al. evaluated the artifact size on three-dimensional MR angiograms as well as the MR safety for 18 different commercially available hemostatic and ligating clips. All of the clips were acceptable or safe at 1.5-Tesla insofar as there was no heating or substantial magnetic field interactions measured for these implants.

Specific MRI-related labeling statements for certain hemostatic clips that require further attention during the pre-MRI screening procedure are, as follows:

Resolution Clip. The Resolution Clip (Boston Scientific Corporation) is indicated for placement within the gastrointestinal tract for the purpose of endoscopic marking or hemostasis. Currently, the Resolution Clip is labeled, as follows: "Do not perform MRI procedures on patients who have had clips placed within their gastrointestinal tract, as this could be harmful to patients."

Long Clip, HX-600-090L. The Long Clip HX-600-090L (Olympus Medical Systems Corporation) is indicated for placement within the gastrointestinal tract for the purpose of endoscopic marking, hemostasis, or closure of GI tract luminal perforations within 20-mm as a supplementary method. Currently, the Long Clip HX-600-090L is labeled, as follows: "Do not perform MRI procedures on patients who have clips placed within their gastrointestinal tracts. This could be harmful to the patient."

Additional information: Olympus endoscopic clips have been shown to remain in the patient an average of 9.4 days, but retention is based on a variety of factors and may result in a longer retention period. Prior to MRI, the physician should confirm there are no residual clips in the GI tract. The following techniques may be used for confirmation:

1) View the lesion under radiologic imaging. Olympus clip fixing devices are radiopaque. By using x-ray, the physician can determine if any residual clips are in the gastrointestinal tract. If no clips are evident under radiologic imaging, MRI may be accomplished.

2) Endoscopically examine the lesion. If no clips remain at the lesion, MRI may be accomplished.

QuickClip2, HX-201LR-135 & HX-201UR-135. The QuickClip2, HX-201LR-135 & HX-201UR-135 (Olympus Medical Systems Corporation) are indicated for placement within the gastrointestinal tract for the purpose of endoscopic marking, hemostasis, or closure of GI tract luminal perforations within 20-mm as a supplementary method. Currently, the QuickClip2 (HX-201LR-135 & HX-201UR-135) is labeled, as follows: "Do not perform MRI procedures on patients who have clips placed within their gastrointestinal tracts. This could be harmful to the patient."

Additional information: Olympus endoscopic clips have been shown to remain in the patient an average of 9.4 days, but retention is based on a variety of factors and may result in a longer retention period. Prior to MRI, the physician should confirm there are no residual clips in the GI tract. The following techniques may be used for confirmation:

1) View the lesion under radiologic imaging. Olympus clip fixing devices are radiopaque. By using x-ray, the physician can determine if any residual clips are in the gastrointestinal tract. If no clips are evident under radiologic imaging, MRI may be accomplished.

2) Endoscopically examine the lesion. If no clips remain at the lesion, MRI may be accomplished.

QuickClip2 Long, HX-201LR-135L & HX-201UR-135L. The QuickClip2 Long, HX-201LR-135L & HX-201UR-135L (Olympus

Medical Systems Corporation) are indicated for placement within the gastrointestinal tract for the purpose of endoscopic marking, hemostasis, or closure of GI tract luminal perforations within 20-mm as a supplementary method. Currently, the QuickClip2 Long (HX-201LR-135L & HX-201UR-135L) is labeled, as follows: "Do not perform MRI procedures on patients who have clips placed within their gastrointestinal tracts. This could be harmful to the patient."

Additional information: Olympus endoscopic clips have been shown to remain in the patient an average of 9.4 days, but retention is based on a variety of factors and may result in a longer retention period. Prior to MRI, the physician should confirm there are no residual clips in the GI tract. The following techniques may be used for confirmation:

1) View the lesion under radiologic imaging. Olympus clip fixing devices are radiopaque. By using x-ray, the physician can determine if any residual clips are in the gastrointestinal tract. If no clips are evident under radiologic imaging, MRI may be accomplished.

2) Endoscopically examine the lesion. If no clips remain at the lesion, MRI may be accomplished.

TriClip Endoscopic Clipping Device. An investigation by Gill et al. involving excised tissue exposed to 1.5-Tesla MR system, reported that the TriClip (TriClip Endoscopic Clipping Device, Wilson-Cook Medical Inc., Winston-Salem, NC) demonstrated "detachment from gastric tissue". Therefore, the TriClip should be considered "*unsafe*" for MRI.

MRI at 3-Tesla and Hemostatic Clips, Other Clips, Fasteners, and Staples. At 3-Tesla, a variety of hemostatic clips, other clips, fasteners, and staples have been evaluated for MRI issues including magnetic field interactions and MRI-related heating. In general, these devices do not present an additional risk to patients undergoing MR procedures. Please refer to **The List** for specific information.

REFERENCES

Brown MA, Carden JA, Coleman RE, et al. Magnetic field effects on surgical ligation clips. Magn Reson Imaging 1987;5:443-453.

Barrafato D, Henkelman RM. Magnetic resonance imaging and surgical clips. Can J Surg 1984;27:509-512.

Gill KR, Pooley RA, Wallace MB. Magnetic resonance imaging compatibility of endoclips. Gastrointest Endosc. 2009;70:532-6.

Raju GS. Endoclips for GI endoscopy. Gastrointestinal Endoscopy 2004; 59:267-279.

Resolution Clip information, http://www.bostonscientific.com/

Shellock FG. Hemostatic Clips and MRI Procedures: Some Safe…Some May Not Be. Signals No. 66, pp. 20-21, 2008.

Shellock FG. Magnetic Resonance Procedures: Health Effects and Safety. CRC Press, LLC, Boca Raton, FL, 2001.

Shellock FG. MR imaging of metallic implants and materials: a compilation of the literature. Am J Roentgenol 1988;151:811-814.

Shellock FG. Biomedical implants and devices: assessment of magnetic field interactions with a 3.0-Tesla MR system. J Magn Reson Imaging 2002;16:721-732.

Shellock FG, Crues JV. High-field strength MR imaging and metallic biomedical implants: an *ex vivo* evaluation of deflection forces. AJR Am J Roentgenol 1988;151:389-392.

Shellock FG, Morisoli S, Kanal E. MR procedures and biomedical implants, materials, and devices: 1993 update. Radiology 1993;189:587-599.

Shellock FG, Swengros-Curtis J. MR imaging and biomedical implants, materials, and devices: an updated review. Radiology 1991;180:541-550.

Weishaupt D, Quick HH, Nanz D, Schmidt M, Cassina PC, Debatin JF. Ligating clips for three-dimensional MR angiography at 1.5-T: *in vitro* evaluation. Radiology 2000;214:902-907.

InSound XT Series and Lyric Hearing Device

MRI Information

For the **InSound XT Series** and **Lyric Hearing Device** (InSound Medical, Newark, CA), each hearing system must be removed prior to an MRI procedure. Furthermore, these devices are not allowed in the MR system room. Each device may be self-removed if an MRI examination is required.

[MR healthcare professionals are advised to contact the manufacturer to ensure that the latest safety information is obtained and carefully followed in order to ensure patient safety relative to the use of an MR procedure.]

REFERENCE

http://www.insoundmedical.com/

Insulin Pumps

An insulin pump allows the replacement of slow-acting insulin for basal needs with a continuous infusion of rapid-acting insulin. By using an insulin pump, the patient can typically match the dosage of insulin to lifestyle and activities, rather than adjusting those to the body's response to insulin injections. The advantages of the using an insulin pump include the fact that it replaces the need for periodic injections by delivering rapid-acting insulin continuously throughout the day via a catheter, which greatly simplifies the management of diabetes.

There are two basic types of insulin pumps, one is used as an external device and the other is implanted internally. Both types currently pose hazards to patients referred to MRI procedures. For an external insulin pump, it may simply need to be removed and kept out of the MRI environment to ensure that there is no adverse impact on the functionality of this device. The information below provides MRI labeling for several commonly used insulin pumps:

Insulin Pumps (Animas Corporation, a Johnson and Johnson Company).

This MRI information pertains to the following insulin pumps from Animas Corporation, a Johnson and Johnson Company:

-Animas 2020 Insulin Pump

-IR Animas 1200

-IR 1000 Insulin Pump

-IR 1100 Insulin Pump

-IR 1200 Insulin Pump

Each insulin pump indicated above should not be exposed to very strong electromagnetic fields, such as MRIs, RF welders, or magnets used to pick up automobiles. Very strong magnetic fields, such as that associated with MRI, can "magnetize" the portion of the insulin pump's motor that regulates insulin delivery and, thus, damage this device.

For the patient: If you plan to undergo an MRI, remove the insulin pump beforehand and keep it outside of the MR system room during the procedure.

If the pump is accidentally allowed into the MR system room, disconnect the pump immediately and contact Animas Pump Support for important instructions.

For the Healthcare Professional: Do not bring the insulin pump into the MR system at any time. If the pump is accidentally allowed into the MR system room, disconnect the pump immediately and contact Animas Pump Support for important instructions.

Cozmo Pump, Infusion Pump

According to the User Manual for the Cozmo Pump (Deltec, Inc., St. Paul, MN), which is a device used to administer insulin, the following is stated regarding Magnetic Resonance Imaging (MRI):
"Caution: Avoid strong electromagnetic fields, like those present with Magnetic Resonance Imaging (MRI) and direct x-ray, as they can affect how the pump works. If you cannot avoid them, you must take the pump off."

Medtronic MiniMed 2007 Implantable Insulin Pump System

The Medtronic MiniMed 2007 Implantable Insulin Pump System (Medtronic Minimed, Northridge, CA) may offer treatment advantages for diabetes patients who have difficulty maintaining consistent glycemic control. Patients that have not responded well to intensive insulin therapy, including multiple daily insulin injections or continuous subcutaneous insulin infusion using an external pump, may be primary candidates for the Medtronic MiniMed 2007 System. The Medtronic MiniMed 2007 System delivers insulin into the peritoneal cavity in short, frequent bursts or "pulses", similar to how pancreatic beta cells secrete insulin.

The Medtronic MiniMed 2007 Implantable Insulin Pump is designed to withstand common electrostatic and electromagnetic interference but must be removed prior to undergoing an MR procedure. Any magnetic field exceeding 600 gauss will interfere with the proper functioning of the pump for as long as the pump remains in that field. Fields much higher than that, such as those emitted by an MR system, may cause irreparable damage to the pump.

By comparison, infusion sets (MMT-11X, MMT-31X, MMT-32X, MMT-37X, MMT-39X) used with this device contain no metallic components and are safe to be used and can remain attached to the patient during an MR procedure. The only exceptions would be Polyfin infusion sets. Polyfin infusion sets (MMT-106 AND MMT-107, MMT-16X, MMT-30X, MMT-36X) have a surgical steel needle that remains in the subcutaneous tissue. These infusion sets should be removed prior to any MR procedure.

MiniMed Paradigm REAL-Time Insulin Pump and Continuous Glucose Monitoring System (522 and 722 Insulin Pumps; Medtronic Minimed, Northridge, CA)

MRI Information for Patients Magnetic fields

Do **not** use pump cases that have a magnetic clasp.

Do **not** expose your insulin pump to MRI equipment or other devices that generate very strong magnetic fields.

The magnetic fields in the immediate vicinity of these devices can damage the part of the pump's motor that regulates insulin delivery, possibly resulting in over-delivery and severe hypoglycemia.

Your pump must be removed and kept outside the room during magnetic resonance imaging (MRI) procedures.

If your pump is inadvertently exposed to a strong magnetic field, discontinue use and contact your local help line or representative for further assistance.

The insulin pump, transmitter, and sensor must be removed prior to entering the MRI environment.

DANA Diabecare IIS Insulin Pump and DANA Diabecare Insulin Infusion Pump (SOOIL Development Co., Ltd. San Diego, CA)

The pump must not be used in the presence of intense electromagnetic fields, such as those generated by certain electrically powered medical devices. The pump should be removed prior to the user having a CT Scan, MRI or X-ray.

[MRI healthcare professionals are advised to contact the respective manufacturer in order to obtain the latest safety information to ensure patient safety relative to the use of an MR procedure.]

REFERENCES

www.animascorp.com
www.cozmore.com
www.minimed.com
www.sooilusa.com

Intrauterine Contraceptive Devices and Other Devices

Intrauterine contraceptive devices (IUD) may be made from nonmetallic materials (e.g., plastic) or a combination of nonmetallic and metallic materials. Copper is typically the metal used in an IUD, however, stainless steel or other metals may also be utilized. The "Copper T" and "Copper 7" both have a fine copper coil wound around a portion of the IUD. Testing conducted to determine MRI issues for the copper IUDs indicated that these objects are safe for patients in the MR environment using MR systems operating at 1.5-Tesla or less. This includes the Multiload Cu375, the Nova T (containing copper and silver), and the Gyne T IUDs. An artifact may be seen for the metallic component of the IUD, however, the extent of this artifact is relatively small because of the low magnetic susceptibility of copper.

Zieman and Kanal (2007) reported 3-Tesla MRI *in vitro* test results for the Copper T 380A IUD. No significant deflection, torque, heating or artifact was found. Thus, this IUD is acceptable for patients undergoing MRI at 3-Tesla or less.

Importantly, stainless steel IUDs exist and, to date, these devices have not undergone testing to determine if they are acceptable for patients in association with MR procedures.

The Mirena intrauterine system (IUS) is a hormone-releasing device that contains levonorgestrel to prevent pregnancy. This T-shaped device is made entirely from nonmetallic materials that include polyethylene, barium sulfate (i.e., which makes it radiopaque), and silicone. Therefore, the Mirena is safe for patients undergoing MR procedures using MR systems operating at all static magnetic field strengths.

The Implanon implant (Etonogestrel) is a single-rod, nonmetallic, subdermal device that offers women up to three years of contraceptive protection. This implant is acceptable for patients undergoing MR procedures at all static magnetic field strengths.

REFERENCES

Hess T, Stepanow B, Knopp MV. Safety of intrauterine contraceptive devices during MR imaging. Eur Radiol 1996;6:66-68.

http://www.implanon.com

http://www.mirena-us.com

Kido A, et al. Intrauterine devices and uterine peristalsis: evaluation with MRI. Magn Reson Imaging. 2008;26:54-8.

Mark AS, Hricak H. Intrauterine contraceptive devices: MR imaging. Radiology 1987;162:311-314.

Mirena (levonorgestrel-releasing intrauterine system (IUS), Product Insert information, Berlex Laboratories, Wayne, NJ

Shellock FG. Magnetic Resonance Procedures: Health Effects and Safety. CRC Press, LLC, Boca Raton, FL, 2001.

Westerway SC, Picker R, Christie J. Implanon implant detection with ultrasound and magnetic resonance imaging. Aust NZ Obstet Gynaecol 2003;43:346-350.

Zhuang LQ, Yang BY. Comparison of clinical effects of stainless steel IUDs with and without copper. Shengzhi Yu biun. 1984;4:48-50.

Zieman M, Kanal E. Copper T 380A IUD and magnetic resonance imaging. Contraception. 2007;75:93-5.

IsoMed Implantable Constant-Flow Infusion Pump

IsoMed: All models beginning with 8472
Medtronic, Inc., Minneapolis, MN

Reference: SynchroMed IsoMed Information for Prescribers Manual

IsoMed pump performance has not been established in >1.5 Tesla (T) magnetic resonance scanners. Patients should not have magnetic resonance imaging (MRI) using >1.5 T scanners.

Exposure of IsoMed pumps to MRI fields of 1.5 T has demonstrated no impact on pump performance and a limited effect on the quality of the diagnostic information.

Testing on the IsoMed pump has established the following with regard to MRI safety and diagnostic issues:

Tissue heating adjacent to implant during MRI scans
Specific absorption rate (SAR) — Presence of the pump can potentially cause a twofold increase of the local temperature rise in tissues near the pump. During a 20-minute pulse sequence in a 1.5 T GE Signa scanner with a whole-body average SAR of 1 W/kg, a temperature rise of 1 degrees C in a static phantom was observed near the pump implanted in the "abdomen" of the phantom. The temperature rise in a static phantom represents a worst case for physiological temperature rise and the 20-minute scan time is representative of a typical imaging session. Implanting the pump in other locations may result in higher temperature rises in tissues near the pump.

In the unlikely event that the patient experiences uncomfortable warmth near the pump, the MRI scan should be stopped and the scan parameters adjusted to reduce the SAR to comfortable levels.

Peripheral Nerve Stimulation during MRI scans
Time-varying gradient magnetic fields — Presence of the pump may potentially cause a two-fold increase of the induced electric field in tissues near the pump. With the pump implanted in the abdomen, using pulse sequences that have dB/dt up to 20 T/ s, the measured induced

electric field near the pump is below the threshold necessary to cause stimulation.

In the unlikely event that the patient reports stimulation during the scan,the proper procedure is the same as for patients without implants— stop the MRI scan and adjust the scan parameters to reduce the potential for nerve stimulation.

Static magnetic field

For magnetic fields up to 1.5 T, the magnetic force and torque on the pump will be less than the force and torque due to gravity.
In the unlikely event that the patient reports a slight tugging sensation at the pump implant site, an elastic garment or wrap may be used to prevent the pump from moving and reduce the sensation the patient may experience.

Image distortion

The IsoMed pump will cause image dropout on MRI images in the region surrounding the pump. The extent of image artifact depends on the pulse sequence chosen with gradient echo sequences generally causing the most image dropout. Spin echo sequences will cause image dropout in a region approximately 50% larger than the pump itself, about 12 cm across, but with little image distortion or artifact beyond that region

Minimizing Image Distortion — MRI image artifact may be minimized by careful choice of pulse sequence parameters and location of the angle and location of the imaging plane. However, the reduction in image distortion obtained by adjustment of pulse sequence parameters will usually be at a cost in signal-to-noise ratio. These general principles should be followed:

- Use imaging sequences with stronger gradients for both slice and read encoding directions. Employ higher bandwidth for both radio-frequency pulse and data sampling.
- Choose an orientation for read-out axis that minimizes the appearance of in-plane distortion.
- Use spin echo or gradient echo MR imaging sequences with a relatively high data sampling bandwidth.
- Use shorter echo time for gradient echo technique, whenever possible.
- Be aware that the actual imaging slice shape can be curved in space due to the presence of the field disturbance of the pump (as stated above).

- Identify the location of the implant in the patient, and when possible, orient all imaging slices away from the implanted pump.

[MR healthcare professionals are advised to contact the respective manufacturer in order to obtain the latest safety information to ensure patient safety relative to the use of an MR procedure.]

REFERENCES

www.Medtronic.com

www.medtronic.com/mrimanuals

Licox CC1.P1 Oxygen and Temperature Probe, Brain Tissue Oxygen Monitoring System

Licox CC1.P1 Oxygen and Temperature Probe, Brain Tissue Oxygen Monitoring System (Integra NeuroSciences, Plainsboro, NJ)

MRI SAFETY OF THE LICOX IT2 COMPLETE BRAIN TUNNELING PROBE KIT INCLUDING THE MODEL CC1.P1 OXYGEN AND TEMPERATURE PROBE AND MODEL VK5.2 PARENTERAL PROBE GUIDE AT 1.5 TESLA

It is important to read and understand this document in its entirety before conducting an MRI (magnetic resonance imaging) procedure on a patient with an implanted Licox CC1.P1 Oxygen and Temperature Probe. Failure to strictly adhere to these guidelines may result in serious injury to the patient.

This information applies to the following Integra products:

- Model IT2 Complete Brain Tunneling Probe Kit, consisting of
- Model CC1.P1 Oxygen and Temperature Probe
- Model VK5.2 Parenteral Probe Guide

WARNINGS

- These guidelines apply to MRI procedures conducted using a 1.5 Tesla MR System, ONLY.
- Testing has not been performed on other MR Systems and therefore should not be used.
- Use only normal operating mode. Do not perform MR scans in the 1st level or higher level control mode.
- Disconnect all cables and patient monitoring devices from the Licox CC1.P1 probe prior to entering the MRI environment. Failure to do so may result in serious injury to the patient. It is not possible to monitor brain oxygen tension during MRI procedures using this device.

- The position or orientation of the Licox CC1.P1 catheter and VK5.2 Parenteral Probe Guide does not impact their MRI safety characteristics.

DO NOT EXCEED AN RF (RADIO FREQUENCY) WHOLE BODY AVERAGED SAR (SPECIFIC ABSORPTION RATE) OF 1.0 W/Kg IN THE HEAD OR BODY DURING THE MRI PROCEDURE.

OVERVIEW

The Licox IT2 Complete Brain Tunneling Probe Kit including the CC1.P1 Oxygen and Temperature Probe and VK5.2 Parenteral Probe Guide were subjected to MRI testing, which included radio frequency induced heating, magnetically induced displacement force and torque to demonstrate that these components were considered "MR Conditional" as defined in ASTM F2503, Standard Practice for Marking Medical Devices and Other Items for Safety in the Magnetic Resonance Environment using a 1.5-Tesla MR system, ONLY. Testing has not been performed on other MR Systems and therefore should not be used.

This document outlines recommended guidelines and specific conditions under which the Licox IT2 Complete Brain Tunneling Probe Kit has been shown to pose minimal risk to a patient undergoing an MRI procedure.

Deviation from these guidelines may increase the potential for serious harm to the patient. MRI conditions utilizing MR systems with higher or lower static magnetic fields have not been assessed for the Licox IT2 Complete Brain Tunneling Probe Kit and, as such, must be avoided to ensure patient safety.

MRI – LICOX IT2 INTERACTIONS

MRI INDUCED HEATING

Under certain conditions, RF fields generated by MRI can induce substantial currents in metallic components contained within medical device products. This may rapidly produce significant heating of a device. Failure to follow the recommendations contained in this communication may result in the generation of thermal lesions and serious patient harm.

MAGNETIC FIELD INTERACTIONS

Magnetic materials contained within an implanted device may experience translational attraction or rotational forces when brought into the static magnetic field of an MR system. The Licox CC1.P1 Probe contains magnetic material and has been shown in safety testing to not be substantially affected by translational attraction and torque related to exposure to a 1.5 Tesla static magnetic field of an MR system.

IMAGE ARTIFACTS

The presence of the Licox CC1.P1 Probe will cause minor artifacts on the MR image. It is up to the discretion of the interpreting physician to determine if the location of the sensor is in the area of imaging interest and whether it will adversely affect the quality of the diagnostic information required from the MRI procedure.

The Licox CC1.P1 connector will cause substantial artifacts and distortion on the MR image. As such, position the connector away from the anatomy of interest during the MRI procedure.

PROCEDURE

In addition to standard safety procedures for MRI, the following precautions must be followed specific to the Licox IT2 product:

1) Inform the patient of the potential risks of undergoing an MRI procedure with this device. Disconnect all cables and patient monitoring devices attached to the Licox IT2 prior to transporting the patient into the MRI environment.
2) Use only the following types of radio frequency (RF) coils for the MRI procedure:
   a) Transmit/receive RF body coil
   b) Transmit body coil/receive-only head coil
   c) Transmit/receive head coil
   d) Transmit/receive lower extremity coil - for imaging of lower extremities only, not for imaging the head of patients.
3) Set MRI parameters to the lowest usable whole body averaged SAR level. **THIS MUST NOT EXCEED A WHOLE BODY AVERAGED SAR OF 1.0 W/kg IN THE HEAD OR BODY** to minimize the risk of excessive heating of device components.
4) Verify that the MR system has appropriately calculated and updated the SAR value after all parameter changes have been made. Ensure that the proper patient weight is used for the SAR calculations.
5) For head scans using the transmit body coil the local SAR must be less than 2.0-W/kg.
6) A knowledgeable MRI expert (e.g., MRI physicist, MRI-trained radiologist) must verify that all set-up steps and settings have been properly implemented and checked prior to performing the MRI procedure.
7) If conscious and alert, provide the patient with a means of alerting the MRI system operator of unusual sensations. Instruct the patient to

watch for sensations such as overheating or shock. Terminate the MRI procedure immediately if so notified by the patient.

8) Monitor the patient continuously during the MRI examination and be prepared to stop and respond in the event of an emergency.

[MR healthcare professionals are advised to contact the respective manufacturer in order to obtain the latest safety information to ensure patient safety relative to the use of an MR procedure.]

REFERENCES

http://www.integralife.com/

Licox MR Safety Fact Sheet: Licox IT2 Complete Brain Oxygen and Temperature Tunneling Probe Kit - 5/06 (Integra NeuroSciences, Plainsboro, NJ)

Magnetically-Activated Implants and Devices

Various types of implants incorporate magnets for a variety of reasons. For example, the magnet may be used to retain the implant in place (e.g., certain prosthetic devices), to guide a ferromagnetic object into a specific position, to permit the functional aspects of the implant, to change the operation of the implant (e.g., adjustable pressure valves), or to program the device. Because there is a high likelihood of perturbing the function, demagnetizing, or displacing these implants, MR procedures typically should not be performed in patients with these implants or devices. However, in some cases, patients with magnetically-activated implants and devices may undergo MR procedures as long as certain precautions are followed. For example, see section entitled **Cerebrospinal Fluid (CSF) Shunt Valves and Accessories**.

Implants and devices that use magnets (e.g., certain types of dental implants, magnetic sphincters, magnetic stoma plugs, magnetic ocular implants, otologic implants, and other prosthetic devices) may be damaged by exposure to MR systems which, in turn, may necessitate surgery to replace or reposition them. For example, Schneider et al. reported that an MR examination is capable of demagnetizing the permanent magnet associated with an otologic implant (i.e., the Audiant magnet). Obviously, this has important implications for patients undergoing MR procedures.

Whenever possible, and if this can be done without risk to the patient, a magnetically-activated implant or device (e.g., an externally applied prosthesis or magnetic stoma plug) should be removed prior to the MR procedure. This will permit the examination to be performed safely. Knowledge of the specific aspects of the magnetically-activated implant or device is essential to recognize potential problems and to guarantee that an MR examination may be performed without risk.

Extrusion of an eye socket magnetic implant in a patient imaged with a 0.5-Tesla MR system has been described. This type of magnetic prosthesis was used in the patient after enucleation. For this prosthesis, a removable eye prosthesis adheres with a magnet of opposite polarity to a permanent implant sutured to the rectus muscles and conjunctiva by magnetic attraction through the conjunctiva. This "magnetic linkage" is intended to permit the eye prosthesis to move in a coordinated fashion with that of eye movement. In the reported incident, the static magnetic field of the MR system produced sufficient attraction of the ferromagnetic portion of the prosthesis to cause serious injury to the patient.

Certain dental prosthetic appliances utilize magnetic forces to retain the implant in place. The magnet may be contained within the prosthesis and attached to a ferromagnetic post implanted in the mandible or the magnetic component may be the implanted component. Therefore, whether or not an MR procedure may be performed without problems depends on the configuration of the magnetically-active dental implant.

REFERENCES

Blankenstein FH, et al. Signal loss in magnetic resonance imaging caused by intraoral anchored dental magnetic materials. Rofo. 2006;178:787-93.

Gaston A, et al. External magnetic guidance of endovascular catheters with a superconducting magnet: preliminary trials. J Neuroradiol 1988;15:137-147.

Grady MS, et al. Nonlinear magnetic stereotaxis: three dimensional *in vivo* remote magnetic manipulation of a small object in canine brain. Med Phys 1990;17:405-415.

Jeon JH, et al. Reversing the polarity of a cochlear implant magnet after magnetic resonance imaging. Auris Nasus Larynx. 2011 Aug 31. [Epub ahead of print]

Majdani O, et al. Artifacts caused by cochlear implants with non-removable magnets in 3-T MRI: phantom and cadaveric studies. Eur Arch Otorhinolaryngol. 2009;266:1885-90.

Majdani O, et al. Demagnetization of cochlear implants and temperature changes in 3.0-T MRI environment. Otolaryngol Head Neck Surg. 2008;139:833-9.

Ranney DF, Huffaker HH. Magnetic microspheres for the targeted controlled release of drugs and diagnostic agents. Ann NY Acad Sci 1987;507:104-119.

Schneider ML, Walker GB, Dormer KJ. Effects of magnetic resonance imaging on implantable permanent magnets. Am J Otol 1995;16:687-689.

Shellock FG. Magnetic Resonance Procedures: Health Effects and Safety. CRC Press, LLC, Boca Raton, FL, 2001.

Shellock FG. Ex vivo assessment of deflection forces and artifacts associated with high-field strength MRI of "mini-magnet" dental prostheses. Magn Reson Imaging 1989;7 (Suppl 1):38.

Young DB, Pawlak AM. An electromagnetically controllable heart valve suitable for chronic implantation. ASAIO Trans 1990;36:M421-M425.

Yuh WTC, et al. Extrusion of an eye socket magnetic implant after MR imaging examination: potential hazard to a patient with eye prosthesis. J Magn Reson Imaging 1991;1:711-713.

Medivance Nasogastric Sump Tube with YSI Series 400 Temperature Sensor

MRI Information. The **Medivance Nasogastric Sump Tube with YSI Series 400 Temperature Sensor**, 18-Fr. (Medivance, Inc., Louisville, CO) was determined to be <u>MR-conditional</u> according to the terminology specified in the American Society for Testing and Materials (ASTM) International, Designation: F2503. Standard Practice for Marking Medical Devices and Other Items for Safety in the Magnetic Resonance Environment.

Non-clinical testing demonstrated that the Medivance Nasogastric Sump Tube with YSI Series 400 Temperature Sensor, 18-Fr. is MR Conditional. A patient with this device can be scanned safely, immediately after placement under the following conditions:

- Static magnetic field of 3-Tesla or less
- Spatial gradient magnetic field of 720-Gauss/cm or less
- Maximum MR system reported whole-body-averaged specific absorption rate (SAR) of 3-W/kg for 15 minutes of scanning.

In non-clinical testing, the Medivance Nasogastric Sump Tube with YSI Series 400 Temperature Sensor, 18-Fr. produced a temperature rise of 0.9°C at a maximum MR system-reported whole body averaged specific absorption rate (SAR) of 3-W/kg for 15-minutes of MR scanning in a 3-Tesla MR system using a transmit/receive body coil (Excite, Software G3.0-052B, General Electric Healthcare, Milwaukee, WI).

MR image quality may be compromised if the area of interest is in the exact same area or relatively close to the position of the Medivance Nasogastric Sump Tube with YSI Series 400 Temperature Sensor, 18-Fr. Therefore, optimization of MR imaging parameters to compensate for the presence of this device may be necessary.

Artifact Information

Pulse Sequence	T1-SE	T1-SE	GRE	GRE
Signal Void Size	10,377-mm^2	90-mm^2	3,992-mm^2	75-mm^2
Plane Orientation	Parallel	Perpendicular	Parallel	Perpendicular

IMPORTANT NOTE: To ensure patient safety during MRI, the Medivance Nasogastric Sump Tube with YSI Series 400 Temperature Sensor, 18-Fr. must be labeled to verify that it is positioned exactly as it was for this MRI assessment: straight down the center of the patient, with the remaining tubing/connector going out the back of the MR system. The Medivance Nasogastric Sump Tube with YSI Series 400 Temperature Sensor, 18-Fr. should NOT be connected to a monitor and there should be NO loops or coils present. See additional information below:

1) The Medivance Nasogastric Sump Tube with YSI Series 400 Temperature Sensor, 18-Fr. must disconnected from the monitor prior to the MRI procedure.

2) Remove all electrically conductive material from the bore of the MR system that is not required for the procedure (i.e., unused surface coils, cables, etc.).

3) Keep electrically conductive material that must remain in the bore of the MR system from directly contacting the patient by placing insulation or space between the conductive material and the patient.

4) Position the Medivance Nasogastric Sump Tube with YSI Series 400 Temperature Sensor, 18-Fr. in a straight configuration to prevent cross points, coils, and loops. The remaining portion of this device, along with the connector should be positioned in a straight line out the BACK of the MR system (i.e., NOT along side the inside of the MR system).

5) Ensure that the Medivance Nasogastric Sump Tube with YSI Series 400 Temperature Sensor, 18-Fr. exiting the patient does not touch the patient.

6) Monitor the patient continuously using a verbal means (e.g., intercom). If the patient reports any unusual sensation, discontinue the MRI procedure immediately. Notably, MRI procedures should not be performed in patients that are unable to communicate (e.g., sedated, anesthetized, etc.).

Miscellaneous Implants and Devices

Many miscellaneous implants, materials, devices, and objects have been tested with regard to MR procedures and the MR environment. For example, various types of firearms have been evaluated in the MR environment. These firearms exhibited strong ferromagnetism. In fact, two of the six firearms that underwent testing discharged in a reproducible manner while in the MR system room. Obviously, firearms should remain outside of the MR environment to prevent problems or possible injuries.

MR-guided biopsy, therapeutic, and minimally invasive surgical procedures are important clinical applications that are performed on conventional, open-architecture, or "double-donut" MR systems specially designed for this work. These procedures present challenges for the instruments and devices that are needed to support these interventions. Metallic surgical instruments and other devices potentially pose hazards (e.g., "missile" effects) or other problems (i.e., image artifacts and distortion that can obscure the area of interest) that must be addressed to apply MR-guided techniques effectively. Various manufacturers have used "weakly" ferromagnetic, nonferromagnetic or nonmetallic materials to make special instruments for interventional MR procedures.

Other medical products and devices have been developed with metallic components that are either entirely nonferromagnetic and non-conducting or made from metals that have a low magnetic susceptibility (e.g., titanium, non-magnetic types of stainless steel, etc.) that are acceptable for use in the MR environment.

MRI at 3-Tesla and Miscellaneous Implants and Devices. Many implants and devices have been tested in association with 3-Tesla MR systems. Refer to **The List** to determine information about specific miscellaneous implants and devices assessed at 3-Tesla.

REFERENCES

Go KG, et al. Interaction of metallic neurosurgical implants with magnetic resonance imaging at 1.5-Tesla as a cause of image distortion and of hazardous movement of the implant. Clin Neurosurg 1989;91:109-115.

Kanal E, Shaibani A. Firearm safety in the MR imaging environment. Radiology 1994;193:875-876.

Lufkin R, Jordan S, Lylyck P, et al. MR imaging with topographic EEG electrodes in place. AJNR Am J Neuroradiol 1988;9:953-954.

Planert J, et al. Measurements of magnetism-forces and torque moments affecting medical instruments, implants, and foreign objects during magnetic resonance imaging at all degrees of freedom. Med. Physics 1996;23:851-856.

Shellock FG. Biomedical implants and devices: assessment of magnetic field interactions with a 3.0-Tesla MR system. J Magn Reson Imaging 2002;16:721-732.

Shellock FG. MR-compatibility of an endoscope designed for use in interventional MR procedures. AJR Am J Roentgenol 1998;71:1297-1300.

Shellock FG. Magnetic Resonance Procedures: Health Effects and Safety. CRC Press, LLC, Boca Raton, FL, 2001.

Shellock FG. MR safety update 2002: Implants and devices. J Magn Reson Imaging 2002;16:485-496.

Shellock FG. Metallic neurosurgical implants: assessment of magnetic field interactions, heating, and artifacts at 1.5-Tesla. Radiology 2001;218:611.

Shellock FG. Surgical instruments for interventional MRI procedures: assessment of MR safety. J Magn Reson Imaging 2001;13:152-157.

Shellock FG, Shellock VJ. Ceramic surgical instruments: evaluation of MR-compatibility at 1.5-Tesla. J Magn Reson Imaging 1996;6:954-956.

Shellock FG, Shellock VJ. Evaluation of MR compatibility of 38 bioimplants and devices. Radiology 1995;197:174.

To SYC, Lufkin RB, Chiu L. MR-compatible winged infusion set. Comput Med Imag Graph 1989;13:469-472.

Zhang J, et al. Temperature changes in nickel-chromium intracranial depth electrodes during MR scanning. AJNR Am J Neuroradiol 1993;14:497-500.

Neurostimulation Systems: General Information

The incidence of patients receiving implanted neurostimulation or neuromodulation systems for treatment of neurological disorders and other conditions is increasing. Because of the inherent design and intended function of neurostimulation systems, [including those used for deep brain stimulation (DBS), spinal cord stimulation (SCS), vagus nerve stimulation (VNS), and other similar devices], the electromagnetic fields used for MR procedures may produce a variety of problems. For example, altered function of a neurostimulation system that results from exposure to the electromagnetic fields of an MR system may cause discomfort, pain, or serious injuries to the patients.

MRI-related heating has been reported to create the greatest concern for various devices used for neuromodulation. Variables that impact heating include, the following:

- The specific type of neuromodulation system
- Electrical characteristics of the specific neuromodulation system
- Field strength and RF wavelength of the MR system
- Type of transmit RF coil (i.e., transmit head vs transmit body RF coil)
- The amount of RF energy delivered-RF power level
- The specific absorption rate (SAR)
- The technique used to calculate or estimate SAR used by the MR system
- The patient's anatomy undergoing MR imaging
- The landmark position or body part undergoing MRI relative to the transmit RF coil
- The orientation and configuration of the implantable pulse generator (IPG), extension (e.g., the cable connecting the pulse generator (PG) to the implanted lead), and the lead relative to the source of RF energy (i.e., the transmit RF coil)

Importantly, the exact criteria for the particular neurostimulation system with regard to the implantable PG, leads, electrodes, and operational aspects of the device and the MR system conditions must be defined by comprehensive testing and carefully followed to ensure patient safety.

On-going investigations continue to define the acceptable criteria to permit MR examinations, including those involving 1.5- and 3-Tesla MR systems, to be performed in patients with implanted neurostimulation systems. Notably, interventional MR procedures have been described recently using real-time MR imaging to place DBS electrodes. The use of MR-guidance results in several advantages including reduced overall procedure times as well as the ability to confirm appropriate electrode placement prior to completing surgery.

[MR healthcare professionals are advised to contact the respective manufacturer in order to obtain the latest safety information to ensure patient safety relative to the use of an MR procedure.]

REFERENCES

Aziz TZ. Current and future directions of post-deep brain stimulation implant magnetic resonance imaging scanning. World Neurosurg. 2011;76:69-70.

Baker K, Nyenhuis JA, Hridlicka G, Rezai AR, Tkach JA, Sharan A, Shellock FG. Neurostimulator implants: assessment of magnetic field interactions associated with 1.5- and 3.0-Tesla MR systems. J Magn Reson Imaging 2005;21:72-77.

Baker KB, Tkach JA, Nyenhuis JA, Phillips M, Shellock FG, Gonzalez-Martinez J, Rezai AR. Evaluation of specific absorption rate as a dosimeter of MRI-Related implant heating. J Magn Reson Imaging 2004;20:315-320.

Baker KB, Tkach J, Hall JD, Nyenhuis JA, Shellock FG, Rezai AR. Reduction of MRI-related heating in deep brain stimulation leads using a lead management system. Neurosurgery 2005;57:392-397.

Baker KB, et al. Variability in RF-induced heating of a deep brain stimulation implant across MR systems. J Magn Reson Imaging 2006;24:1236-42.

Baker KB, et al. Deep brain stimulation for obsessive-compulsive disorder: using functional magnetic resonance imaging and electrophysiological techniques: technical case report. Neurosurgery. 2007;61(5 Suppl 2):E367-8.

Bhidayasiri R, Bronstein JM, Sinha S, Krahl SE, Ahn S, Behnke EJ, Cohen MS, Frysinger R, Shellock FG. Bilateral neurostimulation systems used for deep brain stimulation: *In vitro* study of MRI-related heating at 1.5-Tesla and implications for clinical imaging of the brain. Magnetic Resonance Imaging 2005;23:549-555.

Bronstein JM, et al. Deep brain stimulation for Parkinson disease: an expert consensus and review of key issues. Arch Neurol. 2011;68:165.

Chhabra V, Sung E, et al. Safety of magnetic resonance imaging of deep brain stimulator systems: a serial imaging and clinical retrospective study. J Neurosurg. 2010;112:497-502.

De Andres J, Valia JC, et al. Magnetic resonance imaging in patients with spinal neurostimulation systems. Anesthesiology. 2007;106:779-86.

Dormont D, et al. Chronic thalamic stimulation with three-dimensional MR stereotactic guidance. AJNR Am J Neuroradiol 1997;18:1093-1097.

Elkelini MS, Hassouna MM. Safety of MRI at 1.5-Tesla in patients with implanted sacral nerve neurostimulator. Eur Urol. 2006 Aug;50(2):311-6.

Englot DJ, et al. Abnormal T2-weighted MRI signal surrounding leads in a subset of deep brain stimulation patients. Stereotact Funct Neurosurg. 2011;89:311-317.

Finelli DA, Rezai AR, Ruggieri P, Tkach J, Nyenhuis J, Hridlicka G, Sharan A, Stypulkowski PH, Shellock FG. MR-related heating of deep brain stimulation electrodes: an *in vitro* study of clinical imaging sequences. AJNR Am J Neuroradiol 2002;23:1795-1802.

Fraix V, et al. Effects of magnetic resonance imaging in patients with implanted deep brain stimulation systems. J Neurosurg. 2010;113:1242-5.

Georgi A-C, Stippich C, Tronnier VM, Heiland S. Active deep brain stimulation during MRI: a feasibility study. Magn Reson in Medicine 2003;51:380-388.

Gleason CA, et al. The effect of magnetic resonance imagers on implanted neurostimulators. Pacing Clin Electrophysiol 1992;15:81-94.

Gorny KR, et al. 3 Tesla MRI of patients with a vagus nerve stimulator: initial experience using a T/R head coil under controlled conditions. J Magn Reson Imaging. 2010 ;31:475-81.

Gupte AA, et al. MRI-related heating near deep brain stimulation electrodes: more data are needed. Stereotact Funct Neurosurg. 2011;89:131-40.

Henderson J, Tkach J, Phillips M, Baker K, Shellock FG, Rezai A. Permanent neurological deficit related to magnetic resonance imaging in a patient with implanted deep brain stimulation electrodes for Parkinson's disease: Case report. Neurosurgery 2005;57:E1063.

Kovacs N, Nagy F, Kover F, et al. Implanted deep brain stimulator and 1.0-Tesla magnetic resonance imaging. J Magn Reson Imaging. 2006;24:1409-12.

Larson PS, et al. Magnetic resonance imaging of implanted deep brain stimulators: experience in a large series. Stereotact Funct Neurosurg. 2008;86:92-100.

Liem LA, van Dongen VC. Magnetic resonance imaging and spinal cord stimulation systems. Pain 1997;70:95-97.

Maldonado IL, et al. Magnetic resonance-based deep brain stimulation technique: a series of 478 consecutive implanted electrodes with no perioperative intracerebral hemorrhage. Neurosurgery. 2009;65(6 Suppl):196-201.

Mogilner AY, Rezai AR. Brain stimulation: history, current clinical application, and future prospects. Acta Neurochir Suppl. 2003;87:115-120.

Mohsin SA, Sheikh NM, Saeed U. MRI-induced heating of deep brain stimulation leads. Phys Med Biol. 2008;53:5745-56.

Nazzaro JM, Lyons KE, Wetzel LH, Pahwa R. Use of brain MRI after deep brain stimulation hardware implantation. Int J Neurosci. 2010;120:176-83.

Phillips MD, et al. Parkinson disease: pattern of functional MR imaging activation during deep brain stimulation of subthalamic nucleus--initial experience. Radiology. 2006;239:209-16.

Rezai AR, et al. Thalamic stimulation and functional magnetic resonance imaging: localization of cortical and subcortical activation with implanted electrodes. J Neurosurg 1999;90;583-590.

Rezai AR, Baker K, Tkach J, Phillips M, Hrdlicka G, Sharan A, Nyenhuis J, Ruggieri P, Henderson J, Shellock FG. Is magnetic resonance imaging safe for patients with neurostimulation systems used for deep brain stimulation (DBS)? Neurosurgery 2005;57:1056-1062.

Rezai AR, Finelli D, Ruggieri P, Tkach J, Nyenhuis JA, Shellock FG. Neurostimulators: Potential for excessive heating of deep brain stimulation electrodes during MR imaging. J Magn Reson Imaging 2001;14:488-489.

Rezai AR, Finelli D, Nyenhuis JA, Hrdlick G, Tkach J, Ruggieri P, Stypulkowski PH, Sharan A, Shellock FG. Neurostimulator for deep brain stimulation: Ex vivo evaluation of MRI-related heating at 1.5-Tesla. J Magn Reson Imaging 2002;15:241-250.

Rezai AR, Phillips M, Baker K, Sharan AD, Nyenhuis J, Tkach J, Henderson J, Shellock FG. Neurostimulation system used for deep brain stimulation (DBS): MR safety issues and implications of failing to follow guidelines. Investigative Radiology 2004;39:300-303.

Rise MT. Instrumentation for neuromodulation. Archives Of Medical Research 2000;31:237-247.

Ryu SI, et al. Asymptomatic transient MRI signal changes after unilateral deep brain stimulation electrode implantation for movement disorder. Stereotact Funct Neurosurg. 2004;82:65-9.

Sankar T, Lozano AM. Magnetic resonance imaging and deep brain stimulation: questions of safety. World Neurosurg. 2011;76:71-3.

Shellock FG. MRI Safety and Neuromodulation Systems.In: NEUROMODULATION Krames ES, Peckham PH, Rezai, AR, Editors. Academic Press/Elsevier, New York, 2009.

Shellock FG. MR imaging and electronically-activated devices. Radiology. 219:294-295, 2001.

Shellock FG. Begnaud J, Inman DM. VNS Therapy System: *In vitro* evaluation of MRI-related heating and function at 1.5- and 3-Tesla. Neuromodulation 2006;9:204-213.

Shellock FG, et al. Implantable microstimulator: magnetic resonance safety at 1.5-Tesla. Investigative Radiology 2004;39:591-594.

Shrivastava D, et al. Effect of the extracranial deep brain stimulation lead on radiofrequency heating at 9.4 Tesla (400.2 MHz). J Magn Reson Imaging. 2010;32:600-7.

Smith CD, et al. Chapter 16. Health effects of induced electrical currents: Implications for implants. In: Magnetic resonance: health effects and safety, FG Shellock, Editor, CRC Press, Boca Raton, FL, 2001; pp. 393-413.

Spiegel J, et al. Transient dystonia following magnetic resonance imaging in a patient with deep brain stimulation electrodes for the treatment of Parkinson disease. J Neurosurgery 2003;99:772-774.

Tagliati M, et al. and the National Parkinson Foundation DBS Working Group. Safety of MRI in patients with implanted deep brain stimulation devices. Neuroimage. 2009;47 Suppl 2:T53-7.

Thani NB, et al. Accuracy of postoperative computed tomography and magnetic resonance image fusion for assessing deep brain stimulation electrodes. Neurosurgery. 2011;69:207-14.

Tronnier VM, et al. Magnetic resonance imaging with implanted neurostimulation systems: an in vitro and in vivo study. Neurosurgery 1999;44:118-25.

Ullman M, et al. A pilot study of human brain tissue post-magnetic resonance imaging: information from the National Deep Brain Stimulation Brain Tissue Network (DBS-BTN). Neuroimage. 2011;54 Suppl 1:S233-

Utti RJ, Tsuboi Y, et al, Wharen RE. Magnetic resonance imaging and deep brain stimulation. Neurosurgery 2002;51:1423-1431.

Weise LM, et al. Postoperative MRI examinations in patients treated by deep brain stimulation using a non-standard protocol. Acta Neurochir (Wien). 2010;152:2021-7.

Zonenshayn M, Mogilner AY, Rezai AR. Neurostimulation and functional brain stimulation. Neurological Research 2000;22;318-325.

Zrinzo L, et al. Clinical safety of brain magnetic resonance imaging with implanted deep brain stimulation hardware: large case series and review of the literature. World Neurosurg. 2011;76:164-72.

Neurostimulation Systems: Deep Brain Stimulation

MRI Guidelines for Medtronic Deep Brain Stimulation Systems
Medtronic Inc., Minneapolis, MN

Models:
Kinetra: 7428
Soletra: 7426
Itrel II: 7424
Activa PC Deep Brain Neurostimulator (Model 37601)
Activa RC Deep Brain Neurostimulator (Model 37612)
Activa SC Deep Brain Neurostimulator (Model 37602)
Activa SC Deep Brain Neurostimulator (Model 37603)

MRI and Activa Therapy

Introduction

It is important to read this section in its entirety before conducting an MRI examination on a patient with any implanted Activa System component.

Due to the number and variability of parameters that affect MRI compatibility, the safety of patients or continued functioning of Activa Systems exposed to MRI cannot be absolutely ensured. MRI systems generate powerful electromagnetic fields that can produce a number of interactions with implanted components of the Activa neurostimulation system. Some of these interactions, especially heating, are potentially hazardous and can lead to serious injury or death. However, with appropriate control measures, particularly with respect to the selection of MRI parameters and RF coils, it is generally possible to safely perform an MRI head scan on an Activa patient. In addition, Activa System components can affect the MRI image, potentially impacting the diagnostic use of this modality. The following information describes the potential interactions and control measures that should be taken to minimize the risks from these interactions.

Contraindication

Implantation of an Activa Brain Stimulation System is contraindicated for patients who will be exposed to Magnetic Resonance Imaging (MRI) using a full body transmit radio-frequency (RF) coil, a receive-only head coil, or a head transmit coil that extends over the chest area. Performing MRI with this equipment can cause tissue lesions from component heating, especially at the lead electrodes, resulting in serious and permanent injury including coma, paralysis, or death.

Warnings

- Do not conduct an MRI examination on a patient with any implanted Activa System component until you read and fully understand all the information in this section. Failure to follow all warnings and guidelines related to MRI can result in serious and permanent injury including coma, paralysis, or death.
- In-vitro testing has shown that exposure of the Activa neurostimulator system to MRI at parameters other than those described in this guideline can induce significant heating at the lead electrodes or at breaks in the lead. Excessive heating may occur even if the lead and/or extension are the only part of the Activa System that is implanted. Excessive heating can result in serious and permanent injury including coma, paralysis, or death.
- MRI examinations of patients with an implanted Activa System should only be done if absolutely needed and then only if these guidelines are followed. MRI should not be considered for Activa patients if other potentially safer diagnostic methods such as CT, X-ray, ultrasound, or other methods will provide adequate diagnostic information.
- A responsible individual with expert knowledge about MRI, such as an MRI radiologist or MRI physicist, must assure all procedures in this guidelines are followed and that the MRI scan parameters, especially RF specific absorption rate (SAR) and gradient dB/dt parameters, comply with the recommended settings, both for the pre-scan (tuning) and during the actual MRI examination. The responsible individual must verify that parameters entered into the MRI system meet the guidelines in this section.
- Do not conduct an MRI examination if the patient has any other implants or limiting factors that would prohibit or contraindicate an MRI examination.

Precautions

- The neurostimulator, especially those without filtered feedthroughs such as the Itrel II Model 7424, may be reset or potentially damaged when subjected to an MRI examination. If reset, the neurostimulator must be reprogrammed. If damaged, the neurostimulator must be replaced.
- MRI images may be severely distorted or image target areas can be completely blocked from view near the implanted Activa System components, especially near the neurostimulator. If the MRI targeted image area is near the neurostimulator, it may be necessary to move the neurostimulator to obtain an image, or use alternate imaging techniques. Do not remove the neurostimulator and leave the lead system implanted as this can result in higher than expected lead heating.
- Carefully weigh any decision to perform magnetic resonance imaging (MRI) examinations on patients who require the neurostimulator to control tremor. Image quality during MRI examinations may be reduced, because the tremor may return when the neurostimulator is turned off.
- If possible, do not sedate the patient so that the patient can provide feedback of any problems during the examination.
- Monitor the patient during the MRI examination. Verify that the patient is feeling normal and is responsive between each individual scan sequence of the MRI examination. Discontinue the MRI immediately if the patient becomes unresponsive to questions or experiences any heating, pain, shocking sensations/uncomfortable stimulation, or unusual sensations.

Note: The MRI guidelines provided here may significantly extend the MRI examination time or prevent some types of MRI examinations from being conducted on Activa patients.

General Information on MRI

An MRI system produces three types of electromagnetic fields that may interact with implanted neurostimulation systems. All three of these fields are necessary to produce an MRI image. Each of these fields can also produce specific but different types of interactions with implanted neurostimulator systems. These fields include:

- **Static Magnetic Field.** This is a steady state non-varying magnetic field that is normally always ON, even when no scan is underway. In a 1.5 Tesla MRI system, the static magnetic field is approximately 30,000 times greater than the magnetic field of the earth.

- **Gradient Magnetic Field.** This is a low-frequency pulsed magnetic field that is only present during a scan. The gradient magnetic field can induce voltages onto the lead system that may result in unintended stimulation or functional interactions with the neurostimulator.

- **RF Field.** This is a pulsed radio frequency (RF) field that is only present during a scan. It can be produced by a variety of transmission RF coils such as a whole body transmit coil or an extremity coil such as a transmit/receive head coil. Only a transmit/receive head coil should be used as the other RF coils can expose more of the lead system to RF energy, thereby increasing the risk of excessive heating and thermal lesions possibly resulting in coma, paralysis, or death.

MRI Interactions with Implanted Activa Systems

MRI/neurostimulation system interactions are various, and the risk to the patient can range from minimal to severe. These interactions include the following:

Heating – The MRI RF field induces voltages onto the lead system that can produce significant heating effects at the lead electrode-tissue interface or at the location of any breaks in the neurostimulator lead system. Component heating from the MRI RF field is the most serious risk from MRI exposure. Failure to follow these MRI recommendations can result in thermal lesions possibly resulting in coma, paralysis, or death.

Magnetic Field Interactions – Magnetic field interactions such as force and torque effects are produced by the static magnetic field. Any magnetic material will be attracted to the static magnetic field of the MRI. The force and torque effects may produce movement of the neurostimulator that can be uncomfortable to the patient, open a recent incision, or both. Activa System components are designed with minimal magnetic materials.

Induced Stimulation – Gradient magnetic fields may induce voltages onto the lead system that may cause unintended stimulation. The voltage of the induced stimulation pulses is proportional to the time rate of change (dB/dt) of the gradient pulses, the effective loop area created by the neurostimulator lead system, and the location of the lead system with respect to the gradient coils of the MRI.

Effects on Neurostimulator Function – The static, gradient, and RF fields of the MRI may affect the neurostimulator operation and programming. The static magnetic field may cause the neurostimulator to turn ON or OFF if the neurostimulator uses a magnetically controlled switch that allows the patient to control stimulation by the application of a handheld magnet. Additionally, the MRI RF, static, and gradient fields may temporarily affect or disable other functions, such as telemetry or stimulation pulses. Parameters will need to be reprogrammed if the MRI causes a POR (Power On Reset) of the neurostimulator.

Image Artifacts and Distortion – The neurostimulation system components, particularly the neurostimulator, can cause significant imaging artifacts and/or distortion of the MRI image, particularly if the neurostimulator components contain magnetic material. The neurostimulator can cause the MRI image to be completely blocked from view (i.e., signal loss or signal "void") or severely distorted within several inches of the neurostimulator.

MRI Procedure

Scope

These MRI/neurostimulator exposure guidelines apply to Activa Systems comprising combinations of the following components:

- Neurostimulator Models: Itrel II 7424, Soletra 7426, Kinetra 7428, Activa RC 37612, Activa PC 37601
- Lead Extension Models: 7495, 7482, 7482A, 37085
- Lead Models: DBS 3387, 3389

Supervision

A responsible individual such as an MRI radiologist or MRI physicist must assure these procedures are followed. If the MRI is operated by an MRI technician, it is strongly recommended the responsible individual verifies that the MRI recommendations are followed.

Preparation

Do the following prior to performing an MRI examination on an Activa patient:

1) Inform the patient of the risks of undergoing an MRI.
2) Check if the patient has any other implants or conditions that would prohibit or contraindicate an MRI examination. Do not conduct an MRI examination if any are found.

3) Verify that all proposed MRI examination parameters comply with the "MRI Operation Settings" on Table 2. If not, the parameters must be modified to meet these requirements. If this cannot be done, do not perform an MRI.

4) If the patient has implanted leads but does not have an implanted neurostimulator, perform the following steps:

   - Wrap the external portion of the leads/percutaneous extensions with insulating material.
   - Keep the external portion of the leads/percutaneous extensions out of contact with the patient.
   - Keep the external leads/percutaneous extensions straight, with no loops, and running down the center of the head coil.

5) If the patient has an implanted neurostimulator, perform the following steps:

   - Review the neurostimulator with a clinician programmer and print out a copy of the programmed parameters for reference.
   - Test for possible open circuits by measuring impedance and battery current on all electrodes in unipolar mode (see Table 1). If an open circuit is suspected, obtain an x-ray to identify whether the open circuit is caused by a broken lead wire. If a broken lead wire is found, do not perform an MRI.

Warning: An MRI procedure should not be performed in a patient with an Activa System that has a broken lead wire because higher than normal heating may occur at the break or the lead electrodes which can cause thermal lesions. These lesions may result in coma, paralysis, or death.

Table 1. Measurement Values Indicating Possible Open Circuits

Neurostimulator	Impedance
Itrel II Model 7424	>2000
Soletra Model 7426	>2000
Kinetra Model 7428	>2000
Activa RC Model 37612	>2000
Activa PC Model 37601	>2000

Note: For all devices, any measurement with a value of <250 Ω typically indicates a possible short circuit.

Warning: An MRI procedure should not be performed in a patient with an Activa System that has a broken lead wire because higher than normal heating may occur at the break or the lead electrodes, which can cause thermal lesions. These lesions may result in coma, paralysis, or death.

- If the Activa System is functioning properly and no open or short circuits are found, program the neurostimulator to the settings provided in Table 2.

Table 2. Recommended Neurostimulator Settings (for all programs) for MRI

Parameter	Setting
Stimulation output	OFF
Stimulation mode	Bipolar (Soletra and Itrel II only)
Amplitude	0 Volts (Soletra and Itrel II only)
Magnetic (reed) switch	Disabled (Kinetra Model 7428 only)
Day Cycling	Disabled (Kinetra Model 7428 only)
Other parameters	Do not change

MRI Operation Settings

Prior to the MRI examination, a responsible individual such as an MRI radiologist or MRI physicist must assure the examination will be conducted according to the following MRI requirements. If standard MRI pulse sequences will be used, they must meet these requirements. If they do not, the pulse parameters must be adjusted so that they comply with these requirements:

Warning: In-vitro testing has shown that exposure of the Activa System to MRI under conditions other than described in this guideline can induce excessive heating at the lead electrodes or at breaks in the lead to cause lesions. These lesions may result in coma, paralysis, or death.

- Use only a 1.5 Tesla horizontal bore MRI (do not use open sided or other field strength MRI systems).
- Use only a transmit/receive head coil.

Contraindication: Implantation of an Activa Brain Stimulation System is contraindicated for patients who will be exposed to Magnetic Resonance Imaging (MRI) using a full body transmit radio-frequency (RF) coil, a receive-only head coil, or a head transmit coil that extends over the chest area. Performing MRI with this equipment can cause tissue lesions from component heating, especially at the lead electrodes, resulting in serious and permanent injury including coma, paralysis, or death.

- Enter the correct patient weight into the MRI console to assure the head SAR is estimated correctly.

- Use MRI examination parameters that limit the displayed average head SAR to 1/10 (0.1) W/kg or less for all RF pulse sequences unless the applied SAR is known. If known, an applied SAR up to 1/10 (0.1) W/kg may be used.

Warnings

- Ensure the SAR value is the value for head SAR. Some MRI systems may only display SAR, whole body SAR, or local body SAR. Make sure the value being limited to 1/10 (0.1) W/kg is for head SAR. Excessive heating may occur if the wrong SAR value is used.
- If MRI parameters must be manually adjusted after the initial automatic MRI prescan, do not make any adjustments that will increase the SAR value. Some MRI machines may not automatically update the displayed SAR value if manual adjustments are made. This may lead to higher than expected temperature increases in the Activa System, particularly at the lead electrodes.
- Limit the gradient dB/dt field to 20 Tesla/second or less.

Note: The recommendations provided are based on in-vitro testing and should result in a safe MRI examination of a patient with an implanted Medtronic Activa System. However, due to the many variables that affect safety, Medtronic cannot absolutely ensure safety or that the neurostimulator will not be damaged. The user of this information assumes full responsibility for the consequences of conducting an MRI examination on a patient with an implanted Activa System.

Prior to the MRI Examination

Prior to the scan examination, the responsible individual must verify the MRI examination parameters comply with these guidelines.

- Patients with implanted Activa Systems should be informed of the risks of undergoing an MRI.
- If possible, do not use sedation so the patient can inform the MRI operator of any heating, discomfort, or other problems.
- Instruct the patient to immediately inform the MRI operator if any discomfort, stimulation, shocking, or heating occurs during the examination.

During the MRI Examination

- Monitor the patient both visually and audibly. Check the patient between each imaging sequence. Discontinue the MRI examination immediately if the patient is unable to respond to questions or reports any problems.

- Conduct the examination using only the MRI pulse sequence that the MRI radiologist or physicist has confirmed meets the MRI requirements above.

Post MRI Examination Review

- Verify that the patient is feeling normal.
- Verify that the neurostimulator is functional.
- Reprogram the neurostimulator to pre-MRI settings.

[MR healthcare professionals are advised to contact the respective manufacturer in order to obtain the latest safety information to ensure patient safety relative to the use of an MR procedure.]

REFERENCE

http://www.medtronic.com/

Neurostimulation System: Enterra Therapy, Gastric Electrical Stimulation (GES)

The **Enterra Therapy, Gastric Electrical Stimulation (GES) System** (Medtronic, Inc., Minneapolis, MN), is a neurostimulation system indicated for treatment of patients with chronic, intractable (drug refractory) nausea and vomiting secondary to gastroparesis of diabetic or idiopathic etiology. Enterra Therapy uses mild electrical pulses to stimulate the stomach. This electrical stimulation helps to control the symptoms associated with gastroparesis, including nausea and vomiting.

Enterra Models: 7425G, 3116

Patients with an implanted device should not be exposed to the electromagnetic fields produced by magnetic resonance imaging (MRI). Use of MRI may potentially result in system failure or dislodgment, heating, or induced voltages in the neurostimulator and/or lead. An induced voltage through the neurostimulator or lead may cause uncomfortable, "jolting," or "shocking," levels of stimulation.

Clinicians should carefully weigh the decision to use MRI in patients with an implanted neurostimulation system, and note the following:

- Magnetic and radio-frequency (RF) fields produced by MRI may change the neurostimulator settings, activate the device, and injure the patient.
- Patients treated with MRI should be closely monitored and programmed parameters verified upon cessation of MRI.

[MR healthcare professionals are advised to contact the respective manufacturer in order to obtain the latest safety information to ensure patient safety relative to the use of an MR procedure.]

REFERENCE

http://www.medtronic.com/

Neurostimulation System: InterStim Therapy - Sacral Nerve Stimulation (SNS) for Urinary Control

InterStim Therapy - Sacral Nerve Stimulation (SNS) for Urinary Control (Medtronic, Inc., Minneapolis, MN) is a treatment for urinary urge incontinence, non-obstructive urinary retention, and significant symptoms of urgency-frequency in patients who have failed or could not tolerate more conservative treatments. In properly selected patients, InterStim Therapy can be dramatically successful in reducing or eliminating symptoms. The implantable InterStim System uses mild electrical stimulation of the sacral nerve that influences the behavior of the bladder, sphincter, and pelvic floor muscles.

This information on MRI pertains to the following Medtronic products:
InterStim: Model number 3023
InterStim II: Model number 3058

Magnetic resonance imaging (MRI) – MRI is not recommended for a patient who has any implanted component of a neurostimulation system. Exposing a patient with an implanted neurostimulation system or component to MRI may potentially injure the patient or damage the neurostimulator. Clinicians should carefully weigh the decision to use MRI in patients with an implanted neurostimulation system, and note the following:

Induced electrical currents from the MRI to the neurostimulation system or component may cause heating, especially at the lead electrode site, resulting in tissue damage. Induced electrical currents may also stimulate or shock the patient.

Note: This warning applies even if only a lead or extension is implanted.

Factors that increase the risks of heating and patient injury include, but are not limited to, the following:

- High MRI Specific Absorption Rate (SAR) radio frequency (RF) power levels.
- MRI RF transmit coil that is near or extends over the implanted lead.
- Implanted leads with small surface area electrodes.
- Short distances between lead electrodes and tissue that is sensitive to heat.
- An MRI may permanently damage the neurostimulator, requiring it be removed or replaced.
- An MRI may affect the normal operation of the neurostimulator.
- An MRI can also reset the neurostimulator to power-on-reset values requiring reprogramming by a trained InterStim clinician.
- The neurostimulator can move within the implant pocket and align with the MRI field, resulting in discomfort or reopening of a recent implant incision.

In addition, the image details from MRI may be degraded, distorted, or blocked from view by the implanted neurostimulation system.

Patients treated with MRI should be closely monitored and programmed parameters verified upon cessation of MRI.

[MR healthcare professionals are advised to contact the respective manufacturer in order to obtain the latest safety information to ensure patient safety relative to the use of an MR procedure.]

REFERENCE

http://www.medtronic.com/

Neurostimulation Systems: Spinal Cord Stimulation

St. Jude Medical

Genesis, GenesisXP, GenesisRC, Eon, Eon C, Eon Mini, and Renew

The Genesis, GenesisXP, GenesisRC, Eon, EonC, Eon Mini, and Renew neuromodulation devices (St. Jude Medical) used for spinal cord stimulation are indicated as aids in the management of chronic intractable pain of the trunk and/or limbs including unilateral or bilateral pain associated with any of the following: failed back surgery syndrome, intractable low back and leg pain, as well as for the treatment of other conditions.

MRI Information. The labeling information for these afore-mentioned products states:
"Warnings/Precautions: Diathermy therapy, cardioverter defibrillators, magnetic resonance imaging (MRI), explosive or flammable gases, theft detectors and metal screening devices, lead movement, operation of machinery and equipment, postural changes, pediatric use, pregnancy, and case damage. Patients who are poor surgical risks, with multiple illnesses, or with active general infections should not be implanted."

In addition, the following has been stated:
"Magnetic resonance imaging (MRI). Patients with implanted neurostimulation systems should not be subjected to MRI. The electromagnetic field generated by an MRI may forcefully dislodge implanted components, damage the device electronics, and induce voltage through the lead that could jolt or shock the patient."

Therefore, these devices are currently contraindicated for patients referred for MR procedures.

REFERENCE

http://sjmneuropro.com

Neurostimulation Systems: Spinal Cord Stimulation

Medtronic, Inc

**PrimeAdvanced Spinal Cord Neurostimulator
(PrimeAdvanced, Model 37702)
RestoreAdvanced Spinal Cord Neurostimulator
(RestoreAdvanced, Model 37713)
RestoreUltra Spinal Cord Neurostimulator
(RestoreUltra, Model 37712)**

Models:

**Itrel 3: 7425
Restore: 37711
Synergy: 7427
SynergyPlus: 7479
Synergy Versitrel: 7427V
SynergyCompact: 7479B**

Medtronic, Minneapolis, MN

MRI and Neurostimulation Therapy for Chronic Pain

Medtronic recommends that you do not conduct an MRI examination of any part of the body on a patient using a radio-frequency (RF) transmit body coil. If all of the instructions stated in this section are followed, MRI examinations of the head only using an RF transmit/receive head coil may be safely performed.

It is important to read this information in its entirety before conducting an MRI examination on a patient with any implanted component of a Medtronic neurostimulation system for chronic pain. These instructions do not apply to other implantable products or other devices, products, or items.

Contact Medtronic if you have any questions. www.Medtronic.com

Due to the number and variability of parameters that affect MRI compatibility, the safety of patients or continued functioning of neurostimulation systems exposed to MRI cannot be absolutely ensured. MRI systems generate powerful electromagnetic fields that can produce a number of interactions with implanted components of the neurostimulation system. Some of these interactions, especially heating, are potentially hazardous and can lead to serious injury or death. However, when all instructions stated in this section are followed, MRI examinations of the head only may be safely performed. In addition, neurostimulation system components can affect the MRI image, potentially impacting the diagnostic use of this modality. The following information describes the potential interactions and control measures that should be taken to minimize the risks from these interactions.

The instructions in this section describe how to conduct a head-only MRI examination of a patient with a neurostimulation system implanted for chronic pain, using a transmit/receive head coil of a 1.5-Tesla horizontal bore MRI. MRI examinations of any other part of the body are not recommended, as these require the use of the MRI RF transmit body coil, which may produce hazardous temperatures at the location of the implanted lead electrodes.

Warnings
MRI RF transmit body coil – Medtronic recommends that you do not conduct an MRI examination using an RF transmit body coil on a patient with any implanted neurostimulation system component because the interaction of the MRI with the neurostimulation system may lead to serious injury or death. See the section "Risks associated with MRI examination".

MRI transmit/receive head coil – An MRI examination of the head only (no other part of the body) can be conducted safely using an RF transmit/receive head coil when all instructions in this section are followed.

Limitations

- MRI should not be considered for patients with neurostimulation systems if other potentially safer diagnostic methods such as CT, x-ray, ultrasound, or others will provide adequate diagnostic information.
- These instructions apply only to Medtronic neurostimulation therapies for chronic pain for approved indications.

- The instructions in this section apply to all Medtronic fully implantable neurostimulators, leads, and extensions used for chronic pain therapy.

Note: The instructions contained in this section are not applicable to MRI examinations of patients with radiofrequency (RF) neurostimulators. Medtronic recommends physicians not prescribe MRI for a patient who has an implanted Itrel 3 Model 7425 Neurostimulator. The Itrel 3 Neurostimulator is highly susceptible to reset or damage when subjected to an MRI examination. If reset, the neurostimulator must be reprogrammed. If damaged, the neurostimulator must be replaced. The Itrel 3 Neurostimulator has an increased risk of induced electrical current, which may stimulate or shock the patient.

Contact Medtronic for information about newer models or any updates.

- The RF transmit/receive head coil must not cover any implanted system component.
- If the patient has any other implants or products that prohibit or contraindicate an MRI examination, follow the instructions from the manufacturer. The instructions in this section apply only to the Medtronic products listed above.
- Do not conduct an MRI examination if the patient's neurostimulation system has a broken lead wire, because higher than normal heating may occur at the break or lead electrodes. Excessive heating can cause tissue damage and result in severe injury or death.
- Physicians should not prescribe MRI for patients undergoing trial neurostimulation and having systems that are not fully implanted.

If the MRI targeted image area is near the neurostimulator, it may be necessary to move the neurostimulator to obtain an image, or use alternate imaging techniques. MRI images may be severely distorted or image target areas can be completely blocked from view near the implanted neurostimulation system components, especially near the neurostimulator.

- Do not remove the neurostimulator and leave the lead system implanted as this can result in higher than expected lead heating. Excessive heating can cause tissue damage and result in severe injury or death.

Risks associated with MRI examination – Exposing a patient with an implanted neurostimulation system or component to MRI may potentially injure the patient or damage the neurostimulator. The known potential risks are as follows:

- Induced electrical currents from the MRI to the neurostimulation system or component may cause heating, especially at the lead-electrode site, resulting in tissue damage. Induced electrical currents may also stimulate or shock the patient.

Note: This warning applies even if only a lead or extension is implanted.

Factors that increase the risks of heating and patient injury include, but are not limited to, the following:

- High MRI specific absorption rate (SAR) RF power levels
- Low impedance leads or extensions (Medtronic product names or model numbers designated by a "Z," an "LZ," or "low impedance")
- MRI RF transmit/receive coil that is near or extends over the implanted lead system
- Implanted lead systems with small surface area electrodes
- Short distances between lead electrodes and heat-sensitive tissue
- Exposure to gradients exceeding a dB/dt limit of 20 Tesla per second may result in overstimulation or shocking, particularly for unipolar-capable devices.
- MRI may permanently damage the neurostimulator, requiring explant or replacement.
- MRI may affect the operation of the neurostimulator. The MRI may also reset the parameters to power-on-reset settings, requiring reprogramming with the clinician programmer. The Itrel 3 Model 7425 Neurostimulator is highly susceptible to reset or damage when subjected to an MRI examination. If reset, the neurostimulator must be reprogrammed. If damaged, the neurostimulator must be replaced. An Itrel 3 neurostimulator also might exhibit unpredictable behavior if subjected to an MRI examination.

The neurostimulator may move within the implant pocket and align itself with the MRI field, which may cause patient discomfort or a recent neurostimulator implant incision to open.

Cautions

Patient interaction during MRI – If possible, do not sedate the patient so that the patient can provide feedback of any problems during the examination.

Monitor the patient during the MRI examination. Verify that the patient is feeling normal and is responsive between each individual scan sequence of the MRI examination. Discontinue the MRI immediately if the patient becomes unresponsive to questions or experiences any heating, pain, shocking sensations/ uncomfortable stimulation, or unusual sensations.

MRI procedure using an RF transmit/receive head coil
Supervision
If all of the instructions stated in this section are followed, MRI examinations of the head using an RF transmit/receive head coil may be safely performed.

Prior to the MRI examination, an individual with the proper knowledge of MRI equipment such as an MRI radiologist or MRI physicist must ensure the MRI examination will be conducted according to the information outlined in this section.

Note: Due to the additional requirements in these instructions, MRI examination time maybe significantly extended.

MRI exposure requirements
Prior to an MRI examination, determine whether the patient has multiple active medical device implants (such as deep-brain stimulation systems, implantable cardiac defibrillators, and others). The most restrictive MRI exposure requirements must be used if the patient has multiple active medical device implants. Contact the appropriate manufacturers of the devices if you have questions.

If the following requirements cannot be met, do not proceed with the MRI examination.

- Use only an RF transmit/receive head coil.*
- Use only a 1.5-Tesla horizontal bore MRI (do not use open sided or other field strength MRI systems).
- Enter the correct patient weight into the MRI console to ensure the head SAR is estimated correctly. The MRI scan sequences must meet the following requirements. If they do not, the pulse parameters must be adjusted so that they comply with these requirements.
- Use MRI examination parameters that limit the head SAR to 1.5 W/kg or less for all RF pulse sequences.

- Limit the gradient dB/dt field to 20 Tesla per second or less.

*Important: If you are unsure if your MRI has RF transmit/receive head coil capability or if it displays "head SAR", check with your MRI manufacturer.

Note: The requirements provided are based on *in-vitro* testing and should result in a safe MRI examination of a patient with an implanted Medtronic neurostimulation system when all instructions in this section are followed. However, due to the many variables that affect safety, the safety of patients or continued functionality of neurostimulator systems exposed to MRI cannot be absolutely ensured. The user of this information assumes full responsibility for the consequences of conducting an MRI examination on a patient with an implanted neurostimulation system.

Preparation for the MRI examination
Do the following prior to performing an MRI examination on a patient with an implanted neurostimulation component:

1) Inform the patient of all of the risks of undergoing an MRI examination as stated in this section.
2) If possible, do not use sedation so the patient can inform the MRI operator of any heating, discomfort, or other problems.
3) Instruct the patient to immediately inform the MRI operator if any discomfort, stimulation, shocking, or heating occurs during the examination.
4) Determine if the patient has any other implants or conditions that would prohibit or contraindicate an MRI examination. If you are unclear what implants may be present, perform an x-ray to determine implant type and location. Do not conduct an MRI examination if any conditions or implants that would prohibit or contraindicate an MRI are present.
5) Verify that all proposed MRI examination parameters comply with the "MRI exposure requirements" (see above). If not, the parameters must be modified to meet these requirements. If parameters cannot be modified, do not perform an MRI.
6) If the patient has implanted leads but does not have an implanted neurostimulator, perform the following steps:

   - Wrap the external portion of the leads/percutaneous extensions with insulating material, such as dry gauze.
   - Keep the external portion of the leads/percutaneous extensions out of contact with the patient.

- Keep the external leads/percutaneous extensions straight, with no loops, and running down the center of the head coil.

7) If the patient has an implanted neurostimulator, perform the following steps:

- Review the neurostimulator with a clinician programmer and print out a copy of the programmed parameters for reference.
- Test for possible open circuits by measuring impedance on all electrodes. An impedance measurement greater than 4000 for Synergy Plus, Synergy Compact, Synergy Versitrel, Synergy, or Itrel 3 indicates a possible open circuit. An impedance measurement greater than 3600 for Restore indicates a possible open circuit.
- If an open circuit is suspected, obtain an x-ray to identify whether the open circuit is caused by a broken lead wire. If a broken lead wire is found, do not perform an MRI examination.

Warning: Do not conduct an MRI examination if the patient's neurostimulation system has a broken lead wire, because higher than normal heating may occur at the break or lead electrodes. Excessive heating can cause thermal lesions and result in severe injury or death.

8) If the system is functioning properly and no broken lead wires are found, program the neurostimulator to the settings provided in Table 1.

Table 1. Recommended neurostimulator settings for MRI examinations

Parameter	Setting
Stimulation output	OFF (all programs)
Stimulation mode	Bipolar (all programs)
Amplitude	0 Volts (all programs)
Magnetic (reed) switch	Disabled (Itrel 3 Model 7425 only)
Other parameters	Do not change

During the MRI examination

- Monitor the patient both visually and audibly. Check the patient between each imaging sequence. Discontinue the MRI examination immediately if the patient is unable to respond to questions or reports any problems.

- Conduct the examination using only the MRI pulse sequence that the MRI radiologist or physicist has confirmed meets the "MRI exposure requirements" outlined in this section.

Post-MRI examination review

- Verify that the patient feels normal.
- Verify that the neurostimulator is functional.
- Reprogram the neurostimulator to pre-MRI settings.

Models:
Mattrix: 3272, 3271

Reference: Pain Therapy IFP (221351-001)

Medtronic recommends physicians **not** prescribe an MRI for a patient who has any implanted component of a [Mattrix] system. Exposing a patient with a [Mattrix] system or component to an MRI may potentially injure the patient and/or damage the receiver. The known potential risks are as follows:

- Induced electrical currents from the MRI to the [Mattrix] system or component may cause heating, especially at the lead electrode site, resulting in tissue damage. Induced electrical currents may also stimulate or shock the patient.

Note: This warning applies even if only a lead or extension is implanted.

Heating risks are affected by a number of factors involving the MRI equipment and the implanted [Mattrix] system. Factors that increase the risks of heating and patient injury include, but are not limited to, the following:

- High MRI Specific Absorption Rate (SAR) Radio Frequency (RF) power levels
- Low impedance leads or extensions (Medtronic product names or model numbers designated by a "Z," an "LZ," or "low impedance")
- MRI RF transmit coil that is near or extends over the implanted lead system
- Implanted lead systems with small surface area electrodes
- Short separation distances between lead electrodes and thermally sensitive tissue

- An MRI may permanently damage the receiver, which may require explant or possible replacement.
- An MRI may affect the functional operation of the receiver
- The receiver may move within the implant pocket and align itself with the MRI field, which may cause patient discomfort or a recent receiver implant incision to open.

In addition, the image details from MRI may be degraded, distorted, or blocked from view by the implanted [Mattrix] system.

[MR healthcare professionals are advised to contact the respective manufacturer in order to obtain the latest safety information to ensure patient safety relative to the use of an MR procedure.]

REFERENCE

http://www.medtronic.com/

Neurostimulation System: Vagus Nerve Stimulation

Vagus Nerve Stimulation, Vagal Nerve Stimulator, VNS Therapy, NeuroCybernetic Prosthesis (NCP) System

(Cyberonics, Inc., Houston, TX)

Important Note (12/2011): Cyberonics, Inc. recently received approval from the Food and Drug Administration for expansion of MRI use with VNS Therapy Systems. The expansion includes, the following:
-New MRI labeling: All cylindrical MRI scanners with magnetic field strengths of 3.0 and 1.5- Tesla.
-Previous MRI labeling: GE Signa 1.5-Tesla scanner, only.

-New MRI labeling: MR imaging of the head and extremities, including knees, using transmit/receive RF coils.
-Previous MRI labeling: Head imaging, only, using transmit/receive RF coil

Current MRI information for the Vagus Nerve Stimulator, VNS Therapy, NeuroCybernetic Prosthesis (NCP) System may be found by visiting http://www.cyberonics.com.

Important Note: Highly specific conditions must be followed in order to safety perform MRI in patients with the Vagus Nerve Stimulator, VNS Therapy, NeuroCybernetic Prosthesis (NCP) System.

[MR healthcare professionals are advised to contact the respective manufacturer in order to obtain the latest safety information to ensure patient safety relative to the use of an MR procedure.]

REFERENCES

http://www.cyberonics.com
http://dynamic.cyberonics.com/manuals/

Ocular Implants, Lens Implants, and Devices

Of the different ocular implants, lens implants, and devices tested in the MR environment, the Fatio eyelid spring, the retinal tack made from martensitic (i.e., ferromagnetic) stainless steel (Western European), the Troutman magnetic ocular implant, and the Unitek round wire eyelid spring demonstrated positive magnetic field interactions in association with exposure to 1.5-Tesla MR systems. By comparison, many of the lens implants pose no hazard to the patient during an MRI procedure since they are not made from metallic materials (see **The List**).

A patient with a Fatio eyelid spring or round wire eyelid spring may experience discomfort but would probably not be injured as a result of exposure to an MR system. In fact, patients have undergone MR procedures with eyelid wires after having a protective plastic covering placed around the globe along with a firmly applied eye patch as a precaution.

The retinal tack made from martensitic stainless steel and Troutman magnetic ocular implant may injure a patient undergoing an MR procedure, although no such case has ever been reported.

[For additional information pertaining to ocular related prostheses, see **Glaucoma Drainage Implants (Shunt Tubes)**, **Magnetically-Activated Implants and Devices**, and **Scleral Buckle (Scleral Buckling Procedure**.]

REFERENCES

Albert DW, Olson KR, Parel JM, et al. Magnetic resonance imaging and retinal tacks. Arch Ophthalmol 1990;108:320-321.

de Keizer RJ, Te Strake L. Intraocular lens implants (pseudophakoi) and steelwire sutures: a contraindication for MRI? Doc Ophthalmol 1984;61:281-284.

Joondeph BC, Peyman GA, Mafee MF, et al. Magnetic resonance imaging and retinal tacks [Letter]. Arch Ophthalmol 1987;105:1479-1480.

Marra S, et al. Effect of magnetic resonance imaging on implantable eyelid weights. Ann Otol Rhinol Laryngol 1995;104:448-452.

Roberts CW, Haik BG, Cahill P. Magnetic resonance imaging of metal loop intraocular lenses. Arch Ophthalmol 1990;108:320-321.

Seiff SR, Vestel KP, Truwit CL. Eyelid palpebral springs in patients undergoing magnetic resonance imaging: an area of possible concern [Letter]. Arch Ophthalmol 1991;109:319.

Shellock FG. Magnetic Resonance Procedures: Health Effects and Safety. CRC Press, LLC, Boca Raton, FL, 2001.

Shellock FG, Kanal E. Magnetic Resonance: Bioeffects, Safety, and Patient Management. Second Edition, Lippincott-Raven Press, New York, 1996.

Shellock FG, Myers SM, Schatz CJ. Ex vivo evaluation of ferromagnetism determined for metallic scleral "buckles" exposed to a 1.5-T MR scanner. Radiology 1992;185:288-289.

Orthopedic Implants, Materials, and Devices

Most of the orthopedic implants, materials, and devices evaluated for MRI issues (i.e., magnetic field interactions, heating, and artifacts) are made from nonferromagnetic materials and, therefore, are safe or "MR conditional" according to specific conditions for patients undergoing MR procedures. However, due to the length or formation of a conductive loop, MRI-related heating may be a problem for some orthopedic implants, especially cervical fixation devices or external fixation systems (see below).

The Perfix interference screw used for reconstruction of the anterior cruciate ligament has been found to be highly ferromagnetic. Because this interference screw is firmly imbedded in bone for its specific application, it is held in place with sufficient retentive force to prevent movement or dislodgment. Patients with Perfix interference screws have safely undergone MR procedures using MR systems operating at 1.5-Tesla.

Patients with many of the "MR safe" or "MR conditional" orthopedic implants, materials, and devices indicated in **The List** have undergone MR procedures using MR systems operating at 3-Tesla or less without incident.

External Fixation Systems. External fixation systems comprise specially designed frames, clamps, rods, rod-to-rod couplings, pins, posts, fasteners, wire fixations, fixation bolts, washers, nuts, hinges, sockets, connecting bars, screws and other components used in orthopedic and reconstructive surgery. Indications for external fixation systems are varied and include the following treatment applications:

- Open and closed fracture fixation;
- Pseudoarthroses of long bones (both congenital and acquired);
- Limb lengthening by metaphyseal or epiphyseal distraction;
- Correction of bony or soft tissue defects; and
- Correction of bony or soft tissue deformities.

The assessment of MRI issues for external fixation systems is particularly challenging because of the myriad of possible components (many of which are made from conductive materials) and configurations used for these devices. The primary concern is MRI-related heating which is dependent on particular aspects (e.g., the lengths of the component parts) of the external fixation system. Importantly, the MRI conditions (strength of the static magnetic field, RF field, RF transmit coil, pulse sequence, body part imaged, position of the fixation device relative to the transmit RF coil, etc.) used greatly impacts the safety aspects of scanning patients with external fixation systems.

To ensure patient safety, guidelines are typically applied on a case by case basis and, therefore, MR professionals are referred to product labeling approved by the U.S. Food and Drug Administration for a given external fixation system. Notably, the acceptable MRI conditions typically apply to the specific configuration(s) used in the evaluation of a given fixation device, ONLY. Other configurations may be unsafe.

Vibration Associated With MR Procedures. Graf et al. reported that torque acting on metallic implants or instruments due to eddy-current induction in associated with MR imaging can be considerable. Larger implants (such as fixation devices) made from well-conducting materials are especially affected. Gradient switching was shown to produce fast alternating torque. Significant vibrations at off-center positions of the metal parts may explain why some patients with metallic implants sometimes report feeling heating sensations during MR examinations.

MRI at 3-Tesla and Orthopedic Implants, Materials, and Devices. A variety of orthopedic implants have been evaluated for magnetic field interactions at 3-Tesla (see **The List**). Most of these are considered to be acceptable for patients based on findings for deflection angles, torque, and their intended *in vivo* uses. For some orthopedic implants, MRI-related heating was evaluated and is a concern for certain devices, especially external fixation systems and cervical fixation devices.

[MR healthcare professionals are advised to contact the respective manufacturer in order to obtain the latest safety information to ensure patient safety relative to the use of an MR procedure.]

REFERENCES

Farrelly C, et al. Imaging of soft tissues adjacent to orthopedic hardware: comparison of 3-T and 1.5-T MRI. AJR Am J Roentgenol. 2010;194:W60-4.

Graf H, et al. Metal artifacts caused by gradient switching. Magnetic Resonance in Medicine 2005;54;231-234.

Knott PT, et al. A comparison of magnetic and radiographic imaging artifact after using three types of metal rods: stainless steel, titanium, and vitallium. Spine J. 2010;10:789-94.

Koch KM, et al. Magnetic resonance imaging near metal implants. J Magn Reson Imaging. 2010;32:773-87.

Luechinger R, Boesiger P, Disegi JA. Safety evaluation of large external fixation clamps and frames in a magnetic resonance environment. J Biomed Mater Res B Appl Biomater. 2007;82:17-22.

Lyons CJ, Betz RR, Mesgarzadeh M, et al. The effect of magnetic resonance imaging on metal spine implants. Spine 1989;14:670-672.

McComb C, Allan D, Condon B. Evaluation of the translational and rotational forces acting on a highly ferromagnetic orthopedic spinal implant in magnetic resonance imaging. J Magn Reson Imaging. 2009;29:449-53.

Mechlin M, et al. Magnetic resonance imaging of postoperative patients with metallic implants. AJR Am J Roentgenol 1984;143:1281-1284.

Mesgarzadeh M, et al. The effect on medical metal implants by magnetic fields of magnetic resonance imaging. Skeletal Radiol 1985;14:205-206.

Muranaka H, et al. Evaluation of RF heating on hip joint implant in phantom during MRI examinations. Nippon Hoshasen Gijutsu Gakkai Zasshi. 2010;66:725-33.

Shellock FG. Magnetic Resonance Procedures: Health Effects and Safety. CRC Press, LLC, Boca Raton, FL, 2001.

Shellock FG. Biomedical implants and devices: assessment of magnetic field interactions with a 3.0-Tesla MR system. J Magn Reson Imaging 2002;16:721-732.

Shellock FG, Crues JV. High-field-strength MR imaging and metallic bioimplants: an *in vitro* evaluation of deflection forces and temperature changes induced in large prostheses [Abstract]. Radiology 1987;165:150.

Shellock FG, Kanal E. Magnetic Resonance: Bioeffects, Safety, and Patient Management. Second Edition, Lippincott-Raven Press, New York, 1996.

Shellock FG, Mink JH, Curtin S, et al. MRI and orthopedic implants used for anterior cruciate ligament reconstruction: assessment of ferromagnetism and artifacts. J Magn Reson Imaging 1992;2:225-228.

Shellock FG, Morisoli S, Kanal E. MR procedures and biomedical implants, materials, and devices: 1993 update. Radiology 1993;189:587-599.

Stradiotti P, et al. Metal-related artifacts in instrumented spine. Techniques for reducing artifacts in CT and MRI: state of the art. Eur Spine J. 2009;18 Suppl 1:102-8.

Yang CW, Liu L, et al. Magnetic resonance imaging of artificial lumbar disks: safety and metal artifacts. Chin Med J (Engl). 2009;20;122:911-6.

Otologic Implants

Of the otologic implants evaluated for the presence of magnetic field interactions (note: MRI-related heating is not considered to be an issue for these relatively small implants), the McGee stapedectomy piston prosthesis, made from platinum and chromium-nickel alloy stainless steel, is ferromagnetic. The manufacturer recalled this otologic implant. Patients who received this device have been issued warnings to avoid MR procedures. The specific item and lot numbers of the McGee implants recalled and considered to be a contraindication for MR procedures are as follows (Personal Communication, Winston Geer, Smith & Nephew Richards Inc., Barlett, TN, 1995):

Item No.	Lot Number
14-0330	1W91100, 4UO9690
14-0331	4U09700
14-0332	1W91110, 4U58540, 4U86300
14-0333	4U09710, 1W34390, 2WR4073
14-0334	4U09720, 1W34390, 2WR4073
14-0335	1W34400, 4U09730
14-0336	3U18350, 3U50470, 4UR2889
14-0337	3U18370, 4UR2889
14-0338	3U18390, 4U02900, 4UR1453
14-0339	3U18400, 3U50500
14-0340	3U18410, 3U50500
14-0341	3U41200, 4UR2889

MRI at 3-Tesla and Otologic Implants. Many otologic implants have been evaluated for magnetic field interactions at 3-Tesla (see **The List**). In consideration of the relatively small sizes of these items, MRI-related heating is not a concern at 3-Tesla. For the ones tested, all are considered to be acceptable for patients based on findings for translational attraction, torque, and according to the intended *in vivo* uses of these specific devices.

Otologic Implants, Micromedics, Inc. (Eagan, MN). MRI testing at 3-Tesla was conducted on the following products from Micromedics, Inc:

Stainless Steel Vent Tube & Stainless Steel Wire

Because of the size of the metallic mass associated with these particular products, the MRI test findings (MR Conditional 6, 3-Tesla or less) apply to all of the product families listed below (Micromedics, Inc., Eagan, MN):

VT-0205-, Fluoroplastic with stainless steel wire
VT-0702-, Silicone with stainless steel wire
VT-1402-, Stainless Steel with stainless steel wire
VT-1412-, Titanium with stainless steel wire
VT-1505-, Polyethylene with stainless steel wire

Otologic Implants, Grace Medical (Memphis, TN). The Otologic device families from Grace Medical (Memphis, TN; www.GraceMedical.com) listed below are considered **MR Safe** according to the American Society for Testing and Materials (ASTM) International, Designation: F2503, since these items are made from non-metallic and non-conducting materials:

Device Family	Family Product Number(s)	Device Material(s)
Stapes Prostheses-Pistons	401-XXX, 402-XXX, 403-XXX, 404-XXX, 405-XXX, 406-XXX, 408-XXX	Fluoroplastic
Partial and Total Prostheses	1XX, 190-XXX	hydroxyapatite
Partial and Total Prostheses	2XX, 193	hydroxyapatite, Silicone

The Otologic device families listed below are considered **MR Conditional** according to the American Society for Testing and Materials (ASTM) International, Designation: F2503 and based on MRI tests conducted on selected implants that represented worst case with regard to materials and mass.

Device Family	Family Product Number(s)	Device Material(s)
ALTO Partial and Total Prostheses	6XX	Titanium, Silicone, hydroxyapatite
K-Helix Prostheses	756-XXX, 757-XXX	Titanium
Strasnick Prostheses	220-XXX, 270-XXX	Titanium, Silicone
Precise Prostheses	700-XXX, 705-XXX, 720-XXX, 750-XXX, 765-XXX, 770-XXX	Titanium, hydroxyapatite

Device Family	Family Product Number(s)	Device Material(s)
Stapes Prostheses-Piston	409-XXX, 410-XXX, 411-XXX, 412-XXX, 413-XXX, 415-XXX, 417-XXX, 418-XXX, 419-XXX, 452-XXX, 453-XXX, 465-XXX, 466-XXX, 467-XXX, 468-XXX, 469-XXX	Titanium, Platinum, Stainless Steel, Nitinol, Fluoroplastic
Stapes Prostheses-Buckets	420-XXX, 421-XXX, 422-XXX, 423-XXX, 424-XXX, 425-XXX, 426-XXX, 427-XXX, 428-XXX, 429-XXX, 430-XXX	Titanium, Nitinol

The **MRI Information** is, as follows (3-Tesla, Conditional 6):
Non-clinical testing has demonstrated that patients with these specific Grace Medical ossicular implants can undergo MRI safely, immediately after implantation under the following conditions:

- Static magnetic field of 3-Tesla or less
- Maximum spatial gradient magnetic field of 720-Gauss/cm or less.
- MR system reported, whole-body-averaged specific absorption rate (SAR) of 2.9-W/kg for 15 minutes of scanning (i.e., per pulse sequence).

MRI-Related Heating: Under controlled testing conditions a temperature rise equal to or less than +1.6 °C occurred.

Artifact Information: MR image quality may be compromised if the area of interest is in the exact same area or relatively close to the device. Therefore, optimization of imaging parameters may be necessary.

REFERENCES

Applebaum EL, Valvassori GE. Effects of magnetic resonance imaging fields on stapedectomy prostheses. Arch Otolaryngol 1985;11:820-821.

Applebaum EL, Valvassori GE. Further studies on the effects of magnetic resonance fields on middle ear implants. Ann Otol Rhinol Laryngol 1990;99:801-804.

Bauknecht HC, et al. Behaviour of titanium middle ear implants at 1.5 and 3 Tesla field strength in magnetic resonance imaging. Laryngorhinootologie. 2009;88:236-40.

Fritsch MH. MRI scanners and the stapes prosthesis. Otol Neurotol 2007;28:733-8.

Fritsch MH, Mosier KM. MRI compatibility issues in otology. Curr Opin Otolaryngol Head Neck Surg. 2007;15:335-340.

Fritsch MH, Gutt JJ. Ferromagnetic movements of middle ear implants and stapes prostheses in a 3-T magnetic resonance field. Otol Neurotol. 2005;26:225-230.

Leon JA, Gabriele OF. Middle ear prothesis: significance in magnetic resonance imaging. Magn Reson Imaging 1987;5:405-406.

Martin AD, et al. Safety evaluation of titanium middle ear prostheses at 3.0 Tesla. Otolaryngol Head Neck Surg 2005;132:537-42.

Nogueira M, Shellock FG. Otologic bioimplants: Ex vivo assessment of ferromagnetism and artifacts at 1.5-Tesla. AJR Am J Roentgenol 1995;163:1472-1473.

Shellock FG. Magnetic Resonance Procedures: Health Effects and Safety. CRC Press, LLC, Boca Raton, FL, 2001.

Shellock FG, Morisoli S, Kanal E. MR procedures and biomedical implants, materials, and devices: 1993 update. Radiology 1993;189:587-599.

White DW. Interaction between magnetic fields and metallic ossicular prostheses. Am J Otol 1987;8:290-292.

Wild DC, Head K, Hall DA. Safe magnetic resonance scanning of patients with metallic middle ear implants. Clin Otolaryngol. 2006;31:508-510.

www.gracemedical.com

Oxygen Tanks and Gas Cylinders

According to Chaljub et al., accidents related to ferromagnetic oxygen tanks and other gas cylinders that can become projectiles might be increasing. In fact, missile-related accidents for these objects as well as other items have resulted in at least one fatality, several injuries, damage to MR systems, and down-time (i.e., loss of revenue) for many MRI centers.

Therefore, MRI facilities must implement a policy for safe administration of oxygen to patients undergoing MR procedures. In lieu of utilizing pipes to directly deliver gases to patients, the use of non-magnetic (usually aluminum) gas cylinders is one means of preventing "missile effect" hazards in the MR environment. Non-magnetic oxygen tanks and cylinders for other gases are commercially available from various vendors.

MRI centers should have a sufficient number of nonmagnetic oxygen tanks and strict policies to prevent emergency staff members from introducing ferromagnetic objects into the MR environment. Notably, some hospital-based MR centers have nonmagnetic oxygen tanks used throughout their buildings to prevent projectile accidents.

Nonmagnetic tanks must be prominently labeled and/or color-coded to avoid confusion with magnetic cylinders. Additionally, only regulators tested and demonstrated to be acceptable for use in a high magnetic field environment should be used with the nonmagnetic cylinders. Furthermore, all healthcare workers that work in the MR environment must be informed regarding the fact that only nonmagnetic oxygen and other gas cylinders are allowed into the MR system room.

Nonmagnetic or weakly magnetic (i.e., MR conditional) oxygen regulators, flow meters, cylinder carts, cylinder stands, cylinder holders for wheelchairs, and suction devices are also commercially available to provide safe respiratory support and management of patients in the MR environment and for transfer to and from the MRI facility.

REFERENCES

Chaljub G, et al. Projectile cylinder accidents resulting from the presence of ferromagnetic nitrous oxide or oxygen tanks in the MR suite. American Journal of Roentgenology 2001;177:27-30.

Colletti PM. Size "H" oxygen cylinder: accidental MR projectile at 1.5-Tesla. Journal of Magnetic Resonance Imaging 2004;19:141-143.

ECRI. Patient Death Illustrates the Importance of Adhering to Safety Precautions in Magnetic Resonance Environments. ECRI, Plymouth Meeting, PA, Aug. 6, 2001.

Jolesz FA, et al. Compatible instrumentation for intraoperative MRI: expanding resources. Journal of Magnetic Resonance Imaging, 1998;8:8-11.

Keeler EK, et al. Accessory equipment considerations with respect to MRI compatibility. Journal of Magnetic Resonance Imaging, 1998;8:12-18.

Shellock FG. Magnetic Resonance Procedures: Health Effects and Safety. CRC Press, Boca Raton, FL, 2001.

Palatal System Implant Assembly

The **Palatal System Implant Assembly** (Pavad Medical, Inc., Fremont, CA) is designed to treat sleep disordered breathing.

MRI Information

The Palatal System Implant Assembly was determined to be MR-conditional according to the terminology specified in the ASTM International, Designation: F2503. Standard Practice for Marking Medical Devices and Other Items for Safety in the Magnetic Resonance Environment.

Non-clinical testing demonstrated that the Palatal System Implant Assembly is MR Conditional. A patient with this implant can be scanned safely, immediately after placement under the following conditions:

- Static magnetic field of 1.5-Tesla
- Maximum spatial gradient magnetic field of 250-Gauss/cm
- Maximum MR system reported whole-body-averaged specific absorption rate (SAR) of 3.5-W/kg for 15 minutes of scanning (per pulse sequence)

In non-clinical testing, the Palatal System Implant Assembly produced a temperature rise of 0.8°C at a maximum MR system-reported whole body averaged specific absorption rate (SAR) of 3.5-W/kg for 15-minutes of MR scanning in a 1.5-Tesla MR system using a transmit/receive body coil (1.5-Tesla, Magnetom, Software Numaris/4, Version Syngo MR 2002B DHHS, Siemens Medical Solutions, Malvern, PA).

MR image quality may be compromised if the area of interest is in the exact same area or relatively close to the position of the Palatal System Implant Assembly. Therefore, optimization of MR imaging parameters to compensate for the presence of this implant may be necessary. The following chart provides artifact information for the Palatal System Implant Assembly in relation to different pulse sequences at 1.5-Tesla:

Pulse sequence	Signal Void
T1-weighted spin echo, long axis orientation	2.7-cm^2
T1-weighted spin echo, short axis orientation	2.7-cm^2
Gradient echo, long axis orientation	8.8-cm^2
Gradient echo, short axis orientation	9.6-cm^2

MRI Procedures and Function of the Palatal System Implant Assembly

The effects of MRI procedures on the functional aspects of Palatal System Implant Assembly devices were assessed. *In-vitro* testing was performed on a phantom with six Palatal System Implant Assembly devices placed in various orientations relative to the MR system. MRI was conducted using 1.5-Tesla/64 MHz MR system (transmit/receive RF body coil) to perform 8 different MR imaging pulse sequences, as follows: T1-weighted spin echo, T1-weighted fast spin echo, T2-weighted spin echo, T2- weighted fast spin echo, three dimensional fast gradient echo, turbo/fast gradient echo, turbo/fast spoiled gradient echo, echo planar imaging.

The findings indicated that there was no apparent damage or alteration in the function of the Palatal System Implant Assembly. Thus, the Palatal System Implant Assembly was demonstrated to maintain full functionality after exposure to the MRI conditions indicated above.

Additional guidelines for the Palatal System Implant Assembly include:

- Do not use MR systems other than 1.5 Tesla MR systems.
- Continuously monitor the patients using visual and audio means (i.e., intercom system) throughout the MR procedure
- Instruct the patient to alert the MR system operator of any unusual sensations or problems so the MR system operator can terminate the MRI procedure, if needed.
- Provide the patient with a means to alert the MR system operator of any unusual sensations or problems that may be experienced during the MRI procedure.

Patent Ductus Arteriosus (PDA) Occluders, Atrial Septal Defect (ASD) Occluders, Ventricular Septal Defect (VSD) Occluders, and Patent Foramen Ovale (PFO) Closure Devices

Cardiac occluders and closure devices are implants used to treat patients with patent ductus arteriosus (PDA), atrial septal defect (ASD), ventricular septal defect (VSD), or patent foramen ovale (PFO) heart conditions. For implants that have been evaluated relative to the use of 1.5-T MR systems, as long as the proper size occluder or closure device is used, the amount of retention provided by the folded-back, hinged arms of the implant is sufficient to keep it in place, acutely. Eventually, tissue growth covers the cardiac occluder or closure device and facilitates retention.

Certain metallic PDA, ASD, VSD occluders and PFO closure devices tested for magnetic qualities were made from either 304V stainless steel or MP35N. Occluders made from 304V stainless steel were found to be "weakly" ferromagnetic, whereas those made from MP35N were nonferromagnetic in association with a 1.5-Tesla MR system.

Patients with cardiac occluders made from MP35N (i.e., a nonferromagnetic alloy) may undergo MR procedures at 1.5-Tesla or less any time after placement of these implants. However, patients with cardiac occluders made from 304V stainless steel (i.e., a "weakly ferromagnetic" material) are advised to wait a minimum of six weeks after implantation before undergoing MR procedures. This wait period permits tissue ingrowth to provide additional retentive forces for the occluders made from weakly ferromagnetic materials.

If there is any question about the integrity of the retention aspects of a metallic cardiac occluder made from a ferromagnetic material, the individual or patient should not be allowed into the MR environment or to undergo an MR procedure.

MRI at 3-Tesla and PDA, ASD, VSD Occluders and PFO Closure Devices. Various PDA, ASD, VSD occluders and PFO closure devices have been evaluated at 3-Tesla (see **The List**). All of these tested to date are considered to be acceptable for patients referred for MR examinations based on findings for deflection angles, torque, MRI-related heating and the intended *in vivo* uses of these specific devices.

REFERENCES

Shellock FG, Morisoli SM. Ex vivo evaluation of ferromagnetism and artifacts for cardiac occluders exposed to a 1.5-Tesla MR system. J Magn Reson Imaging 1994;4:213-215.

Shellock FG. Magnetic Resonance Procedures: Health Effects and Safety. CRC Press, LLC, Boca Raton, FL, 2001.

Shellock FG, Valencerina S. Septal repair implants: evaluation of MRI safety at 3-Tesla. Magnetic Resonance Imaging 2005;23:1021-1025.

Pellets and Bullets

The majority of pellets and bullets tested in the MR environment were found to be composed of nonferromagnetic materials, however, these items are often "contaminated" by ferromagnetic metals. Ammunition that proved to be ferromagnetic tended to be manufactured in foreign countries and/or used for military applications. Shrapnel typically contains steel and, therefore, presents a potential hazard for patients undergoing MR procedures.

Because pellets, bullets, and shrapnel are frequently contaminated with ferromagnetic materials, the risk versus benefit of performing an MR procedure should be carefully considered. Additional consideration must be given to whether the metallic object is located near or in a vital anatomic structure, with the assumption that the object is likely to be ferromagnetic and can potentially move.

In an effort to reduce lead poisoning in "puddling" type ducks, the federal government requires many of the eastern United States to use steel shotgun pellets instead of lead. The presence of steel shotgun pellets presents a potential hazard to patients undergoing MR procedures and causes substantial imaging artifacts at the immediate position of these metallic objects.

In one case, a small metallic BB located in a subcutaneous site caused painful symptoms in a patient exposed to an MR system, although no serious injury occurred. In consideration of this information, MR healthcare professionals should exercise caution when deciding to perform MR procedures in patients with pellets, bullets, shrapnel or other similar ballistic objects.

Smugar et al. conducted an investigation to determine whether neurological problems developed in patients with intraspinal bullets or bullet fragments in association with MR imaging performed at 1.5-Tesla. Patients were queried during scanning for symptoms of discomfort, pain, or changes in neurological status. Additionally, detailed neurological examinations were performed prior to MRI, post MRI, and at the patients' discharge. Based on these findings, Smugar et al. concluded that patients with complete spinal cord injury may undergo MR imaging if they have intraspinal bullets or fragments without concern for affects on their physical or neurological status. Thus, metallic fragments in the spinal canals of paralyzed patients are believed to represent only a relative contraindication to MR procedures.

Eshed et al. (2010) conducted a retrospective investigation of the potential hazards for patients undergoing MRI at 1.5-Tesla with retained metal fragments from combat and terrorist attacks. Metal fragments in 17 patients were in ranged in size between one and 10-mm. One patient reported a superficial migration of a 10-mm fragment after MRI. No other adverse reactions were reported. The authors concluded that 1.5T MRI examinations are safe in patients with retained metal fragments from combat and terrorist attacks not in the vicinity of vital organs. However, caution is advised as well as an assessment of risk:benefit for the patient.

REFERENCES

Eshed I, et al. Is magnetic resonance imaging safe for patients with retained metal fragments from combat and terrorist attacks? Acta Radiol. 2010;51:170-4.

Shellock FG. Magnetic Resonance Procedures: Health Effects and Safety. CRC Press, LLC, Boca Raton, FL, 2001.

Shellock FG, Kanal E. Magnetic Resonance: Bioeffects, Safety, and Patient Management. Second Edition, Lippincott-Raven Press, New York, 1996.

Smugar SS, Schweitzer ME, Hume E. MRI in patients with intraspinal bullets. J Magn Reson Imaging 1999;9:151-153.

Teitelbaum GP. Metallic ballistic fragments: MR imaging safety and artifacts [Letter]. Radiology 1990;177:883.

Teitelbaum GP, Yee CA, Van Horn DD, et al. Metallic ballistic fragments: MR imaging safety and artifacts. Radiology 1990;175:855-859.

Penile Implants

Several types of penile implants and prostheses have been evaluated for magnetic field interactions associated with MR systems. Of these, two (i.e., the Duraphase and Omniphase models) demonstrated substantial ferromagnetic qualities when exposed to a 1.5-Tesla MR system. Fortunately, it is unlikely for a penile implant to severely injure a patient undergoing an MR procedure because of the degree of magnetic field interactions associated with the 1.5-Tesla MR system. This is especially true when one considers the manner in which this device is utilized. Nevertheless, it would be uncomfortable for a patient with a ferromagnetic penile implant to undergo an MR examination. For this reason, subjecting a patient with the Duraphase or Omniphase penile implant to the MR environment or an MR procedure is inadvisable.

MRI at 3-Tesla and Penile Implants. Several different penile implants have been tested in association with 3-Tesla MR systems. Findings for these specific penile implants indicated that they either exhibited no magnetic field interactions or relatively minor or "weak" magnetic field interactions. Accordingly, these specific penile implants are considered acceptable for patients undergoing MR procedures using MR systems operating at 3-Tesla or less and according to the MR conditional labeling (see **The List**).

REFERENCES

Shellock FG. Magnetic Resonance Procedures: Health Effects and Safety. CRC Press, LLC, Boca Raton, FL, 2001.

Shellock FG, Crues JV, Sacks SA. High-field magnetic resonance imaging of penile prostheses: *in vitro* evaluation of deflection forces and imaging artifacts [Abstract]. In: Book of Abstracts, Society of Magnetic Resonance in Medicine. Berkeley, CA: Society of Magnetic Resonance in Medicine, 1987;3:915.

Shellock FG, Kanal E. Magnetic Resonance: Bioeffects, Safety, and Patient Management. Second Edition, Lippincott-Raven Press, New York, 1996.

Pessaries

A pessary is a relatively small medical device that is inserted into the vagina or rectum and held in place by the pelvic floor musculature. In some instances, a pessary may contain metal to permit forming it into a shape to facilitate proper fit and retention. Typically, the pessary is a firm ring or similar structure that presses against the wall of the vagina and urethra to help decrease urinary leakage or other condition. Indications for the pessary include pelvic support defects, such as uterine prolapse and vaginal prolapse, as well as stress urinary incontinence.

MRI Information. A wide variety of pessary styles exist, including those made entirely from nonmetallic, nonconducting materials (e.g., plastic, silicone, or latex) as well as those that have metallic components. Pessaries made from nonmetallic, nonconducting materials pose no problems for patients undergoing MR procedures. However, pessaries that have metallic components may cause substantial artifacts and/or may pose risks to patients undergoing MR examinations. As such, a patient with a pessary that contains metal should be given additional consideration prior to the MR examination. Notably, to date, there is no report of injury or other significant problem related to performing MR examinations in patients with these devices.

REFERENCES

Brubacker L. The vaginal pessary. In: Friedman AJ, ed. American Urogynecologic Society Quarterly Report 1991.

Davila GW. Vaginal prolapse: management with nonsurgical techniques. Postgrad Med 1996;99: 171-6,181,184-5.

Deger RB, Menzin AW, Mikuta JJ. The vaginal pessary: past and present. Postgrad Obstet Gynecol 1993;13:1-8.

Komesu YM, et al. Restoration of continence by pessaries: magnetic resonance imaging assessment of mechanism of action. Am J Obstet Gynecol. 2008;198:563.e1-6.

Miller DS. Contemporary use of the pessary. In: Sciarra JJ, ed. Gynecology and obstetrics. Revised 1997 ed. Philadelphia: Lippencott-Raven, 1997:1-12.

Zeitlin MP, Lebherz TB. Pessaries in the geriatric patient. J Am Geriatr Soc 1992;40:635-9.

PillCam Capsule Endoscopy Device

The PillCam (Including the following: M2A, PillCam SB, PillCam SB2, PillCam ESO, PillCam ESO2, PillCam COLON 2) Capsule Endoscopy Device (Given Imaging Inc., Norcross, GA) is an ingestible device for use in the gastrointestinal tract. Peristalsis moves the PillCam Capsule smoothly and painlessly throughout the gastrointestinal tract, transmitting color video images as it passes. The procedure allows patients to continue daily activities during the endoscopic examination. The PillCam Capsule Endoscopy Device is a first-line tool in the detection of abnormalities of the small bowel.

The PillCam Capsule Endoscopy Device has been utilized to diagnose diseases of the small intestine including Crohn's Disease, celiac disease and other malabsorption disorders, benign and malignant tumors of the small intestine, vascular disorders and medication related small bowel injuries.

MRI Information

The User Manual for the PillCam Capsule Endoscopy Device states:

"Undergoing an MRI while the capsule is inside the patient's body may result in serious damage to his/her intestinal tract or abdominal cavity. If the patient did not positively verify the excretion of the PillCam Capsule from his/her body, he/she should contact the physician for evaluation and possible abdominal X-ray before undergoing an MRI examination."

This information applies to all versions/models of the PillCam devices.

[Reprinted with permission from Given Imaging Inc., Norcross, GA]

REFERENCE

www.givenimaging.com

RF BION Microstimulator

Surgically implanted neurostimulators and electrodes are utilized to provide functional electrical stimulation of the affected site. However, these devices may be associated with considerable surgical morbidity and expense. As such, there has been an on-going effort to develop technology that combines the reliability of using an implanted device with a low morbidity and low cost procedure. This effort has yielded a miniaturized, implantable device designed for functional electrical stimulation.

In 1988, Heetderks first demonstrated the feasibility of using a millimeter-sized, neuromodulation or neural prosthetic implant. Over the years, this so-called "microstimulator" evolved to its present form. The microstimulator now exists as a relatively small, wireless, digitally controlled stimulator that is implanted using a minimally invasive procedure to provide electrical pulses to a muscle or nerve. This device receives power and command signals by inductive coupling from an externally worn device that generates a radiofrequency magnetic field. The microstimulator is undergoing clinical trials to assess its therapeutic effect on a variety of neurological disorders including urinary incontinence, shoulder subluxation, drop foot, ventilator-dependant respiratory deficiencies, and sleep apnea.

RF BION Microstimulator. The implantable RF BION Microstimulator (Alfred E. Mann Foundation for Scientific Research, Valencia, CA and Advanced Bionics Corporation, Valencia, CA) is a wireless device designed for functional electrical stimulation of the peripheral nervous system. This hermetically-sealed implant is a small, lightweight, cylindrical-shaped device (length, 16.6-mm; diameter-2.4 mm; mass, 0.265-g). The active electrodes are welded on each end cap: an iridium disk on the cathodal side and a platinum-iridium eyelet on the anodal side.

The microstimulator receives power and digital commands via a 2-MHz radiofrequency magnetic field link generated from an external coil that is worn by the patient. Because of the small size of this microstimulator, it may be implanted through a specially designed, trocar-based 12- or 14-gauge implant tool or via a small surgical opening for placement near a nerve or at the motor unit of a muscle. A suture passed through one of the end caps allows the microstimulator to be maintained in a properly implanted position.

MRI and the RF BION Microstimulator

Safety information for the use of a magnetic resonance imaging (MRI) procedure (i.e., imaging, angiography, functional imaging, spectroscopy, etc.) in a patient with the RF BION Microstimulator is highly specific to the type of MR system and conditions used to determine safety criteria for this implant. Safety information for MR procedures described herein pertains to the use of a 1.5-Tesla MR system, gradient magnetic fields of 20-Tesla/second or less, and a whole body averaged specific absorption rate (SAR) of 2.0 W/kg or less for 15-minutes of imaging (i.e., per pulse sequence).

Warning: The effects on the RF BION Microstimulator of performing MRI procedures using other MR systems and other conditions have not been determined.

The following information describes testing that was performed on the effect of magnetic resonance imaging (MRI) procedures on an implanted RF BION Microstimulator.

MR procedures MUST ONLY be performed according to the following information:

Magnetic Field Interactions. Magnetic field interactions (translational attraction and torque) were assessed for the RF BION Microstimulator in association with exposure to a 1.5-Tesla MR system. The RF BION Microstimulator displays relatively moderate magnetic field interactions. [The deflection angle measured for the RF BION Microstimulator was 58 degrees. Thus, the magnetic force is 1.6 times the gravitational force (0.42 g). The maximal magnetic torque was calculated to be equal to 3.9 times the "gravity torque", the product of the implant's length and weight. Therefore, torque can be viewed as a force equivalent to 0.98 g acting on one end of the RF BION Microstimulator with the other end fixed.] Because of the presence of the ferrite material (mass of 32 mg), the intended *in vivo* use of this implant must be considered.

Notably, tissue encapsulation around the RF BION Microstimulator is a major factor that will retain this implant *in situ*. *In vivo* research demonstrated that counter-forces provided by encapsulation (i.e., fibrous tissue) that occurs 2 to 3 weeks after implantation will prevent the RF BION Microstimulator from being moved or dislodged in association with the exposure to a 1.5-Tesla MR system. Therefore, considering that the mass of the RF BION Microstimulator is relatively small (0.25 g), and this implant does not contain any sharp ends, magnetic field interactions associated with exposure to a 1.5-Tesla MR system will not move or dislodge this implant after a conservative post-op waiting period of 6 to 8 weeks.

Interactions with Time-Varying Magnetic Fields. The potential interactions of the RF BION Microstimulator with magnetic resonance imaging (MRI)-related time-varying magnetic fields (gradient and RF) were theoretically and experimentally investigated with respect to a 1.5-Tesla/64-MHz MR system.

Effects of Radiofrequency Fields. Based on theoretical analysis and *in vitro* experiments, the presence of the RF BION Microstimulator in a patient undergoing an MRI procedure at a whole-body-averaged specific absorption rate (SAR) of 2-W/kg for 15-min.(i.e., per pulse sequence) will not result in a substantial increase in temperature. Therefore, a patient with the RF BION Microstimulator is not at increased risk with respect to MRI-related heating of this implant under the conditions used for this assessment.

Effects of Gradient Fields. The electric field in the body induced by the MRI pulsed gradient magnetic fields may exceed 5 V/m. Given the size and shape of the RF BION Microstimulator, this field intensity induces minimal voltage (95 mV) along the length of the implant. Importantly, concentration of the gradient currents will be no greater than that resulting from the concentration rising from bones surrounded by tissue. Therefore, no physiological impact is expected by the interaction between the RF BION Microstimulator with the gradient currents in the tissue of a patient with this implant undergoing an MR procedure at 1.5-Tesla/64 MHz. Accordingly, a patient with the RF BION Microstimulator may safely be exposed to the gradient magnetic fields (dB/dt) at levels that are currently allowed for 1.5-Tesla MR systems operating with conventional pulse sequences and standard accessories (e.g., surface RF coils).

Warning: Unconventional or non-standard MR techniques have not been assessed for the RF BION Microstimulator and, therefore, must be avoided.

MRI Procedures and Function of the RF BION Microstimulator. The effects of MRI procedures on the functional aspects of the RF BION System were assessed. *In vitro* testing was performed on a phantom with nine RF BION devices placed in various orientations relative to the MR system.

MR imaging was conducted using a 1.5-Tesla/64-MHz MR system (transmit/receive RF body coil) to perform 15 different MR imaging pulse sequences, as follows: (1) T1-weighted, spin echo pulse sequence, (2) T1-weighted, fast spin echo pulse sequence, (3) T2-weighted, spin echo pulse sequence, (4) T2-weighted, fast spin echo pulse sequence, (5) Gradient echo, two dimensional pulse sequence, (6) Gradient echo, three dimensional pulse sequence, (7) Fast gradient echo, two dimensional pulse sequence, (8) Fast gradient echo, three dimensional pulse sequence, (9) Fast spoiled gradient echo, two dimensional pulse, sequence, (10) Fast spoiled gradient echo, three dimensional pulse sequence, (11) T1-weighted, spin echo pulse sequence with high whole-body averaged specific absorption rate (1.1 W/kg), (12) T1-weighted, fast spin echo pulse sequence with high whole-body averaged specific absorption rate (1.1 W/kg), (13) T2-weighted, spin echo pulse sequence with high whole body averaged specific absorption rate (1.1 W/kg), (14) T2-weighted, fast spin echo pulse sequence with high whole-body averaged specific absorption rate (1.1 W/kg), and (15) Gradient echo, three dimensional pulse sequence with magnetization transfer contrast with high whole-body averaged specific absorption rate (1.1 W/kg)

The findings indicated that there was no apparent damage or alteration in the functional aspects of the RF BION Microstimulators. Thus, the RF BION Microstimulator was demonstrated to maintain full functionality after exposure to the MR imaging conditions indicated above.

Warning: The effect of using any other MR imaging pulse sequence or procedure on the RF BION Microstimulator is unknown.

Additional MRI Safety Guidelines for the RF BION Microstimulator

- DO NOT use MR systems other than 1.5 Tesla MR systems.
- Continuously monitor the patient using visual and audio means (i.e., intercom system) throughout the MR procedure.
- Instruct the patient to alert the MR system operator of any unusual sensations or problems so the MR system operator can terminate the MRI procedure, if needed.
- Provide the patient with a means to alert the MR system operator of any unusual sensations or problems that may be experienced during the MR procedure.

Post-MRI Procedure Recommendations for the RF BION Microstimulator. After undergoing an MRI procedure, the RF BION Microstimulator should be checked to ensure that it is working properly. To do so, stimulation threshold measurements should be obtained and compared to pre-MRI procedure threshold levels.

[For additional information about this product, including safety guidelines, contact the Alfred E. Mann Foundation, Valencia, CA; http://www.aemf.org and Advanced Bionics Corporation, Sylmar, CA; http://www.advancedbionics.com/]

[MR healthcare professionals are advised to contact the respective manufacturer in order to obtain the latest safety information to ensure patient safety relative to the use of an MR procedure.]

REFERENCES

Arcos, I, Davis R, Fey K, Mishler D, Sanderson D, Tanacs C, Vogel MJ, Wolf R, Zilberman Y, Schulman J. Second-generation microstimulator. Artificial Organs 2002;26:228-231.

Cameron T, Loeb GE, Peck RA, Schulman JH, Strojnik P, Troyk PR. Micromodular implants to provide electrical stimulation of paralyzed muscles and limbs. IEEE Trans Biomed Eng 1997; 44:781-90.

Heetderks, WJ. RF powering of millimeter- and submillimeter-sized neural prosthetic implants. IEEE Trans Biomed Eng 1988;35:323-327.

Loeb GE, Peck RA, Moore WH, Hood K. BION system for distributed neural prosthetic interfaces. Med Eng Phys. 2001;23:9-18.

Shellock FG, Cosendai G, Park S-M, Nyenhuis JA. Implantable microstimulator: magnetic resonancesafety at 1.5-Tesla. Investigative Radiology 2004;39:591-594.

Walter JS, Riedy L, King W, Wheeler JS, Najafi K, Anderson CL, Gudausky TM, Dokmeci M. Short-term bladder-wall response to implantation of microstimulators. J Spinal Cord Med. 1997;20:319-23.

Zealear DL, Garren KC, Rodriguez RJ, Reyes JH, Huang S, Dokmeci MR, Najafi K. The biocompatibility, integrity, and positional stability of an injectable microstimulator for reanimation of the paralyzed larynx. IEEE Trans Biomed Eng. 2001;48:890-7.

Reveal Plus Insertable Loop Recorder

The 9526 Reveal Plus Insertable Loop Recorder (ILR, Medtronic, Inc., Minneapolis, MN) is an implantable, single-use, programmable device containing two surface electrodes for continuous recording of the patient's subcutaneous electrocardiogram. This device is used to record the electrocardiogram subcutaneously and is indicated for patients who experience transient symptoms that may suggest a cardiac arrhythmia and patients with clinical syndromes or situations at increased risk of cardiac arrhythmias.

MRI and the Reveal Plus Insertable Loop Recorder

The Reveal Plus Insertable Loop Recorder contains no lead wires or large loops of electrically conductive material. The electromagnetic fields produced during magnetic resonance imaging may adversely affect the data stored by the Reveal Plus Insertable Loop Recorder. Therefore, consideration must be given to interrogating the Reveal Plus Insertable Loop Recorder in order to save the data that could become corrupted or erased. Accordingly, careful planning in conjunction with the physician responsible for the patient's Reveal Plus Insertable Loop Recorder is necessary.

Also, since this device contains ferromagnetic components, strong magnetic fields associated with the MR system may apply a mechanical force on the Reveal Plus Insertable Loop Recorder. Accordingly, the patient may feel slight movement of this device. While this does not represent a safety hazard, the patient must be informed of this possibility to avoid undue concern.

Additional information may be found in the Reveal Plus 9526 Insertable Loop Recorder System Product Information Manual, as follows:

- For information on how to interrogate and save data, refer to "How to Interrogate the ILR" and " How to Save To Disk," both in Chapter 3.
- For information on resetting collection data/parameters, refer to "Clearing Memory Without Changing Gain and Sensitivity Settings" in Chapter 2.

- For testing patient triggered storage integrity, refer to "Storing an Event in a Clinical Setting" in Chapter 2.

[Information provided with permission, Medtronic, Inc., Minneapolis, MN]

[MR healthcare professionals are advised to contact the respective manufacturer in order to obtain the latest safety information to ensure patient safety relative to the use of an MR procedure.]

REFERENCES

Gimbel JR, Wilkoff BL. Artefact mimicking tachycardia during magnetic resonance imaging in a patient with an implantable loop recorder. Heart. 2003;89:e10

Gimbel JR. Magnetic resonance imaging of implantable cardiac rhythm devices at 3.0 Tesla. Pacing Clin Electrophysiol. 2008;31:795-801.

http://www.medtronic.com/

Krahn A, et al. Final results from a pilot study with an implantable loop recorder to determine the etiology of syncope in patients with negative non-invasive and invasive testing. American Journal of Cardiology 82:117-119, 1998.

Reveal Syncope Validation Project (RSVP) Clinical Summary. Medtronic data on file.

Shellock FG, et al. Cardiac pacemakers, ICDs, and loop recorder: Evaluation of translational attraction using conventional ("long-bore") and "short-bore" MR systems at 1.5- and 3-Tesla. Journal of Cardiovascular Magnetic Resonance 2003;5:387-397.

Shellock FG. MR Safety and the Reveal Insertable Loop Recorder. Signals, No. 49, Issue 3, pp. 8, 2004.

Wong JA, et al. Feasibility of magnetic resonance imaging in patients with an implantable loop recorder. Pacing Clin Electrophysiol. 2008;31:333-7.

Reveal DX 9528 and Reveal XT 9529, Insertable Cardiac Monitors

Reveal DX 9528 Insertable Cardiac Monitor
Magnetic Resonance Imaging (MRI) – The Reveal DX is MR Conditional. It has been demonstrated to pose no known hazards in a specified MR environment with the conditions of use specified in the product manual. These conditions are quite extensive and must be reviewed carefully.

To download the manual for the **Reveal DX 9528 Insertable Cardiac Monitor** please visit www.medtronic.com/mrimanuals and enter the Model number for this product (i.e., 9528).

Reveal XT 9529 Insertable Cardiac Monitor
Magnetic Resonance Imaging (MRI) – The Reveal XT is MR Conditional. It has been demonstrated to pose no known hazards in a specified MR environment with the conditions of use specified in the product manual. These conditions are quite extensive and must be reviewed carefully.

To download the manual for the **Reveal XT 9529 Insertable Cardiac Monitor** please visit www.medtronic.com/mrimanuals and enter the Model number for this product (i.e., 9529).

[Information provided with permission, Medtronic, Inc., Minneapolis, MN]

[MR healthcare professionals are advised to contact the respective manufacturer in order to obtain the latest safety information to ensure patient safety relative to the use of an MR procedure.]

REFERENCES

www.medtronic.com
www.medtronic.com/mrimanuals

St. Jude Medical (SJM) Confirm, Implantable Cardiac Monitor

Implantable Cardiac Monitor, St. Jude Medical, Sylmar, CA

The St. Jude Medical (SJM) Confirm Implantable Cardiac Monitor (ICM) (St. Jude Medical, Sylmar, CA) is designed to monitor and store ECG data and to communicate with the St. Jude Medical, Merlin Patient Care System and the SJM Confirm external patient activator. The SJM Confirm ICM is an implantable patient-activated and automatically-activated monitoring system that records subcutaneous ECG and is indicated in the following cases:

-Patients with clinical syndromes or situations at increased risk of cardiac arrhythmias
-Patients who experience transient symptoms that may suggest a cardiac arrhythmia

The following information was provided by St. Jude Medical for the Confirm ICM:

Effects of Magnetic Resonance Imaging (MRI) on SJM Confirm Implantable Cardiac Monitors

This letter is being provided in response to your request for information about Magnetic Resonance Imaging and SJM Confirm implantable cardiac monitors.

Background. Magnetic Resonance Imaging (MRI) is a medical imaging technique used in radiology to visualize detailed internal structures. MRI is contraindicated by MRI manufacturers for patients with implantable cardiac monitors (ICMs). (*NOTE: This statement by SJM is incorrect.*) It is important to note that the SJM Confirm provides no therapy to the patient and is a cardiac diagnostic monitor only. It contains no lead wires.

Potential Effects. St. Jude Medical has not performed any formal testing on the effects of MRI exposure upon SJM Confirm ICMs. SJM Confirm is a diagnostic monitor and therefore only diagnostic data collection would be affected in the event one of these rare effects occurs.

A summary of potential effects is provided in the table below and is based on clinical experience and a review of the scientific literature.

Potential Effect	Estimated Frequency
Noisy EGM recordings	Common
Corruption of saved data	Rare
Backup operation	Rare
Component damage	Rare

Recommendations. Clinicians should carefully weigh the decision to use MRI with SJM Confirm patients. If MRI must be performed, the following should be considered:

-Consideration should be given to interrogating the SJM Confirm prior to MRI exposure in order to save any data that has been recorded in the device. Accordingly, planning in conjunction with the physician responsible for the patient's SJM Confirm is necessary.

-If there is any concern with the SJM Confirm following MRI exposure, the device operation may be assessed by the patient's following physician.

If you have any questions on this topic, please contact St. Jude Medical Technical Services at 800-722-3774.

[MR healthcare professionals are advised to contact the respective manufacturer in order to obtain the latest safety information to ensure patient safety relative to the use of an MR procedure.]

REFERENCE

www.sjm.com/professional.aspx

SAM Sling

The SAM Sling (SAM Medical Products, Newport, OR) is a force-controlled circumferential pelvic belt designed to provide safe and effective reduction and stabilization of open-book pelvic fractures. Pelvic ring fractures are devastating injuries, accompanied by extensive internal bleeding that can often be fatal. Since the mid-nineteenth century, the standard first-aid protocol has been to wrap a bedsheet or belt around the victim's hips, cinch it tight, and hope for the best. This technique works, even for the worst type of pelvic fractures, known as open-book fractures because the pelvic ring has sprung open, like the pages of a book. Compression "closes the book," reduces pain, slows bleeding, and promotes clot formation as the patient is transported to an emergency department.

Researchers determined that the optimum safe pressure for closing unstable open-book fractures falls in a range centered on approximately 150 Newtons, or 33 pounds. That finding allowed the creation of the SAM Sling's patented "autostop" buckle, which has spring-loaded prongs that lock the buckle in place when the right amount of force is applied.

MRI Information. Based on in vitro testing, the SAM Sling will not present a hazard or risk to a patient undergoing an MRI procedure using an MR system operating at 3-Tesla or less. The SAM Sling contains ferromagnetic springs in the buckle. Therefore, it is important to ensure that the SAM Sling is firmly applied to the patient prior to entry into the MRI environment (as stated in the labeling for this device). Accordingly, there will be no hazard or risk to a patient undergoing an MRI procedure. The SAM Sling should not be removed from the patient while in the MR system or in the MR system room. This product is not recommended for use on children.

REFERENCE

SAM Medical Products, http://www.sammedical.com

Scleral Buckle
(Scleral Buckling Procedure)

The application of a scleral buckle (note, this is a procedure not an implant) or "scleral buckling" is a surgical technique used to repair retinal detachments and was first used experimentally by ophthalmic surgeons in 1937. By the early 1960s, scleral buckling became the method of choice when the development of new materials, particularly silicone, offered surgeons better opportunities to improve patient care.

The buckling element is usually left in place permanently. The element pushes in, or "buckles," the sclera toward the middle of the eye. This buckling effect on the sclera relieves the traction on the retina, allowing the retinal tear to settle against the wall of the eye. The buckle effect may cover only the area behind the detachment or it may encircle the eyeball like a ring. This procedure effectively holds the retina against the sclera until scarring seals the tear and prevents fluid leakage, which could cause further retinal detachment. Scleral buckles come in many shapes and sizes. The encircling band is usually a thin silicone band sewn around the circumference of the sclera of the eye. In rare instances, a metallic clip may be used. Some metallic clips may pose a risk to patients undergoing MRI procedures.

Tantalum Clips
Tantalum clips were found to be less bulky than sutures, allowing the surgeon to adjust the tension of the circling band for the scleral buckle. These clips did not cause tissue reaction and did not harbor infection. Because tantalum is a nonmagnetic metal, these clips are considered to be acceptable for patients undergoing MRI procedures.

REFERENCES

Bakshandeh H, Shellock FG, Schatz CJ, Morisoli SM. Metallic clips used for scleral buckling: ex vivo evaluation of ferromagnetism at 1.5 T. J Magn Reson Imaging. 1993;3:559.

Lincoff H. Radial buckling in the repair of retinal detachment. Int Ophthalmol Clin. 1976;16:127-34.

Michels RG. Scleral buckling methods for rhegmatogenous retinal detachment. Retina. 1986;6:1-49.

Sleuth Implantable ECG Monitoring System

The Sleuth Implantable ECG Monitoring System (Sleuth and Sleuth AT, Models 2010 and 2020, Transoma Medical, St. Paul, MN) is an implantable, patient-activated and automatically-activated cardiac monitoring system that records the electrocardiogram (ECG) subcutaneously. This device is indicated for patients with clinical syndromes or situations at increased risk of cardiac arrhythmias and for patients who experience transient symptoms that may suggest a cardiac arrhythmia.

MRI INFORMATION
MR Conditional: 1.5-T MRI

NOTE: The monitoring system does not need to be adjusted during MR scanning. However, MR scanning may cause electromagnetic interference that may cause the system to record ECG events. MR scanning may also interfere with the quality of the ECG signal. Therefore, ECG data acquired during an MR scan may be inaccurate or unusable.

The Sleuth IMD (Models 2010 and 2020) was determined to be MR conditional based on information provided in the following document: American Society for Testing and Materials (ASTM) International, Designation: F2503. Standard Practice for Marking Medical Devices and Other Items for Safety in the Magnetic Resonance Environment. ASTM International, West Conshohocken, Pennsylvania, 2005.

Non-clinical testing has demonstrated the Sleuth IMD is MR conditional. It can be scanned safely under:

- static magnetic field of 1.5-Tesla
- spatial gradient magnetic field of 250 Gauss/cm
- maximum MR system reported whole-body-averaged specific absorption rate (SAR) of 3.5 W/kg for 15 minutes of scanning (per pulse sequence)

In non-clinical testing in a phantom, the device produced a temperature rise of less than or equal to 1.3 degrees C at a maximum whole-body-averaged specific absorption rate (SAR) of 3.5 W/kg for 15 minutes of MR scanning in a 1.5-Tesla MR system (Magnetom, Siemens Medical Solutions, Malvern, PA, Software Numaris/4, Version Syngo MR 2002B DHHS Active-shielded, horizontal field scanner).

The maximum whole body averaged specific absorption rate (SAR) reported was measured by the MR system. MR image quality may be compromised if the area of interest is in the same area or relatively close to the position of the Sleuth IMD. The table below provides maximum signal voids (artifact size) for the standard imaging pulse sequences at 1.5 Tesla per ASTM F2119:

Signal Void	Pulse Sequence	Imaging Plane
115 cm^2	T1-weighted spin echo	Parallel
68 cm^2	T1-weighted spin echo	Perpendicular
162 cm^2	Gradient echo	Parallel
280 cm^2	Gradient echo	Perpendicular

The effect of performing MRI procedures using higher static magnetic field or higher levels of RF energy on a patient with the IMD has not been determined. MRI healthcare professionals are advised to contact Transoma Medical to ensure that the latest safety information is obtained and carefully followed to ensure patient safety relative to the use of an MR procedure.

Note: Magnetic forces may act on the housing of the implanted IMD and result in a tugging sensation that patients may feel. This force does not pose a safety hazard, but to mitigate patient alarm, patients should be made aware of the possibility of such a sensation.

[*The information for the Sleuth was reprinted with permission by Transoma Medical, St. Paul, MN]

[MR healthcare professionals are advised to contact the manufacturer to ensure that the latest safety information is obtained and carefully followed in order to ensure patient safety relative to the use of an MR procedure.]

REFERENCE

www.transoma.com

Surgical Instruments and Devices

Interventional magnetic resonance (MR) techniques have evolved into clinically viable surgical and therapeutic applications. This has resulted in the development and performance of innovative procedures that include percutaneous biopsy (e.g., breast, bone, brain, abdominal, etc.), endoscopic surgery of the abdomen, spine, and sinuses, neurosurgical procedures, and MR-guided monitoring of thermal therapies (i.e., laser-induced, RF-induced, and cryomediated procedures).

Surgical instruments and devices are an important necessity for interventional MR. Besides the typical MRI issues, there are possible hazards in the interventional MR environment related to the surgical instruments and devices that must be addressed to ensure the safety of healthcare practitioners and patients. Many of the conventional instruments and devices are made from metallic materials that can create substantial problems in association with interventional MR.

The interventional MR safety issues that exist for surgical instruments and devices include unwanted movement caused by magnetic field interactions (e.g., the "missile effect", translational attraction, torque), issues related to eddy currents, and heat generated by RF power deposition. Furthermore, the operational aspects of various instruments may be adversely impacted by the electromagnetic fields used for MR imaging. Artifacts associated with the use of a surgical instrument or device can be particularly problematic if in the imaging area of interest during its intended use. To address these problems, various surgical instruments and devices have been developed that do not present an additional risk or problem to the patient or MR healthcare practitioner in the interventional MR environment.

REFERENCES

Hinks RS, Bronskill MJ, Kucharczyk W, Bernstein M, Collick BD, Henkelman RM. MR systems for image-guided therapy. J Magn Reson Imaging 1998;8:19-25.

Jolesz FA. Interventional and intraoperative MRI: a general overview of the field. J Magn Reson Imaging 1998;3-7.

Jolesz FA. Image-guided procedures and the operating room of the future. Radiology 1997; 204:601-612.

Jolesz FA, et al. Compatible instrumentation for intraoperative MRI: expanding resources. J Magn Reson Imaging 1998;8:8-11.

Maldonado IL, et al. Magnetic resonance-based deep brain stimulation technique: a series of 478 consecutive implanted electrodes with no perioperative intracerebral hemorrhage. Neurosurgery. 2009;65(6 Suppl):196-201.

Shellock FG. Compatibility of an endoscope designed for use in interventional MR imaging procedures. AJR Amer J Roentgenol 1998;171:1297-1300.

Shellock FG. Metallic surgical instruments for interventional MRI procedures: evaluation of MR safety. J Magn Reson Imaging 2001;13:152-157.

Shellock FG. MRI safety of instruments designed for interventional MRI: assessment of ferromagnetism, heating, and artifacts. Workshop on New Insights into Safety and Compatibility Issues Affecting In Vivo MR, Syllabus, International Society of Magnetic Resonance in Medicine, Berkeley, 1998; pp. 39.

Shellock FG, Shellock VJ. Ceramic surgical instruments: Evaluation of MR-compatibility at 1.5 Tesla. J Magn Reson Imaging 1996;6:954-956.

Thomas C, Wojtczyk H, et al. Carbon fibre and nitinol needles for MRI-guided interventions: First in vitro and in vivo application. Eur J Radiol. 2011;79:353-358

Sutures

Sutures are made from a variety of materials, including those that are nonmetallic and metallic. Various sutures *with the needles removed* have been testing at 1.5- and 3-Tesla. For the thirteen different sutures evaluated at 1.5-Tesla, all were shown to be acceptable for patients.

MRI at 3-Tesla and Sutures. At 3-Tesla, most of the sutures evaluated displayed no magnetic field interactions, while two (Flexon suture and Steel suture, United States Surgical, North Haven, CT) showed minor deflection angles and torque. For these two sutures, the *in situ* application of these materials provides sufficient counter-forces to prevent movement or dislodgment. Therefore, in consideration of the intended *in vivo* use of these materials, all of the sutures with the needles removed tested to date are acceptable at 3-Tesla.

REFERENCES

American Society for Testing and Materials (ASTM) Designation: F 2052. Standard test method for measurement of magnetically induced displacement force on passive implants in the magnetic resonance environment. In: Annual Book of ASTM Standards, Section 13, Medical Devices and Services, Volume 13.01 Medical Devices; Emergency Medical Services. West Conshohocken, PA, 2002, pp. 1576-1580.

Shellock FG. Biomedical implants and devices: assessment of magnetic field interactions with a 3.0-Tesla MR system. J Magn Reson Imaging J Magn Reson Imaging 2002;16:721-732.

SynchroMed, SynchroMed EL, and SynchroMed II Drug Infusion Systems

The Effects of Magnetic Resonance Imaging (MRI) on Medtronic Drug Infusion Systems

For SynchroMed pump models 8615, 8616, 8617 and 8618 please refer to the MRI Information for the SynchroMed EL Pump.

Before any medical procedure is begun, patients must always inform any health care personnel that they have an implanted drug infusion system and share this information about MRI with them.

MRI Information for the SynchroMed EL Pump
Models: SynchroMed EL: All models beginning with 8626, 8627
Reference: SynchroMed IsoMed Information for Prescribers Manual

Introduction

SynchroMed EL pump performance has not been established for greater than 3.0 Tesla (T) horizontal, closed-bore MRI scanners. SynchroMed EL pump performance has not been established using other types of MRI scanners such as open-sided or standing MRI.

Temporary motor stall and stall recover

The magnetic field of the MRI scanner will temporarily stop the rotor of the SynchroMed EL pump motor and suspend drug infusion for the duration of the MRI exposure. The pump should resume normal operation upon termination of MRI exposure; however, there is the potential for an extended delay in pump recovery after exiting the MRI magnetic field because exposure to the MRI magnetic field may cause the motor gears within the pump to bind temporarily without permanent damage. This is caused by the potential for backward rotation of the pump rotor magnet when it aligns with the MRI magnetic field. This temporary binding may delay the return of proper infusion after the pump is removed from the MRI magnetic field. While extended delays in pump recovery are unlikely, reports have indicated that there is the potential for a two to twenty-four hour delay in return to proper drug infusion after completion of an MRI scan.

Warning: Patients receiving intrathecal baclofen therapy (e.g. Lioresal Intrathecal) are at higher risk for adverse events, as baclofen withdrawal can lead to a life threatening condition if not treated promptly and effectively. For complete product information, refer to the Lioresal Intrathecal (baclofen injection) Package Insert. For information on other drugs, please refer to the product labeling for the drug being administered.

Potential for permanent motor stall

Ninety (90) degrees alignment of an implanted pump with the z axis of 1.5 T and 3.0 T horizontal, closed-bore magnetic resonance imaging (MRI) scanners can cause MRI-induced demagnetization of the internal pump motor magnets, which can result in permanent, nonrecoverable stoppage of the pump. This is due to the orientation of the pump with respect to the magnetic field of a horizontal, closed-bore MRI system. SynchroMed EL pump performance has not been established using other types of MRI scanners such as open-sided or standing MRI.

Note: If the pump face is oriented at 90 degrees to the z-axis, the refill port would be facing towards the patient's feet or head.

Preparation for the MRI examination

Prior to MRI, the physician should ensure the pump is not oriented 90 degrees with respect to the z-axis of the MRI scanner. The physician should also determine if the patient implanted with a SynchroMed EL pump can safely be deprived of drug delivery. If the patient cannot be safely deprived of drug delivery, alternative delivery methods for the drug can be used during the time required for the MRI scan. If there is concern that depriving the patient of drug delivery may be unsafe for the patient during the MRI procedure, medical supervision should be provided while the MRI is conducted.

Note: Prior to the MRI scan, confirm that the pump program settings are documented in case reprogramming is required after the scan.

Post-MRI examination review

Upon completion of the MRI scan, or shortly thereafter, the SynchroMed EL pump must be interrogated using the clinician programmer in order to confirm that electromagnetic interference from the MRI has not affected the pump status. If interrogation using the clinician programmer shows that a "Pump Memory Error" occurred, the physician must reprogram the pump in order for proper drug infusion to resume. A Pump Memory Error Alarm (double tone) will accompany a Pump Memory Error. If this occurs, notify:

- US only: Medtronic Technical Services at 1-800-707-0933.

The SynchroMed EL pump does not detect or alarm for motor stalls. A physician should confirm a SynchroMed EL pump has resumed proper drug infusion after an MRI by performing a pump roller study. If a pump roller study cannot be performed, patients must be closely monitored for return of underlying symptoms to confirm the pump has resumed proper drug infusion after an MRI. The duration of monitoring depends on the drug and the delivery rate. Consult the patient's providing physician for likely time period for return of symptoms in the event of a pump stoppage.

Additional safety and diagnostic issues

Testing on the SynchroMed EL pump has established the following with regard to other MRI safety and diagnostic issues:

Tissue heating adjacent to implant during MRI scans

Specific absorption rate (SAR) — Presence of the pump can potentially cause an increase of the local temperature in tissues near the pump. During a 20-minute pulse sequence in a 1.5 T GE Signa scanner with a whole-body average SAR of 1 W/kg, a temperature increase of 1 degrees C in a static phantom was observed near the pump implanted in the "abdomen" of the phantom. The 20-minute scan time is representative of a typical imaging session. Implanting the pump more lateral to the midline of the abdomen may result in greater temperature increases in tissues near the pump.

Testing in a 3.0 T GE Signa scanner using transmit-receive RF body coil (at an MR system reported whole body averaged SAR of 3.0 W/kg and a spatial peak SAR of 5.9 W/kg) resulted in maximum heating of 1.7 degrees C for the SynchroMed EL pump.

In the unlikely event that the patient experiences uncomfortable warmth near the pump, the MRI scan should be stopped and the scan parameters adjusted to reduce the SAR to comfortable levels.

Peripheral nerve stimulation during MRI scans

Time-varying gradient magnetic fields — Presence of the pump may potentially cause a two-fold increase of the induced electric field in tissues near the pump. With the pump implanted in the abdomen, using pulse sequences that have dB/dt up to 20 T/s, the measured induced electric field near the pump is below the threshold necessary to cause stimulation.

In the unlikely event that the patient reports stimulation during the scan, the proper procedure is the same as for patients without implants—stop the MRI scan and adjust the scan parameters to reduce the potential for nerve stimulation.

Static magnetic field

For magnetic fields up to 3.0 T, the magnetic force and torque on the pump will be less than the force and torque due to gravity. The patient may experience a slight tugging sensation at the pump implant site. An elastic garment or wrap will prevent the pump from moving and reduce the sensation the patient may experience.

Image distortion

The pump contains ferromagnetic components that will cause image distortion and image dropout in areas around the pump. The severity of image artifact is dependent on the MR pulse sequence used. For spin echo pulse sequences, the area of significant image artifact may be 20-25 cm across. Images of the head or lower extremities should be largely unaffected.

Minimizing image distortion — Careful choice of pulse sequence parameters and location of the angle and location of the imaging plane may minimize MR image artifact; however, the reduction in image distortion obtained by adjustment of pulse sequence parameters will usually be at a cost in signal-to-noise ratio. The following general principles should be followed:

- Use imaging sequences with stronger gradients for both slice and read encoding directions. Employ higher bandwidth for both radio-frequency pulse and data sampling.
- Choose an orientation for read-out axis that minimizes the appearance of in-plane distortion.
- Use spin echo or gradient echo MR imaging sequences with a relatively high data sampling bandwidth.

- Use shorter echo time for gradient echo technique, whenever possible.
- Be aware that the actual imaging slice shape can be curved in space due to the presence of the field disturbance of the pump (as stated above).
- Identify the location of the implant in the patient, and when possible, orient all imaging slices away from the implanted pump.

MRI Information for SynchroMed II Pump
Models: SynchroMed II: All models beginning with 8637
Reference: SynchroMed IsoMed Information for Prescribers Manual

Introduction

SynchroMed II pump performance has not been established for greater than 3.0 Tesla (T) horizontal, closed-bore MRI scanners. SynchroMed II pump performance has not been established using other types of MRI scanners such as open-sided or standing MRI.

Temporary motor stall and stall recovery

The magnetic field of the MRI scanner will temporarily stop the rotor of the SynchroMed II pump motor and suspend drug infusion for the duration of the MRI exposure. The pump should resume normal operation upon termination of MRI exposure; however, there is the potential for an extended delay in pump recovery after exiting the MRI magnetic field because exposure to the MRI magnetic field may cause the motor gears within the pump to bind temporarily without permanent damage. This is caused by the potential for backward rotation of the pump rotor magnet when it aligns with the MRI magnetic field. This temporary binding may delay the return of proper infusion after the pump is removed from the MRI magnetic field. While extended delays in pump recovery are unlikely, reports have indicated that there is the potential for a two to twenty-four hour delay in return to proper drug infusion after completion of an MRI scan.

Warning: Patients receiving intrathecal baclofen therapy (e.g. Lioresal Intrathecal) are at higher risk for adverse events, as baclofen withdrawal can lead to a life threatening condition if not treated promptly and effectively. For complete product information, refer to the Lioresal Intrathecal (baclofen injection) Package Insert. For information on other drugs, please refer to the product labeling for the drug being administered.

Time required for stall and recovery detection

The SynchroMed II pump detects motor stall and motor stall recovery. Medtronic does not recommend programming the SynchroMed II pump to "stopped pump mode" prior to an MRI because of the possibility of an increased delay in the detection of an extended motor stall. Motor stall events are recorded in the pump event log and can be reviewed using the clinician programmer. A motor stall will also cause the pump alarm to sound (two tone alarm). The slower the programmed delivery rate, the longer it may take for the stall detection algorithm to log motor stall and motor stall recovery. For pumps programmed to deliver at least 0.048 ml/day, the motor stall detection (with audible alarm) should occur within 20 minutes of exposure to the MRI magnetic field. Stall recovery detection should occur within 20 minutes of exiting the MRI magnetic field. The detection of a motor stall and detection of motor stall recovery may each take up to 90 minutes if the pump is programmed to minimum rate mode (0.006 ml/day).

Potential for delay in logging motor stall events

In some cases, electromagnetic interference (EMI) from an MRI scan can interfere with normal event logging. If this occurs, it may cause the pump to switch into the telemetry mode. 'Telemetry mode' is a special state in which the pump is able to communicate with the clinician programmer. While in this state, the pump infuses normally; however, some error logging and the audible alarm for motor stall are suspended. If the pump switches into telemetry mode due to EMI, the pump resumes drug delivery after leaving the MRI magnetic field; however, pump motor stall and motor stall recovery detection function is not active until the post-MRI pump interrogation ends telemetry mode (refer to "Post-MRI examination review"). Due to this issue, if the interrogation is not performed upon completion of the MRI scan or shortly thereafter, review of the pump logs may indicate that the pump ceased drug delivery for an extended period of time, when in fact it had recovered normally. In this scenario, you may receive an erroneous "stopped pump period may exceed tube set" error message.

Note: In some cases, the SynchroMed II pump event log may not register motor stall recovery until after the pump has been interrogated a second time due to the effect of electromagnetic interference on the pump.

Potential for permanent motor stall

Ninety (90) degrees alignment of an implanted pump with the z axis of 1.5 T and 3.0 T horizontal, closed-bore magnetic resonance imaging

(MRI) scanners can cause MRI-induced demagnetization of the internal pump motor magnets, which can result in permanent, nonrecoverable stoppage of the pump. This is due to the orientation of the pump with respect to the magnetic field of a horizontal, closed-bore MRI system. SynchroMed II pump performance has not been established using other types of MRI scanners such as open-sided or standing MRI.

Note: If the pump face is oriented at 90 degrees to the z-axis, the refill port would be facing towards the patient's feet or head.

Preparation for the MRI examination

Prior to MRI, the physician should ensure the pump is not oriented 90 degrees with respect to the z axis of the MRI scanner. The physician should also determine if the patient implanted with a SynchroMed II pump can safely be deprived of drug delivery. If the patient cannot be safely deprived of drug delivery, alternative delivery methods for the drug can be used during the time required for the MRI scan. If there is concern that depriving the patient of drug delivery may be unsafe for the patient during the MRI procedure, medical supervision should be provided while the MRI is conducted.

Post-MRI examination review

Upon completion of the MRI scan, or shortly thereafter, the physician must confirm that therapy has properly resumed by interrogating the SynchroMed II pump with the clinician programmer. For pumps programmed to deliver at least 0.048 ml/day, the detection of the motor stall should occur within 20 minutes of MRI exposure.

Detection of the motor stall: Recovery and recording of the recovery in the pump event log will typically occur within 20 minutes of the removal of the pump from the MRI magnetic field.

Note: Both the detection of the motor stall and detection of the motor stall recovery may each take up to 90 minutes if the pump is programmed to minimum rate mode (0.006 ml/day). In the unlikely event that electromagnetic interference from the MRI scan causes a change to "safe state", the pump will automatically switch to minimum rate mode (infusion at 0.006 ml/day). The pump must be reprogrammed in order for proper infusion to resume.

The following pump interrogation guidelines should be used to determine whether the pump has resumed proper function (refer to the SynchroMed

II Programming Guide for information about how to interrogate the pump and view event logs).

1) At least 20 minutes after completing MRI exposure, interrogate the pump using the clinician programmer and select the check box to download event logs. If the event log states "Motor Stall Occurred" and "Motor Stall Recovery Occurred", normal function of the pump has returned.

2) If event log **does not** show stall and recovery, wait 20 minutes after the initial interrogation, re-interrogate the pump using the clinician programmer, and review the event logs again. (This will address the potential for event logging delays due to electromagnetic interference from the MRI magnetic field.)

If the event log states "Motor Stall Occurred" and **does not** state "Motor Stall Recovery Occurred", there is a potential for an extended motor stall due to temporary gear binding. Contact:

- US only: Medtronic Technical Services at 1-800-707-0933.
- In all other cases, the pump has resumed its normal operation.

Additional safety and diagnostic issues

Testing on the SynchroMed II pump has established the following with regard to other MRI safety and diagnostic issues:

Tissue heating adjacent to implant during MRI scans

Specific absorption rate (SAR) — Presence of the pump can potentially cause an increase of the local temperature in tissues near the pump. During a 20-minute pulse sequence in a 1.5 T GE Signa scanner with a whole-body average SAR of 1 W/kg, a temperature increase of 1 degrees C in a static phantom was observed near the pump implanted in the "abdomen" of the phantom. The 20-minute scan time is representative of a typical imaging session. Implanting the pump more lateral to the midline of the abdomen may result in greater temperature increases in tissues near the pump. Testing in a 3.0 T GE Signa scanner using transmit-receive RF body coil (at an MR system reported whole body averaged SAR of 3.0 W/kg and a spatial peak SAR of 5.9 W/kg) resulted in maximum heating of 2.7 degrees C for the SynchroMed II pump.

- In the unlikely event that the patient experiences uncomfortable warmth near the pump, the MRI scan should be stopped and the scan parameters adjusted to reduce the SAR to comfortable levels.

Peripheral nerve stimulation during MRI scans

Time-varying gradient magnetic fields — Presence of the pump may potentially cause a two-fold increase of the induced electric field in tissues near the pump. With the pump implanted in the abdomen, using pulse sequences that have dB/dt up to 20 T/s, the measured induced electric field near the pump is below the threshold necessary to cause stimulation. In the unlikely event that the patient reports stimulation during the scan, the proper procedure is the same as for patients without implants—stop the MRI scan and adjust the scan parameters to reduce the potential for nerve stimulation.

Static magnetic field

For magnetic fields up to 3.0 T, the magnetic force and torque on the pump will be less than the force and torque due to gravity. The patient may experience a slight tugging sensation at the pump implant site. An elastic garment or wrap will prevent the pump from moving and reduce the sensation the patient may experience.

Image distortion

The pump contains ferromagnetic components that will cause image distortion and image dropout in areas around the pump. The severity of image artifact is dependent on the MR pulse sequence used. For spin echo pulse sequences, the area of significant image artifact may be 20-25 cm across. Images of the head or lower extremities should be largely unaffected.

Minimizing image distortion — Careful choice of pulse sequence parameters and location of the angle and location of the imaging plane may minimize MR image artifact; however, the reduction in image distortion obtained by adjustment of pulse sequence parameters will usually be at a cost in signal-to-noise ratio. The following general principles should be followed:

- Use imaging sequences with stronger gradients for both slice and read encoding directions. Employ higher bandwidth for both radio-frequency pulse and data sampling.
- Choose an orientation for read-out axis that minimizes the appearance of in-plane distortion.
- Use spin echo or gradient echo MR imaging sequences with a relatively high data sampling bandwidth.
- Use shorter echo time for gradient echo technique, whenever possible.

- Be aware that the actual imaging slice shape can be curved in space due to the presence of the field disturbance of the pump (as stated above).
- Identify the location of the implant in the patient, and when possible, orient all imaging slices away from the implanted pump.

[MR healthcare professionals are advised to contact the respective manufacturer in order to obtain the latest safety information to ensure patient safety relative to the use of an MR procedure.]

REFERENCE

http://www.medtronic.com

TheraSeed Radioactive Seed Implant

The TheraSeed radioactive seed implant (Theragenics Corporation, Buford, GA) is used to deliver low-level radiation to the prostate to treat cancer. The TheraSeed radioactive seed is a relatively small implant comprised of a titanium tube with two graphite pellets and a lead marker inside. The outside dimensions of tube are approximately length 0.177" in length with a diameter of 0.032".

Palladium-103 is the isotope contained in the TheraSeed implant. Because the radiation is so low and the seeds are placed so precisely, virtually all the radiation is absorbed by the prostate. Treatments with the TheraSeed implant may involve placement in the prostate of from 80 to 120 of these devices. These "seeds" are implanted with "spacers" between them and placed according to treatment plans, so that they do not contact one another during their intended "*in vivo*" use.

Magnetic resonance tests (magnetic field interactions, heating, induced currents, and artifacts) conducted on the TheraSeed revealed that this implant is acceptable for patients undergoing MR procedures at 3-Tesla or less.

REFERENCE

http://www.theraseed.com/

Transdermal Medication Patches and Other Drug Delivery Patches

A transdermal patch allows continuous and prolonged drug delivery that may be more effective and safer than oral medication. In addition, patches offer the potential to deliver medications that would otherwise require injections. Future advances in technology will expand the utilization of drug patches. For example, researchers are currently working on various technologies to "force" larger molecules through the skin. These so-called "active patches" may permit the delivery of insulin to diabetics, as well as the administration of red-cell stimulating erythropoietin for treatment of anemic patients without injections.

Several anecdotal reports have indicated that transdermal medication patches that contain aluminum foil or other similar metallic component may cause excessive heating or a burn in a patient undergoing an MR procedure. For example, a Deponit (nitroglycerin transdermal delivery system) patch that contains an aluminum foil component, was worn by a patient during MR imaging. This patient received a second-degree burn during the examination that was performed using conventional pulse sequences and standard imaging procedures (Personal communication, Robert E. Mucha, Schwarz Pharma, Milwaukee, WI; 1995). This injury was likely due to MRI-related heating of the metallic foil associated with this transdermal patch.

The U.S. Food and Drug Administration is aware of at least two other adverse events in which patients wearing nicotine transdermal patches during MRI examinations experienced burns. In one case, the patient was wearing a nicotine (Habitrol) transdermal patch. When the patient was removed from the scanner at the completion of the MRI procedure, he stated that his arm was "burning". Upon examination, his upper left arm appeared to be mildly erythematous and there was a small blister where the patch was located. In another case, a patient underwent a brief MRI examination of the lumbar spine while wearing a nicotine transdermal patch. Later, the patient complained of burn lines on his upper arms that were associated with this patch.

In consideration of the above, a patient wearing a transdermal patch that has a metallic component must be identified prior to undergoing an MR procedure. The patient's physician should be contacted to determine if it is possible to temporarily remove the medication patch to prevent excessive heating and burns. After the MR examination, a new patch should be applied following the directions of the prescribing physician (Personal communication, Robert E. Mucha, Schwarz Pharma, Milwaukee, WI; 1995). Importantly, this procedure should be conducted in consultation with the physician responsible for prescribing the transdermal patch or otherwise responsible for the management of the patient.

The Institute for Safe Medical Practices has stated that medication patches such as ANDRODERM, TRANSDERM-NITRO, DEPONIT, NICODERM, NICOTROL, CATAPRES-TTS, and possibly others should be removed prior to an MR examination. In addition, other patches to be aware of include the nicotine patch marketed as Habitrol and its "private label" equivalents and Scopolamine\Hyoscine HydroBromide, marketed as TransDerm Scop (Personal Communication, 05/19/04, Crispin C. Fernandez, M.D. Medical Affairs, Novartis Consumer Health, Inc. Parsippany, NJ).

Notably, not all transdermal medication patches contain a metallic component and, therefore, these patches do not need to be removed from the patient for the MRI examination. Furthermore, if the body part with the patch is not within the transmit RF coil (e.g., performing MRI of the brain using a transmit/receive head coil in a patient with a transdermal medication patch applied to the torso), there is no risk to the patient.

ActiPatch
ActiPatch (BioElectronics, Frederick, MD) is a medical, drug-free device that delivers pulsed electromagnetic frequency therapies to accelerate healing of soft tissue injuries. The ActiPatch has an embedded battery-operated microchip that delivers continuous pulsed therapy to reduce pain and swelling.

MRI and the ActiPatch. The ActiPatch must be removed prior to performing an MRI procedure to prevent possible damage to this device and the potential risk of excessive heating.

REFERENCES

http://www.bielcorp.com

Institute for Safe Medical Practices, Medication Safety Alert! Burns in MRI patients wearing transdermal patches. Vol. 9, Issue 7, April 8, 2004. http://www.ismp.org/msaarticles/burnsprint.htm

Kanal E, Barkovich AJ, Bell C, et al. ACR guidance document for safe MR practices: 2007. AJR Am J Roentgenol. 2007;188:1447-1474.

Kuehn BM. FDA warning: remove drug patches before MRI to prevent burns to skin. JAMA. 2009;301:1328.

FDA Public Health Advisory: Risk of Burns during MRI Scans from Transdermal Drug Patches with Metallic Backings
[Reprinted with permission.]

The FDA has been made aware of information about certain transdermal patches (medicated patches applied to the skin) that contain aluminum or other metals in the backing of the patches. Patches that contain metal can overheat during an MRI scan and cause skin burns in the immediate area of the patch.

Transdermal patches slowly deliver medicines through the skin. Some patches contain metal in the layer of the patch that is not in contact with the skin (the backing). The metal in the backing of these patches may not be visible. The labeling for most of the medicated patches that contain metal in the backing provides a warning to patients about the risk of burns if the patch is not removed before an MRI scan. However, not all transdermal patches that contain metal have this warning for patients in the labeling.

The FDA is in the process of reviewing the labeling and composition of all medicated patches to ensure that those made with materials containing metal provide a warning about the risk of burns to patients who wear the patches during an MRI scan.

Until this review is complete, FDA recommends that healthcare professionals referring patients to have an MRI scan identify those patients who are wearing a patch before the patients have the MRI scan. The healthcare professional should advise these patients about the procedures for removing and disposing of the patch before the MRI scan, and replacing the patch after the MRI scan. MRI facilities should follow published safe practice recommendations concerning patients who are wearing patches (1, 2).

Until this safety issue is resolved, FDA recommends that patients who use medicated patches (including nicotine patches) do the following:

- Tell the doctor referring you for an MRI scan that you are using a patch and why you are using it (such as, for pain, smoking cessation, hormones)
- Ask your doctor for guidance about removing and disposing of the patch before having an MRI scan and replacing it after the procedure.

- Tell the MRI facility that you are using a patch. You should do this when making your appointment and during the health history questions you are asked when you arrive for your appointment.

The FDA urges health care professionals and patients to report possible cases of skin burns while wearing patches during an MRI to the FDA through the MedWatch program by phone (1-800-FDA-1088) or by the Internet at http://www.fda.gov/medwatch/index.html.

(1) Kanal, et. al, "ACR Guidance Document for Safe MR Practices: 2007," AJR 2007; 188:1–27.

(2) Guidelines for Screening Patients For MR Procedures and Individuals for the MR Environment, Institute for Magnetic Resonance Safety, Education, and Research, www.imrser.org, 2010.

FDA Update: (03/09/2009)

FDA has evaluated the composition of available patches to determine which of them contain metal components and to assure that this information is included in their labeling. Based on current information from this evaluation, FDA is working with the manufacturers of the following patches to update the labeling to include adequate warnings to patients about the risk of burns to the skin if the patch is worn during an MRI scan. It should be noted that some of the drugs listed may have a generic equivalent and more than one size and strength of patch. FDA will update this posting as information becomes available.

Proprietary Name Generic/Established Name

Catapres TTS / Clonidine
Neupro / Rotigotine
Lidopel / Lidocaine HCl and epinephrine
Synera / Lidocaine/Tetracaine
Transderm-Scop / Scopolamine
Prostep / Nicotine transdermal system
Habitrol / Nicotine transdermal system
Nicotrol TD / Nicotine transdermal system
Androderm / Testosterone transdermal system
Fentanyl / Fentanyl
Salonpas Power Plus / Methyl Salicylate/Menthol

Vascular Access Ports, Infusion Pumps*, and Catheters

Vascular access ports, infusion pumps, and catheters are implants and devices commonly used to provide long-term vascular administration of chemotherapeutic agents, antibiotics, analgesics and other medications (also, see information pertaining to the **AccuRx Constant Flow Implantable Pump, Ambulatory Infusion Pumps, Insulin Pumps,** the **IsoMed Implantable Constant-Flow Infusion Pump**, and the **SynchroMed, SynchroMED EL,** and **SynchroMed II Drug Infusion Systems**). Vascular access ports are usually implanted in a subcutaneous pocket over the upper chest wall with the catheters inserted in the jugular, subclavian, or cephalic vein.

Vascular access ports have a variety of similar features (e.g., a reservoir, central septum, and catheter) and may be constructed from different materials including stainless steel, titanium, silicone, and plastic. Because of the widespread use of vascular access ports and associated catheters and the high probability that patients with these devices may require MR procedures, it has been important to characterize the MRI issues for these implants.

Three of the implantable vascular access ports and catheters evaluated for safety with MR procedures showed measurable magnetic field interactions during exposure to the MR systems (typically 1.5-Tesla) used for testing, but the interactions were minor relative to the *in vivo* applications of these implants. Therefore, an MR procedure is acceptable at 1.5-Tesla or less in a patient that has one of the vascular access ports or catheters shown in **The List**.

With respect to MR imaging and artifacts, in general, vascular access ports that produce the least amount of artifact are made entirely from nonmetallic materials. The ones that produce the largest artifacts are composed of metal(s) or have metal in an unusual shape (e.g., the OmegaPort Access Devices).

Even vascular access ports made entirely from nonmetallic materials are seen on the MR images because they contain silicone. The septum portion vascular access ports is typically made from silicone. Using MR imaging, the Larmor precessional frequency of fat is close to that of silicone (i.e.,

100 Hz at 1.5-T). Therefore, silicone used in the construction of a vascular access port may be observed on MR images with varying degrees of signal intensity depending on the pulse sequence that is used.

If a radiologist did not know that this type of vascular access port was present in a patient, the MR signal produced by the silicone component of the device could be considered an abnormality, or at the very least, present a confusing image. For example, this may cause a diagnostic problem in a patient evaluated for a rupture of a silicone breast implant, because silicone from the vascular access port may be misinterpreted as an "extracapsular silicone implant rupture."

MRI at 3-Tesla and Vascular Access Ports and Catheters. For the vascular access ports assessed for magnetic field interactions at 3-Tesla, these did not exhibit substantial magnetic field interactions and, therefore, will not move or dislodge in this MR environment. For the accessories, some showed measurable magnetic field interactions (see **The List**). However, during the *intended uses* of these accessories, it is unlikely that they will present a problem in the 3-Tesla MR environment considering that the simple application of a small piece of adhesive tape or other appropriate means of retention effectively counterbalances the magnetic qualities of these devices (Unpublished Observations, F.G. Shellock).

REFERENCES

Shellock FG. Magnetic Resonance Procedures: Health Effects and Safety. CRC Press, LLC, Boca Raton, FL, 2001.

Shellock FG. Biomedical implants and devices: assessment of magnetic field interactions with a 3.0-Tesla MR system. J Magn Reson Imaging J Magn Reson Imaging 2002;16:721-732.

Shellock FG, Nogueira M, Morisoli S. MR imaging and vascular access ports: *ex vivo* evaluation of ferromagnetism, heating, and artifacts at 1.5-T. J Magn Reson Imaging 1995;4:481-484.

Shellock FG, Shellock VJ. Vascular access ports and catheters tested for ferromagnetism, heating, and artifacts associated with MR imaging. Magn Reson Imaging 1996;14:443-447.

VeriChip Microtransponder

The VeriChip Microtransponder is a miniaturized, implantable radio frequency identification device (RFID). This is a passive device that contains an electronic circuit, which is activated externally by a low-power electro-magnetic field emitted by a battery powered scanner. The Microtransponder is implanted subcutaneously.

With regard to MRI procedures, the labeling for this device states: Patients with the VeriChip Microtransponder may safely undergo MRI diagnostics in up to 7-Tesla cylindrical systems. See section below.

INSTRUCTIONS FOR PATIENTS UNDERGOING MRI

- The patient should be monitored continuously throughout the MRI procedure using visual and audio means (e.g., intercom system).
- Instruct the patient to alert the MR system operator of any unusual sensations or problems so that, if necessary, the MR system operator can immediately terminate the procedure.
- Provide the patient with a means to alert the MR system operator of any unusual sensations or problems.
- Do not perform MRI if the patient is sedated, anesthetized, confused or otherwise unable to communicate with the MR system operator.

REFERENCE

http://www.verichipcorp.com

VOCARE Bladder System, Implantable Functional Neuromuscular Stimulation

The NeuroControl VOCARE Bladder System [also referred to as the FineTech-Brindley Bladder System, Finetech Medical LTD] is a radiofrequency (RF) powered motor control neuroprosthesis or neurostimulation system that consists of both implanted and external components. The VOCARE Bladder System delivers low levels of electrical stimulation to a spinal cord injured patient's intact sacral spinal nerve roots to elicit functional contraction of the muscles innervated by them. The NeuroControl VOCARE Bladder System consists of the following subsystems:

- The **Implanted Components** include the Implantable Receiver-Stimulator and Extradural Electrodes.
- The **External Components** include the External Controller, External Transmitter, External Cable, Transmitter Tester, Battery Charger and Power Cord.
- The **Surgical Components** include the Surgical Stimulator, Intradural Surgical Probe, Extradural Surgical Probe, Surgical Test Cable, and Silicone Adhesive.

The NeuroControl VOCARE Bladder System is indicated for the treatment of patients who have clinically complete spinal cord lesions (ASIA Classification) with intact parasympathetic innervation of the bladder and are skeletally mature and neurologically stable, to provide urination on demand and to reduce post-void residual volumes of urine. Secondary intended use is to aid in bowel evacuation.

CONTRAINDICATIONS

The NeuroControl VOCARE Bladder System is contraindicated for patients with the following characteristics:

- Poor or inadequate bladder reflexes
- Active or recurrent pressure ulcers
- Active sepsis
- Implanted cardiac pacemaker

WARNINGS

The NeuroControl VOCARE Bladder System may only be prescribed, implanted, or adjusted by clinicians who have been trained and certified in its implementation and use.

PRECAUTIONS

- **X-rays, Diagnostic Ultrasound**: X-ray imaging, and diagnostic ultrasound have not been reported to affect the function of the Implantable Receiver-Stimulator or Extradural Electrodes. However, the implantable components may obscure the view of other anatomic structures.

- **MRI**: Testing of the VOCARE Bladder System in a 1.5-Tesla scanner with a maximum spatial gradient of 450 gauss/cm or less, exposed to an average Specific Absorption Rate (SAR) of 1.1 W/kg, for a 30 minute duration resulted in localized temperature rises up to 5.5 degrees C in a gel phantom (without blood flow) and translational force less than that of a 12 gram mass and torque of 0.47 N-cm (less than that produced by the weight of the device). A patient with a VOCARE Bladder System may undergo an MR procedure using a shielded or unshielded MR system with a static magnetic field of 1.5-Tesla only and a maximum spatial gradient of 450 gauss/cm or less. The implantable components may obscure the view of other nearby anatomic structures. Artifact size is dependent on variety of factors including the type of pulse sequence used for imaging (e.g. larger for gradient echo pulse sequences and smaller for spin echo and fast spin echo pulse sequences), the direction of the frequency encoding, and the size of the field of view used for imaging. The use of non-standard scanning modes to minimize image artifact or improve visibility should be applied with caution and with the Specific Absorption Rate (SAR) not to exceed an average of 1.1 W/kg and gradient magnetic fields no greater than 20 Tesla/sec. The use of Transmit RF Coils other than the scanner's Body RF Coil or a Head RF Coil is prohibited. Testing of the function of each electrode should be conducted prior to MRI scanning to ensure no leads are broken. Do not expose patients to MRI if any lead is broken or if integrity cannot be established as excessive heating may result in a broken lead. Patients should be advised to empty their bladder or bowel prior to MRI scanning as a precaution. The external components of the VOCARE Bladder System must be removed prior to MRI scanning. Patients must be continuously observed during the MRI procedure and instructed to report any unusual sensations (e.g., warming, burning, or neuromuscular stimulation). Scanning must be discontinued immediately if any unusual sensation occurs. Contact NeuroControl Corporation for additional information.

[Excerpted with permission from VOCARE Bladder System Implantable Functional Neuromuscular Stimulator, NeuroControl Corporation, Valley View, OH]

[MR healthcare professionals are advised to contact the respective manufacturer in order to obtain the latest safety information to ensure patient safety relative to the use of an MR procedure.]

REFERENCE

http://www.finetech-medical.co.uk/

The List – Information and Terminology

The List contains information for thousands of implants, devices, materials, and other products. The objects in **The List** are divided into general categories to facilitate access and review of pertinent information.

To properly utilize **The List**, particular attention must be given to the information indicated for the highest static magnetic **Field Strength** used for testing and the **Status** information indicated for a given **Object**. The "default" **Field Strength** indicated for an *MR Safe* implant is 1.5-Tesla. *Note:* These specific terms correspond to the column headings for information compiled in **The List**. In addition, for certain objects (e.g., those designated as *Conditional 5)*, it may be necessary to refer to specific recommendations or guidelines in **SECTION II** of this textbook or to contact the manufacturer of the implant or device for the latest MRI labeling information, particularly if the implant/device in question is electronically-activated or otherwise an "active" implant. Frequently, specific MRI information is found at the implant/device company's website. See **Appendix III** for a list of company websites.

The relevant terminology for **The List** is, as follows:

Object: This is the implant, device, material, or product that underwent evaluation relative to an MR procedure or the MR environment. Information is provided for the material(s) used to make the object and the manufacturer of the object, if known. The term "SS" refers to stainless steel. Note that there are magnetic and nonmagnetic forms of stainless steel.

Status: This information pertains to the results of the tests conducted for the object. Testing typically included an assessment of magnetic field interactions (i.e., deflection and/or torque) and MRI-related heating, as needed. In some cases, medical products were assessed for induced electrical currents and the impact of an MR procedure or the MR environment on the functional or operational aspects of the object.

Information for each object has been specifically categorized using a **Status** designation, which indicates the object to be **Safe, Conditional,** or **Unsafe**, as follows (***IMPORTANT NOTE***: See the section entitled *Terminology Applied to Implants and Devices)**:

Safe – The object is considered to be safe for the patient undergoing an MR procedure or an individual in the MR environment, with special reference to the highest static magnetic field strength that was used for the evaluation. The object has undergone testing to demonstrate that it is safe or it is made from material(s) considered to be safe with regard to the MR environment (e.g., plastic, silicone, glass, etc.) or an MR procedure. Refer to additional information for the particular object indicated in the text of **SECTION II** of this textbook (see **Table of Contents**).

Terminology from the American Society for Testing and Materials (ASTM) International and utilized by the Food and Drug Administration refers to __MR safe__ as an item that poses no known hazards in all MRI environments. Using the current terminology, MR safe items include non-conducting, non-metallic, non-magnetic items such as a plastic Petri dish.

Conditional – The object may or may not be safe for the patient undergoing an MR procedure or an individual in the MR environment, depending on the specific conditions that are present.

Current terminology from the American Society for Testing and Materials (ASTM) International and utilized by the Food and Drug Administration refers to __MR conditional__ as an item that has been demonstrated to pose no known hazards in a specified MRI environment with specified conditions of use. Field conditions that define the MRI environment include static magnetic field strength, highest spatial gradient of the magnetic field*, dB/dt (time varying magnetic fields), radio frequency (RF) fields, and specific absorption rate (SAR). Additional conditions, including specific configurations of the item (e.g., the routing of leads used for a neurostimulation system), may be required.

[Please review: Commentary - Regarding the Value Reported for the Term "Spatial Gradient Magnetic Field" and How This Information Is Applied to Labeling of Medical Implants and Devices, Shellock FG, Kanal E, Gilk, TB. American Journal of Roentgenology, **2011;196:142-145.** To obtain this article, please visit *www.IMRSER.org*.]

The MR conditional information has been sub-categorized to indicate specific recommendations for the particular object, as follows:

Conditional 1 – The object is acceptable for the patient or individual in the MR environment, despite the fact that it showed positive findings for magnetic field interactions during testing. Notably, the object is considered to be "weakly" ferromagnetic, *only.*

In general, the object is safe because the magnetic field interactions were characterized as "mild" or "weak" relative to the *in vivo* forces or counter-forces present for the object. For example, certain prosthetic heart valve prostheses and annuloplasty rings showed measurable magnetic field interactions during exposure to the MR systems used for testing, but the magnetic field interactions were less than the forces exerted on the implants by the beating heart.

Additionally, there may be substantial "retentive" or counter-forces provided by the presence of sutures or other means of fixation (e.g., screws, cement, etc.), tissue ingrowth, scarring, or granulation that serve to prevent the object from presenting a risk or hazard to the patient undergoing an MR procedure or an individual in the MR environment.

For a device or product that is used for an MR-guided procedure (e.g., laryngoscope, endoscope, etc.), there may be minor magnetic field interactions in association with the MR system. Eddy currents may also be present. However, the device or product is considered to be acceptable if it is used in its "intended" manner, as specified by the manufacturer. Special attention should be given to the strength of the static magnetic field used for testing the device or product. Functional or operational aspects may need to be considered.

Additionally, specific recommendations for the use of the device or product in the MR environment or during an MR procedure (i.e., typically presented in the Product Insert or Instructions for Use) should be followed carefully. See also **Conditional 7** information below.

Conditional 2 – These particular "weakly" ferromagnetic objects – including coils, filters, stents, clips, cardiac occluders, or other implants - typically become firmly incorporated into the tissue six weeks following placement. Therefore, it is unlikely that these objects will be moved or dislodged by interactions with the magnetic fields of MR systems operating at the static magnetic field strength used for testing. Furthermore, to date, there has been no report of an injury to a patient or individual in association with an MR procedure for these coils, stents, filters, cardiac occluders or other similar implants designated as "**Conditional 2**".

Of note is that if the implant is made from a nonmagnetic material (e.g., Phynox, Elgiloy, Titanium, Titanium alloy, MP35N, Nitinol, etc.), it is *not* necessary to wait a minimum of six weeks before performing and MR procedure using an MR system operating at 1.5-Tesla or less. In some cases, this may also apply to 3-Tesla MR systems.

Special Note: If there is any concern regarding the integrity of the implant or the integrity of the tissue with regard to its ability to retain the object in place during an MR procedure or during exposure to the MR environment, the patient or individual should not be allowed into the MR environment.

Conditional 3 – Certain transdermal patches with metallic foil (e.g., Deponit, nitroglycerin transdermal delivery system) or other metallic components, although not attracted to an MR system, have been reported to heat excessively during MR procedures. This excessive heating may produce discomfort or burn a patient or individual wearing a transdermal patch with a metallic component. Therefore, it is recommended that the patch be removed prior to the MR procedure. A new patch should be applied immediately after the examination. This procedure should only be done in consultation with the patient's or individual's personal physician responsible for prescribing the transdermal medication patch.

Conditional 4 - This halo vest or cervical fixation device may have ferromagnetic component parts, however, the magnetic field interactions have not been determined. Nevertheless, there has been no report of patient injury in association with the presence of this device in the MR environment at the static magnetic field strength used for MR safety testing. Issues may still be present with regard to MRI-related heating. As such, guidelines provided in the *Product Insert* or *Instructions for Use* for a given halo vest or cervical fixation device should be carefully followed. Halo vests and cervical fixation devices made from conducting metals may heat excessively during an MR procedure, resulting in serious patient injury. Contact the manufacturer for further information. Also, refer to the latest information for cervical fixation devices, as several products have now been evaluated at 3-Tesla.

Conditional 5 - This object is acceptable for a patient undergoing an MR procedure or an individual in the MR environment *only* if specific guidelines or recommendations are followed. See specific information for a given object in **SECTION II** and contact the manufacturer for further information, as needed. Please refer to the specific criteria for performing the MR procedure by reviewing the information for the object in this textbook. Consult the manufacturer of the particular device for the latest safety information. Frequently, this information is best found at the company's website. *A list of biomedical company websites is provided in Appendix III.*

Conditional 6 - This implant/device was determined to be MR-conditional according to the terminology specified in the American Society for Testing and Materials (ASTM) International, Designation: F2503. Standard Practice for Marking Medical Devices and Other Items for Safety in the Magnetic Resonance Environment.

Non-clinical testing demonstrated that the implant/device is MR Conditional. A patient with this implant/device can be scanned safely immediately after placement under the following conditions:

- Static magnetic field of 3-Tesla or less
- Maximum spatial gradient magnetic field of 720-Gauss/cm or less
- Maximum MR system reported whole-body-averaged specific absorption rate (SAR) of 3-W/kg for 15 minutes of scanning (per pulse sequence)

In non-clinical testing, the implant/device produced a temperature rise of less than or equal to 3.0 degrees C at a maximum MR system-reported whole body averaged specific absorption rate (SAR) of 3-W/kg for 15-minutes of MR scanning in a 3-Tesla MR system using a transmit/receive body coil (Excite, Software G3.0-052B, General Electric Healthcare, Milwaukee, WI).

MR image quality may be compromised if the area of interest is in the exact same area or relatively close to the position of the implant/device. Therefore, optimization of MR imaging parameters to compensate for the presence of this implant/device may be necessary.

Attention: Contact the manufacturer of this implant/device for further information, as needed.

Conditional 7 - *Important Note:* This device is not intended for use during the operation of an MR system for an MR procedure. That is, this device should not be *inside of the bore* of the MR system, exposing this device to the time-varying and RF fields that are present during an MR procedure.

Attention: Contact the manufacturer of this implant/device for further information.

Conditional 8 – Note: This information pertains to an implant/device that has MRI labeling at 1.5-Tesla and 3-Tesla, only. In some cases, it may pertain to a single and two-overlapped version of a stent. Contact the manufacturer for additional MRI information, as needed.

The implant/device was determined to be MR-conditional according to the terminology specified in the American Society for Testing and Materials (ASTM) International, Designation: F2503. Standard Practice for Marking Medical Devices and Other Items for Safety in the Magnetic Resonance Environment.

Non-clinical testing demonstrated that the implant/device is MR Conditional. A patient with this implant/device can be scanned safely immediately after placement under the following conditions:

For magnetic field interactions,

-Static magnetic field of 3-Tesla or less

-Maximum spatial gradient magnetic field of 720-Gauss/cm or less

MRI-Related Heating

In non-clinical testing, the implant/device produced the following temperature rises during MRI performed for 15-min (per pulse sequence) in 1.5-Tesla (1.5-Tesla/64-MHz, Magnetom, Siemens Medical Solutions, Malvern, PA. Software Numaris/4, Version Syngo MR 2002B DHHS) and 3-Tesla (3-Tesla/128-MHz, Excite, Software G3.0-052B, General Electric Healthcare, Milwaukee, WI) MR systems, using MR system reported, whole body averaged SAR of 3-W/kg or less, as follows:

Highest temperature change	*MRI Condition*
Less than or equal to 4.0 degrees C	1.5-T/64-MHz
Less than or equal to 4.0 degrees C	3-T/128-MHz

Artifact Information

MR image quality may be compromised if the area of interest is in the exact same area or relatively close to the position of the implant/device. Therefore, optimization of MR imaging parameters to compensate for the presence of this implant/device may be necessary.

Attention: Contact the manufacturer of this implant/device for further information.

Terminology from the American Society for Testing and Materials (ASTM) International and utilized by the Food and Drug Administration refers to MR Unsafe as an item that is known to pose hazards in all MRI environments. MR Unsafe items include magnetic items such as a pair of ferromagnetic scissors.

Unsafe 1 – The object is considered to pose a potential or realistic risk or hazard to a patient or individual in the MR environment primarily as the result of movement or dislodgment of the object. Other hazards may also exist. Therefore, in general, the presence of this object is considered to be a contraindication for an MR procedure and/or for an individual to enter the MR environment.

Note that the "default" static magnetic field strength for an *MR unsafe* implant or device is 1.5-Tesla.

Unsafe 2 – This object displays only minor magnetic field interactions which, in consideration of the *in vivo* application of this object, is unlikely to pose a hazard or risk in association with movement or dislodgment. Nevertheless, the presence of this object is considered to be a contraindication for an MR procedure or for an individual in the MR environment. Potential risks of performing an MR procedure in a patient or individual with this object are related to possible induced currents, excessive heating, or other potentially hazardous conditions. Therefore, it is inadvisable to perform an MR procedure in a patient or individual with this object.

For example, although certain cardiovascular catheters and accessories typically do not exhibit magnetic field interactions, there are other mechanisms whereby these devices may pose a hazard to the patient or individual or in the MR environment (e.g., excessive MRI-related heating).

The Swan-Ganz thermodilution catheter (and other similar catheters) displays no attraction to the MR system. However, there has been a report of a Swan-Ganz catheter that "melted" in a patient during an MR procedure. Therefore, the presence of this cardiovascular catheter and/or other similar device is considered to be a contraindication for a patient undergoing an MR procedure.

Field Strength – This is the highest strength of the static magnetic field of the MR system that was used for the evaluation of the object. In most cases, a 1.5-Tesla MR system was used for testing. However, there are some objects that were tested at field strengths lower (e.g., 0.15-Tesla) or higher (e.g., 3-Tesla) than 1.5-Tesla.

Note that the "default" field strength for an *MR unsafe* implant or device is 1.5-Tesla.

There are MR systems with static magnetic field strengths that exceed 3.0-Tesla (i.e., as high as 8-Tesla or 9.4-Tesla). Some objects have been assessed to determine the relative amount of magnetic field interactions in association with these very high-field-strength MR systems.

Important Note: An object that exhibits only "mild" or "weak" magnetic field interactions in association with exposure to a 1.5-Tesla MR system may be attracted with sufficient force by a higher field strength scanner (e.g., 3-Tesla), potentially posing a risk to a patient or individual. Therefore, careful consideration must be given to each object relative to the static magnetic field strength of the MR system used for testing as well as the conditions that are present for the patient or individual under consideration prior to exposure to the MR environment.

Furthermore, for implants and devices that have an elongated shape or form a loop of a certain diameter, MRI-related heating may be of concern. Please refer to **3-Tesla MR Safety Information for Implants and Devices** in this textbook for additional guidance and recommendations.

Reference – This is the peer-reviewed publication or other documentation used for the MRI safety information indicated for a particular object.

*Terminology Applied to Implants and Devices

IMPORTANT NOTE: See the section in this textbook entitled, **Terminology Applied to Implants and Devices,** for a full explanation of the proper terms used for MRI labeling.

Also, for a comprehensive explanation, see Shellock FG, Woods TO, Crues JV. MRI labeling information for implants and devices: Explanation of terminology. Radiology 2009;253:26-30 (available as a PDF file on *www.IMRSER.org*)

Use of Terminology

The current MRI labeling terminology is intended to help elucidate matters related to biomedical implants and devices to ensure the safe use of MRI technology. Notably, this terminology (i.e., MR safe, MR conditional, and MR unsafe) has not been applied *retrospectively* to implants and devices that previously received U.S. Food and Drug Administration (FDA) approved labeling using the older terms "MR safe" or "MR compatible" (i.e., this applies to those objects tested prior to 2005). Accordingly, this should be understood to avoid undue confusion regarding the matter of MRI-related labeling for "older" vs. "newer" implants, or those that have undergone retesting for MRI issues.

REFERENCES

American Society for Testing and Materials (ASTM) International, Designation: F2503. Standard Practice for Marking Medical Devices and Other Items for Safety in the Magnetic Resonance Environment. ASTM International, West Conshohocken, PA.

Shellock FG, Kanal E, Gilk T. Regarding the value reported for the term "spatial gradient magnetic field" and how this information is applied to labeling of medical implants and devices. American Journal of Roentgenology. 2011;196:142-145.

Shellock FG, Woods TO, Crues JV. MRI labeling information for implants and devices: Explanation of terminology. Radiology 2009;253:26-30.

Woods TO. Standards for medical devices in MRI: present and future. J Magn Reson Imaging. 2007;26:1186-9.

Woods TO. Guidance for Industry and FDA Staff - Establishing Safety and Compatibility of Passive Implants in the Magnetic Resonance (MR) Environment. Document issued on: August 21, 2008; http://www.fda.gov/cdrh/osel/guidance/1685.html

Object	Status	Field Strength (T)	Reference

Aneurysm Clips

Object	Status	Field Strength (T)	Reference
Aesculap AVM clip *Curved, Phynox* *Aesculap, Inc., www.aesculapusa.com*	Safe	1.5, 3	
Aesculap AVM clip *curved, Phynox* *Aesculap, Inc., www.aesculapusa.com*	Safe	1.5, 3	
Aesculap AVM clip *straight, Phynox* *Aesculap, Inc., www.aesculapusa.com*	Safe	1.5, 3	
Codman AVM Micro Clip *Codman, www.depuy.com*	Conditional 6	3	116
Codman Slim-Line Aneurysm Clip *Codman, www.depuy.com*	Conditional 6	3	116
Codman Slim-Line Aneurysm Clip Graft *Codman, www.depuy.com*	Conditional 6	3	116
Codman Slim-Line Mini Aneurysm Clip *Codman, www.depuy.com*	Conditional 6	3	116
Codman Slim-Line Temporary Vessel Aneurysm Clip *Codman, www.depuy.com*	Conditional 6	3	116
Downs Multi-Positional, Aneurysm Clip *17-7PH*	Unsafe 1	1.39	1
Drake (DR 14, DR 21), Aneurysm Clip *Edward Weck, Triangle Park, NJ*	Unsafe 1	1.39	1
Drake (DR 16), Aneurysm Clip *Edward Weck, Triangle Park, NJ*	Unsafe 1	0.147	1
Drake Aneurysm Clip, 301 SS *Edward Weck, Triangle Park, NJ*	Unsafe 1	1.5	2
GIANT L-Aneurysm Clip, TITANIUM Permanent *aneurysm clip, 40-mm straight blade* *Peter Lazic Mikrochirurgische, www.lazic.de*	Conditional 6	3	
Heifetz Aneurysm Clip, 17-7PH *Edward Weck, Triangle Park, NJ*	Unsafe 1	1.89	4
Heifetz Aneurysm Clip, Elgiloy *Edward Weck, Triangle Park, NJ*	Safe	1.89	2
Housepian Aneurysm Clip	Unsafe 1	0.147	1
Kapp Aneurysm Clip, 405 SS *V. Mueller*	Unsafe 1	1.89	2
Kapp, Curved Aneurysm Clip, 404 SS *V. Mueller*	Unsafe 1	1.39	1
Kapp, Straight Aneurysm Clip, 404 SS *V. Mueller*	Unsafe 1	1.39	1
Kopitnik AVM Microclips, All FE Models *Aesculap, Inc., www.aesculapusa.com*	Safe	3	
Kopitnik AVM Microclip, aneurysm clip *Peter Lazic Mikrochirurgische, www.lazic.de*	Safe	1.5	
L-Aneurysm Clip System, Titanium *Peter Lazic GmbH, www.lazic.de*	Safe	3	

Object	Status	Field Strength (T)	Reference
L-Aneurysm Clip *20 degree Angle, 5-mm, 7.5-mm, 10-mm, Titanium* *Peter Lazic Mikrochirurgische, www.lazic.de*	Conditional 6	3	
L-Aneurysm Clip *45 degree Angle, 5-mm, 7.5-mm, 10-mm, Titanium* *Peter Lazic Mikrochirurgische, www.lazic.de*	Conditional 6	3	
L-Aneurysm Clip *90 degree Angle, 5-mm, 7.5-mm, 10-mm, Titanium* *Peter Lazic Mikrochirurgische, www.lazic.de*	Conditional 6	3	
L-Aneurysm Clip *Angle with radius, 7.5-mm, 10-mm, Titanium* *Peter Lazic Mikrochirurgische, www.lazic.de*	Conditional 6	3	
L-Aneurysm Clip *Bayonet, 7-mm, 10-mm, 12-mm, Titanium* *Peter Lazic Mikrochirurgische, www.lazic.de*	Conditional 6	3	
L-Aneurysm Clip *Curved, 7-mm, 9-mm, 12-mm, 15-mm, Titanium* *Peter Lazic Mikrochirurgische, www.lazic.de*	Conditional 6	3	
L-Aneurysm Clip *Fenestrated 3.5-mm 45 degree Angle, 5-mm, 7.5-mm, 10-mm, Titanium* *Peter Lazic Mikrochirurgische, www.lazic.de*	Conditional 6	3	
L-Aneurysm Clip *Fenestrated 3.5-mm 90 degree Angle, 5-mm, 7.5-mm, 10-mm, Titanium* *Peter Lazic Mikrochirurgische, www.lazic.de*	Conditional 6	3	
L-Aneurysm Clip *Fenestrated 3.5-mm Straight, 4-mm, 6-mm, 9-mm, Titanium* *Peter Lazic Mikrochirurgische, www.lazic.de*	Conditional 6	3	
L-Aneurysm Clip *Fenestrated 5-mm 45 degree Angle, 5-mm, 7.5-mm, 10-mm Titanium* *Peter Lazic Mikrochirurgische, www.lazic.de*	Conditional 6	3	
L-Aneurysm Clip *Fenestrated 5-mm 90 degree Angle, 5-mm, 7.5-mm, 10-mm, Titanium* *Peter Lazic Mikrochirurgische, www.lazic.de*	Conditional 6	3	
L-Aneurysm Clip *Fenestrated 5-mm Straight, 4-mm, 6-mm, 9-mm, 12-mm Titanium* *Peter Lazic Mikrochirurgische, www.lazic.de*	Conditional 6	3	
L-Aneurysm Clip *Giant Aneurysm Clip Bayonet, 21-mm, Titanium* *Peter Lazic Mikrochirurgische, www.lazic.de*	Conditional 6	3	
L-Aneurysm Clip *Giant Aneurysm Clip Straight, 21-mm, 25-mm, 30-mm, 35-mm, 40-mm, Titanium* *Peter Lazic Mikrochirurgische, www.lazic.de*	Conditional 6	3	
L-Aneurysm Clip *J Curved, 7-mm, 9-mm, 11-mm, Titanium* *Peter Lazic Mikrochirurgische, www.lazic.de*	Conditional 6	3	

Object	Status	Field Strength (T)	Reference
L-Aneurysm Clip *Mini Clip Angle and Curved, 5-mm, Titanium* *Peter Lazic Mikrochirurgische, www.lazic.de*	Conditional 6	3	
L-Aneurysm Clip *Mini Clip Angle, 7-mm, Titanium* *Peter Lazic Mikrochirurgische, www.lazic.de*	Conditional 6	3	
L-Aneurysm Clip *Mini Clip Bayonet, 4-mm, 7-mm, Titanium* *Peter Lazic Mikrochirurgische, www.lazic.de*	Conditional 6	3	
L-Aneurysm Clip *Mini Clip Curved Narrow Jaw, 4-mm, Titanium* *Peter Lazic Mikrochirurgische, www.lazic.de*	Conditional 6	3	
L-Aneurysm Clip *Mini Clip Curved, 4-mm, 5-mm, Titanium* *Peter Lazic Mikrochirurgische, www.lazic.de*	Conditional 6	3	
L-Aneurysm Clip *Mini Clip Sideward Angle, 5-mm, Titanium* *Peter Lazic Mikrochirurgische, www.lazic.de*	Conditional 6	3	
L-Aneurysm Clip *Mini Clip Sideward Curved, 6-mm, Titanium* *Peter Lazic Mikrochirurgische, www.lazic.de*	Conditional 6	3	
L-Aneurysm Clip *Mini Clip Slightly Curved Narrow Jaw, 3-mm, 4-mm, Titanium* *Peter Lazic Mikrochirurgische, www.lazic.de*	Conditional 6	3	
L-Aneurysm Clip *Mini Clip Slightly Curved, 4-mm, 5-mm, 7-mm, Titanium* *Peter Lazic Mikrochirurgische, www.lazic.de*	Conditional 6	3	
L-Aneurysm Clip *Mini Clip Straight Narrow Jaw, 3-mm, 5-mm, Titanium* *Peter Lazic Mikrochirurgische, www.lazic.de*	Conditional 6	3	
L-Aneurysm Clip *Mini Clip Straight, 3-mm, 5-mm, 7-mm, Titanium* *Peter Lazic Mikrochirurgische, www.lazic.de*	Conditional 6	3	
L-Aneurysm Clip *Sideward Angle, 8-mm, 12-mm, Titanium* *Peter Lazic Mikrochirurgische, www.lazic.de*	Conditional 6	3	
L-Aneurysm Clip *Sideward curved, 9-mm, Titanium* *Peter Lazic Mikrochirurgische, www.lazic.de*	Conditional 6	3	
L-Aneurysm Clip *Slightly curved, 7-mm, 9-mm, 12-mm, 15-mm, 18-mm, Titanium* *Peter Lazic Mikrochirurgische, www.lazic.de*	Conditional 6	3	
L-Aneurysm Clip *Straight, 7-mm, 9-mm, 12-mm, 15-mm, 18-mm, Titanium* *Peter Lazic Mikrochirurgische, www.lazic.de*	Conditional 6	3	
Mayfield Aneurysm Clip, 301 SS *Codman, www.depuy.com*	Unsafe 1	1.5	3
Mayfield Aneurysm Clip, 304 SS *Codman, www.depuy.com*	Unsafe 1	1.89	5
McFadden Aneurysm Clip, 301 SS *Codman, www.depuy.com*	Unsafe 1	1.5	2

Object	Status	Field Strength (T)	Reference
McFadden Vari-Angle, Aneurysm Clip *micro clip, fenestrated, 9-mm straight blade, MP35N* *Codman, www.depuy.com*	Safe	1.5	
McFadden Vari-Angle, Aneurysm Clip *micro clip, 9-mm straight blade, MP35N,* *Codman, www.depuy.com*	Safe	1.5	
Olivercrona *Aneurysm Clip*	Safe	1.39	1
Perneczky Aneurysm Clip *curved, 20-mm* *Zeppelin Chirurgische Instrumente, Germany*	Safe	1.5	
Perneczky Aneurysm Clip *curved, 9-mm* *Zeppelin Chirurgische Instrumente, Germany*	Safe	1.5	
Perneczky Aneurysm Clip *straight, 2-mm blade, SS alloy* *Zeppelin Chirurgische Instrumente, Germany*	Safe	1.5, 3	82
Perneczky Aneurysm Clip *straight, 3-mm* *Zeppelin Chirurgische Instumente, Germany*	Safe	1.5	
Perneczky Aneurysm Clip *straight, 6-mm blade, SS alloy* *Zeppelin Chirurgische Instrumente, Germany*	Safe	1.5, 3	82
Perneczky Aneurysm Clip *straight, 7-mm blade, SS alloy* *Zeppelin Chirurgische Instrumente, Germany*	Safe	1.5, 3	82
Perneczky Aneurysm Clip *straight, 9-mm* *Zeppelin Chirurgische Instrumente, Germany*	Safe	1.5	
Pivot Aneurysm Clip *17-7PH*	Unsafe 1	1.89	5
R. Spetzler Titanium Aneurysm Clip *for Permanent Occlusion, 5-mm Fenestrated Bayonet* *11-mm blade length (M-9248), Ti6Al4V (Titanium alloy)* *Allegiance Healthcare Corporation, V. Mueller Neuro/Spine,* *San Carlos, CA*	Safe	1.5, 3	
R. Spetzler Titanium Aneurysm Clip *for Permanent Occlusion, 5-mm Fenestrated Straight* *12-mm blade length (M-9227), Ti6Al4V (Titanium alloy)* *Allegiance Healthcare Corporation, V. Mueller Neuro/Spine,* *San Carlos, CA*	Safe	1.5, 3	
R. Spetzler Titanium Aneurysm Clip *for Permanent Occlusion, Mini 40 degree Side* *5-mm blade length (M-9450), Ti6Al4V (Titanium alloy)* *Allegiance Healthcare Corporation, V. Mueller Neuro/Spine,* *San Carlos, CA*	Safe	1.5, 3	
R. Spetzler Titanium Aneurysm Clip *for Permanent Occlusion, Standard Bayonet* *12-mm blade length (M-9152), Ti6Al4V (Titanium alloy)* *Allegiance Healthcare Corporation, V. Mueller Neuro/Spine,* *San Carlos, CA*	Safe	1.5, 3	

Object	Status	Field Strength (T)	Reference
R. Spetzler Titanium Aneurysm Clip *for Permanent Occlusion, Standard Straight* *15-mm blade length (M-9113), Ti6Al4V (Titanium alloy)* *Allegiance Healthcare Corporation, V. Mueller Neuro/Spine,* *San Carlos, CA*	Safe	1.5, 3	
Scoville Aneurysm Clip *EN58J* *Downs Surgical, Inc., Decatur, GA*	Safe	1.89	2
Slim-Line Aneurysm Clip *Fenestrated Straight, 4-mm opening, 6-mm blade, MP35N* *Codman, www.depuy.com*	Safe	1.5, 3	
Spetzler Pure Titanium Aneurysm Clip *Model C-2200, straight, 5-mm blade, C.P. Titanium* *NMT Neurosciences, Duluth, Georgia*	Safe	1.5, 3	82
Spetzler Pure Titanium Aneurysm Clip *Model C-2203, straight, 11-mm blade, C.P. Titanium* *NMT Neurosciences, Duluth, Georgia*	Safe	1.5, 3	82
Spetzler Pure Titanium Aneurysm Clip *Model C-2212, curved, 7-mm blade, C.P. Titanium* *NMT Neurosciences, Duluth, Georgia*	Safe	1.5, 3	82
Spetzler Pure Titanium Aneurysm Clip *Model C-2214, curved, 11-mm blade, C.P. Titanium* *NMT Neurosciences, Duluth, Georgia*	Safe	1.5, 3	82
Spetzler Pure Titanium Aneurysm Clip *Model C-2224, straight, 11-mm/3.5-mm fenestrated blade* *C.P. Titanium* *NMT Neurosciences, Duluth, Georgia*	Safe	1.5, 3	82
Spetzler Pure Titanium Aneurysm Clip *Model C-2526, straight, 11-mm blade, C.P. Titanium* *NMT Neurosciences, Duluth, Georgia*	Safe	1.5, 3	82
Spetzler Pure Titanium Aneurysm Clip *straight, 9-mm blade, C. P. Titanium* *Elekta Instruments, Atlanta, GA*	Safe	1.5, 3	82
Spetzler Titanium Aneurysm Clip *straight, 13-mm blade, double turn, C.P. Titanium* *Elekta Instruments, Inc., Atlanta, GA*	Safe	1.5	68
Spetzler Titanium Aneurysm Clip *straight, 13-mm blade, single turn, C.P. Titanium* *Elekta Instruments, Inc., Atlanta, GA*	Safe	1.5, 3	68, 82
Spetzler Titanium Aneurysm Clip *straight, 9-mm blade, double turn, C.P. Titanium* *Elekta Instruments, Inc., Atlanta, GA*	Safe	1.5	68
Spetzler Titanium Aneurysm Clip *straight, 9-mm blade, single turn, C.P. Titanium* *Elekta Instruments, Inc., Atlanta, GA*	Safe	1.5, 3	68, 82
Stevens Aneurysm Clip, silver alloy	Safe	0.15	6
Sugita Aneurysm Clip, Elgiloy *Downs Surgical, Inc., Decatur, GA*	Safe	1.89	2
Sugita Aneurysm Clip *Fenestrated large, bent, 7.5-mm, Elgiloy,* *Mizhuo America, Inc., www.mizuho.com*	Safe	1.5, 3	82

Object	Status	Field Strength (T)	Reference
Sugita Titanium Aneurysm Clip *mini temporary, angled, 5-mm blade, Titanium alloy* *Mizhuo America, Inc., www.mizuho.com*	Safe	1.5	
Sugita Titanium Aneurysm Clip *mini temporary, straight large, 6-mm blade, Titanium alloy* *Mizhuo America, Inc., www.mizuho.com*	Safe	1.5	
Sugita Titanium Aneurysm Clip *mini temporary, straight slim, 6-mm blade, Titanium alloy* *Mizhuo America, Inc., www.mizuho.com*	Safe	1.5	
Sugita Titanium Aneurysm Clip *mini, angled, 5-mm blade, Titanium alloy* *Mizhuo America, Inc., www.mizuho.com*	Safe	1.5	
Sugita Titanium Aneurysm Clip *mini, angled, 7-mm blade, Titanium alloy* *Mizhuo America, Inc., www.mizuho.com*	Safe	1.5	
Sugita Titanium Aneurysm Clip *mini, bayonet, 5-mm blade, Titanium alloy* *Mizhuo America, Inc., www.mizuho.com*	Safe	1.5	
Sugita Titanium Aneurysm Clip *mini, curved slim, 5.2-mm blade, Titanium alloy* *Mizhuo America, Inc., www.mizuho.com*	Safe	1.5	
Sugita Titanium Aneurysm Clip *mini, curved slim, 6.7-mm blade, Titanium alloy* *Mizhuo America, Inc., www.mizuho.com*	Safe	1.5	
Sugita Titanium Aneurysm Clip *mini, curved slim, 8.2-mm blade, Titanium alloy* *Mizhuo America, Inc., www.mizuho.com*	Safe	1.5	
Sugita Titanium Aneurysm Clip *mini, curved, 4.5-mm blade, Titanium alloy* *Mizhuo America, Inc., www.mizuho.com*	Safe	1.5	
Sugita Titanium Aneurysm Clip *mini, curved, 5.5-mm blade, Titanium alloy* *Mizhuo America, Inc., www.mizuho.com*	Safe	1.5	
Sugita Titanium Aneurysm Clip *mini, curved, 5-mm blade, Titanium alloy* *Mizhuo America, Inc., www.mizuho.com*	Safe	1.5	
Sugita Titanium Aneurysm Clip *mini, side curved, 7-mm blade, Titanium alloy* *Mizhuo America, Inc., www.mizuho.com*	Safe	1.5	
Sugita Titanium Aneurysm Clip *mini, straight large, 6-mm blade, Titanium alloy* *Mizhuo America, Inc., www.mizuho.com*	Safe	1.5	
Sugita Titanium Aneurysm Clip *mini, straight slim, 4-mm blade, Titanium alloy* *Mizhuo America, Inc., www.mizuho.com*	Safe	1.5	
Sugita Titanium Aneurysm Clip *mini, straight slim, 6-mm blade, Titanium alloy* *Mizhuo America, Inc., www.mizuho.com*	Safe	1.5	
Sugita Titanium Aneurysm Clip *mini, straight small, 4-mm blade, Titanium alloy* *Mizhuo America, Inc., www.mizuho.com*	Safe	1.5	

Object	Status	Field Strength (T)	Reference
Sugita Titanium Aneurysm Clip *Standard, 1/4 curved, 11-mm blade, Titanium alloy* *Mizhuo America, Inc., www.mizuho.com*	Safe	1.5	
Sugita Titanium Aneurysm Clip *Standard, 1/4 curved, large, 8.6-mm blade, Titanium alloy* *Mizhuo America, Inc., www.mizuho.com*	Safe	1.5	
Sugita Titanium Aneurysm Clip *Standard, 1/4 curved, small, 7.6-mm blade, Titanium alloy* *Mizhuo America, Inc., www.mizuho.com*	Safe	1.5	
Sugita Titanium Aneurysm Clip *Standard, 45 degree curved, large, 10-mm blade, Titanium alloy* *Mizhuo America, Inc., www.mizuho.com*	Safe	1.5	
Sugita Titanium Aneurysm Clip *Standard, 45 degree curved, medium, 7.5-mm blade,* *Titanium alloy* *Mizhuo America, Inc., www.mizuho.com*	Safe	1.5	
Sugita Titanium Aneurysm Clip *Standard, 45 degree curved, small, 5-mm blade, Titanium alloy* *Mizhuo America, Inc., www.mizuho.com*	Safe	1.5	
Sugita Titanium Aneurysm Clip *Standard, angled, 12-mm blade, Titanium alloy* *Mizhuo America, Inc., www.mizuho.com*	Safe	1.5	
Sugita Titanium Aneurysm Clip *Standard, angled, 8-mm blade, Titanium alloy* *Mizhuo America, Inc., www.mizuho.com*	Safe	1.5	
Sugita Titanium Aneurysm Clip *Standard, bayonet large, 12-mm blade, Titanium alloy* *Mizhuo America, Inc., www.mizuho.com*	Safe	1.5	
Sugita Titanium Aneurysm Clip *Standard, bayonet small, 10-mm blade, Titanium alloy* *Mizhuo America, Inc., www.mizuho.com*	Safe	1.5	
Sugita Titanium Aneurysm Clip *Standard, bayonet, 7-mm blade, Titanium alloy* *Mizhuo America, Inc., www.mizuho.com*	Safe	1.5	
Sugita Titanium Aneurysm Clip *Standard, curved (155 g), 9-mm blade, Titanium alloy* *Mizhuo America, Inc., www.mizuho.com*	Safe	1.5	
Sugita Titanium Aneurysm Clip *Standard, curved (160 g), 9-mm blade, Titanium alloy* *Mizhuo America, Inc., www.mizuho.com*	Safe	1.5	
Sugita Titanium Aneurysm Clip *Standard, for Permanent Occlusion, 45 degree angled,* *19-mm, serrated blade, Titanium alloy* *Mizhuo America, Inc., www.mizuho.com*	Safe	1.5, 3	82
Sugita Titanium Aneurysm Clip *Standard, J-angled, large, 9-mm blade, Titanium alloy* *Mizhuo America, Inc., www.mizuho.com*	Safe	1.5	
Sugita Titanium Aneurysm Clip *Standard, J-angled, medium, 7.5-mm blade, Titanium alloy* *Mizhuo America, Inc., www.mizuho.com*	Safe	1.5	

Object	Status	Field Strength (T)	Reference
Sugita Titanium Aneurysm Clip *Standard, J-angled, small, 6-mm blade, Titanium alloy* *Mizhuo America, Inc., www.mizuho.com*	Safe	1.5	
Sugita Titanium Aneurysm Clip *Standard, L-angled, large, 10-mm blade, Titanium alloy* *Mizhuo America, Inc., www.mizuho.com*	Safe	1.5	
Sugita Titanium Aneurysm Clip *Standard, L-angled, medium, 7.5-mm blade, Titanium alloy* *Mizhuo America, Inc., www.mizuho.com*	Safe	1.5	
Sugita Titanium Aneurysm Clip *Standard, L-angled, small, 5-mm blade, Titanium alloy* *Mizhuo America, Inc., www.mizuho.com*	Safe	1.5	
Sugita Titanium Aneurysm Clip *Standard, L-curved, large, 10-mm blade, Titanium alloy* *Mizhuo America, Inc., www.mizuho.com*	Safe	1.5	
Sugita Titanium Aneurysm Clip *Standard, L-curved, small, 7.5-mm blade, Titanium alloy* *Mizhuo America, Inc., www.mizuho.com*	Safe	1.5	
Sugita Titanium Aneurysm Clip *Standard, side angled, 12-mm blade, Titanium alloy* *Mizhuo America, Inc., www.mizuho.com*	Safe	1.5	
Sugita Titanium Aneurysm Clip *Standard, side angled, 8-mm blade, Titanium alloy* *Mizhuo America, Inc., www.mizuho.com*	Safe	1.5	
Sugita Titanium Aneurysm Clip *Standard, side curved bayonet, 8.5-mm blade, Titanium alloy* *Mizhuo America, Inc., www.mizuho.com*	Safe	1.5	
Sugita Titanium Aneurysm Clip *Standard, side curved, 9-mm blade, Titanium alloy* *Mizhuo America, Inc., www.mizuho.com*	Safe	1.5	
Sugita Titanium Aneurysm Clip *Standard, slight curved bayonet, 12-mm blade, Titanium alloy* *Mizhuo America, Inc., www.mizuho.com*	Safe	1.5	
Sugita Titanium Aneurysm Clip *Standard, slightly angled, 8-mm blade, Titanium alloy* *Mizhuo America, Inc., www.mizuho.com*	Safe	1.5	
Sugita Titanium Aneurysm Clip *Standard, slightly curved (165), 11-mm blade, Titanium alloy* *Mizhuo America, Inc., www.mizuho.com*	Safe	1.5	
Sugita Titanium Aneurysm Clip *standard, slightly curved (170), 11-mm blade, Titanium alloy* *Mizhuo America, Inc., www.mizuho.com*	Safe	1.5	
Sugita Titanium Aneurysm Clip *Standard, slightly curved, 18-mm blade, Titanium alloy* *Mizhuo America, Inc., www.mizuho.com*	Safe	1.5	
Sugita Titanium Aneurysm Clip *Standard, slightly curved, 9-mm blade, Titanium alloy* *Mizhuo America, Inc., www.mizuho.com*	Safe	1.5	
Sugita Titanium Aneurysm Clip *Standard, slightly curved, small, 14-mm blade, Titanium alloy* *Mizhuo America, Inc., www.mizuho.com*	Safe	1.5	

Object	Status	Field Strength (T)	Reference
Sugita Titanium Aneurysm Clip *Standard, small curved, 9-mm blade, Titanium alloy* *Mizhuo America, Inc., www.mizuho.com*	Safe	1.5	
Sugita Titanium Aneurysm Clip *Standard, staight (small), 12-mm blade, Titanium alloy* *Mizhuo America, Inc., www.mizuho.com*	Safe	1.5	
Sugita Titanium Aneurysm Clip *Standard, straight large, 18-mm blade, Titanium alloy* *Mizhuo America, Inc., www.mizuho.com*	Safe	1.5	
Sugita Titanium Aneurysm Clip *Standard, straight medium, 15-mm blade, Titanium alloy* *Mizhuo America, Inc., www.mizuho.com*	Safe	1.5	
Sugita Titanium Aneurysm Clip *Standard, straight, large, 10-mm blade, Titanium alloy* *Mizhuo America, Inc., www.mizuho.com*	Safe	1.5	
Sugita Titanium Aneurysm Clip *Standard, straight, small, 7-mm blade, Titanium alloy* *Mizhuo America, Inc., www.mizuho.com*	Safe	1.5	
Sugita Titanium Aneurysm Clip *Temporary, bayonet, 7-mm blade, Titanium alloy* *Mizhuo America, Inc., www.mizuho.com*	Safe	1.5	
Sugita Titanium Aneurysm Clip *Temporary, curved, 8-mm blade, Titanium alloy* *Mizhuo America, Inc., www.mizuho.com*	Safe	1.5	
Sugita Titanium Aneurysm Clip *Temporary, slightly curved, 11-mm blade, Titanium alloy* *Mizhuo America, Inc., www.mizuho.com*	Safe	1.5	
Sugita Titanium Aneurysm Clip *Temporary, straight large, 10-mm blade, Titanium alloy* *Mizhuo America, Inc., www.mizuho.com*	Safe	1.5	
Sugita Titanium Aneurysm Clip *Temporary, straight small, 7-mm blade, Titanium alloy* *Mizhuo America, Inc., www.mizuho.com*	Safe	1.5	
Sugita, AVM Micro Clip *Aneurysm Clip, Elgiloy* *Mizhuo America, Inc., www.mizuho.com*	Safe	1.5	
Sugita, bent, mini aneurysm clip *for temporary occlusion, Elgiloy* *Mizhuo America, Inc., www.mizuho.com*	Safe	1.5	
Sugita, bent, standard aneurysm clip *for temporary occlusion, Elgiloy* *Mizhuo America, Inc., www.mizuho.com*	Safe	1.5	
Sugita, sideward CVD bayonet, standard *aneurysm clip for permanent occlusion* *Mizhuo America, Inc., www.mizuho.com*	Safe	1.5	
Sugita, straight, large *aneurysm clip for permanent occlusion, Elgiloy* *Mizhuo America, Inc., www.mizuho.com*	Safe	1.5	

Object	Status	Field Strength (T)	Reference
Sugita *Fenestrated Large Fujita, Blade Deflected Type* *Aneurysm Clip for Permanent Occlusion* *angled, 10-mm serrated blade, Elgiloy* *Mizhuo America, Inc., www.mizuho.com*	Safe	1.5, 3	82
Sugita *Fenestrated large, bent, Aneurysm Clip for permanent occlusion* *Elgiloy* *Mizhuo America, Inc., www.mizuho.com*	Safe	1.5	
Sugita *Large Aneurysm Clip for Permanent Occlusion* *straight, 21-mm serrated blade, Elgiloy* *Mizhuo America, Inc., www.mizuho.com*	Safe	1.5, 3	82
Sugita *Long Aneurysm Clip for Permanent Occlusion* *straight, 19-mm nonserration blade, Elgiloy* *Mizhuo America, Inc., www.mizuho.com*	Safe	1.5, 3	82
Sugita *Standard bent, Aneurysm Clip, 8-mm blade, Elgiloy* *Mizhuo America, Inc., www.mizuho.com*	Safe	1.5, 3	82
Sugita *Standard curved, Aneurysm Clip, 6-mm blade, Elgiloy* *Mizhuo America, Inc., www.mizuho.com*	Safe	1.5, 3	82
Sugita *Temporary Mini, Aneurysm Clip, bent, 7-mm blade, Elgiloy* *Mizhuo America, Inc., www.mizuho.com*	Safe	1.5, 3	82
Sugita *Temporary standard straight Aneurysm Clip, 7-mm blade, Elgiloy* *Mizhuo America, Inc., www.mizuho.com*	Safe	1.5, 3	82
Sundt AVM Micro Aneurysm Clip System *MP35N, Codman,* *www.depuy.com*	Conditional 6	3	
SUNDT AVM MICRO CLIP *# 3, MP35N* *Codman, www.depuy.com*	Safe	1.5, 3	
SUNDT AVM MICRO CLIP *# 4, MP35N* *Codman, www.depuy.com*	Safe	1.5, 3	
SUNDT AVM MICRO CLIP *# 5, MP35N* *Codman, www.depuy.com*	Safe	1.5, 3	
Sundt AVM, Micro Clip *aneurysm clip, MP35N* *Codman, www.depuy.com*	Safe	1.5	
SUNDT SLIM-LINE ANEURYSM CLIP *# 6, Bayonet, MP35N* *Codman, www.depuy.com*	Safe	1.5, 3	
SUNDT SLIM-LINE ANEURYSM CLIP *# 6, Forward Angle, MP35N* *Codman, www.depuy.com*	Safe	1.5, 3	

Object	Status	Field Strength (T)	Reference
SUNDT SLIM-LINE ANEURYSM CLIP *Fenestrated Bayonet, Straight, 6-mm opening, 15-mm blade,* *MP35N* *Codman, www.depuy.com*	Safe	1.5, 3	
SUNDT SLIM-LINE ANEURYSM CLIP *Fenestrated Straight, 4-mm opening, 24-mm blade, MP35N* *Codman, www.depuy.com*	Safe	1.5, 3	
SUNDT SLIM-LINE ANEURYSM CLIP *Sharp Right Angle, 12-mm blade, MP35N* *Codman, www.depuy.com*	Safe	1.5, 3	
SUNDT SLIM-LINE MINI ANEURYSM CLIP *# 6, Right Angle, MP35N* *Codman, www.depuy.com*	Safe	1.5, 3	
SUNDT SLIM-LINE MINI ANEURYSM CLIP *# 6, Straight, MP35N* *Codman, www.depuy.com*	Safe	1.5, 3	
SUNDT SLIM-LINE MINI ANEURYSM CLIP *# 7, Right Angle, MP35N* *Codman, www.depuy.com*	Safe	1.5, 3	
Sundt Slim-Line Mini Aneurysm Clip *also known as Slimline, MP35N* *Codman, www.depuy.com*	Conditional 6	3	
Sundt Slim-Line Temporary Vessel Aneurysm Clip *also known as Slimline, MP35N* *Codman, www.depuy.com*	Conditional 6	3	
Sundt Slim-Line, Graft Clip *Aneurysm Clip, MP35N* *Codman, www.depuy.com*	Safe	1.5	
Sundt Slim-Line, Temporary Aneurysm Clip *10-mm blade, MP35N* *Codman, www.depuy.com*	Safe	1.5	
Sundt-Kees Multi-Angle *Aneurysm Clip, 17-7PH* *Downs Surgical, Inc., Decatur, GA*	Unsafe 1	1.89	2
Sundt-Kees Slim-Line Aneurysm Clip *also known as Slimline, 30 Degree Forward Angle, MP35N* *Codman, www.depuy.com*	Conditional 6	3	
Sundt-Kees Slim-Line Aneurysm Clip *also known as Slimline, 30 Degree Forward Curve, MP35N* *Codman, www.depuy.com*	Conditional 6	3	
Sundt-Kees Slim-Line Aneurysm Clip *also known as Slimline Bayonet,* *30 Degree Curved Forward-Left, MP35N* *Codman, www.depuy.com*	Conditional 6	3	
Sundt-Kees Slim-Line Aneurysm Clip *also known as Slimline Bayonet,* *30 Degree Curved Forward-Right, MP35N* *Codman, www.depuy.com*	Conditional 6	3	
Sundt-Kees Slim-Line Aneurysm Clip *also known as Slimline Bayonet, Straight, MP35N* *Codman, www.depuy.com*	Conditional 6	3	

Object	Status	Field Strength (T)	Reference
Sundt-Kees Slim-Line Aneurysm Clip *also known as Slimline Curved, MP35N* *Codman, www.depuy.com*	Conditional 6	3	
Sundt-Kees Slim-Line Aneurysm Clip *also known as Slimline Fenestrated 45 Degree Angle,* *6-mm Opening, MP35N* *Codman, www.depuy.com*	Conditional 6	3	
Sundt-Kees Slim-Line Aneurysm Clip *also known as Slimline Fenestrated 45 Degree Angle* *4-mm Opening, 30 Degree, MP35N* *Codman, www.depuy.com*	Conditional 6	3	
Sundt-Kees Slim-Line Aneurysm Clip *also known as Slimline Fenestrated 90 Degree Angle,* *4-mm Opening, MP35N* *Codman, www.depuy.com*	Conditional 6	3	
Sundt-Kees Slim-Line Aneurysm Clip *also known as Slimline Fenestrated 90 Degree Angle,* *6-mm Opening, MP35N* *Codman, www.depuy.com*	Conditional 6	3	
Sundt-Kees Slim-Line Aneurysm Clip *also known as Slimline Fenestrated Bayonet Straight,* *6-mm Opening, MP35N* *Codman, www.depuy.com*	Conditional 6	3	
Sundt-Kees Slim-Line Aneurysm Clip *also known as Slimline Fenestrated Straight,* *3-mm Extended Tandem, 6-mm, MP35N* *Codman, www.depuy.com*	Conditional 6	3	
Sundt-Kees Slim-Line Aneurysm Clip *also known as Slimline Fenestrated Straight,* *4-mm Opening, MP35N* *Codman, www.depuy.com*	Conditional 6	3	
Sundt-Kees Slim-Line Aneurysm Clip *also known as Slimline Fenestrated Straight,* *5-mm Extended Tandem, 6-mm, MP35N* *Codman, www.depuy.com*	Conditional 6	3	
Sundt-Kees Slim-Line Aneurysm Clip *also known as Slimline Fenestrated Straight,* *6-mm Opening, MP35N* *Codman, www.depuy.com*	Conditional 6	3	
Sundt-Kees Slim-Line Aneurysm Clip *also known as Slimline Graft,* *4-mm Diameter, MP35N* *Codman, www.depuy.com*	Conditional 6	3	
Sundt-Kees Slim-Line Aneurysm Clip *also known as Slimline Reinforcing 30 Degree Angle,* *6-mm Wide, MP35N* *Codman, www.depuy.com*	Conditional 6	3	
Sundt-Kees Slim-Line Aneurysm Clip *also known as Slimline Reinforcing 60 Degree Angle,* *6-mm Wide, MP35N* *Codman, www.depuy.com*	Conditional 6	3	

Object	Status	Field Strength (T)	Reference
Sundt-Kees Slim-Line Aneurysm Clip *also known as Slimline Reinforcing Zero Degree Angle,* *6-mm Wide, MP35N* *Codman, www.depuy.com*	Conditional 6	3	
Sundt-Kees Slim-Line Aneurysm Clip *also known as Slimline Right Angle,MP35N* *Codman, www.depuy.com*	Conditional 6	3	
Sundt-Kees Slim-Line Aneurysm Clip *also known as Slimline Sharp Right Angle, MP35N* *Codman, www.depuy.com*	Conditional 6	3	
Sundt-Kees Slim-Line Aneurysm Clip *also known as Slimline Sideward Angle, MP35N* *Codman, www.depuy.com*	Conditional 6	3	
Sundt-Kees Slim-Line Aneurysm Clip *also known as Slimline Slightly curved, MP35N* *Codman, www.depuy.com*	Conditional 6	3	
Sundt-Kees Slim-Line Aneurysm Clip *also known as Slimline Straight, MP35N* *Codman, www.depuy.com*	Conditional 6	3	
Sundt-Kees Slim-Line Aneurysm Clip *also known as Slimline Super Bayonet, MP35N* *Codman, www.depuy.com*	Conditional 6	3	
Sundt-Kees Slim-Line *fenestrated, aneurysm clip, 9-mm blade, MP35N* *Codman, www.depuy.com*	Safe	1.5	
Sundt-Kees, Slim-Line *9-mm blade, MP35N, aneurysm clip* *Codman, www.depuy.com*	Safe	1.5	
Vari-Angle Aneurysm Clip *17-7PH* *Codman, www.depuy.com*	Unsafe 1	1.89	5
Vari-Angle McFadden Aneurysm Clip *MP35N* *Codman, www.depuy.com*	Safe	1.89	2
Vari-Angle Micro Aneurysm Clip *17-7PH* *Codman, www.depuy.com*	Unsafe 1	0.15	2
Vari-Angle Spring Aneurysm Clip *17-7PH* *Codman, www.depuy.com*	Unsafe 1	0.15	2
Yasargil Aneurysm Clip *All "FD" Models, per the manufacturer* *Aesculap, Inc., www.aesculapusa.com*	Unsafe 1	1.5	
Yasargil Aneurysm Clip *All "FE" Models per the manufacturer* *Aesculap, Inc., www.aesculapusa.com*	Safe	3	
Yasargil Aneurysm Clip *All "FT" Models, per the manufacturer* *Aesculap, Inc., www.aesculapusa.com*	Safe	3	
Yasargil Aneurysm Clip *316L SS* *Aesculap, Inc., www.aesculapusa.com*	Safe	1.89	5

Object	Status	Field Strength (T)	Reference
Yasargil Aneurysm Clip *Model FD* *Aesculap, Inc., www.aesculapusa.com*	Unsafe 1	1.5	
Yasargil Aneurysm Clip *Model FE 720T, mini, permanent, 7-mm blade, Titanium alloy* *Aesculap, Inc., www.aesculapusa.com*	Safe	1.5	
Yasargil Aneurysm Clip *Model FE 740T, standard, permanent, 7-mm blade, Titanium alloy* *Aesculap, Inc., www.aesculapusa.com*	Safe	1.5	
Yasargil Aneurysm Clip *Model FE 748, standard, 9-mm blade, bayonet, Phynox* *Aesculap, Inc., www.aesculapusa.com*	Safe	1.5	
Yasargil Aneurysm Clip *Model FE 750, 9-mm blade, straight, Phynox* *Aesculap, Inc., South Francisco, CA*	Safe	1.5	
Yasargil Aneurysm Clip *Model FE 750T, standard, permanent, 9-mm blade, Titanium alloy* *Aesculap, Inc., www.aesculapusa.com*	Safe	1.5	
Yasargil Aneurysm Clip *Model FE* *Aesculap, Inc., www.aesculapusa.com*	Safe	1.5	
Yasargil *Mini Clip, Titanium, Aneurysm Clip, Model FT728T* *bayonet, 7-mm blade, Titanium alloy* *Aesculap, Inc., www.aesculapusa.com*	Safe	1.5, 3	82
Yasargil Phynox Aneurysm Clip *Aneurysm Clip, All FE Models* *Aesculap, Inc., www.aesculapusa.com*	Safe	3	
Yasargil, Standard Aneurysm Clip Titanium *Model FT740T, straight, 7-mm blade, Titanium alloy* *Aesculap, Inc., www.aesculapusa.com*	Safe	1.5, 3	82
Yasargil, Standard Aneurysm Clip Titanium *Model FT758T, bayonet, 12-mm blade, Titanium alloy* *Aesculap, Inc., www.aesculapusa.com*	Safe	1.5, 3	82
Yasargil, Standard Aneurysm Clip Titanium *Model FT760T, 11-mm blade, Titanium alloy* *Aesculap, Inc., www.aesculapusa.com*	Safe	1.5, 3	82
Yasargil, Standard Aneurysm Clip Titanium *Model FT790T, straight, 20-mm blade, Titanium alloy* *Aesculap, Inc., www.aesculapusa.com*	Safe	1.5, 3	82
Yasargil, Standard Aneurysm Clip, Permanent *Model FE660K, straight, 12-mm blade, Phynox, SN FYA21* *Aesculap, Inc., www.aesculapusa.com*	Safe	3	
Yasargil, Standard Aneurysm Clip, Permanent *Model FE660K, straight, 12-mm blade, Phynox, SN FYA46* *Aesculap, Inc., www.aesculapusa.com*	Safe	3	
Yasargil, Standard Aneurysm Clip, Permanent *Model FE662K, angled, 10-mm blade, Phynox, SN FKJ41* *Aesculap, Inc., www.aesculapusa.com*	Safe	3	
Yasargil, Standard Aneurysm Clip, Permanent *Model FE662K, angled, 10-mm blade, Phynox, SN FUJ53* *Aesculap, Inc., www.aesculapusa.com*	Safe	3	

Object	Status	Field Strength (T)	Reference
Yasargil, Standard Aneurysm Clip, Permanent *Model FE840K, straight, 25-mm blade, Phynox, SN FYR65* *Aesculap, Inc., www.aesculapusa.com*	Safe	3	
Yasargil, Standard Aneurysm Clip, Permanent *Model FE840K, straight, 25-mm blade, Phynox, SN FYS01* *Aesculap, Inc., www.aesculapusa.com*	Safe	3	
Yasargil, Standard Aneurysm Clip, Permanent *Model FT650T, straight, 9-mm blade, Titanium alloy, SN CQY63* *Aesculap, Inc., www.aesculapusa.com*	Safe	3	
Yasargil, Standard Aneurysm Clip, Permanent *Model FT650T, straight, 9-mm blade, Titanium alloy, SN CQY83* *Aesculap, Inc., www.aesculapusa.com*	Safe	3	
Yasargil, Standard Aneurysm Clip, Permanent *Model FT662T, angled, 10-mm blade, Titanium alloy, SN CLU37* *Aesculap, Inc., www.aesculapusa.com*	Safe	3	
Yasargil, Standard Aneurysm Clip, Permanent *Model FT662T, angled, 10-mm blade, Titanium alloy, SN CLU54* *Aesculap, Inc., www.aesculapusa.com*	Safe	3	
Yasargil, Standard Aneurysm Clip, Permanent *Model FTD790D, straight, 20-mm blade, Titanium alloy,* *SN CTW58* *Aesculap, Inc., www.aesculapusa.com*	Safe	3	
Yasargil, Standard Aneurysm Clip, Permanent *Model FTD790D, straight, 20-mm blade, Titanium alloy,* *SN CTW73* *Aesculap, Inc., www.aesculapusa.com*	Safe	3	
Yasargil, Standard Aneurysm Clip *Model FE750, straight, 9-mm blade, Phynox* *Aesculap, Inc., www.aesculapusa.com*	Safe	1.5, 3	82
Yasargil, Standard Aneurysm Clip *Model FE780, straight, 14-mm blade, Phynox* *Aesculap, Inc., www.aesculapusa.com*	Safe	1.5, 3	82
Yasargil, Standard Aneurysm Clip *Model FE786, curved, 15.3-mm blade, Phynox* *Aesculap, Inc., www.aesculapusa.com*	Safe	1.5, 3	82
Yasargil, Standard Aneurysm Clip *Model FE790K, straight, 20-mm blade, Phynox* *Aesculap, Inc., www.aesculapusa.com*	Safe	1.5, 3	82
Yasargil, Standard Aneurysm Clip *Model FE798, bayonet, 20-mm blade, Phynox* *Aesculap, Inc., www.aesculapusa.com*	Safe	1.5, 3	82
Yasargil, Standard Aneurysm Clip *Model FE798, bayonet, 20-mm blade, Phynox* *Aesculap, Inc., www.aesculapusa.com*	Safe	1.5, 3	82
Yasargil, Standard Aneurysm Clip *Model FE887, 7-mm blade, Phynox* *Aesculap, Inc., www.aesculapusa.com*	Safe	1.5, 3	82
Yasargil Clip Standard Permanent *aneurysm clip, Phynox, 25-mm straight blade* *Peter Lazic Mikrochirurgische, www.lazic.de*	Conditional 6	3	

Object	Status	Field Strength (T)	Reference
Yasargil Clip Standard Permanent *aneurysm clip, Phynox, 90 degree Angle, 5-mm, 7-mm, 10-mm* *Peter Lazic Mikrochirurgische, www.lazic.de*	Conditional 6	3	
Yasargil Clip Standard Permanent *aneurysm clip, Phynox, Angle with Radius, 8-mm, 10-mm* *Peter Lazic Mikrochirurgische, www.lazic.de*	Conditional 6	3	
Yasargil Clip Standard Permanent *aneurysm clip, Phynox, Bayonet 45 degree Angle* *5-mm, 7-mm, 9-mm, 11-mm* *Peter Lazic Mikrochirurgische, www.lazic.de*	Conditional 6	3	
Yasargil Clip Standard Permanent *aneurysm clip, Phynox, Bayonet Angle,* *5-mm, 2.5-mm, 3.5-mm, 4.5-mm* *Peter Lazic Mikrochirurgische, www.lazic.de*	Conditional 6	3	
Yasargil Clip Standard Permanent *aneurysm clip, Phynox, Bayonet Angle, 5-mm* *Peter Lazic Mikrochirurgische, www.lazic.de*	Conditional 6	3	
Yasargil Clip Standard Permanent *aneurysm clip, Phynox, Bayonet,* *7-mm, 10-mm, 12-mm, 17-mm, 20-mm* *Peter Lazic Mikrochirurgische, www.lazic.de*	Conditional 6	3	
Yasargil Clip Standard Permanent *aneurysm clip, Phynox, Curved and Angle, 8-mm* *Peter Lazic Mikrochirurgische, www.lazic.de*	Conditional 6	3	
Yasargil Clip Standard Permanent *aneurysm clip, Phynox, Curved,* *7-mm, 9-mm, 11-mm, 15-mm, 17-mm* *Peter Lazic Mikrochirurgische, www.lazic.de*	Conditional 6	3	
Yasargil Clip Standard Permanent *aneurysm clip, Phynox, Fenestrated 3.5-mm 45 degree Angle* *5-mm, 7-mm, 11-mm* *Peter Lazic Mikrochirurgische, www.lazic.de*	Conditional 6	3	
Yasargil Clip Standard Permanent *aneurysm clip, Phynox, Fenestrated 3.5-mm 90 degree Angle* *5-mm, 7-mm, 11-mm* *Peter Lazic Mikrochirurgische, www.lazic.de*	Conditional 6	3	
Yasargil Clip Standard Permanent *aneurysm clip, Phynox, Fenestrated 3.5-mm Straight* *3-mm, 4-mm, 5-mm, 7-mm, 9-mm, 12-mm* *Peter Lazic Mikrochirurgische, www.lazic.de*	Conditional 6	3	
Yasargil Clip Standard Permanent *aneurysm clip, Phynox, Fenestrated 5-mm 45 degree Angle* *Opening Sideward Left, 5-mm, 7-mm* *Peter Lazic Mikrochirurgische, www.lazic.de*	Conditional 6	3	
Yasargil Clip Standard Permanent *aneurysm clip, Phynox, Fenestrated 5-mm 45 degree Angle* *Opening Sideward Right, 5-mm, 7-mm* *Peter Lazic Mikrochirurgische, www.lazic.de*	Conditional 6	3	
Yasargil Clip Standard Permanent *aneurysm clip, Phynox, Fenestrated 5-mm 45 degree Angle* *5-mm, 7-mm, 11-mm* *Peter Lazic Mikrochirurgische, www.lazic.de*	Conditional 6	3	

Object	Status	Field Strength (T)	Reference
Yasargil Clip Standard Permanent *aneurysm clip, Phynox, Fenestrated 5-mm 90 degree Angle Jaw Curved Left, 5-mm, 7-mm, 10-mm* *Peter Lazic Mikrochirurgische, www.lazic.de*	Conditional 6	3	
Yasargil Clip Standard Permanent *aneurysm clip, Phynox, Fenestrated 5-mm 90 degree Angle Jaw Curved Right, 5-mm, 7-mm, 10-mm* *Peter Lazic Mikrochirurgische, www.lazic.de*	Conditional 6	3	
Yasargil Clip Standard Permanent *aneurysm clip, Phynox, Fenestrated 5-mm 90 degree Angle Opening Sideward Left, 5-mm, 7-mm* *Peter Lazic Mikrochirurgische, www.lazic.de*	Conditional 6	3	
Yasargil Clip Standard Permanent *aneurysm clip, Phynox, Fenestrated 5-mm 90 degree Angle Opening Sideward Right, 5-mm, 7-mm* *Peter Lazic Mikrochirurgische, www.lazic.de*	Conditional 6	3	
Yasargil Clip Standard Permanent *aneurysm clip, Phynox, Fenestrated 5-mm 90 degree Angle 5-mm, 7-mm, 11-mm* *Peter Lazic Mikrochirurgische, www.lazic.de*	Conditional 6	3	
Yasargil Clip Standard Permanent *aneurysm clip, Phynox, Fenestrated 5-mm Bayonet 5-mm, 7-mm, 11-mm* *Peter Lazic Mikrochirurgische, www.lazic.de*	Conditional 6	3	
Yasargil Clip Standard Permanent *aneurysm clip, Phynox Fenestrated 5-mm Straight Opening Sideward Right 5-mm, 7-mm, 10-mm* *Peter Lazic Mikrochirurgische, www.lazic.de*	Conditional 6	3	
Yasargil Clip Standard Permanent *aneurysm clip, Phynox, Fenestrated 5-mm Straight 3-mm, 4-mm, 5-mm, 7-mm, 9-mm, 12-mm* *Peter Lazic Mikrochirurgische, www.lazic.de*	Conditional 6	3	
Yasargil Clip Standard Permanent *aneurysm clip, Phynox, J Curved, 7-mm, 9-mm, 11-mm* *Peter Lazic Mikrochirurgische, www.lazic.de*	Conditional 6	3	
Yasargil Clip Standard Permanent *aneurysm clip, Phynox, Mini Clip Angle and Curved, 5-mm* *Peter Lazic Mikrochirurgische, www.lazic.de*	Conditional 6	3	
Yasargil Clip Standard Permanent *aneurysm clip, Phynox, Mini Clip Angle, 7-mm* *Peter Lazic Mikrochirurgische, www.lazic.de*	Conditional 6	3	
Yasargil Clip Standard Permanent *aneurysm clip, Phynox, Mini Clip Bayonet, 4-mm, 7-mm* *Peter Lazic Mikrochirurgische, www.lazic.de*	Conditional 6	3	
Yasargil Clip Standard Permanent *aneurysm clip, Phynox, Mini Clip Curved Narrow Jaw, 4-mm* *Peter Lazic Mikrochirurgische, www.lazic.de*	Conditional 6	3	
Yasargil Clip Standard Permanent *aneurysm clip, Phynox, Mini Clip Curved, 4-mm, 5-mm* *Peter Lazic Mikrochirurgische, www.lazic.de*	Conditional 6	3	

Object	Status	Field Strength (T)	Reference
Yasargil Clip Standard Permanent *aneurysm clip, Phynox, Mini Clip Sideward Angle, 5-mm* *Peter Lazic Mikrochirurgische, www.lazic.de*	Conditional 6	3	
Yasargil Clip Standard Permanent *aneurysm clip, Phynox, Mini Clip Sideward Curved, 6-mm* *Peter Lazic Mikrochirurgische, www.lazic.de*	Conditional 6	3	
Yasargil Clip Standard Permanent *aneurysm clip, Phynox, Mini Clip Slightly Curved Narrow Jaw* *3-mm, 4-mm* *Peter Lazic Mikrochirurgische, www.lazic.de*	Conditional 6	3	
Yasargil Clip Standard Permanent *aneurysm clip, Phynox, Mini Clip Slightly Curved,* *4-mm, 5-mm, 7-mm* *Peter Lazic Mikrochirurgische, www.lazic.de*	Conditional 6	3	
Yasargil Clip Standard Permanent *aneurysm clip, Phynox, Mini Clip Straight Narrow Jaw* *3-mm, 5-mm* *Peter Lazic Mikrochirurgische, www.lazic.de*	Conditional 6	3	
Yasargil Clip Standard Permanent *aneurysm clip, Phynox, Mini Clip Straight, 3-mm, 5-mm, 7-mm* *Peter Lazic Mikrochirurgische, www.lazic.de*	Conditional 6	3	
Yasargil Clip Standard Permanent *aneurysm clip, Phynox, Sideward Angle, 7-mm, 11-mm* *Peter Lazic Mikrochirurgische, www.lazic.de*	Conditional 6	3	
Yasargil Clip Standard Permanent *aneurysm clip, Phynox, Sideward Curved, 9-mm* *Peter Lazic Mikrochirurgische, www.lazic.de*	Conditional 6	3	
Yasargil Clip Standard Permanent *aneurysm clip, Phynox, Slightly Curved* *7-mm, 9-mm, 11-mm, 15-mm, 17-mm, 20-mm* *Peter Lazic Mikrochirurgische, www.lazic.de*	Conditional 6	3	
Yasargil Clip Standard Permanent *aneurysm clip, Phynox, Straight with Radius, 9-mm, 10-mm* *Peter Lazic Mikrochirurgische, www.lazic.de*	Conditional 6	3	
Yasargil Clip Standard Permanent *aneurysm clip, Phynox, Straight* *7-mm, 8-mm, 11-mm, 15-mm, 17-mm, 20-mm, 25-mm* *Peter Lazic Mikrochirurgische, www.lazic.de*	Conditional 6	3	
Yasargil Clip Standard Permanent *aneurysm clip, Phynox, Tangential Angle, 13-mm* *Peter Lazic Mikrochirurgische, www.lazic.de*	Conditional 6	3	
Yasargil *T-Bar Aneurysm Clip, Permanent, Model FE853K* *45 degree angle, 9-mm blade, Phynox* *Aesculap, Inc., www.aesculapusa.com*	Safe	3	
Yasargil *T-Bar Aneurysm Clip, Permanent, Model FE856K* *90 degree angle, 13-mm blade, Phynox* *Aesculap, Inc., www.aesculapusa.com*	Safe	3	
Yasargil *T-Bar Aneurysm Clip, Permanent, Model FT853T* *45 degree angle, 9-mm blade, Titanium* *Aesculap, Inc., www.aesculapusa.com*	Safe	3	

Object	Status	Field Strength (T)	Reference
Yasargil *T-Bar Aneurysm Clip, Permanent, Model FT856T* *90 degree angle, 13-mm blade, Titanium* *Aesculap, Inc., www.aesculapusa.com*	Safe	3	
Yasargil Titanclip *Standard Permanent, aneurysm clip, Titanium* *25-mm straight blade* *Peter Lazic Mikrochirurgische, www.lazic.de*	Conditional 6	3	
Yasargil Titanclip *Standard Permanent, aneurysm clip, Titanium* *45 degree Angle, 5-mm, 7-mm, 9-mm, 11-mm* *Peter Lazic Mikrochirurgische, www.lazic.de*	Conditional 6	3	
Yasargil Titanclip *Standard Permanent, aneurysm clip, Titanium* *90 degree Angle, 5-mm, 7-mm, 10-mm* *Peter Lazic Mikrochirurgische, www.lazic.de*	Conditional 6	3	
Yasargil Titanclip *Standard Permanent, aneurysm clip, Titanium* *Angle with Radius, 8-mm, 10-mm* *Peter Lazic Mikrochirurgische, www.lazic.de*	Conditional 6	3	
Yasargil Titanclip *Standard Permanent, aneurysm clip, Titanium* *Bayonet Angle, 2.5-mm, 3.5-mm, 4.5-mm* *Peter Lazic Mikrochirurgische, www.lazic.de*	Conditional 6	3	
Yasargil Titanclip *Standard Permanent, aneurysm clip, Titanium* *Bayonet Angle, 5-mm* *Peter Lazic Mikrochirurgische, www.lazic.de*	Conditional 6	3	
Yasargil Titanclip *Standard Permanent, aneurysm clip, Titanium* *Bayonet, 7-mm, 10-mm, 12-mm, 17-mm, 20-mm* *Peter Lazic Mikrochirurgische, www.lazic.de*	Conditional 6	3	
Yasargil Titanclip *Standard Permanent, aneurysm clip, Titanium* *Curved and Sideward Angle, 8-mm* *Peter Lazic Mikrochirurgische, www.lazic.de*	Conditional 6	3	
Yasargil Titanclip *Standard Permanent, aneurysm clip, Titanium* *Curved, 7-mm, 9-mm, 11-mm, 15-mm, 17-mm* *Peter Lazic Mikrochirurgische, www.lazic.de*	Conditional 6	3	
Yasargil Titanclip *Standard Permanent, aneurysm clip, Titanium* *Fenestrated 3.5-mm 45 degree Angle* *5-mm, 7-mm, 11-mm* *Peter Lazic Mikrochirurgische, www.lazic.de*	Conditional 6	3	
Yasargil Titanclip *Standard Permanent, aneurysm clip, Titanium* *Fenestrated 3.5-mm 90 degree Angle, 5-mm, 7-mm, 11-mm* *Peter Lazic Mikrochirurgische, www.lazic.de*	Conditional 6	3	

Object	Status	Field Strength (T)	Reference
Yasargil Titanclip *Standard Permanent, aneurysm clip, Titanium* *Fenestrated 3.5-mm Straight* *3-mm, 4-mm, 5-mm, 7-mm, 9-mm, 12-mm* *Peter Lazic Mikrochirurgische, www.lazic.de*	Conditional 6	3	
Yasargil Titanclip *Standard Permanent, aneurysm clip, Titanium* *Fenestrated 45 degree Opening Sideward Left, 5-mm, 7-mm* *Peter Lazic Mikrochirurgische, www.lazic.de*	Conditional 6	3	
Yasargil Titanclip *Standard Permanent, aneurysm clip, Titanium* *Fenestrated 45 degree Opening Sideward Right, 5-mm, 7-mm* *Peter Lazic Mikrochirurgische, www.lazic.de*	Conditional 6	3	
Yasargil Titanclip *Standard Permanent, aneurysm clip, Titanium* *Fenestrated 5-mm 45 degree Angle, 5-mm, 7-mm, 11-mm* *Peter Lazic Mikrochirurgische, www.lazic.de*	Conditional 6	3	
Yasargil Titanclip *Standard Permanent, aneurysm clip, Titanium* *Fenestrated 5-mm 90 degree Angle Jaw Curved Left* *5-mm, 7-mm, 10-mm* *Peter Lazic Mikrochirurgische, www.lazic.de*	Conditional 6	3	
Yasargil Titanclip *Standard Permanent, aneurysm clip, Titanium* *Fenestrated 5-mm 90 degree Angle Jaw Curved Right* *5-mm, 7-mm, 10-mm* *Peter Lazic Mikrochirurgische, www.lazic.de*	Conditional 6	3	
Yasargil Titanclip *Standard Permanent, aneurysm clip, Titanium* *Fenestrated 5-mm 90 degree Angle, 5-mm, 7-mm, 11-mm* *Peter Lazic Mikrochirurgische, www.lazic.de*	Conditional 6	3	
Yasargil Titanclip *Standard Permanent, aneurysm clip, Titanium* *Fenestrated 5-mm Bayonet, 5-mm, 7-mm, 11-mm* *Peter Lazic Mikrochirurgische, www.lazic.de*	Conditional 6	3	
Yasargil Titanclip *Standard Permanent, aneurysm clip, Titanium* *Fenestrated 5-mm Straight Opening Sideward Right,* *5-mm, 7-mm, 10-mm* *Peter Lazic Mikrochirurgische, www.lazic.de*	Conditional 6	3	
Yasargil Titanclip *Standard Permanent, aneurysm clip, Titanium* *Fenestrated 5-mm Straight* *3-mm, 4-mm, 5-mm, 7-mm, 9-mm, 12-mm* *Peter Lazic Mikrochirurgische, www.lazic.de*	Conditional 6	3	
Yasargil Titanclip *Standard Permanent, aneurysm clip, Titanium* *Fenestrated 90 degree Opening Sideward Left, 5-mm, 7-mm* *Peter Lazic Mikrochirurgische, www.lazic.de*	Conditional 6	3	
Yasargil Titanclip *Standard Permanent, aneurysm clip, Titanium* *Fenestrated 90 degree Opening Sideward Right, 5-mm, 7-mm* *Peter Lazic Mikrochirurgische, www.lazic.de*	Conditional 6	3	

Object	Status	Field Strength (T)	Reference
Yasargil Titanclip *Standard Permanent, aneurysm clip, Titanium* *J Curved, 7-mm, 9-mm, 11-mm* *Peter Lazic Mikrochirurgische, www.lazic.de*	Conditional 6	3	
Yasargil Titanclip *Standard Permanent, aneurysm clip, Titanium* *Mini Clip Angle and Curved, 5-mm* *Peter Lazic Mikrochirurgische, www.lazic.de*	Conditional 6	3	
Yasargil Titanclip *Standard Permanent, aneurysm clip, Titanium* *Mini Clip Angle, 7-mm* *Peter Lazic Mikrochirurgische, www.lazic.de*	Conditional 6	3	
Yasargil Titanclip *Standard Permanent, aneurysm clip, Titanium* *Mini Clip Bayonet, 4-mm, 7-mm* *Peter Lazic Mikrochirurgische, www.lazic.de*	Conditional 6	3	
Yasargil Titanclip *Standard Permanent, aneurysm clip, Titanium* *Mini Clip Curved Narrow Jaw, 4-mm* *Peter Lazic Mikrochirurgische, www.lazic.de*	Conditional 6	3	
Yasargil Titanclip *Standard Permanent, aneurysm clip, Titanium* *Mini Clip Curved, 4-mm, 5-mm* *Peter Lazic Mikrochirurgische, www.lazic.de*	Conditional 6	3	
Yasargil Titanclip *Standard Permanent, aneurysm clip, Titanium* *Mini Clip Sideward Angle, 5-mm* *Peter Lazic Mikrochirurgische, www.lazic.de*	Conditional 6	3	
Yasargil Titanclip *Standard Permanent, aneurysm clip, Titanium* *Mini Clip Sideward Curved, 6-mm* *Peter Lazic Mikrochirurgische, www.lazic.de*	Conditional 6	3	
Yasargil Titanclip *Standard Permanent, aneurysm clip, Titanium* *Mini Clip Slightly Curved Narrow Jaw, 3-mm, 4-mm* *Peter Lazic Mikrochirurgische, www.lazic.de*	Conditional 6	3	
Yasargil Titanclip *Standard Permanent, aneurysm clip, Titanium* *Mini Clip Slightly Curved, 4-mm, 5-mm, 7-mm* *Peter Lazic Mikrochirurgische, www.lazic.de*	Conditional 6	3	
Yasargil Titanclip *Standard Permanent, aneurysm clip, Titanium* *Mini Clip Straight Narrow Jaw, 3-mm, 5-mm* *Peter Lazic Mikrochirurgische, www.lazic.de*	Conditional 6	3	
Yasargil Titanclip *Standard Permanent, aneurysm clip, Titanium* *Mini Clip Straight, 3-mm, 5-mm, 7-mm* *Peter Lazic Mikrochirurgische, www.lazic.de*	Conditional 6	3	
Yasargil Titanclip *Standard Permanent, aneurysm clip, Titanium* *Sideward Angle, 7-mm, 11-mm* *Peter Lazic Mikrochirurgische, www.lazic.de*	Conditional 6	3	

Object	Status	Field Strength (T)	Reference
Yasargil Titanclip *Standard Permanent, aneurysm clip, Titanium* *Sideward Curved, 9-mm* *Peter Lazic Mikrochirurgische, www.lazic.de*	Conditional 6	3	
Yasargil Titanclip *Standard Permanent, aneurysm clip, Titanium, Slightly Curved* *7-mm, 9-mm, 11-mm, 15-mm, 17-mm, 20-mm* *Peter Lazic Mikrochirurgische, www.lazic.de*	Conditional 6	3	
Yasargil Titanclip *Standard Permanent, aneurysm clip, Titanium* *Straight with Radius, 9-mm, 11-mm* *Peter Lazic Mikrochirurgische, www.lazic.de*	Conditional 6	3	
Yasargil Titanclip *Standard Permanent, aneurysm clip, Titanium, Straight* *7-mm, 9-mm, 11-mm, 15-mm, 17-mm, 20-mm, 25-mm* *Peter Lazic Mikrochirurgische, www.lazic.de*	Conditional 6	3	
Yasargil Titanclip *Standard Permanent, aneurysm clip, Titanium,* *Tangential Angle, 13-mm* *Peter Lazic Mikrochirurgische, www.lazic.de*	Conditional 6	3	
Yasargil Titanium Aneurysm Clips *All FT Models* *Aesculap, Inc., www.aesculapusa.com*	Safe	3	

Object	Status	Field Strength (T)	Reference

Biopsy Needles, Markers, and Devices

Object	Status	Field Strength (T)	Reference
Adjustable, Automated Aspiration Biopsy Gun *10, 15, and 20-mm, 304 SS, MD Tech* *Watertown, MA*	Unsafe 1	1.5	7
Adjustable, Automated Biopsy Gun *6, 13, and 19-mm, 304 SS, MD Tech* *Watertown, MA*	Unsafe 1	1.5	7
AOS Marker Seed *Alpha-Omega Services, Inc.* *Bellflower, CA*	Conditional 6	3	
ASAP 16, Automatic 16 G Core Biopsy System *19-cm length, 304 SS*	Unsafe 1	1.5	7
AspirationNeedle MRI *MRI Devices Corporation, Waukesha, WI*	Safe	1.5	
ATEK TriMark, Biopsy Marker *Hologic, www.hologic.com*	Conditional 5	3	
Automatic Cutting Needle with Depth Markings *14 G, 10-cm length, 304 SS, biopsy needle* *Manan, Northbrook, IL*	Unsafe 1	1.5	7
Automatic Cutting Needle with Ultrasound Tip *& Depth Markings 18 G, 16-cm length, 304 SS, biopsy needle* *Manan, Northbrook, IL*	Unsafe 1	1.5	7
Automatic Cutting Needle with Ultrasound Tip & Depth Markings *18 G, 20-cm length, 304 SS, biopsy needle* *Manan, Northbrook, IL*	Unsafe 1	1.5	7
Basic II Hookwire Breast Localization Needle *304 SS* *MD Tech, Watertown, MA*	Unsafe 1	1.5	7
Beaded Breast Localization Wire Set *19 G, 3-1/2 inch needle with 7-7/8 inch wire, 304 SS* *Inrad, Grand Rapids, MI*	Unsafe 1	1.5	7
Beaded Breast Localization Wire Set *20 G, 2 inch needle with 5-7/8 inch wire, 304 SS* *Inrad, Grand Rapids, MI*	Unsafe 1	1.5	7
Biopsy Gun *13-mm, biopsy needle* *Meadox, Oakland, NJ*	Unsafe 1	1.5	7
Biopsy Gun *25-mm, biopsy needle* *Meadox, Oakland, NJ*	Unsafe 1	1.5	7
Biopsy Needle *17 G, 10-cm length* *Meadox, Oakland, NJ*	Unsafe 1	1.5	7
Biopsy Needle *20 G, 15-cm length* *Meadox, Oakland, NJ*	Unsafe 1	1.5	7
Biopsy Needle *22 G, 15-cm length* *Cook Medical, Inc., www.cookmedical.com*	Unsafe 1	1.5	7

Object	Status	Field Strength (T)	Reference
Biopsy Needle *22 G, 15-cm length* *Meadox, Oakland, NJ*	Unsafe 1	1.5	7
Biopty-Cut Biopsy Needle *14 G, 10-cm length, 304 SS* *C.R. Bard, Inc., Covington, GA*	Unsafe 1	1.5	7
Biopty-Cut Biopsy Needle *16 G, 16-cm length, 304 SS* *C.R. Bard, Inc., Covington, GA*	Unsafe 1	1.5	7
Biopty-Cut Biopsy Needle *18 G, 18-cm length, 304 SS* *C.R. Bard, Inc., Covington, GA*	Unsafe 1	1.5	7
Biopty-Cut Biopsy Needle *18 G, 20-cm length, 304 SS* *C.R. Bard, Inc., Covington, GA*	Unsafe 1	1.5	7
BoneBiopsy Set MRI *manual version, includes trocar, stylet, drill and ejector* *MRI Devices Corporation, Waukesha, WI*	Safe	1.5	
Breast Localization Needle *20 G, 5-cm length, 304 SS* *Manan, Northbrook, IL*	Unsafe 1	1.5	7
Breast Localization Needle *20 G, 7-cm length, 304 SS* *Manan, Northbrook, IL*	Unsafe 1	1.5	7
Chiba Needle and HiLiter *Ultrasound Enhancement, 22 G, 3-7/8 inch biopsy needle, 304 SS* *Inrad, Grand Rapids, MI*	Unsafe 1	1.5	7
Coaxial Needle Set Chiba-type *22 G, 5-7/8 inch biopsy needle, 304 SS* *Inrad, Grand Rapids, MI*	Unsafe 1	1.5	7
Coaxial Needle Set Introducer *19G, 2-15/16 inch biopsy needle, 304 SS* *Inrad, Grand Rapids, MI*	Unsafe 1	1.5	7
CoaxNeedle MRI *MRI Devices Corporation, Waukesha, WI*	Safe	1.5	
CorMark *Tissue Marker, 14 gauge* *Ethicon Endosurgery, Cincinnati, OH*	Safe	3	
Cutting Needle & Gun *18 G, 155-mm length, biopsy needle* *Meadox, Oakland, NJ*	Unsafe 1	1.5	7
Cutting Needle *14 G, 9-cm length, biopsy needle* *West Coast Medical, Laguna Beach, CA*	Unsafe 1	1.5	7
Cutting Needle *16 G, 17-mm length, 304 SS, biopsy needle* *BIP USA, Inc., Niagara Falls, NY*	Unsafe 1	1.5	7
Cutting Needle *16 G, 19-mm length, 304 SS, biopsy needle* *BIP USA, Inc., Niagara Falls, NY*	Unsafe 1	1.5	7

Object	Status	Field Strength (T)	Reference
Cutting Needle *18 G, 100-mm length, biopsy needle* *Meadox, Oakland, NJ*	Unsafe 1	1.5	7
Cutting Needle *18 G, 15-cm length, biopsy needle* *West Coast Medical, Laguna Beach, CA*	Unsafe 1	1.5	7
Cutting Needle *18 G, 150-mm length, biopsy needle* *Meadox, Oakland, NJ*	Unsafe 1	1.5	7
Cutting Needle *18 G, 9-cm length, biopsy needle* *West Coast Medical, Laguna Beach, CA*	Unsafe 1	1.5	7
Cutting Needle *19 G, 15-cm length, biopsy needle* *West Coast Medical, Laguna Beach, CA*	Unsafe 1	1.5	7
Cutting Needle *19 G, 6-cm length, biopsy needle* *West Coast Medical, Laguna Beach, CA*	Unsafe 1	1.5	7
Cutting Needle *19 G, 9-cm length, biopsy needle* *West Coast Medical, Laguna Beach, CA*	Unsafe 1	1.5	7
Cutting Needle *20 G, 15-cm length, biopsy needle* *West Coast Medical, Laguna Beach, CA*	Unsafe 1	1.5	7
Cutting Needle *20 G, 20-cm length, biopsy needle* *West Coast Medical, Laguna Beach, CA*	Unsafe 1	1.5	7
Cutting Needle *20 G, 9-cm length, biopsy needle* *West Coast Medical, Laguna Beach, CA*	Unsafe 1	1.5	7
Echotip Ultra Fiducial Marker *Cook Medical, www.cookmedical.com*	Conditional 6	3	
Fully Automatic BiopsyGun MRI *MRI Devices Corporation, Waukesha, WI*	Safe	1.5	
Hawkins Blunt Needle *304 SS, biopsy needle,* *MD Tech, Watertown, MA*	Unsafe 1	1.5	7
Hawkins III Breast Localization Needle *MD Tech, Watertown, MA*	Unsafe 1	1.5	7
HydroMark Breast Biopsy Site Marker *Stainless Steel and Titanium,* *Biopsy Sciences, Tucson, AZ*	Conditional 6	3	
KMD-Mark1 *marker* *Kent Medical Devices, Inc., Minneapolis, MN*	Conditional 6	3	
LeLoc MRI *Tumor Localizer* *MRI Devices Corporation, Waukesha, WI*	Safe	1.5	
Lufkin Aspiration Cytology Needle *20 G, 5-cm length, biopsy needle, high nickel alloy* *E-Z-Em, Inc., Westbury, NY*	Safe	1.5	9

Object	Status	Field Strength (T)	Reference
Lufkin Biopsy Needle *18 G, 15-cm length, high nickel alloy* *E-Z-Em, Inc., Westbury, NY*	Safe	1.5	8
Lufkin Biopsy Needle *18 G, 5-cm length, high nickel alloy* *E-Z-Em, Inc., Westbury, NY*	Safe	1.5	8
Lufkin Biopsy Needle *22 G, 10-cm length, high nickel alloy* *E-Z-Em, Inc., Westbury, NY*	Safe	1.5	8
Lufkin Biopsy Needle *22 G, 15-cm length, high nickel alloy* *E-Z-Em, Inc., Westbury, NY*	Safe	1.5	8
Lufkin Biopsy Needle *22 G, 5-cm length, high nickel alloy* *E-Z-Em, Inc., Westbury, NY*	Safe	1.5	8
MammoMark *Tissue Marker, 8 gauge* *Ethicon Endosurgery, Cincinnati, OH*	Safe	3	
MammoMark *Tissue Marker Deployment Device, 8 gauge* *Ethicon Endosurgery, Cincinnati, OH*	Safe	3	
MammoMark *Tissue Marker, 11 gauge* *Ethicon Endosurgery, Cincinnati, OH*	Safe	3	
MammoMark *Tissue Marker Deployment Device, 11 gauge* *Ethicon Endosurgery, Cincinnati, OH*	Safe	3	
MammoMark II *Tissue Marker, 11 gauge* *Ethicon Endosurgery, Cincinnati, OH*	Safe	3	
MammoMark II *Tissue Marker Deployment Device, 11 gauge* *Ethicon Endosurgery, Cincinnati, OH*	Safe	3	
Micromark Clip, marking clip *316L SS,* *Biopsys Medical, Irvine, CA*	Safe	1.5	61
MicroMark II Clip *316L SS* *Ethicon Endosurgery, Cincinnati, OHio*	Safe	1.5, 3	
MReye Chiba Biopsy Needle *William Cook Europe A/S, Bjaeverskov, Denmark*	Safe	1.5	
MReye Franseen Lung Biopsy Needle *William Cook Europe A/S, Bjaeverskov, Denmark*	Safe	1.5	
MReye Interventional Needle *biopsy needle* *William Cook Europe A/S, Bjaeverskov, Denmark*	Safe	1.5	
MReye Kopans Breast Lesion *Localization Needles, (21, 20, 19 gauges; 5.0, 9.0, 15.0 lengths)* *William Cook Europe A/S, Bjaeverskov, Denmark*	Safe	1.5	
MR Ghiatas Beaded *Breast Localization Wire Set, needle and wire* *Inrad Inc., Kentwood, MI*	Conditional 6	3	

Object	Status	Field Strength (T)	Reference
MR Ghiatas *Breast Localization Wire Sets, Inconel Alloy* *C. R. Bard, Inc., Murray Hill, NJ*	Conditional 6	3	
MRI BioGun *18 G, 10-cm length, high nickel alloy, biopsy needle* *E-Z-Em, Inc., Westbury, NY*	Safe	1.5	8
MRI BiopsyKit *MRI Devices Corporation, Waukesha, WI*	Safe	1.5	
MRI Histology Needle *18 G, 15-cm length, high nickel alloy, biopsy needle* *E-Z-Em, Inc., Westbury, NY*	Safe	1.5	7
MRI Histology Needle *18 G, 5-cm length, high nickel alloy, biopsy needle* *E-Z-Em, Inc., Westbury, NY*	Safe	1.5	8
MRI Histology Needle *20 G, 10-cm length, high nickel alloy, biopsy needle* *E-Z-Em, Inc., Westbury, NY*	Safe	1.5	8
MRI Histology Needle *20 G, 15-cm length, high nickel alloy, biopsy needle* *E-Z-Em, Inc., Westbury, NY*	Safe	1.5	8
MRI Histology Needle *20 G, 5-cm length, high nickel alloy, biopsy needle* *E-Z-Em, Inc., Westbury, NY*	Safe	1.5	7
MRI Histology Needle *20 G, 7.5-cm length, high nickel alloy, biopsy needle* *E-Z-Em, Inc., Westbury, NY*	Safe	1.5	8
MRI Lesion Marking System *20 G, 7.5-cm length, high nickel alloy* *E-Z-Em, Inc., Westbury, NY*	Safe	1.5	8
MRI Needle, 20-gauge, 9-cm *QSUM Biopsy Disposables LLC, www.qsum.net*	Conditional 7	3	
MRI Needle, surgical grade SS *biopsy needle* *Cook Medical, Inc., www.cookmedical.com*	Safe	1.5	7
mrt Biopsy Needle *all sizes, Titanium alloy* *Daum Medical, Baltimore, MD and Schwerin, Germany*	Safe	1.5	
NeuroCut Needle MRI *MRI Devices Corporation, Waukesha, WI*	Safe	1.5	
NeuroGate Set MRI *MRI Devices Corporation, Waukesha, WI*	Safe	1.5	
NeuroPunctureNeedle MRI *MRI Devices Corporation, Waukesha, WI*	Safe	1.5	
Percucut Biopsy Needle and Stylet *19.5 gauge x 10-cm, 316L SS* *E-Z-Em, Inc., Westbury, NY*	Unsafe 1	1.5	7
Percucut Biopsy Needle and Stylet *21 gauge x 10-cm, 316L SS* *E-Z-Em, Inc., Westbury, NY*	Unsafe 1	1.5	7
PunctureNeedle MRI *MRI Devices Corporation, Waukesha, WI*	Safe	1.5	

Object	Status	Field Strength (T)	Reference
Sadowsky Breast Marking System *20 G, 5-cm length needle and 7 inch hook wire, 316L SS* *Ranfac Corporation, Avon, MA*	Unsafe 1	1.5	7
SecureMark, Biopsy Marker *Hologic, www.hologic.com*	Conditional 5	3	
Semi-Automatic BiopsyGun MRI *MRI Devices Corporation, Waukesha, WI*	Safe	1.5	
SenoMark UltraCor MRI *SS, M shaped breast biopsy marker, clip* *SenoRx, Aliso Viejo, CA*	Conditional 6	3	
SenoMark UltraCor MRI *Titanium, X shaped breast biopsy marker, clip* *SenoRx, Aliso Viejo, CA*	Conditional 6	3	
Single Loop Titanium Marker *Tissue Marker, Titanium alloy* *RUBICOR Medical Inc., Redwood City, CA*	Conditional 6	3	
SmartGuide CT/MRI *MRI Devices Corporation, Waukesha, WI*	Safe	1.5	
Soft Tissue Biopsy Needle Gun & biopsy needle *304 SS* *Anchor Products Co., Addison, IL*	Unsafe 1	1.5	7
Spirotome Single Use 10 Standard *receiving needle, plastic trocar, Inox trocar, cutting cannula* *biopsy device* *MEDINVENTS, Belgium*	Conditional 5	3	
Surgical Mesh with X-Ray Marker *NuVasive, Inc., San Diego, CA*	Conditional 6	3	
TargoGrid *positioning grid for biopsies and punctures* *MRI Devices Corporation, Waukesha, WI*	Safe	1.5	
Trocar Needle *304 SS, biopsy needle* *BIP USA, Inc., Niagara Falls, NY*	Unsafe 1	1.5	7
Trocar Needle, Disposable *SS, biopsy needle* *Cook Medical, Inc., www.cookmedical.com*	Unsafe 1	1.5	7
TumoLoc MRI *Tumor Localizer* *MRI Devices Corporation, Waukesha, WI*	Safe	1.5	
UltraClip II *MR Tissue Marker Device, tissue marker* *Inrad Inc., Kentwood, MI*	Conditional 6	3	
UltraClip II *MR Tissue Marker Device, Titanium Alloy* *C. R. Bard, Inc., Murray Hill, NJ*	Conditional 6	3	
UltraClip II *Tissue Markers, Clips Only, Titanium Alloy, PVA, Inconel Alloy,* *BioDur Alloy* *C. R. Bard, Inc., Murray Hill, NJ*	Conditional 6	3	
Ultra-Core, biopsy needle *16 G, 16-cm length, 304 SS*	Unsafe 1	1.5	7

Object	Status	Field Strength (T)	Reference

Breast Tissue Expanders and Implants

Object	Status	Field Strength (T)	Reference
Becker Expander/Mammary Mentor H/S *Prosthesis, 316L SS, breast implant* *Santa Barbara, CA*	Safe	1.5	10
Breast Tissue Expander *Style 133 FV with MAGNA-SITE Injection Site, magnetic port* *McGhan Medical/INAMED Aesthetics, Santa Barbara, CA*	Unsafe 1	1.5	86
Breast Tissue Expander *Style 133 LV with MAGNA-SITE Injection Site, magnetic port* *McGhan Medical/INAMED Aesthetics, Santa Barbara, CA*	Unsafe 1	1.5	86
Breast Tissue Expander *Style 133 MV with MAGNA-SITE Injection Site, magnetic port* *McGhan Medical/INAMED Aesthetics, Santa Barbara, CA*	Unsafe 1	1.5	86
Breast Tissue Expander *STYLE 133V (133 V) Series, MAGNA-SITE Injection Site* *Allergan, Inc., www.allergan.com*	Unsafe 1	1.5	
Breast Tissue Expander *STYLE 133 FV, MAGNA-SITE Injection Site* *Allergan, Inc., www.allergan.com*	Unsafe 1	1.5	
Breast Tissue Expander *STYLE 133 FX, MAGNA-SITE Injection Site* *Allergan, Inc., www.allergan.com*	Unsafe 1	1.5	
Breast Tissue Expander *STYLE 133 LV, MAGNA-SITE Injection Site* *Allergan, Inc., www.allergan.com*	Unsafe 1	1.5	
Breast Tissue Expander *STYLE 133 MV, MAGNA-SITE Injection Site* *Allergan, Inc., www.allergan.com*	Unsafe 1	1.5	
Breast Tissue Expander *STYLE 133 MX, MAGNA-SITE Injection Site* *Allergan, Inc., www.allergan.com*	Unsafe 1	1.5	
Breast Tissue Expander *STYLE 133 SV, MAGNA-SITE Injection Site* *Allergan, Inc., www.allergan.com*	Unsafe 1	1.5	
Breast Tissue Expander *STYLE 133 SX, MAGNA-SITE Injection Site* *Allergan, Inc., www.allergan.com*	Unsafe 1	1.5	
CONTOUR PROFILE Tissue Expander *Mentor, www.mentorwwllc.com*	Unsafe 1	1.5	
CPX2 Tissue Expander *Mentor, www.mentorwwllc.com*	Unsafe 1	1.5	
CPX3 Tissue Expander *Mentor, www.mentorwwllc.com*	Unsafe 1	1.5	
Double Chamber Breast Tissue Expander *Model 20739-400,* *SILIMED, Inc., Dallas, TX*	Unsafe 1	1.5	
Infall, breast implant (inflatable with magnetic port) *3101198 Model, breast implant* *Heyerschultzz*	Unsafe 1	1.5	
MemoryGel Breast Implant *Mentor, www.mentorwwllc.com*	Safe	1.5, 3	

Object	Status	Field Strength (T)	Reference
MemoryGel SILTEX Breast Implant *Mentor, www.mentorwwllc.com*	Safe	1.5, 3	
Radovan Tissue Expander *316L SS, Mentor H/S* *Santa Barbara, CA*	Safe	1.5	10
SILTEX CONTOUR PROFILE *Breast Implant, Adjustable* *Mentor, www.mentorwwllc.com*	Safe	1.5, 3	
SILTEX CONTOUR PROFILE *Saline Breast Implant* *Mentor, www.mentorwwllc.com*	Safe	1.5, 3	
SILTEX CONTOUR PROFILE Tissue Expander *Mentor, www.mentorwwllc.com*	Unsafe 1	1.5	
SILTEX Low, Medium, and Tall Height Tissue Expander *Style 6100* *Mentor, www.mentorwwllc.com*	Unsafe 1	1.5	
SILTEX Round Saline Breast Implant *Mentor, www.mentorwwllc.com*	Safe	1.5, 3	
SILTEX SPECTRUM *Breast Implant, Adjustable* *Mentor, www.mentorwwllc.com*	Safe	1.5, 3	
Siltex Spectrum Post-Operatively *Adjustable Saline-Filled Mammary Prosthesis, 316L SS* *Mentor H/S, Santa Barbara, CA*	Safe	1.5	10
SPECTRUM Breast Implant, Adjustable *Mentor, www.mentorwwllc.com*	Safe	1.5, 3	
Tissue expander with magnetic port *breast implant* *McGhan Medical Corporation, Santa Barbara, CA*	Unsafe 1	1.5	

	Status	Field Strength (T)	Reference

Cardiac Pacemakers, ICDs, and Cardiac Monitors

Object	Status	Field Strength (T)	Reference
Accent MRI and Accent ST MRI Cardiac Pacemaker Systems *Models PM1224, PM2224, PM1226, PM2226, PM1124 PM2124* *St. Jude Medical, www.sjmprofessional.com/MRI*	Conditional 5	1.5	
Advisa MRI SureScan Pacing System *Advisa DR MRI SureScan Pacing System* *Medtronic, Inc., www.Medtronic.com*	Conditional 5	1.5	
AngelMed Guardian, Implantable Cardiac Monitor *Angel Medical Systems, Shrewsbury, NJ*	Unsafe 1	1.5	
Cosmos, Model 283-01, Pacemaker *Intermedics, Inc., Freeport, TX*	Unsafe 1	3	85
Cosmos II, Model 283-03, Pacemaker *Intermedics, Inc., Freeport, TX*	Unsafe 2	3	85
Cosmos II, Model 284-05, Pacemaker *Intermedics, Inc., Freeport, TX*	Unsafe 1	3	85
Delta TRS, Type DDD, Model 0937 *Pacemaker* *Cardiac Pacemakers, Inc., St. Paul, MN*	Unsafe 1	3	85
EnRhythm MRI SureScan Pacing System *Cardiac Pacemaker* *Medtronic, Inc., www.Medtronic.com*	Conditional 5	1.5	
Ensura DR MRI SureScan Pacing System *Medtronic, Inc., www.Medtronic.com*	Conditional 5	1.5	
GEM DR 7271, Dual Chamber Implantable *Cardioverter Defibrillator* *Medtronic, Inc., www.Medtronic.com*	Unsafe 1	3	85
GEM II DR 7273, Dual Chamber Implantable *Cardioverter Defibrillator* *Medtronic, Inc., www.Medtronic.com*	Unsafe 1	3	85
KAPPA DR403, Dual Chamber Rate *Responsive Pacemaker* *Medtronic, Inc., www.Medtronic.com*	Unsafe 2	3	85
KAPPA DR706, Dual Chamber Rate *Responsive Pacemaker* *Medtronic, Inc., www.Medtronic.com*	Unsafe 1	3	85
MARQUIS DR 7274 *Implantable Cardioverter Defibrillator* *Medtronic, Inc., www.Medtronic.com*	Unsafe 1	3	85
MICRO JEWEL II 7223CX *Implantable Cardioverter Defibrillator* *Medtronic, Inc., www.Medtronic.com*	Unsafe 1	3	85
Nova *Model 281-01* *Intermedics, Inc., Freeport, TX*	Unsafe 1	3	85
Nova II *Model 281-05, Pacemaker* *Intermedics, Inc., Freeport, TX*	Unsafe 2	3	85
Nova II *Model 282-04, Pacemaker* *Intermedics, Inc., Freeport, TX*	Unsafe 2	3	85

Object	Status	Field Strength (T)	Reference
ProMRI Pacing System, Cardiac Pacemaker *BIOTRONIK, www.biotronik.com/en/de/28956*	Conditional 5	1.5	
Quantum *Model 253-19, Pacemaker* *Intermedics, Inc., Freeport, TX*	Unsafe 1	3	85
Reveal Plus Insertable Loop Recorder (ILR) *9526 Reveal Plus Insertable Loop Recorder* *Insertable Cardiac Monitor* *Medtronic, Inc., www.Medtronic.com*	Conditional 5	1.5	90, 91
Reveal DX 9528 *Insertable Cardiac Monitor* *Medtronic, Inc., www.Medtronic.com*	Conditional 5	1.5, 3	
Reveal XT 9529 *Insertable Cardiac Monitor* *Medtronic, Inc., www.Medtronic.com*	Conditional 5	1.5, 3	
Relay *Model 294-03, Pacemaker* *Intermedics, Inc., Freeport, TX*	Unsafe 1	3	85
Res-Q ACE *Model 101-01, Pacemaker* *Intermedics, Inc., Freeport, TX*	Unsafe 1	3	85
SJM Confirm *Model DM2100, Implantable Cardiac Monitor* *St. Jude Medical, www.sjmprofessional.com*	Unsafe 1	1.5	
SIGMA SDR306 *Dual Chamber Rate, Responsive Pacemaker* *Medtronic, Inc., www.Medtronic.com*	Unsafe 1	3	85
THERA VDD 8968I *Dual Chamber Atrial Sensing, Ventricular Sensing,* *Pacing Pacemaker* *Medtronic, Inc., www.Medtronic.com*	Unsafe 2	3	85

Object	Status	Field Strength (T)	Reference

Cardiovascular Catheters and Accessories

Object	Status	Field Strength (T)	Reference
Apollo Micro Catheter *15-mm Tip,* *ev3 Inc., Irvine, CA*	Conditional 8	1.5, 3	
Apollo Micro Catheter *70-mm Tip, Nitinol, Platinum Alloy, Teflon, Polyether Amide* *ev3 Inc., Irvine, CA*	Conditional 8	1.5, 3	
Arrow You-Bend *Two Lumen Hemodialysis Catheter* *Arrow International Inc., Reading, PA*	Conditional 6	3	
AVA 3xi Catheter, All Models *Edwards Lifesciences, www.edwards.com*	Safe	1.5, 3	
AVA 3xi Introducer Valve, All Models *Edwards Lifesciences, www.edwards.com*	Safe	1.5, 3	
AVA HF Catheter, All Models *Edwards Lifesciences, www.edwards.com*	Safe	1.5, 3	
Bactiseal Endoscopic Ventricular Catheter *Codman, www.DePuy.com*	Safe	1.5, 3	
Cannon II Plus Chronic Hemodialysis Catheter (CHDC) *Arrow International, www.arrowintl.com*	Conditional 6	3	
CliniCath Catheter *Smiths Medical, St. Paul, MN*	Safe	3	
Codman SureStream Intraspinal Catheter *0-degree connector, 90-degree connector* *Codman, www.depuy.com*	Conditional 6	3	
Chronic Catheter *COVIDIEN, www.covidien.com*	Conditional 6	3	
Dura-Flow Chronic Dialysis Catheter *Angiodynamics, Inc., www.Angiodynamics.com*	Safe	1.5, 3	
DuraMax Chronic Dialysis Catheter *Angiodynamics, Inc., www.Angiodynamics.com*	Safe	1.5, 3	
EVENMORE Chronic Dialysis Catheter *Angiodynamics, Inc., www.Angiodynamics.com*	Safe	1.5, 3	
FlexTip Plus Epidural Catheter *Regional Anesthesia Device* *Teleflex Medical, Wyomissing, PA*	Conditional 5	1.5, 3	
IntroFlex Catheter, All Models *Edwards Lifesciences, www.edwards.com*	Safe	1.5, 3	
LifeJet VP VascPak *Angiodynamics, Inc., www.Angiodynamics.com*	Safe	1.5, 3	
Morpheus Smart PICC *Angiodynamics, Inc., www.Angiodynamics.com*	Safe	1.5, 3	
MultiMed CVC Catheter, All Models *Edwards Lifesciences, www.edwards.com*	Safe	1.5, 3	
NeoStar Triple Lumen Catheter *Angiodynamics, Inc., www.Angiodynamics.com*	Safe	1.5, 3	
NextStep Retrograde Catheter *Arrow International, www.arrowintl.com*	Conditional 6	3	
Opticath Catheter, Model U400, catheter *Abbott Laboratories, Morgan Hill, CA*	Unsafe 2	1.5	60

Object	Status	Field Strength (T)	Reference
Opticath PA Catheter with extra port *Abbott Laboratories, Morgan Hill, CA*	Unsafe 2	1.5	60
Opticath PA Catheter with RV Pacing Port *Abbott Laboratories, Morgan Hill, CA*	Unsafe 2	1.5	60
Opti-Q SvO2/CCO *catheter* *Abbott Laboratories, Morgan Hill, CA*	Unsafe 2	1.5	60
Oximetric 3, SO2 *Optical Module* *Abbott Laboratories, Morgan Hill, CA*	Unsafe 2	1.5	60
Palindrome Sapphire HD Catheter *Covidien, www.covidien.com*	Conditional 6	3	
PediaSat Oximetry Catheter, All Models *Edwards Lifesciences, www.edwards.com*	Safe	1.5, 3	
PICC Catheter *Angiodynamics, Inc., www.Angiodynamics.com*	Safe	1.5, 3	
PolyFlow Peripherally Inserted Catheter *Smiths Medical, St. Paul, MN*	Safe	3	
PreSep Oximetry Catheter, All Models *Edwards Lifesciences, www.edwards.com*	Safe	1.5, 3	
Quadrathane Cannon II Plus Catheter *Arrow International, www.arrowintl.com*	Conditional 6	3	
Quadrathane NextStep Retrograde Catheter *Arrow International, www.arrowintl.com*	Conditional 6	3	
RV Pacing Lead *Abbott Laboratories, Morgan Hill, CA*	Unsafe 2	1.5	60
SCHON Chronic Hemodialysis Catheter *Angiodynamics, Inc., www.Angiodynamics.com*	Safe	1.5, 3	
SCHON XL Acute Hemodialysis Catheter *Angiodynamics, Inc., www.Angiodynamics.com*	Safe	1.5, 3	
SecurACath, PICC Catheter with Nitinol Securement *Interrad Medical, Inc., St. Paul, MN*	Conditional 5	3	
StimuCath Continuous Peripheral Nerve Block (CPNB) Catheter *Regional Anesthesia Device* *Teleflex Medical, Wyomissing, PA*	Conditional 5	1.5, 3	
Swan-Ganz Flow Directed Catheter, Models 111F7, 115F7 *Edwards Lifesciences, www.edwards.com*	Safe	1.5, 3	
Swan-Ganz Pediatric Catheter, Oximetry without Thermistor, Models 040F4, 040HF4, 015F4, 015HF4 *Edwards Lifesciences, www.edwards.com*	Safe	1.5, 3	
Swan-Ganz Thermodilution Catheter *American Edwards Laboratories, Irvine, CA*	Unsafe 2	1.5	57
Swan-Ganz Triple-lumen Thermodilution Catheter *American Edwards Laboratories, Irvine, CA*	Unsafe 2	1.5	60
TD Thermodilution Catheter *Flow-directed thermodilution pulmonary artery catheter* *Abbott Laboratories, Morgan Hill, CA*	Unsafe 2	1.5	60
TDQ CCO Catheter *Flow-directed thermodilution continuous* *cardiac output pulmonary artery catheter* *Abbott Laboratories, Morgan Hill, CA*	Unsafe 2	1.5	60

Object	Status	Field Strength (T)	Reference
Torque-Line Flow-directed *thermodilution pulmonary artery catheter* *Abbott Laboratories, Morgan Hill, CA*	Unsafe 2	1.5	60
Total Abscession Drainage Catheter *Angiodynamics, Inc., www.Angiodynamics.com*	Safe	1.5, 3	
Transpac IV *Abbott Laboratories, Morgan Hill, CA*	Safe	1.5	60
TruFlow Hemodialysis Catheter *Smiths Medical, St. Paul, MN*	Safe	3	
VAMP, All Models *Edwards Lifesciences, www.edwards.com*	Safe	3	
VAMP Flex, All Models *Edwards Lifesciences, www.edwards.com*	Safe	3	
VAMP Jr., All Models *Edwards Lifesciences, www.edwards.com*	Safe	3	
Vantex CVC Catheter, All Models *Edwards Lifesciences, www.edwards.com*	Safe	3	
VLVCVT5, VolumeView Thermistor Manifold *Edwards Lifesciences, www.edwards.com*	Conditional 7	3	
VLVK520, VolumeView Femoral Catheter *Edwards Lifesciences*	Conditional 8	1.5, 3	
VP1, VAMP Plus *Edwards Lifesciences, www.edwards.com*	Conditional 7	3	
VENTRA Percutaneous Intravenous Catheter *Smiths Medical, St. Paul, MN*	Safe	3	

Object	Status	Field Strength (T)	Reference
Carotid Artery Vascular Clamps			
Crutchfield	Conditional 1	1.5	11
SS, carotid artery vascular clamp			
Codman, www.depuy.com			
Kindt	Conditional 1	1.5	11
SS, carotid artery vascular clamp			
V. Mueller			
Poppen-Blaylock	Unsafe 1	1.5	11
SS, carotid artery vascular clamp			
Codman, www.depuy.com			
Salibi	Conditional 1	1.5	11
SS, carotid artery vascular clamp			
Codman, www.depuy.com			
Selverstone	Conditional 1	1.5	11
SS, carotid artery vascular clamp			
Codman, www.depuy.com			

Object	Status	Field Strength (T)	Reference
Cerebrospinal Fluid (CSF) Shunt Valves and Accessories			
AccuDrain External CSF Drainage System(s) *Integra NeuroSciences, www.integralife.com*	Safe	3	
ACCU FLO Connector *Right Angle, 316L SS* *Codman, www.depuy.com*	Conditional 6	3	
ACCU FLO Connector *Right Angle, Plastic* *Codman, www.depuy.com*	Safe	3	
ACCU-FLO Connector *Straight, 316L SS* *Codman, www.depuy.com*	Conditional 6	3	
ACCU-FLO Connector *Straight, Plastic* *Codman, www.depuy.com*	Safe	3	
ACCU-FLO Connector *Three Way, 316L SS* *Codman, www.depuy.com*	Conditional 6	3	
ACCU-FLO Connector *Three Way, Plastic* *Codman, www.depuy.com*	Safe	3	
Accura II *Adult Integral Shunt System* *Phoenix Biomedical Corporation, Valley Forge, PA*	Safe	1.5	103
Accura II *Pediatric Integral Shunt System* *Phoenix Biomedical Corporation, Valley Forge, PA*	Safe	1.5	102
Anti-Siphon Device *NL8501415* *Integra NeuroSciences, www.integralife.com*	Safe	3	
Burr Hole Valve System(s) *15527, 15539, 12837, 15530, 12834, 12838, 15533, 12835, 12839, 15536, 12836* *Integra NeuroSciences, www.integralife.com*	Safe	3	
BUS Device *Ventriculo-peritoneal shunt* *Codman, www.depuy.com*	Conditional 6	3	
Catheter(s), Integra *NL8501200, NL8501376, NL8501328, NL8501201, NL8501380, NL8501515, NL8501202, NL8501381, NL8501517, NL8501220, NL8501382, NL8501519, NL8501221, NL8501228, NL8501390, NL8501222, NL8501504, NL8501391, NL8501375, NL8501229, NL8501392, NL8501415* *Integra NeuroSciences, www.integralife.com*	Safe	3	
Cerebral ventricular shunt tube connector, *Accu-flow right angle* *Codman, www.depuy.com*	Safe	1.5	3, 94, 95
Cerebral ventricular shunt tube connector, *Accu-Flow, straight* *Codman, www.depuy.com*	Safe	1.5	3, 94, 95

Object	Status	Field Strength (T)	Reference
Cerebral ventricular shunt tube connector, *Accu-flow, T-connector* *Codman, www.depuy.com*	Safe	1.5	3, 94, 95
Connector(s), Integra *NL8501902, NL8501911, NL8501913, NL8501908, NL8501919* *Integra NeuroSciences, www.integralife.com*	Safe	3	
Codman ACCU-FLO Straight Connector *316 SS* *Codman, www.depuy.com*	Conditional 6	3	
Codman ACCU-FLO Straight Connector *Plastic* *Codman, www.depuy.com*	Safe	1.5, 3	
Codman ACCU-FLO Three Way Connector *Plastic* *Codman, www.depuy.com*	Safe	1.5, 3	
Codman ACCU-FLO Three Way Connector *316 SS* *Codman, www.depuy.com*	Conditional 6	3	
Codman ACCU FLO Right Angle Connector *Codman, www.depuy.com*	Conditional 6	3	
Codman Certas Programmable Valve *Programmable CSF Shunt Valve* *Codman, www.depuy.com*	Conditional 5	1.5, 3	119
Codman EDS CSF *External Drainage System* *Codman, www.depuy.com*	Safe	1.5, 3	103
CODMAN HAKIM Precision Pressure Valve *Fixed Pressure CSF Shunt Valve* *Codman, www.DePuy.com*	Conditional 6	3	
Codman HAKIM Programmable Valve *Codman, www.depuy.com*	Conditional 5	1.5, 3	110
Codman Holter Cerebral Catheter-Reservoir *LeRoy Design* *Codman, www.depuy.com*	Conditional 6	1.5, 3	
Codman Holter In-Line Shunt *Filter, Hoffman Design* *Codman, www.depuy.com*	Conditional 6	1.5, 3	
Codman Hydrocephalus Shunt *System Connector* *Codman, www.depuy.com*	Conditional 6	1.5, 3	
CODMAN MEDOS Right Angle Connector *also known as CODMAN Hakim Right Angle Connector* *Codman, www.depuy.com*	Conditional 6	3	
CODMAN MEDOS Straight Connector *also known as CODMAN Hakim Straight Connector* *Codman, www.depuy.com*	Conditional 6	3	
Connector(s), Integra *991002, 999410, 999412, 999415, 999411, 999414, 9MZ500* *Integra NeuroSciences, www.integralife.com*	Safe	3	

Object	Status	Field Strength (T)	Reference
Contour-Flex Valve System(s) *11811, 12507, 14085, 11812, 12508,* *14086, 11813, 12509, 14087, 11814,* *12510, 16254, 11815, 14085, 16255,* *11854, 14086, CFRH, 11855, 14087,* *CFRL, 11856, 14161, CFRM, 12505,* *14162, CFSH, 12506, 14163, CFSL,* *16256, CFSM* *Integra NeuroSciences, www.integralife.com*	Safe	3	
CRx valve *cerebral spinal fluid (CSF), shunt valve* *Sophysa, www.sophysa.com*	Safe	1.5, 3	
CRx Universal Shunt *cerebral spinal fluid (CSF), shunt valve* *Sophysa, www.sophysa.com*	Safe	1.5, 3	
Delta Shunt Assembly *Medtronic, Inc., www.medtronic.com*	Safe	3	96, 103
Diamond valve *cerebral spinal fluid (CSF), shunt valve* *Sophysa, www.sophysa.com*	Safe	1.5, 3	
Diamond II model valve *cerebral spinal fluid (CSF), shunt valve* *Sophysa, www.sophysa.com*	Safe	1.5, 3	
EDM ventricular catheter *External CSF Drainage Product* *Medtronic, Inc., www.medtronic.com*	Safe	3	103
EDS 2 CSF External Drainage System *Codman, www.depuy.com*	Safe	3	103
EDS 3 CSF External Drainage System *Codman, www.depuy.com*	Safe	3	103
Edwards-Barbaro Shunt *Integra NeuroSciences, www.integralife.com*	Safe	3	
Equi-Flow Valve System(s) *15174, SLRKL, SLSKLL, 15175, SLRKLL, SLSKLM, 15179,* *SLRKLM, SLSKM, 15185, SLRKM, SLSL, 15549, SLRL, SLSLL,* *15551, SLRLL, SLSLM, 15552, SLRLM, SLSM, 15554, SLRM,* *15181, 15555, SLSKL* *Integra NeuroSciences, www.integralife.com*	Safe	3	
HOLTER Cerebral Catheter-Reservoir *LeRoy Design, Codman, www.depuy.com*	Conditional 6	3	
HOLTER In Line Shunt Filter *Codman, www.depuy.com*	Conditional 5	3	
HOLTER In Line Shunt Filter *Hoffman Design, Codman, www.depuy.com*	Conditional 6	3	
HOLTER Reservoir *316L SS* *Codman, www.depuy.com*	Conditional 6	3	
HOLTER Rickham Reservoir *316L SS* *Codman, www.depuy.com*	Conditional 6	3	

Object	Status	Field Strength (T)	Reference
HOLTER Rickham Reservoir *Plastic* *Codman, www.depuy.com*	Safe	3	
HOLTER Salmon-Rickham Ventriculostomy Reservoir *316L SS* *Codman, www.depuy.com*	Conditional 6	3	
HOLTER Salmon-Rickham Ventriculostomy Reservoir *Plastic* *Codman, www.depuy.com*	Safe	3	
HOLTER Selker Ventriculostomy Reservoir *Plastic* *Codman, www.depuy.com*	Safe	3	
HOLTER Type A Connector *Codman, www.depuy.com*	Conditional 6	3	
HOLTER Type B Connector *Codman, www.depuy.com*	Conditional 6	3	
HOLTER Ventricular Catheter *Codman, www.depuy.com*	Conditional 6	3	
HOLTER, Selker Valve *316L SS* *Codman, www.depuy.com*	Conditional 6	3	
Integra NPH Valve System(s) *909500, 909507, 909515, 909501, 909507S, 909518, 909502,* *909508, 909520, 909503, 909508S, 909521, 909504, 909512,* *90S512, 909505, 909513, 90S521, 909506, 909514, 90S5211* *Integra NeuroSciences, www.integralife.com*	Safe	3	
LPVII Valve System(s) *NL8509810, NL8509830, NL8509850, NL8509811, NL8509831,* *NL8509851, NL8509820, NL8509840, NL8509860, NL8509821* *NL8509841 NL8509861* *Integra NeuroSciences, www.integralife.com*	Safe	3	
Mishler Valve System(s) *NL8500311, NL8500313, NL8500315, NL8500312,* *NL8500314* *Integra NeuroSciences, www.integralife.com*	Safe	3	
Multi Purpose On-Off Valve System(s) *NL8500108 NL8500125 NL8500128* *Integra NeuroSciences, www.integralife.com*	Safe	3	
Novus Valve System(s) *NL8509010, NL8509021, NL8509610, NL8509011, NL8509311* *NL8509620, NL8509020, NL8509321* *Integra NeuroSciences, www.integralife.com*	Safe	3	
One Piece Shunt Valve System(s) *NL8506102, NL8506302, NL8506403, NL8506201* *NL8506401, NL8506501, NL8506202, NL8506402* *Integra NeuroSciences, www.integralife.com*	Safe	3	
OSV II Low Flow Lumbar *Valve System(s) 909522, 909523* *Integra NeuroSciences, www.integralife.com*	Safe	3	
OSV II Low Pro Valve System(s) *909702P, 909712P, 909700P* *Integra NeuroSciences, www.integralife.com*	Safe	3	

Object	Status	Field Strength (T)	Reference
OSV II Lumbar Valve System(s) *909722, 909723* *Integra NeuroSciences, www.integralife.com*	Safe	3	
OSV II Smart Valve *Integra NeuroSciences, www.integralife.com*	Safe	3	
OSV II Valve System(s) *909700, 909707, 909718, 909701, 909707S, 909719, 909702,* *909708, 909720, 909703, 909708S, 909721, 909704, 909712,* *90S702, 909705, 909713, 90S712, 909706, 909714, 909702P,* *909712P, 909700P* *Integra NeuroSciences, www.integralife.com*	Safe	3	
POLARIS Adjustable Pressure Valve *Sophysa USA, Inc., Costa Mesa, CA*	Conditional 5	3	97, 103
proGAV Adjustable Valve *Aesculap, Inc., www.aesculapusa.com*	Conditional 5	3	104
PS Medical CSF-Flow Control Valve *Medtronic, Inc., www.medtronic.com*	Safe	1.5	96
PS Medical CSF-Ventricular Access Port *Medtronic, Inc., www.medtronic.com*	Safe	1.5	96
PS Medical CSF-Ventricular Reservoir *Medtronic, Inc., www.medtronic.com*	Safe	1.5	96
PS Medical CSF-Ventriculostomy Reservoir *Medtronic, Inc., www.medtronic.com*	Safe	1.5	96
PS Medical Strata Valve *adjustable cerebral spinal fluid valve* *Medtronic, Inc., www.medtronic.com*	Conditional 5	1.5	96
Pudenz Valve System(s) *NL8501330, NL8501358, NL8501411, NL8501331, NL8501359,* *NL8501412, NL8501356, NL8501410, NL8501413, NL8501357* *NL8501414* *Integra NeuroSciences, www.integralife.com*	Safe	3	
Pulsar Valve *Sophysa USA, Inc., Costa Mesa, CA*	Safe	1.5	97
Reservoir(s), Integra *NL8501210, NL8501214, NL8501121, NL8501211,* *NL8501215 NL8501132, NL8501212, NL8500150,* *NL8501192, NL8501213, NL8500155 NL8501195* *Integra NeuroSciences, www.integralife.com*	Safe	3	
Reservoir(s), Integra *999015, 999112, 999303, 999016, 999113, 999304, 999017,* *999301, 951305, 999110, 999302, 951307, 999111* *Integra NeuroSciences, www.integralife.com*	Safe	3	
Rickham Reservoir *316L SS* *Codman, www.depuy.com*	Conditional 6	3	
Right Angle Connector *Nylon* *Codman, www.depuy.com*	Safe	3	
Selker Valve *316L SS* *Codman, www.depuy.com*	Conditional 6	3	

Object	Status	Field Strength (T)	Reference
Selker Valve *Nylon* *Codman, www.depuy.com*	Safe	3	
Shunt valve, Holter-Hausner type *Holter-Hausner, Inc., Bridgeport, PA*	Safe	1.5	55
Shunt valve, Holtertype *The Holter Co., Bridgeport, PA*	Unsafe 1	1.5	55
Single Valve *cerebral spinal fluid (CSF), shunt valve* *Sophysa, www.sophysa.com*	Safe	1.5, 3	
Sophy Adjustable Pressure Valve *Model SP3* *Sophysa, Orsay, France*	Conditional 5	1.5	97
Sophy Adjustable Pressure Valve *Model SU8* *Sophysa, Orsay, France*	Conditional 5	1.5	97
SOPHY Adjustable Pressure Valve *Sophysa USA, Inc., Costa Mesa, CA*	Conditional 5	1.5	97
Sophy Mini Monopressure Valve *Sophysa USA, Inc., Costa Mesa, CA*	Safe	1.5	97
Straight Connector *Nylon* *Codman, www.depuy.com*	Safe	3	
Strata II *Programmable CSF Shunt Valve* *Medtronic, Inc., www.medtronic.com*	Conditional 5	3	
Strata NSC *Programmable CSF Shunt Valve* *Medtronic, Inc., www.medtronic.com*	Conditional 5	3	
Strata *Programmable CSF Shunt Valve* *Medtronic, Inc., www.medtronic.com*	Conditional 5	3	
Suture Tubing Clamp(s), Integra *999004, 999005, 999007* *Integra NeuroSciences, www.integralife.com*	Safe	3	
Three Way Connector *Silicone, Nylon* *Codman, www.depuy.com*	Safe	3	
UltraVS Valve System(s) *NL8501109, NL8501115, NL8501127, NL8501110, NL8501123,* *NL8501128, NL8501111, NL8501124, NL8501129, NL8501113,* *NL8501125, NL8501130, NL8501114, NL8501126, NL8501131* *Integra NeuroSciences, www.integralife.com*	Safe	3	
Ventricular Catheter(s), Peritoneal Catheter(s), *Atrial Catheter(s) 953100, 951102A, 9MZ207, 9MZ100, 9MD1022,* *9MZ208, 953101, 9MD102A, 9MZ209, 9MZ101, 9MD102B,* *9MZ210, 9MZ1011, 9MZ203, 9MZ211, PC1, 9MZ204, VC1,* *951101, 9MZ205, 999013, 951101A, 9MZ206, 999014, 951102* *Integra NeuroSciences, www.integralife.com*	Safe	3	

Object	Status	Field Strength (T)	Reference
Coils, Stents, Filters, and Grafts			
AAA Endograft	Conditional 6	3	
TriVascular2, Inc., Santa Rosa, CA			
Absolute Biliary Stent	Conditional 5	3	
Abbott Vascular, www.abbottvascular.com			
Absolute .035 Biliary Self-Expanding Stent	Conditional 5	3	
Abbott Vascular, www.AbbotVascular.com			
Absolute Pro .035 Biliary Self-Expanding Stent	Conditional 5	3	
Abbott Vascular, www.AbbotVascular.com			
Absolute Pro Stent	Conditional 6	3	
Nickel titanium with nickel titanium platinum markers			
8-mm x 120-mm, Single version			
Abbott Vascular, www.abbottvascular.com			
Absolute Pro Stent	Conditional 6	3	
Nickel titanium with nickel titanium platinum markers			
8-mm x 348-mm, three overlapped version			
Abbott Vascular, www.abbottvascular.com			
Absolute Pro Peripheral Stent	Condiitional 5	3	
Abbott Vascular, www.abbottvascular.com			
Acculink Carotid Stent	Conditional 5	3	
Abbott Vascular, www.abbottvascular.com			
ACS MULTI-LINK Coronary Stent	Conditional 5	3	
Abbott Vascular, www.abbottvascular.com			
ACS Multi-Link RX Duet, 18 x 3.0-mm	Safe	1.5	72
stent, 316L SS			
Abbott Vascular, www.abbottvascular.com			
ACS MULTI-LINK DUET Coronary Stent	Conditional 5	3	
Abbott Vascular, www.abbottvascular.com			
ACS MULTI-LINK TRISTAR Coronary Stent	Conditional 5	3	
Abbott Vascular, www.abbottvascular.com			
ACS MULTI-LINK ULTRA Coronary Stent	Conditional 5	3	
Abbott Vascular, www.abbottvascular.com			
ACS RX Multi-Link	Safe	1.5	72
15 x 3.0-mm, stent, 316L SS			
Abbott Vascular, www.abbottvascular.com			
ACS RX Multi-Link	Safe	1.5	72
15 x 4.0-mm, stent, 316L SS			
Abbott Vascular, www.abbottvascular.com			
ACS RX Multi-Link	Safe	1.5	72
25 x 3.0-mm, stent, 316L SS			
Abbott Vascular, www.abbottvascular.com			
ACS Stent, 316L SS	Safe	1.5	
Abbott Vascular, www.abbottvascular.com			
ACURATE Stent	Conditional 6	3	
Symetis SA, Switzerland			
Adapt Carotid Stent	Conditional 6	3	
carotid artery stent, Nitinol, Tantalum			
Endotex Interventional Systems, Inc., Cupertino, CA			
Advanta V12 Stent	Conditional 6	3	
Atrium Medical Corporation, Hudson, New Hampshire			

Object	Status	Field Strength (T)	Reference
AERO Tracheobronchial Stent *Merit Endotek* *Merit Medical, www.merit.com*	Conditional 6	3	
Aero Tracheal Stent *18-mm x 80-mm, Nickel Titanium with a polyurethane cover* *Alveolus, Inc., Charlotte, NC*	Conditional 6	3	
Aero Tracheal Stent *Nitinol with Polyurethane Cover* *Alveolus, Inc., Charlotte, NC*	Conditional 6	3	
ALIMAXX-B Biliary Stent *Uncovered Biliary Stent* *Merit Endotek* *Merit Medical, www.merit.com*	Conditional 6	3	
ALIMAXX-B Covered Biliary Stent *10-mm x 80-mm, Nickel Titanium with a Silicone covering* *Alveolus, Inc., Charlotte, NC*	Conditional 6	3	
ALIMAXX-B Uncovered Biliary Stent *10-mm x 80-mm, Nickel Titanium* *Alveolus, Inc. Charlotte, NC*	Conditional 6	3	
ALIMAXX-ES Stent *Merit Medical, www.merit.com*	Conditional 8	1.5, 3	
ALIMAXX-ES Esophageal Stent *Merit Endotek* *Merit Medical, www.merit.com*	Conditional 6	3	
ALN Vena Cava Filter *316L SS* *ALN Implants, Chirurgicaux, France*	Conditional 6	3	
Amplatzer Vascular Graft (AVG) *AGA Medical Corporation, www.sjm.com/aga-medical*	Conditional 8	1.5, 3	
Amplatz IVC filter *Cook Medical, Inc., www.cookmedical.com*	Safe	4.7	21
Anaconda Endovascular Device *Nitinol* *Vascutek Ltd.*	Conditional 6	3	
ANCURE Endograft Stent	Safe	1.5	
AneuRx AAA Stent Grafts System *Medtronic, Inc., www.Medtronic.com*	Conditional 6	3	
AneuRx AAAdvantage Stent Grafts System *Medtronic, Inc., www.Medtronic.com*	Safe	3	
AneuRx II Bifurcation Stent Graft *Medtronic, Inc., www.Medtronic.com*	Safe	3	
Angiomed Memotherm Femoral Stent *4-mm x 120-mm, Nitinol* *C.R. Bard, Inc., Billerica, MA*	Safe	1.5	
Angiomed Memotherm Femoral Stent *5-mm x 20-mm, Nitinol* *C.R. Bard, Inc., Billerica, MA*	Safe	1.5	
Angiomed Memotherm Iliac Stent *12-mm x 110-mm, Nitinol* *C.R. Bard, Inc., Billerica, MA*	Safe	1.5	

Object	Status	Field Strength (T)	Reference
Angiomed Memotherm Iliac Stent *8-mm x 20-mm, Nitinol* *C.R. Bard, Inc., Billerica, MA*	Safe	1.5	
AngioStent Stent, 15-mm *Platinum, iridium, Angiodynamics* *Queensbury, NY*	Safe	1.5	
Aorfix Bifurcated Stent Graft system *Lombard Medical, www.LombardMedical.com*	Conditional 5	3	
APOLLO Cerebral Stent *316LVM SS* *MicroPort Medical, www.microport.com.cn/english*	Conditional 6	3	
Apollo Intracranial Stent *MicroPort Medical, www.microport.com.cn/english*	Conditional 8	1.5, 3	
aSpire Covered Stent *100 x 14-mm, Nitinol, nickel, Titanium* *Vascular Architects, Portola, CA*	Safe	1.5	
aSpire II stent *Nitinol with an ePTFE covering* *Vascular Architects, Inc., San Jose, CA*	Safe	3	
Assurant Cobalt Iliac Stent *single and two overlapped versions* *Medtronic, Inc., www.Medtronic.com*	Conditional 8	1.5, 3	
Astron Stent *Nitinol, gold markers* *BIOTRONIK*	Conditional 6	3	
AVE GFX Stent, 316L SS *Arterial Vascular Engineering, Santa Rosa, CA*	Safe	1.5	69
AVE Micro I Stent, 316L SS *Arterial Vascular Engineering, Santa Rosa, CA*	Safe	1.5	69
AVE Micro II Stent, 316L SS *Arterial Vascular Engineering, Santa Rosa, CA*	Safe	1.5	69
AXIOS Stent *Xlumena, Inc., www.xlumena.com*	Conditional 6	3	
AXIUM Detachable Coil, embolization coil *ev3, Inc., www.ev3.net*	Condiitional 5	3	
Axium Detachable Implant for *Neurovascular Malformation* *Embolization coil* *ev3 Neurovascular, Irvine, CA*	Conditional 6	3	
Axxess Biolimus A9 Eluting Bifurcation Stent *coronary artery stent, Nitinol* *Devax, Inc., Irvine, CA*	Conditional 6	3	
Axxess Stent, coronary artery stent *Devax, Inc., Irvine, CA*	Safe	3	
Azur Peripheral Endovascular *Embolization Coil System, Azur Detachable* *MicroVention, Inc., Tustin, CA*	Conditional 6	3	
BARD CONFORMEXX, Biliary Stent *12 x 120-mm, Nitinol* *C. R. Bard* *Angiomed GmbH & Co. Medizintechnik KG* *Karlsruhe, Germany*	Safe	1.5, 3	83

Object	Status	Field Strength (T)	Reference
Bard DeBakey Woven Graft *PET Polyester* *Bard Peripheral Vascular, www.bardpv.com*	Safe	3	
Bard ELUMINEXX Vascular Stent *Bard Peripheral Vascular, www.bardpv.com*	Condiitional 5	3	
Bard LifeStent FlexStar XL Stent *Bard Peripheral Vascular, www.bardpv.com*	Conditional 5	1.5, 3	
Bard LUMINEXX 3 *Biliary and Vascular Stent, Nitinol, tantalum, 14-mm x 120-mm* *C. R. Bard* *Angiomed GmbH & Co. Medizintechnik KG* *Karlsruhe, Germany*	Safe	1.5, 3	
BARD LUMINEXX *Biliary and Vascular Stent, 12 x 120-mm, Nitinol, tantalum* *C. R. Bard* *Angiomed GmbH & Co. Medizintechnik KG* *Karlsruhe, Germany*	Safe	1.5, 3	83
Bard Stent, bifurcated *36 x 20-mm, Nitinol*	Safe	1.5	70
Bard ViVEXX Carotid Stent *Nitinol* *C. R. Bard* *Angiomed GmbH & Co. Medizintechnik KG* *Karlsruhe, Germany*	Safe	3	
Bard XT Stent *15 x 3.0-mm, 316 LVM* *Bard Interventional Products, Billerica, MA*	Safe	1.5	72
Bard XT Stent *316 LVM* *Bard Limited, Ireland*	Safe	1.5	69
Berenstein Hydroflex Embolization Coil *embolization coil* *MicroVention, Inc., www.microvention.com*	Conditional 6	3	
BeStent, 15 x 3.0-mm *316L SS, stent* *Medtronic, Inc., www.Medtronic.com*	Safe	1.5	72
BeStent, 25 x 3.0-mm *316L SS, stent* *Medtronic, Inc., www.Medtronic.com*	Safe	1.5	72
BeStent, MR-safe SS *stent* *Medtronic, Inc., www.Medtronic.com*	Safe	1.5	69
Bifurcated EXCLUDER Endoprosthesis *Nitinol, stent* *W.L. Gore and Associates, Inc., www.goremedical.com*	Safe	1.5	
BIOFLEX Stent *coronary artery stent, 316L SS* *Biosensors International, La Jolla, CA*	Safe	3	
BioMatrix Flex Stent *Biosensors International - USA, La Jolla, CA*	Conditional 8	1.5, 3	
Black Silicone Filiform Double Pigtail Ureteral Stent *Cook Urological, www.cookmedical.com*	Conditional 6	3	

Object	Status	Field Strength (T)	Reference
Blazer Stent *OrbusNeich, www.orbusneich.com*	Conditional 6	3	
Bridge Constant Stent *cobalt alloy, stent* *Medtronic, Inc., www.Medtronic.com*	Safe	3	
BX Stent *316L SS* *Cordis, Miami Lakes, FL*	Safe	1.5	69
BX Velocity Balloon-Expander *Intracranial Intravascular stent, 4.0-mm x 8-mm* *Cordis, www.depuy.com*	Safe	1.5, 3	83
Carbostent Isthmus Iliac Stent *CID, cidvascular.com*	Conditional 8	1.5, 3	
Carotid WALLSTENT Endoprosthesis *Boston Scientific, www.bostonscientific.com*	Conditional 5	3	
CASHMERE Microcoil *embolization coil* *Micrus Endovascular, www.micrusendovascular.com*	Conditional 5	3	
Castor Branched Aortic Stent Graft *MicroPort Medical, www.microport.com.cn/english*	Conditional 8	1.5, 3	
Celect Vena Cava Filter *Cook Medical, Inc., www.cookmedical.com*	Conditional 6	3	
CenterFlex Vascular Graft *Carbon-impregnated ePTFE* *Bard Peripheral Vascular, Tempe, AZ*	Safe	3	
Chromaxx BX Stent *Cobalt Chromium Alloy (Phynox)* *Angiomed GmbH & Co., Karlsruhe, Germany*	Conditional 6	3	
CHOOSTENT *M.I. Tech Co., Ltd., Seoul, Korea*	Conditional 8	1.5, 3	
Cinatra Cobalt-Chromium *coronary artery stent* *Atrium Medical Corporation, Hudson, NH*	Conditional 8	1.5, 3	
Cobra BMS *Bare Metal Stent, L605 Cobalt Chrome* *Medlogics Device Corporation, Santa Rosa, CA*	Conditional 6	3	
Cobra Stent *MEDLOGICS Device Corporation, Santa Rosa, CA*	Conditional 6	3	
Coherex FlatStent EF *Coherex Medical, Salt Lake City, UT*	conditional 6	3	
Complete SE Stent *Nitinol, Tantalum* *Medtronic, Inc., www.Medtronic.com*	Conditional 6	3	
Cook Celect Vena Cava Filter *Cook Medical, Inc., www.cookmedical.com*	Conditional 5	3	
Cook occluding spring embolization coil *MWCE- 338-5-10* *Cook Medical, Inc., www.cookmedical.com*	Conditional 2	1.5	
Cook-Z Stent *Gianturco-Rosch Biliary Design, 10-mm x 30-mm* *Cook Medical, Inc., www.cookmedical.com*	Conditional 2	1.5	

Object	Status	Field Strength (T)	Reference
Cook-Z Stent *Gianturco-Rosch Tracheobronchial Design, 20-mm x 5-cm* *Cook Medical, Inc., www.cookmedical.com*	Conditional 2	1.5	
CORDIS ENTERPRISE Vascular Reconstruction Device *Cordis, www.depuy.com*	Conditional 5	3	
CoRectCoil *Nitinol, stent* *Intratherapeutics, Inc., St. Paul, MN*	Safe	1.5	
Corvita Endoluminal *Graft for Abdominal Aortic Aneurysm, 27-mm x 120-mm* *Schneider (USA) Inc.* *Pfizer Medical Technology Group, Minneapolis, MN*	Safe	1.5	64
CoStar *Coronary Stent, Cobalt Chromium* *Conor Medsystems, Menlo Park, CA*	Safe	3	
CoStar *Paclitaxel-Eluting Coronary Stent* *Conor Medsystems, Menlo Park, CA*	Safe	3	
Covered UltraFlex Esophageal Stent *23-mm diameter x 12-cm length* *Nitinol stent with polyurethane covering* *Boston Scientific, www.bostonscientific.com*	Safe	1.5	
Covered WallFlex Biliary RX Stent *Boston Scientific, www.bostonscientific.com*	Conditional 6	3	
cPAX Embolization Material *NeuroVASx, Inc., Maple Grove, MN*	Safe	1.5, 3	
Cragg Nitinol Spiral Filter	Safe	4.7	21
Cristallo Ideale Carotid Self-Expanding Stent *Conical version, Nitinol* *Invatec Technology Center GmbH, Thurgau, Switzerland*	Conditional 6	3	
Cristallo Ideale Carotid Self-Expanding Stent *Cylindrical version, Nitinol* *Invatec Technology Center GmbH, Thurgau, Switzerland*	Conditional 6	3	
Crossflex Stent *316L SS* *Cordis, www.depuy.com*	Safe	1.5	69
Crown Stent *316L SS* *Cordis, www.depuy.com*	Safe	1.5	69
Crux Filter *Vena cava filter, Nitinol* *Crux Biomedical, Inc., Portola Valley, CA*	Conditional 6	3	
Cypher Select *Sirolimus-Eluting Stent* *Cordis, www.depuy.com*	Conditional 5	3	
CYPHER Sirolimus-eluting Coronary Stent *Cordis, www.cordis.com*	Conditional 5	3	
DELTAPAQ Microcoil, embolization coil *Micrus Endovascular, www.micrusendovascular.com*	Conditional 5	3	
Detach Embolization Coil System *Cook Medical, Inc., www.cookmedical.com*	Conditional 6	3	

Object	Status	Field Strength (T)	Reference
Diamond Colonic Stent *26-mm diameter x 10-cm length* *Boston Scientific, www.bostonscientific.com*	Safe	1.5	
Distaflo Bypass Graft *Carbon-impregnated ePTFE* *Bard Peripheral Vascular, www.bardpv.com*	Safe	3	
DISTAFLO Bypass Graft *Carbon-impregnated ePTFE* *Bard Peripheral Vascular, www.bardpv.com*	Safe	3	
Diverter Stent *8-mm x 32-mm, Elgiloy (Conichrome), Tantalum* *MindGuard, Ltd., Israel*	Safe	1.5	
Double-J Closed Tip *Ureteral Stent, Silicone* *Gyrus ACMI, Inc., www.gyrusacmi.com*	Safe	3	
Double-J II Closed Tip *Ureteral Stent, Polyurethane* *Gyrus ACMI, Inc., www.gyrusacmi.com*	Safe	3	
Double Pigtail Ureteral Stent *Polyurethane* *Gyrus ACMI, Inc., www.gyrusacmi.com*	Safe	3	
Double Pigtail Ureteral Stent *Polyurethane* *Gyrus ACMI, Inc., www.gyrusacmi.com*	Safe	3	
Driver Sprint Stent *Medtronic, Inc., www.Medtronic.com*	Conditional 5	3	
Driver Stent, Including Driver RX, Driver MXII *MicroDriver, MicroDriver MXII, MicroDriver RX* *Coronary Stent* *Medtronic, Inc., www.Medtronic.com*	Conditional 5	3	
Duraflex SE Stent *Nickel Titanium alloy, Tantalum* *Flexible Stenting Solutions, Inc., Eatontown, NJ*	Conditional 8	1.5, 3	
Dynaflo Bypass Graft *Bard Peripheral Vascular, www.bardpv.com*	Safe	1.5	
Dynalink Biliary Stent *Abbott Vascular, www.abbottvascular.com*	Conditional 5	3	
DYNALINK Stent *10-mm x 100-mm, Nickel/Titanium*	Safe	1.5, 3	
DYNALINK Stent *5-mm x 100-mm, Nickel/Titanium*	Safe	1.5, 3	
DYNALINK Stent, 5 to 10-mm (OTW), Nitinol	Safe	1.5	
DYNALINK E Stent, drug eluting stent	Conditional 6	3	
Dynamic Stent *BIOTRONIK*	Conditional 6	3	
Dynamic Renal Stent *BIOTRONIK*	Conditional 6	3	
Eclipse Filter, vena cava filter *Bard Peripheral Vascular, www.bardpv.com*	Conditional 5	3	

Object	Status	Field Strength (T)	Reference
Embolization Coil *IMWCE-38-15-15, Inconel* *Cook Medical, Inc., www.cookmedical.com*	Safe	3	
Embolization Coil *IMWCE-38-20-15, Inconel* *Cook Medical, Inc., www.cookmedical.com*	Safe	3	
Embolization Coil *MWCE-38-14-12 NESTER, Platinum, Inconel* *Cook Medical, Inc., www.cookmedical.com*	Safe	3	
Embolization Coil, Stainless Steel *Cook Medical, Inc., www.cookmedical.com*	Unsafe 1	1.5	
Endeavor Drug Eluting Stent *cobalt alloy* *Medtronic, Inc., www.Medtronic.com*	Conditional 5	3	88
Endeavor Resolute Zotarolimus-Eluting Coronary Stent *Medtronic, Inc., www.Medtronic.com*	Conditional 5	3	
Endeavor Stent, Including Endeavor Sprint *Endeavor MXII, Endeavor Zotarolimus Eluting Coronary Stent* *Medtronic, Inc., www.Medtronic.com*	Conditional 5	3	
EndoCoil Stent *Intratherapeutics, Inc., St. Paul, MN*	Safe	1.5	
EndoCoil-T Stent *Intratherapeutics, Inc., St. Paul, MN*	Safe	1.5	
EndoFit Endoluminal Stent Graft *Cuff(C)* *ENDOMED, Inc., Phoenix, AZ*	Safe	1.5	
EndoFit Endoluminal Stent Graft *Extender (E)* *ENDOMED, Inc., Phoenix, AZ*	Safe	1.5	
EndoFit Endoluminal Stent Graft *Occluder (O)* *ENDOMED, Inc., Phoenix, AZ*	Safe	1.5	
EndoFit Endoluminal Stent Graft *Tapered Aortomonoiliac (A)* *ENDOMED, Inc., Phoenix, AZ*	Safe	1.5	
EndoFit Endoluminal Stent Graft *Thoracic (T)* *ENDOMED, Inc., Phoenix, AZ*	Safe	1.5	
EndoMAXX Stent *Merit Medical, www.merit.com*	Conditional 8	1.5, 3	
Endurant Stent Graft *Medtronic, Inc., www.Medtronic.com*	Conditional 5	1.5, 3	
Enforcer Stent *Cardiovascular Dynamics, Inc.*	Safe	1.5	
Enovus AAA Bifurcated Stent Graft *TriVascular, Inc., Santa Rosa, CA*	Safe	3	
Enovus Iliac Stent Graft *Boston Scientific, www.bostonscientific.com*	Conditional 6	3	
Enterprise Stent *Nitinol with tantalum markers* *Cordis, www.depuy.com*	Safe	3	

Object	Status	Field Strength (T)	Reference
Epic Stent *Boston Scientific, www.bostonscientific.com*	Conditional 5	1, 3	
EsophaCoil-S Stent *Intratherapeutics, Inc., St. Paul, MN*	Safe	1.5	
Esophageal Stent, Niti-S & Comvi Model E2423 *TaeWoong Medical Co., Ltd., www.stent.net*	Conditional 8	1.5, 3	
Eta-2 TA Stent *Nitinol, Tantalum* *Angiomed GmbH & Co., Germany*	Conditional 6	3	
Evolution Biliary Stent *Cook Medical, Inc., www.cookmedical.com*	Conditional 8	1.5, 3	
Evolution Colonic Stent *Cook Medical, Inc., www.cookmedical.com*	Conditional 8	1.5, 3	
Evolution Colonic Stent *Nitinol wire, Tantalum marker bands* *Cook Medical, www.cookmedical.com*	Conditional 6	3	
Evolution Duodenal Stent *Cook Medical, Inc., www.cookmedical.com*	Conditional 8	1.5, 3	
Evolution Esophageal Stent *Nitinol* *Cook Endoscopy, Winston-Salem, NC*	Conditional 8	1.5, 3	
EXCLUDER Bifurcated Endoprosthesis, Stent Graft *W.L. Gore and Associates, www.goremedical.com*	Conditional 8	1.5, 3	
Exhale Drug Eluting Stent *Broncus Technologies, Inc., Mountain View, CA*	Conditional 6	3	
Exponent Carotid Stent *Medtronic, Inc., www.Medtronic.com*	Safe	3	
Express Biliary SD Stent *Boston Scientific, www.bostonscientific.com*	Conditional 5	3	
Express LD Stent 316L SS *Boston Scientific, www.bostonscientific.com*	Conditional 5	3	
Express SD Stent, 316L SS *Boston Scientific, www.bostonscientific.com*	Conditional 5	3	
Express2 Coronary Stent *Boston Scientific, www.bostonscientific.com*	Conditional 5	3	
Fanelli Laparoscopic Endobiliary Stent *Stent* *Cook Surgical Products, Bloomington, IN*	Safe	1.5	
Filiform Double Pigtail *Silicone Stent* *Cook Urological, Inc., Spencer, IN*	Safe	1.5	
Firebird2 Coronary Artery Stent *MicroPort Medical, www.microport.com.cn/english*	Conditional 8	1.5, 3	
FLAIR Endovascular Stent Graft *Bard Peripheral Vascular, www.bardpv.com*	Conditional 5	3	
Flamingo Wallstent Esophageal Endoprosthesis *Elgiloy* *Schneider GmbH, Bulach, Switzerland*	Safe	1.5	
FlexStent, Stent *Flexible Stenting Solutions, www.flexiblestent.com*	Conditional 8	1.5, 3	

Object	Status	Field Strength (T)	Reference
Flower Embolization Microcoil *Platinum* *Target Therapeutics, San Jose, CA*	Safe	1.5	22
FLUENCY Plus Tracheobronchial Stent Graft *Nitinol with tantalum markers* *C. R. Bard* *Angiomed GmbH & Co. Medizintechnik KG, Karlsruhe, Germany*	Safe	3	
FLUENCY Plus Vascular Stent Graft *Nitinol with tantalum markers* *C. R. Bard* *Angiomed GmbH & Co. Medizintechnik KG, Karlsruhe, Germany*	Safe	3	
FLUENCY Vascular and Tracheobronchial Stent Grafts *10-mm x 80-mm, Nitinol* *C. R. Bard* *Angiomed GmbH & Co. Medizintechnik KG, Karlsruhe, Germany*	Safe	1.5	
Formula Stent *Including Formula Renal Stent and Formula 414 Rx Renal Stent* *Cook Medical, Inc., www.cookmedical.com*	Conditional 6	3	
Formula 418 Balloon Expandable Biliary Stent *Cook Medical, Inc., www.cookmedical.com*	Conditional 5	3	
Formula 535 Vascular Stent *Cook Medical, www.cookmedical.com*	Conditional 8	1.5, 3	
Fusion Zilver Biliary Stent System *Cook Medical, www.cookmedical.com*	Conditional 5	3	
G2 Express Vena Cava Filter *Bard Peripheral Vascular, www.bardpv.com*	Conditional 6	3	
G2 Filter *Vena Cava Filter, Femoral Vein* *Bard Peripheral Vascular, www.bardpv.com*	Conditional 5	1.5	
G2 X Vena Cava Filter *Bard Peripheral Vascular, www.bardpv.com*	Conditional 5	3	
G2 X Filter Vena Cava Filter, Femoral Vein *Bard Peripheral Vascular, www.bardpv.com*	Conditional 5	3	
G2 X Filter Vena Cava Filter, Jugular Vein *Bard Peripheral Vascular, www.bardpv.com*	Conditional 5	3	
GDC 3D Shape, various sizes, Platinum *Boston Scientific/Target, Wayne, NJ*	Safe	1.5	
GDC Detachable Coil *GDC 10-3D, 3-D Shape, Platinum alloy* *Boston Scientific Corporation, www.bostonscientific.com*	Safe	3	
GDC Detachable Coil *GDC 10-Soft, Platinum alloy* *Boston Scientific Corporation, www.bostonscientific.com*	Safe	3	
GDC Detachable Coil *GDC 10-Standard, Platinum alloy* *Boston Scientific Corporation, www.bostonscientific.com*	Safe	3	
GDC Detachable Coil *GDC 18-2D, 2 Diameter, Platinum alloy* *Boston Scientific Corporation, www.bostonscientific.com*	Safe	3	
GDC Detachable Coil *GDC 18-3D, 3-D Shape, Platinum alloy* *Boston Scientific Corporation, www.bostonscientific.com*	Safe	3	

Object	Status	Field Strength (T)	Reference
GDC Detachable Coil *GDC 18-Soft, Platinum alloy* *Boston Scientific Corporation, www.bostonscientific.com*	Safe	3	
GDC Detachable Coil *GDC 18-Standard, Platinum alloy* *Boston Scientific Corporation, www.bostonscientific.com*	Safe	3	
GDC Detachable Coil *GDC 2D, 2 Diameter, Platinum alloy* *Boston Scientific Corporation, www.bostonscientific.com*	Safe	3	
GDC TriSpan Coil *14-mm, Nitinol, Platinum* *Boston Scientific Corporation-Target, Fremont, CA*	Safe	1.5, 3	
GDC TriSpan Coil *16-mm, Nitinol, Platinum* *Boston Scientific Corporation-Target, Fremont, CA*	Safe	1.5, 3	
GDC 18-Fibered VortX Shape *Platinum alloy* *Boston Scientific Corporation, www.bostonscientific.com*	Safe	3	
GDC Stretch Resistant Detachable Coil *GDC 10-Soft 2D SR, Platinum alloy* *Boston Scientific Corporation, www.bostonscientific.com*	Safe	3	
GDC Stretch Resistant Detachable Coil *GDC 10-Soft SR, Platinum alloy* *Boston Scientific Corporation, www.bostonscientific.com*	Safe	3	
GDC Stretch Resistant Detachable Coil *GDC 10-UltraSoft SR, Platinum alloy* *Boston Scientific Corporation, www.bostonscientific.com*	Safe	3	
GDC TriSpan Coil *Platinum alloy, Nitinol* *Boston Scientific Corporation, www.bostonscientific.com*	Safe	3	
GFS Stent *Medtronic, Inc., www.Medtronic.com*	Conditional 5	3	
GFX (DOW, DGFW, DFW) Stent *Medtronic, Inc., www.Medtronic.com*	Conditional 5	3	
Genous Bio-Engineered R Stent *316L SS* *OrbusNeich Medical, Inc., Fort Lauderdale, FL*	Conditional 6	3	
Genous Bio-engineered R Stent *coronary artery stent* *OrbusNeich Medical, Inc., Fort Lauderdale, FL*	Conditional 6	3	
Gianturco bird nest IVC filter *Cook Medical, Inc., www.cookmedical.com*	Conditional 2	1.5	21
Gianturco zig-zag stent *Cook Medical, Inc., www.cookmedical.com*	Conditional 2	1.5	21
Gianturco-Roehm Bird's Nest Vena Cava Filter *Cook Medical, Inc., www.cookmedical.com*	Conditional 6	3	
Gianturco-Roubin II *20 x 3.0-mm, stent, 316L SS* *Cook, Bloomington, IN*	Safe	1.5	72
Gianturco-Roubin Flex Stent *Coronary Artery Stent* *Cook Medical, Inc., www.cookmedical.com*	Conditional 5	3	

Object	Status	Field Strength (T)	Reference
Gianturco-Roubin Stent *316L SS,* *Cook, Bloomington, IN*	Safe	1.5	69
Goldvalve Detachable Balloon *Coils, Filters, Stents* *NFocus Neuromedical, Palo Alto, CA*	Conditional 6	3	
GORE EXCLUDER AAA Endoprosthesis *Stent Graft* *W.L. Gore and Associates, Inc., www.goremedical.com*	Conditional 8	1.5, 3	
GORE Intering Vascular Graft *W.L. Gore & Associates, www.goremedical.com*	Safe	1.5	
GORE MYCROMESH Biomaterial *W.L. Gore & Associates, www.goremedical.com*	Safe	1.5	
GORE MYCROMESH PLUS Biomaterial *W.L. Gore & Associates, www.goremedical.com*	Safe	1.5	
GORE PRECLUDE Pericardial Membrane *W.L. Gore & Associates, www.goremedical.com*	Safe	1.5	
GORE PROPATEN Vascular Graft *W.L. Gore & Associates, www.goremedical.com*	Safe	1.5	
Gore TAG Thoracic Endoprosthesis *W. L. Gore & Associates, Inc., www.goremedical.com*	Conditional 8	1.5, 3	
GORE-TEX Stretch Vascular Graft *W.L. Gore & Associates, www.goremedical.com*	Safe	1.5	
GORE-TEX Vascular Graft *W.L. Gore & Associates, www.goremedical.com*	Safe	1.5	
Gore TIPS Endoprosthesis *W. L. Gore & Associates, Inc., www.goremedical.com*	Safe	1.5	
Greenfield vena cava filter *MD Tech, Watertown, MA*	Conditional 2	1.5	21
Greenfield vena cava filter, Titanium alloy *Ormco, Glendora, CA*	Safe	1.5	21
GTX Coronary Artery Stent, CoCr *Global Therapeutics, Broomfield, CO*	Conditional 8	1.5, 3	
Guglielmi detachable coil, Platinum *Target Therapeutics, San Jose, CA*	Safe	1.5	25
Gunther IVC Filter *William Cook, Europe*	Conditional 2	1.5	21
Gunther Tulip Vena Cava Filter *Cook Medical, Inc., www.cookmedical.com*	Conditional 6	3	
Gunther Tulip Vena Cava Filter *Conichrome* *Cook Incorporated, Bloomington, IN*	Conditional 5	3	
Gunther Tulip Vena Cava MReye Filter *Conichrome* *Cook Incorporated, Bloomington, IN*	Conditional 5	3	
HANAROSTENT *M.I. Tech Co., Ltd., Seoul, Korea*	Conditional 8	1.5, 3	
HANAROSTENT Esophagus ST (CCN) *Seoul, Korea*	Conditional 8	1.5, 3	

Object	Status	Field Strength (T)	Reference
HELIPAQ Microcoil *embolization coil* *Micrus Endovascular, www.micrusendovascular.com*	Conditional 5	3	
Hercules Bifurcated Main Body Stent Graft *MicroPort Medical, www.microport.com.cn/english*	Conditional 8	1.5, 3	
Hercules Tubular Stent Graft *MicroPort Medical, www.microport.com.cn/english*	Conditional 8	1.5, 3	
HERCULINK ELITE *Stent*	Conditional 5	3	
Herculink Elite Biliary Stent *Abbott Vascular, www.abbottvascular.com*	Conditional 5	3	
Herculink Plus Biliary Stent *Abbott Vascular, www.abbottvascular.com*	Conditional 5	3	
Hilal Embolization Microcoils *Cook Medical, Inc., www.cookmedical.com*	Conditional 5	3	
Horizon Prostatic Stent, Nitinol *Endocare, Irvine, CA*	Safe	1.5	
HydroCoil Embolic System *embolization coil* *MicroVention, Inc., www.microvention.com*	Conditional 6	3	
HydroCoil Embolic System (HES) Implant *Microvention, www.microvention.com*	Conditional 6	3	
iCast *Atrium Medical Corporation, www.atriummed.com*	Conditional 8	1.5, 3	
Iliac Wallgraft Endoprosthesis *12 x 90* *Schneider (USA) Inc.* *Pfizer Medical Technology Group, Minneapolis, MN*	Safe	1.5	64
Iliac Wallstent Endoprosthesis *5 x 80* *Schneider (USA) Inc.* *Pfizer Medical Technology Group, Minneapolis, MN*	Safe	1.5	64
Iliac Wallstent Endoprosthesis *6 X 90* *Schneider (USA) Inc.* *Pfizer Medical Technology Group, Minneapolis, MN*	Safe	1.5	64
IMPRA Carboflo Vascular Graft *Carbon-impregnated ePTFE* *Bard Peripheral Vascular, www.bardpv.com*	Safe	3	
IMPRA CenterFlex Vascular Graft *Carbon-impregnated ePTFE* *Bard Peripheral Vascular, www.bardpv.com*	Safe	3	
Inflow Gold *15 x 3.0-mm, 316L SS, gold plate, stent* *Inflow Dynamics, Munich, Germany*	Safe	1.5	72
Inflow Gold *9 x 3.0-mm, 316L SS, gold plate, stent* *Inflow Dynamics, Munich, Germany*	Safe	1.5	72
Inflow Stent *316L SS, stent* *Inflow Dynamics, Munich, Germany*	Safe	1.5	69

Object	Status	Field Strength (T)	Reference
Inflow *15 x 3.0-mm, 316L SS, stent* *Inflow Dynamics, Munich, Germany*	Safe	1.5	72
Integrity Coronary Stent *Medtronic, Inc., www.Medtronic.com*	Conditional 5	3	
INTERPAQ Microcoil *embolization coil* *Micrus Endovascular, www.micrusendovascular.com*	Conditional 5	3	
IntraCoil Bronchial Endoprosthesis, stent *Intratherapeutics, Inc., St. Paul, MN*	Safe	1.5	
IntraStent Biliary Endoprosthesis, stent *Intratherapeutics, Inc., St. Paul, MN*	Safe	1.5	
IntraStent DoubleStrut Biliary Endoprosthesis *stent* *Intratherapeutics, Inc., St. Paul, MN*	Safe	1.5	
IntraStent LP Biliary Endoprosthesis *stent* *Intratherapeutics, Inc., St. Paul, MN*	Safe	1.5	
IntraStent Max LD Biliary Stent *ev3, Inc., www.ev3.net*	Conditional 5	1.5	
IntraStent Mega LD Biliary Stent *ev3, Inc., www.ev3.net*	Conditional 5	1.5	
Isthmus Logic Carbostent *CID, cidvascular.com*	Conditional 8	1.5, 3	
Jostent, 316L SS *Jomed, Helsingborg, Sweden*	Safe	1.5	69
Kaneka Stent, Model GGH008 *coronary artery stent* *Kaneka Corporation, Japan*	Conditional 6	3	
L605 Stent *Promed Medical Tech, China*	Conditional 6	3	
Large Diameter Covered Stent *Atrium Medical Corporation, www.atriummed.com*	Conditional 8	1.5, 3	
LEO Plus Next Generation Self-Expanding Intracranial Stent *BALT, France*	Conditional 5	1.5, 3	
LGM IVC Filter, Phynox *B. Braun Vena Tech, Evanston, IL*	Safe	1.5	26
Liberte Coronary Artery Stent *316L SS* *Boston Scientific Corporation, Maple Grove, MN*	Conditional 5	3	
LifeStent FlexStar Stent *Edwards Lifesciences, www.Edwards.com*	Conditional 6	3	
LifeStent FlexStar XL Stent, Nitinol *Edwards Lifesciences, www.Edwards.com*	Conditional 6	3	
LifeStent XL Balloon Expandable Stent *biliary and peripheral vascular stent, 316L SS* *Edwards Lifesciences, www.Edwards.com*	Conditional 6	3	
LithoStent Ureteral Stent, Polyurethane *Gyrus ACMI, Inc., www.gyrusacmi.com*	Safe	3	
Low Profile Covered Stent *Atrium Medical Corporation, www.atriummed.com*	Conditional 8	1.5, 3	

Object	Status	Field Strength (T)	Reference
LPS Stent, bifurcated *36 x 20-mm, Nitinol* *World Medical Manufacturing Corp., Sunrise, FL*	Safe	1.5	70
LPS Thoracic Stent, 46mm, Nitinol *World Medical Manufacturing Corp., Sunrise, FL*	Safe	1.5	70
Lubri-Flex Open Tip Ureteral Stent *Polyurethane* *Gyrus ACMI, Inc., www.gyrusacmi.com*	Safe	3	
LUNA Aneurysm Embolization System *NFOCUS Neuromedical, Inc., Palo Alto, CA*	Conditional 6	3	
Maas Helical Endovascular Stent *Medinvent, Lausanne, Switzerland*	Safe	4.7	21
Maas Helical IVC Filter *Medinvent, Lausanne, Switzerland*	Safe	4.7	21
MAC-Stent, 17 x 3-mm *316L SS* *AMG, Munich, Germany*	Safe	1.5	72
Magic Wallstent *Platinum and cobalt-alloy, stent* *Schneider, Bulach, Switzerland*	Safe	1.5	69
Mardis Ureteral Stent With *Hydro Plus Coating, Mardis Soft Stent* *Boston Scientific, www.bostonscientific.com*	Safe	1.5, 3	
Matrix Detachable Coil *Matrix Extra Firm-2D, Platinum alloy* *Boston Scientific Corporation, www.bostonscientific.com*	Safe	3	
Matrix Detachable Coil *Matrix Extra Firm-3D, Platinum alloy* *Boston Scientific Corporation, www.bostonscientific.com*	Safe	3	
Matrix Detachable Coil *Matrix Firm-2D, Platinum alloy* *Boston Scientific Corporation, www.bostonscientific.com*	Safe	3	
Matrix Detachable Coil *Matrix Firm-3D, Platinum alloy* *Boston Scientific Corporation, www.bostonscientific.com*	Safe	3	
Matrix Detachable Coil *Matrix Soft Helical, Platinum alloy* *Boston Scientific Corporation, www.bostonscientific.com*	Safe	3	
Matrix Detachable Coil *Matrix Soft-2D, Platinum alloy* *Boston Scientific Corporation, www.bostonscientific.com*	Safe	3	
Matrix Detachable Coil *Matrix Standard-2D, Platinum alloy* *Boston Scientific Corporation, www.bostonscientific.com*	Safe	3	
Matrix Detachable Coil *Matrix Standard-3D, Platinum alloy* *Boston Scientific Corporation, www.bostonscientific.com*	Safe	3	
Matrix Stretch Resistant Detachable Coil *Matrix Soft-SR 2D, Platinum alloy* *Boston Scientific Corporation, www.bostonscientific.com*	Safe	3	

Object	Status	Field Strength (T)	Reference
Matrix Stretch Resistant Detachable Coil *Matrix Soft-SR, Platinum alloy* *Boston Scientific Corporation, www.bostonscientific.com*	Safe	3	
Matrix Stretch Resistant Detachable Coil *Matrix Standard-SR 2D, Platinum alloy* *Boston Scientific Corporation, www.bostonscientific.com*	Safe	3	
Matrix Stretch Resistant Detachable Coil *Matrix UltraSoft-SR, Platinum alloy* *Boston Scientific Corporation, www.bostonscientific.com*	Safe	3	
Medtronic AVE Stent, 316L SS, gold *Medtronic, Inc., www.medtronic.com*	Safe	1.5	70
Megalink Biliary Stent *Abbott Vascular, www.abbottvascular.com*	Conditional 5	3	
Mercury Carotid Artery Stent, Nitinol *MicroPort Medical Co., Ltd., People's Republic of China*	Conditional 6	3	
Merlin MD Aneurysm Occlusion Device (AOD) *316L SS, gold markers, polyurethane* *Merlin MD Pte Ltd, Singapore*	Conditional 6	3	
MicroStent II, 316L SS *Medtronic, Inc., www.Medtronic.com*	Safe	1.5	72
Micro-Driver Coronary Stent *Medtronic, Inc., www.Medtronic.com*	Conditional 6	3	
Micro-Driver *MP35N, stent* *Medtronic, Inc., www.Medtronic.com*	Conditional 5	3	
MicroNester *Cook Medical, Inc., www.cookmedical.com*	Conditional 5	3	
MicroPlex Coil System *embolization coil* *MicroVention, Inc., Tustin, CA*	Conditional 6	3	
Microvention Flow Diverter and Coil-Assist Stent *Microvention, www.microvention.com*	Conditional 8	1.5, 3	
MICRUSPHERE Microcoil *embolization coil* *Micrus Endovascular, www.micrusendovascular.com*	Conditional 5	3	
Mini-Crown Stent *316L SS* *Cordis, www.depuy.com*	Safe	1.5	69
Misago Stent *Terumo Medical Corporation, www.terumomedical.com*	Conditional 8	1.5, 3	
Misago Peripheral Stent *Terumo Medical Corporation, www.terumomedical.com*	Conditional 5	1.5, 3	
MiStent Drug-Eluting Coronary Stent *Micell Technologies, Inc., www.micell.com*	Conditional 8	1.5, 3	
Mobin-Uddin IVC/umbrella filter *American Edwards, Santa Ana, CA*	Safe	4.7	21
Mobius O, Type E Stent *Vascular Dynamics, Israel*	Conditional 6	3	
MREYE Embolization Coil *Cook Medical, Inc., www.cookmedical.com*	Conditional 6	3	

Object	Status	Field Strength (T)	Reference
MReye Flipper Detachable Embolization Coils *Cook Medical, Inc., www.cookmedical.com*	Conditional 5	3	
Multi-Flex Open Tip *Ureteral Stent, Polyurethane* *Gyrus ACMI, Inc., www.gyrusacmi.com*	Safe	3	
MULTI-LINK DUET *Stent, 2.5 to 4.0-mm (RX and OTW), 316L SS* *Abbott Vascular, www.abbottvascular.com*	Conditional 5	3	
MULTI-LINK MINI VISION Coronary Stent *Abbott Vascular, www.abbottvascular.com*	Conditional 5	3	
MULTI-LINK PENTA Coronary Stent *Abbott Vascular, www.abbottvascular.com*	Conditional 5	3	
MULTI-LINK PIXEL Coronary Stent *Abbott Vascular, www.abbottvascular.com*	Conditional 5	3	
MULTI-LINK TETRA Coronary Stent *Abbott Vascular, www.abbottvascular.com*	Conditional 5	3	
MULTI-LINK TRISTAR Stent *Abbott Vascular, www.abbottvascular.com*	Conditional 5	3	
MULTI-LINK VISION Coronary Stent *Abbott Vascular, www.abbottvascular.com*	Conditional 5	3	
MULTI-LINK ULTRA Stent *Abbott Vascular, www.abbottvascular.com*	Conditional 5	3	
MULTI-LINK ZETA Coronary Stent *Abbott Vascular, www.abbottvascular.com*	Conditional 5	3	
MULTI-LINK Stent, 2.5 to 4.0-mm (RX and OTW) *316L SS* *Abbott Vascular, www.abbottvascular.com*	Conditional 5	3	
NEC Hemi Device *Coils, Filters, Stents* *NFocus Neuromedical, Palo Alto, CA*	Conditional 6	3	
Nellix AAA Endoprosthesis *Nellix Endovascular, Palo Alto, CA*	Conditional 8	1.5, 3	
Nester Embolization Coil *Cook Medical, Inc., www.cookmedical.com*	Conditional 6	3	
Neuroform Stent *Boston Scientific, www.bostonscientific.com*	Conditional 5	3	108
Neuroform3 Stent *Boston Scientific, www.bostonscientific.com*	Conditional 5	3	
Neurolink Stent *Abbott Vascular, www.abbottvascular.com*	Conditional 5	1.5	
Neurostring Embolization Coil *Biomerix Corporation, Fremont, CA*	Conditional 6	3	
NEVO Sirolimus-eluting *Coronary Artery Stent* *Cordis Corporation*	Conditional 8	1.5, 3	
New retrievable IVC filter *Thomas Jefferson University, Philadelphia, PA*	Conditional 2	1.5	21
NexStent Carotid Stent *Nitinol, stent* *EndoTex Interventional Solutions, Cupertino, CA*	Safe	3	

Object	Status	Field Strength (T)	Reference
Nexus Detachable Coil *embolization coil* *ev3, Inc., www.ev3.net*	Conditional 5	3	
Nexus Embolization Coil *Nexus X-10-20-T10-TC, Platinum-Iridium, Nitinol* *Micro Therapeutics, Inc., Irvine, CA*	Conditional 6	3	
NIR Stent *MR-safe metal* *Medinol Ltd., Jerusalem, Israel*	Safe	1.5	69
NIR Royal Advance Stent *Boston Scientific, www.bostonscientific.com*	Conditional 5	1.5	
Nitinol Braided Neuro Coil Assist Stent *MicroVention, Inc., www.microvention.com*	Conditional 6	3	
Non-Vascular Stent, Double Spherical, Covered, 38-mm x 200-mm *Micro-Tech, www.stent.cc*	Conditional 8	1.5, 3	
Non-Vascular Stent, Double Spherical, 38-mm x 200-mm *Micro-Tech, www.stent.cc*	Conditional 8	1.5, 3	
Non-Vascular Stent, 10-mm x 120-mm, Straight *Micro-Tech, www.stent.cc*	Conditional 8	1.5, 3	
Non-Vascular Stent, Y-shape *Micro-Tech, www.stent.cc*	Conditional 8	1.5, 3	
Nuloy Stent *Coronary Artery Stent* *Icon Interventional Systems, Inc., Cleveland, OH*	Conditional 6	3	
NXT Detachable Coil *embolization coil* *ev3, Inc., www.ev3.net*	Conditional 5	3	
NXT Tetris Detachable Coil *embolization coil* *ev3, Inc., www.ev3.net*	Conditional 5	3	
Omnilink Elite Stent *Abbott Vascular Instruments Deutschland GmbH, Germany*	Conditional 8	1.5, 3	
Omnilink Biliary Stent *Abbott Vascular, www.abbottvascular.com*	Conditional 5	3	
OPTEASE Retrievable Vena Cava Filter *Cordis, www.depuy.com*	Conditional 5	3	
Optimized Flair Endovascular Stent Graft *9-mm x 50-mm* *Bard Peripheral Vascular, www.bardpv.com*	Conditional 6	3	
Option Vena Cava Filter *REX MEDICAL, Conshohocken, PA*	Conditional 5	3	
Orbit Galaxy Embolization Coil *Codman, www.depuy.com*	Conditional 6	3	
Ovation Abdominal Stent Graft *Trivascular, www.Trivascular.com*	Conditional 6	3	
Ovation Thoracic Stent Graft *Trivascular, www.Trivascular.com*	Conditional 6	3	
PALMAZ BLUE Stent *Cordis, www.depuy.com*	Conditional 5	3	
PALMAZ BLUE Transhepatic Biliary Stent *Cordis, www.depuy.com*	Conditional 5	3	

Object	Status	Field Strength (T)	Reference
Palmaz Endovascular Stent *Cordis, www.depuy.com*	Conditional 5	3	
PALMAZ Genesis Stent *Cordis, www.depuy.com*	Conditional 5	3	
Palmaz Genesis Peripheral Stent *316L SS* *Cordis, www.depuy.com*	Conditional 5	3	
Palmaz Genesis Transhepatic Biliary Stent *316L SS* *Cordis, www.depuy.com*	Conditional 5	3	
Palmaz-Schatz Stent *15 x 3.0-mm, 316L SS* *Cordis, www.depuy.com*	Safe	1.5	72
Palmaz-Schatz Stent *P-S 153, 316L SS* *Cordis, www.depuy.com*	Safe	1.5	69
Palmaz-Schatz Stent *P-S 154, 316L SS* *Cordis, www.depuy.com*	Safe	1.5	69
Palmaz-Shatz *balloon-expandable stent* *Cordis, www.depuy.com*	Conditional 2	1.5	
ParaMount Mini Biliary Stent *ev3, Inc., www.ev3.net*	Conditional 5	1.5	
Passager Stent *tantalum, 10-mm x 30-mm* *Meadox Surgimed, Oakland, NJ*	Safe	1.5	
Passager Stent *tantalum, 4-mm x 30-mm* *Meadox Surgimed, Oakland, NJ*	Safe	1.5	
Penumbra Embolization Coil *Penumbra Inc., Alameda, CA*	Conditional 6	3	
Percuflex Plus *Stent Graft with Suprarenal, Ureteral Stent* *4.8 Fr. (1.6-mm x 220-mm)* *Boston Scientific Corporation, Watertown, MA*	Safe	1.5, 3	83
Percuflex Plus Ureteral Stent *With Hydro Plus Coating* *Boston Scientific, www.bostonscientific.com*	Safe	1.5, 3	
Percuflex Ureteral Stent *Boston Scientific, www.bostonscientific.com*	Safe	1.5, 3	
PHAROS Stent, carotid artery stent *BIOTRONIK*	Conditional 6	3	
Pipeline Embolization Device, PED *embolization coil* *ev3, Inc., www.ev3.com*	Conditional 5	3	
Polaris Loop Ureteral Stent *Boston Scientific, www.bostonscientific.com*	Safe	1.5, 3	
Polaris Ultra *Dual Durometer Ureteral Stent* *Boston Scientific, www.bostonscientific.com*	Safe	1.5, 3	

Object	Status	Field Strength (T)	Reference
Polaris Ultra Ureteral Stent *Boston Scientific, www.bostonscientific.com*	Safe	1.5, 3	
Polyflex Airway Stent *Silicone and polyester* *Boston Scientific, www.bostonscientific.com*	Safe	1.5	
Powerlink Suprarenal *Bifurcated Stent Graft, Model 34-16-175RBL* *Endologix, Irvine, CA*	Conditional 8	1.5, 3	
PowerLink *cobalt-alloy* *Endologix, Inc., Irvine, CA*	Safe	1.5	70
PowerWeb, Model 1 *cobalt-alloy* *Endologix, Inc., Irvine, CA*	Safe	1.5	70
PowerWeb *cobalt-alloy* *Endologix, Inc., Irvine, CA*	Safe	1.5	70
Precedent Stent *Nitinol, Platinum* *Boston Scientific, Wayne, NJ*	Safe	1.5	70
Precise Microvascular Anastomotic Device (MACD) *316L SS*	Safe	1.5	71
Precise Nitinol Stent, Carotid *Cordis, www.depuy.com, www.cordislabeling.com com*	Conditional 5	1.5	
Precise Pro RX Nitinol Stent *Cordis, www.depuy.com, www.cordislabeling.com com*	Conditional 5	1.5	
Precise RX Nitinol Stent *Cordis, www.depuy.com, www.cordislabeling.com com*	Conditional 5	1.5	
PRESIDIO Microcoil *embolization coil* *Micrus Endovascular, www.micrusendovascular.com*	Conditional 5	3	
Presillion Stent *Medinol, www.medinol.com*	Conditional 8	1.5, 3	
PRIMUS Biliary Stent *ev3, Inc., www.ev3.net*	Conditional 5	1.5	
PRO-Kinetic Energy Stent *BIOTRONIK*	Conditional 6	3	
PRO-Kinetic Stent *coronary artery stent* *BIOTRONIK*	Conditional 6	3	
PROMUS Everolimus-Eluting Coronary Stent *PROMUS Stent* *Boston Scientific, www.bostonscientific.com*	Conditional 5	3	
ProPass Stent *Vascular Innovations, Inc., Freemont, CA*	Conditional 6	3	
Protege EverFlex Self-Expanding Biliary Stent *ev3, Inc., www.ev3.net*	Conditional 5	1.5	
Protege EverFlex Self-Expanding Stent *ev3 Inc., Plymouth, MN*	Conditional 5	1.5, 3	
Protege GPS Carotid Stent *ev3, Inc., www.ev3.net*	Conditional 5	3	

Object	Status	Field Strength (T)	Reference
Protege GPS Self-Expanding Stent *ev3 Inc., www.ev3.net*	Conditional 8	1.5, 3	
Protege GPS Self-Expanding Biliary Stent *ev3, Inc., www.ev3.net*	Conditional 5	1.5	
Protege RX Carotid Stent *ev3, Inc., www.ev3.net*	Conditional 5	3	
Quadra-coil Ureteral Stent *Polyurethane* *Gyrus ACMI, Inc., www.gyrusacmi.com*	Safe	3	
R Stent *316 LVM SS* *Spectranetics Corporation, Colorado Springs, CO*	Safe	1.5	
R Stent, 316L SS *Orbus Medical Technologies, Fort Lauderdale, FL*	Safe	1.5	
Racer Biliary Stent System *cobalt alloy, stent* *Medtronic, Inc., www.Medtronic.com*	Safe	3	
Radius Stent, 4.0-mm x 31-mm, Nitinol *Boston Scientific, www.bostonscientific.com*	Safe	1.5, 3	
Radius Stent, Nitinol *Boston Scientific, wwww.bostonscientific.com*	Safe	1.5	69
Recovery G2 Filter, Vena Cava Filter *Femoral Vein* *Bard Peripheral Vascular, www.bardpv.com*	Conditional 5	1.5	
Recovery Nitinol Filter, Nitinol *Bard Peripheral Vascular, www.bardpv.com*	Safe	3	
Relay Plus Stent Graft *Bolton Medical, Inc., www.boltonmedical.com*	Conditional 8	1.5, 3	
Resonance Double Pigtail Ureteral Stent, MP35N *Cook Medical, www.cookmedical.com*	Conditional 6	3	
RX HERCULINK ELITE, Biliary Stent, 316L SS	Conditional 6	3	
S3 Stent, L605 Cobalt-Chrome *Medlogics Device Corporation, Santa Rosa, CA*	Conditional 6	3	
S540 Stent *Medtronic, Inc., www.Medtronic.com*	Conditional 5	3	
S660 Stent *Medtronic, Inc., www.Medtronic.com*	Conditional 5	3	
S670, 4.0-mm x 30-mm, 316L SS, stent *Medtronic, Inc., www.Medtronic.com*	Safe	3	
S7, 4.0-mm x 30-mm, 316L SS, stent *Medtronic, Inc., www.Medtronic.com*	Safe	3	
SafeFlo IVC Filter *inferior vena cava filter, Nitinol, Titanium* *Rafael Medical Technologies, Inc., Israel*	Conditional 6	3	
Sapphire Detachable Coil *embolization coil, platinum alloy* *ev3, Inc. Neurovascular Division, ev3.net*	Conditional 5	1.5	
Scuba Stent, Scuba Co-Cr Peripheral Stent *Invatec/Medtronic, www.invatec.com*	Conditional 8	1.5, 3	
Seaquence stent, 316L SS *Nycomed Amersham, Princeton, NJ*	Safe	1.5	72

Object	Status	Field Strength (T)	Reference
Self-expanding Neuroendograft Stent *Surpass Medical Ltd., www.surpass-med.com*	Conditional 6	3	
Silhouette Ureteral Patency Device *MRI information applies to all Silhouette Devices* *Applied Medical Resources, Rancho Santa Margarita, CA*	Conditional 8	1.5, 3	
Silk Artery Reconstruction Device *stent* *BALT, France*	Conditional 8	1.5, 3	
Single-J Urinary *Diversion Specialty Stent, Silicone* *Gyrus ACMI, Inc., www.gyrusacmi.com*	Safe	3	
Simon Nitinol Filter *vena cava filter* *C.R. Bard, Tempe, AZ*	Conditional 6	3	
S.M.A.R.T. CONTROL Nitinol Stent *Transhepatic Biliary System* *Cordis, www.depuy.com*	Conditional 6	3	
S.M.A.R.T. *Shape Memory Alloy Recoverable Technology, Nitinol Stent* *Cordis, www.depuy.com*	Conditional 6	3	
S.M.A.R.T. Nitinol Stent *Transhepatic Biliary System* *Cordis, www.depuy.com*	Conditional 5	3	
Sof-Curl Ureteral Stent *Polyurethane* *Gyrus ACMI, Inc., www.gyrusacmi.com*	Safe	3	
SOLITAIRE AB Neurovascular Remodeling Device *ev3, Inc., www.ev3.com*	Conditional 5	3	
Solitaire Flow Restoration Stent *Nitinol, SS, Platinum* *ev3 Inc., Irvine, CA*	Conditional 8	1.5, 3	
Solus Double Pigtail Stent *Cook Medical, Inc., www.cookmedical.com*	Conditional 6	3	
St. Jude Carotid Stent *10-7 x 40-mm taper stent, two-overlapped version* *St. Jude Medical, www.sjmprofessional.com*	Conditional 6	3	
St. Jude Carotid Stent *10-7 x 50-mm taper stent, single version* *St. Jude Medical, www.sjmprofessional.com*	Conditional 6	3	
Standard Embolization Coil *MWCE-52-15-20, Stainless Steel* *Cook Medical, www.cookmedical.com*	Unsafe 1	1.5	
Strecker stent *tantalum* *MD Tech, Watertown, MA*	Safe	1.5	27
Stentys Bifurcation Stent *Stentys Inc., www.stentys.com*	Conditional 6	3	
Stentys Coronary Stent *Stentys Inc., www.stentys.com*	Conditional 8	1.5, 3	
Stretch VL Flexima Ureteral Stent *With Hydro Plus Coating* *Boston Scientific, www.bostonscientific.com*	Safe	1.5, 3	

Object	Status	Field Strength (T)	Reference
Strider Stent *biliary artery, iliac artery, Nitinol with tantalum markers* *Medtronic, Inc., www.Medtronic.com*	Safe	3	
SUPERA Biliary Stent *IDEV Technologies, Inc., www.idevmd.com*	Conditional 5	1.5, 3	
Supera Stent *IDEV Technologies, Inc., www.idevmd.com*	Conditional 5	1.5, 3	
Svelte Bare Metal Stent *single and two overlapped versions* *Svelte Medical Systems, New Providence, NJ*	Conditional 8	1.5, 3	
TAA Endograft *TriVascular2, Inc., Santa Rosa, CA*	Conditional 6	3	
Taarget Stent Graft *LeMaitre Vascular, Burlington, MA*	Conditional 6	3	
TAG Endoprosthesis *thoracic aneurysm stent graft, 45-mm x 20-cm endoprostheses* *W.L. Gore & Associates, www.goremedical.com*	Conditional 5	3	
Talent Abdominal Stent Graft *Medtronic, Inc., www.Medtronic.com* *http://manuals.medtronic.com/en/index.htm*	Conditional 5	3	
Talent Graft Stent *bare spring model, 16 x 8-mm, Nitinol* *World Medical Manufacturing Corp., Sunrise, FL*	Safe	1.5	
Talent Graft Stent *bare spring model, 36 x 20-mm, Nitinol* *World Medical Manufacturing Corp., Sunrise, FL*	Safe	1.5	
Talent Graft Stent *open web model, 16 x 8-mm, Nitinol* *World Medical Manufacturing Corp., Sunrise, FL*	Safe	1.5	
Talent Graft Stent *open web model, 36 x 20-mm, Nitinol* *World Medical Manufacturing Corp., Sunrise, FL*	Safe	1.5	
Talent Thoracic Graft *Medtronic, Inc., www.Medtronic.com* *http://manuals.medtronic.com/en/index.htm*	Conditional 5	3	
TAXUS Element Stent *Boston Scientific, www.bostonscientific.com*	Conditional 5	3	
TAXUS Express *Paclitaxel-Eluting Coronary Stent, 316L SS* *Boston Scientific, www.bostonscientific.com*	Conditional 5	3	
TAXUS Express2 Atom Stent *Boston Scientific, www.bostonscientific.com*	Conditional 5	3	
TAXUS Express2 Atom Paclitaxel-eluting Coronary Stent *Boston Scientific, www.bostonscientific.com*	Conditional 5	3	
TAXUS Liberte *Paclitaxel-Eluting Coronary Stent, 316L SS* *Boston Scientific, www.bostonscientific.com*	Conditional 5	3	
TAXUS Liberte Atom Paclitaxel-Eluting Coronary Stent *TAXUS Liberte Atom Stent* *Boston Scientific, www.bostonscientific.com*	Conditional 5	3	

Object	Status	Field Strength (T)	Reference
TAXUS Liberte Long Paclitaxel-Eluting Coronary Stent *TAXUS Liberte Long Stent Boston Scientific,* *www.bostonscientific.com*	Conditional 5	3	
Thoraflex Device *Stent Graft* *Vascutek Ltd., www.vascutek.com*	Conditional 8	1.5, 3	
Tornado Embolization Coils *Cook Medical, Inc., www.cookmedical.com*	Conditional 5	3	
Tracheobronchial *Wallstent Endoprosthesis, 14 x 80, stent* *Schneider (USA) Inc.* *Pfizer Medical Technology Group, Minneapolis, MN*	Safe	1.5	64
Tracheobronchial *Wallstent Endoprosthesis, 24 x 70, stent* *Schneider (USA) Inc.* *Pfizer Medical Technology Group, Minneapolis, MN*	Safe	1.5	64
TRAPEASE Permanent Vena Cava Filter *Cordis, www.depuy.com*	Conditional 5	3	
Treovance Abdominal Stent Graft *Bolton Medical, Inc., Sunrise, FL*	Conditional 8	1.5, 3	
TriMaxx Coronary Stent *SS-Tantalum composite, stent* *Abbott Vascular Devices, Redwood City, CA*	Safe	3	
Tryton Side Branch Stent *Tryton Medical, www.trytonmedical.com*	Conditional 6	3	
TRUFILL DCS ORBIT Detachable Coil *embolization coil, Platinum, Tungsten* *Cordis, www.depuy.com*	Safe	3	87
TRUFILL Pushable Coils *Vascular Occlusion System, Platinum* *Cordis, www.depuy.com*	Safe	1.5	
Ultraflex *stent, Titanium alloy*	Safe	1.5	73
Uncovered WallFlex Biliary RX Stent System *Boston Scientific, www.bostonscientific.com*	Conditional 6	3	
Uro-Guide Open Tip *Ureteral Stent, Silicone* *Gyrus ACMI, Inc., www.gyrusacmi.com*	Safe	3	
ULTIPAQ Microcoil *embolization coil* *Micrus Endovascular, www.micrusendovascular.com*	Conditional 5	3	
V12 Renal Covered Stent *Atrium Medical Corporation, www.atriummed.com*	Conditional 8	1.5, 3	
Valecor Platinum Stent *coronary artery stent, CoCr L605, Platinum* *Cornova, Inc., Burlington, MA*	Conditional 8	1.5, 3	
Valeo Biliary Stent *Bard Peripheral Vascular, Inc., www.bardpv.com*	Conditional 6	3	
Valiant Thoracic Stent Graft *Medtronic, Inc., www.Medtronic.com*	Safe	3	

Object	Status	Field Strength (T)	Reference
Vanguard Stent *Nitinol, Platinum* *Boston Scientific, Wayne, NJ*	Safe	1.5	70
VascuFlex SE Stent *B. Braun, www.bbraunusa.com*	Conditional 5	1.5, 3	
VascuFlex SEC Stent *B. Braun, www.bbraunusa.com*	Conditional 5	1.5, 3	
VBS Stent (also known as the Verdi Stent) *Synthes GmbH, Switzerland*	Conditional 6	3	
Vectra VAG *Vascular Access Graft* *Thoralon* *Bard Peripheral Vascular, www.bardpv.com*	Safe	3	
VENAFLO II Vascular Graft *Carbon-impregnated ePTFE* *Bard Peripheral Vascular, www.bardpv.com*	Safe	3	
VENAFLO Vascular Graft *Carbon-impregnated ePTFE* *Bard Peripheral Vascular, www.bardpv.com*	Safe	3	
VenaTech Convertible, Vena Cava Filter *B. Braun, www.bbraunusa.com*	Conditional 5	3	
VenaTech LGM Vena Cava Filter *B. Braun, www.bbraunusa.com*	Conditional 5	1.5, 3	
VenaTech LP Vena Cava Filter *B. Braun, www.bbraunusa.com*	Conditional 5	1.5, 3	
VeriFLEX (Liberte) Stent *Boston Scientific, www.bostonscientific.com*	Conditional 5	1.5, 3	
VIABAHN Endoprosthesis *13-mm x 10-cm, Nitinol* *W. L. Gore & Associates, Inc., www.goremedical.com*	Conditional 5	1.5, 3	
VIABAHN Endoprosthesis *8-mm x 25-cm, single version, Nitinol* *W.L. Gore & Associates, www.goremedical.com*	Conditional 5	1.5, 3	
VIABAHN Endoprosthesis *8-mm x 25-cm, two-overlapped version, Nitinol* *W.L. Gore & Associates, www.goremedical.com*	Conditional 5	1.5, 3	
VIABAHN Endoprosthesis *9-mm x 15-cm, Nitinol* *W. L. Gore & Associates, Inc., www.goremedical.com*	Conditional 5	1.5, 3	
VIABAHN Endoprosthesis *W.L. Gore and Associates, Inc., www.goremedical.com*	Conditional 5	1.5, 3	
VIABIL Biliary Endoprosthesis *W.L. Gore and Associates, Inc., www.goremedical.com*	Conditional 5	3	
VIATORR Endoprosthesis *Stent, Nitinol* *W.L. Gore and Associates, Inc., www.goremedical.com*	Conditional 5	1.5	
VIATORR TIPS Endoprosthesis *W.L. Gore and Associates, Inc., www.goremedical.com*	Conditional 5	3	
Valiant Thoracic Stent Graft *Medtronic, Inc., www.Medtronic.com*	Conditional 5	3	

Object	Status	Field Strength (T)	Reference
Vena Tech LP *vascular filter* *B. Braun, www.bbraunusa.com*	Conditional 5	1.5	
Visi-Pro Balloon Expandable Stent *ev3 Inc., www.ev3.net*	Conditional 8	1.5, 3	
Visi-Pro Biliary Stent *ev3, Inc., www.ev3.net*	Conditional 5	3	
VIVAL Coronary Stent *Avantec Vascular, Sunnyvale, CA*	Conditional 6	3	
vProtect Luminal Shield *Nitinol, Tantalum, Stent* *Prescient Medical, Inc., Doylestown, PA*	Conditional 8	1.5, 3	
V-Track Embolization Coil, HydroCoil *MicroVention, Inc., www.microvention.com*	Conditional 6	3	
V-Track Embolization Coil, MultiPlex *MicroVention, Inc., www.microvention.com*	Conditional 6	3	
V-Trak, HydroCoil, MicroCoil *Embolic Coil(s), Embolization Coil(s)* *Microvention, www.microvention.com*	Conditional 8	1.5, 3	
WallFlex Biliary RX Stent *Boston Scientific, www.bostonscientific.com*	Conditional 5	3	
WallFlex Biliary Stent *covered version* *Boston Scientific, www.bostonscientific.com*	Safe	3	
WallFlex Biliary Stent *uncovered version* *Boston Scientific, www.bostonscientific.com*	Safe	3	
WallFlex Enteral Colonic Stent with Anchor Lock Delivery System *Nitinol* *Boston Scientific, www.bostonscientific.com*	Safe	3	
WallFlex Enteral Duodenal Stent with Anchor Lock Delivery System *Nitinol* *Boston Scientific, www.bostonscientific.com*	Safe	3	
WallFlex Partially Covered Esophageal Stent *Boston Scientific, www.bostonscientific.com*	Conditional 5	3	
WallGraft *Elgiloy* *Boston Scientific, www.bostonscientific.com*	Safe	3	
WallStent biliary endoprosthesis *stent, high nickle SS* *Schneider USA, Plymouth, MN*	Safe	1.5	28
WALLSTENT Endoprosthesis *Boston Scientific, www.bostonscientific.com*	Conditional 5	3	
WallStent Endoprosthesis *Magic Wallstent, 3.5 x 25, stent* *Schneider (USA) Inc.* *Pfizer Medical Technology Group, Minneapolis, MN*	Safe	1.5	64
WallStent Endoprosthesis *With Permalume covering, 8 x 80, stent* *Schneider (USA) Inc.* *Pfizer Medical Technology Group, Minneapolis, MN*	Safe	1.5	64

Object	Status	Field Strength (T)	Reference
WallStent Esophageal II Endoprosthesis *20 x 130, stent* *Schneider (USA) Inc.* *Pfizer Medical Technology Group, Minneapolis, MN*	Safe	1.5	64
WallStent *carotid artery stent* *Boston Scientific, www.bostonscientific.com*	Safe	3	
WallStent *Platinum and cobalt-alloy* *Schneider, Bulach, Switzerland*	Safe	1.5	69
WALLSTENT RX Biliary Endoprosthesis *Boston Scientific, www.bostonscientific.com*	Conditional 5	3	
WEB Aneurysm Embolization Device *Sequent Medical, Inc., Aliso Viejo, CA*	Conditional 6	3	
Wiktor coronary artery stent *Medtronic, Inc. www.Medtronic.com*	Safe	1.5	
Wiktor GX Stent *Medtronic, Inc., www.Medtronic.com*	Safe	1.5	72
Willis Stent *MicroPort Medical, www.microport.com.cn/english*	Conditional 8	1.5, 3	
Wilson-Cook Pancreatic Stent *Wilson-Cook Medical, Inc., Winston-Salem, NC*	Safe	1.5	
Wilson-Cook Pancreatic Wedge Stent *Wilson-Cook Medical, Inc., Winston-Salem, NC*	Safe	1.5	
Wingspan Stent System *Boston Scientific, www.bostonscientific.com*	Safe	3	
Xact Stent, Nitinol *Abbott Vascular, www.abbottvascular.com*	Safe	3	
XactfleX Carotid Stent, Nitinol *Abbott Vascular, www.abbottvascular.com*	Safe	3	
Xceed Biliary Stent *Abbott Vascular, www.abbottvascular.com*	Conditional 5	3	
XIENCE PRIME Stent *Abbott Vascular, www.abbottvascular.com*	Conditional 5	3	
XIENCE V Everolimus Eluting Coronary Stent *Abbott Vascular, www.abbottvascular.com*	Conditional 5	3	
XIENCE V Stent *Abbott Vascular, www.abbottvascular.com*	Conditional 5	3	
Xpert Biliary Stent *Abbott Vascular, www.abbottvascular.com*	Conditional 5	3	
Xpert Stent *Nitinol* *Abbott Vascular, www.abbottvascular.com*	Conditional 6	3	
X-Suit NIR Biliary Metallic Stent *Olympus and Medinol, www.medinol.com*	Conditional 5	1.5, 3	
XSuit-NIR Covered Biliary Stent *Medinol Ltd., Israel*	Conditional 8	1.5, 3	
XTENT Customizable Stent *Coronary Artery Stent* *XTENT, Inc., Menlo Park, CA*	Conditional 6	3	

Object	Status	Field Strength (T)	Reference
X-Trode, 3 segment *stent, 316 SS* *C.R. Bard, Inc., Billerica, MA*	Safe	1.5	
X-Trode, 9 segment *stent, 316 SS* *C.R. Bard, Inc., Billerica, MA*	Safe	1.5	
Zenith AAA Endovascular Graft, Ancillary Components *Stent* *Cook Medical, www.cookmedical.com*	Conditional 5	1.5, 3	
Zenith AAA Endovascular Grafts, Bifurcated, Stent *Cook Medical, www.cookmedical.co*	Conditional 5	1.5, 3	
Zenith AAA Endovascular Graft *Zenith Flex AAA, Stent* *Including starting with prefix TFB, TFFB, TFLE, ELSE,* *ESBE, ESC, ESP, ZIP, AX1, RX1* *Cook Medical* *www.cookmedical.com/di/productMri.doc*	Conditional 5 *Conditional 5*	3	
Zenith AAA Spiral, Z Iliac Leg Graft, Stent *Cook Medical, Inc., www.cookmedical.com*	Conditional 5	1.5, 3	
Zenith Renu AAA Ancillary Grafts, Stent *Cook Medical, www.cookmedical.com*	Conditional 5	1.5, 3	
Zenith TX2 Low-Profile TAA Endovascular Graft, Stent *Cook Medical, Inc., www.cookmedical.com*	Conditional 5	1.5, 3	
Zenith TX2 TAA Endovascular Graft *Cook Medical, Inc., www.cookmedical.com*	Conditional 8	1.5, 3	
Zilver 6 Fr Flex Stent *Cook Medical, Inc., www.cookmedical.com*	Conditional 8	1.5, 3	
Zilver Flex 35 Biliary Stent *Cook Medical, Inc., www.cookmedical.com*	Conditional 8	1.5, 3	
ZILVER FLEX 35 Vascular Stent *Cook Medical, Inc., www.cookmedical.com*	Conditional 8	1.5, 3	
Zilver 518 Vascular *Cook Medical, Inc., www.cookmedical.com*	Conditional 5	3	
Zilver 518 Biliary *Cook Medical, Inc., www.cookmedical.com*	Conditional 5	3	
Zilver 635 Vascular *Cook Medical, Inc., www.cookmedical.com*	Conditional 5	3	
Zilver 635 Biliary *Cook Medical, Inc., www.cookmedical.com*	Conditional 5	3	
Zilver PTX Drug Eluting Peripheral Stent *Cook Medical, Inc., www.cookmedical.com*	Conditional 8	1.5, 3	
Zilver Stent, Iliac artery *Cook Medical, Inc., www.cookmedical.com*	Conditional 5	3	
Zilver Stent, Nitinol, gold *Cook Medical, Inc., www.cookmedical.com*	Conditional 5	3	
Zilver Self-Expanding Stent *Cook Medical, Inc., www.cookmedical.com*	Conditional 5	3	
Zimmon Pancreatic Stent *Cook Medical, Inc., www.cookmedical.com*	Conditional 8	1.5, 3	

Object	Status	Field Strength (T)	Reference
Dental Implants, Devices, and Materials			
Brace band, SS, dental	Conditional 1	1.5	3
American Dental, Missoula, MT			
Brace wire, chrome alloy	Conditional 1	1.5	3
dental			
Ormco Corp., San Marcos, CA			
Castable alloy, dental	Conditional 1	1.5	12
Golden Dental Products, Inc., Golden, CO			
Cement-in keeper, dental	Conditional 1	1.5	12
Solid State Innovations, Inc., Mt. Airy, NC			
Dental amalgam	Safe	1.39	1
dental material			
GDP Direct Keeper, Pre-formed post, dental	Conditional 1	1.5	12
Golden Dental Products, Inc., Golden, CO			
Gutta Percha Points	Safe	1.5	
dental device			
Indian Head Real Silver Points, dental	Safe	1.5	
Union Broach Co., Inc., New York, NY			
Keeper, pre-formed post, dental	Conditional 1	1.5	1
Parkell Products, Inc., Farmingdale, NY			
Magna-Dent, large indirect keeper, dental	Conditional 1	1.5	1
Dental Ventures of America, Yorba Linda, CA			
Palladium clad magnet, dental	Unsafe 1	1.5	13
Parkell Products, Inc., Farmingdale, NY			
Palladium/palladium keeper, dental	Conditional 1	1.5	13
Parkell Products, Inc., Farmingdale, NY			
Palladium/Platinum casting alloy, dental	Conditional 1	1.5	13
Parkell Products, Inc., Farmingdale, NY			
Permanent crown	Safe	1.5	3
amalgam, dental			
Ormco Corp.			
Silver point, dental	Safe	1.5	3
Union Broach Co., Inc., New York, NY			
Stainless steel clad magnet, dental	Unsafe 1	1.5	13
Parkell Products, Inc., Farmingdale, NY			
Stainless steel keeper, dental	Conditional 1	1.5	13
Parkell Products, Inc., Farmingdale, NY			
Titanium clad magnet, dental	Unsafe 1	1.5	13
Parkell Products, Inc., Farmingdale, NY			

Object	Status	Field Strength (T)	Reference
ECG Electrodes			
Accutac, ECG electrode *ConMed Corp., Utica, NY*	Safe	1.5	
Accutac, ECG electrode *Diaphoretic* *ConMed Corp., Utica, NY*	Safe	1.5	
Adult Cloth, ECG electrode *ConMed Corp., Utica, NY*	Safe	1.5	
Adult ECG, ECG electrode *Electrode 3-Pack* *ConMed Corp., Utica, NY*	Safe	1.5	
Adult Foam, ECG electrode *ConMed Corp., Utica, NY*	Safe	1.5	
Cardiac Monitoring ECG Electrode, 2244 *3M, www.3m.com*	Conditional 5	3	
Cardiac Monitoring ECG Electrode, 2570 *3M, www.3m.com*	Conditional 5	3	
Cardiac Monitoring ECG Electrode, 2660 *3M, www.3m.com*	Conditional 5	3	
Cardiac Monitoring ECG Electrode, 2670 *3M, www.3m.com*	Conditional 5	3	
Cleartrace 2, ECG electrode *ConMed Corp., Utica, NY*	Safe	1.5	
Dyna/Trace Diagnostic *ECG Electrode* *ConMed Corp., Utica, NY*	Safe	1.5	
Dyna/Trace Mini, ECG electrode *ConMed Corp., Utica, NY*	Safe	1.5	
Dyna/Trace Stress, ECG electrode *ConMed Corp., Utica, NY*	Safe	1.5	
Dyna/Trace, ECG electrode *ConMed Corp., Utica, NY*	Safe	1.5	
High Demand, ECG electrode *ConMed Corp., Utica, NY*	Safe	1.5	
Holtrode, ECG electrode *ConMed Corp., Utica, NY*	Safe	1.5	
HP M2202A Radio-lucent, ECG electrode *Monitoring Electrode, Ag/AgCl* *Hewlett-Packard, Andover, MA*	Safe	1.5	
Invisatrace Adult, ECG electrode *ConMed Corp., Utica, NY*	Safe	1.5	
Pediatric Foam, ECG electrode *ConMed Corp., Utica, NY*	Safe	1.5	
Plia Cell Diagnostic, ECG electrode *ConMed Corp., Utica, NY*	Safe	1.5	
Plia-Cell Diaphoretic, ECG electrode *ConMed Corp., Utica, NY*	Safe	1.5	
Plia-Cell, ECG electrode *ConMed Corp., Utica, NY*	Safe	1.5	

Object	Status	Field Strength (T)	Reference
Quadtrode MRI, ECG electrode *InVivo Research, Inc., Orlando, FL*	Safe	1.5	
Silvon Adult ECG Electrode *ConMed Corp., Utica, NY*	Safe	1.5	
Silvon Diaphoretic, ECG electrode *ConMed Corp., Utica,NY*	Safe	1.5	
Silvon Stress, ECG electrode *ConMed Corp., Utica, NY*	Safe	1.5	
Silvon, ECG electrode *ConMed Corp., Utica, NY*	Safe	1.5	
Snaptrace, ECG electrode *ConMed Corp., Utica, NY*	Safe	1.5	
SSE Radiotransparent ECG Electrode *ConMed Corp., Utica, NY*	Safe	1.5	
SSE, ECG electrode *ConMed Corp., Utica, NY*	Safe	1.5	

Object	Status	Field Strength (T)	Reference

Foley Catheters With and Without Temperature Sensors

Object	Status	Field Strength (T)	Reference
Bardex I.C. Foley *Catheter with silver and hydrogel coating,16Fr.* *Bard Medical Division, Covington, GA*	Conditional 5	1.5	
Bardex I.C. Temperature Sensing Foley Catheter *with a 6 foot cable, 16 Fr.* *Bard Medical Division, Covington, GA*	Conditional 5	1.5	
Bardex Latex-Free Temperature Sensing 400-Series Foley Catheter *C.R.Bard, Inc., Covington, GA*	Conditional 5	1.5, 3	
Bardex Lubricath Temperature Sensing *Urotrack Plus Foley Catheter with a 6 foot cable, 16 Fr* *Bard Medical Division, Covington, GA*	Conditional 5	1.5	
Bardex Pediatric Temperature Sensing 400-Series *Urotrack Foley Catheter with a detachable cable,12 Fr.* *Bard Medical Division, Covington, GA*	Conditional 5	1.5	
DeRoyal Foley Catheter With Temperature Sensor *18-Fr, REF 81-080718* *DeRoyal Industries, www.DeRoyal.com*	Conditional 5	3	
Extension cable for Foley Catheter *with temperature sensor, 10 feet* *RSP Respiratory Support Products, Inc.* *Smiths Industries, Irvine, CA*	Unsafe 2	1.5	
Foley catheter *Bard Medical Division, Covington, GA*	Safe	1.5	
Foley Catheter *SilverTouch Catheter* *Medline Industries, Inc., Mundelein, IL*	Conditional 6	3	
Foley Catheter with Temperature Sensor, 10 Fr. *RSP Respiratory Support Products, Inc.* *Smiths Industries, Irvine, CA*	Conditional 5	1.5	
Foley Catheter with *Temperature Sensor, 18 Fr.* *RSP Respiratory Support Products, Inc.* *Smiths Industries, Irvine, CA*	Conditional 5	1.5	
Lubri-Sil I.C. Foley Catheter, Non metal version *C.R.Bard, Inc., Covington, GA*	Safe	3	
Lubri-Sil I.C. Foley Catheter *Temperature Sensing 400-Series Foley Catheter* *C.R.Bard, Inc., Covington, GA*	Conditional 6	1.5, 3	

Object	Status	Field Strength (T)	Reference

Halo Vests and Cervical Fixation Devices

Object	Status	Field Strength (T)	Reference
Ambulatory Halo System *halo and cervical fixation*	Conditional 4	1.5	14
Bremer 3D Halo Crown System *with Bremer Air Flo Vest and Titanium Skull Pins* *Cervical Fixation Device* *DePuy Spine Inc., Raynham, MA*	Conditional 6	3	
Bremer Halo Crown System *with Bremer Air Flo Vest and Titanium Skull Pins* *Cervical Fixation Device* *DePuy Spine Inc., Raynham, MA*	Conditional 6	3	
Closed-back halo *Titanium, halo and cervical fixation* *DePuy ACE Medical Co., El Segundo, CA*	Safe	1.5	16
Closed Back Halo *OSSUR Reykjavik, Iceland, OSSUR AMERICAS, Aliso Viejo, CA*	Unsafe 1	1.5	
EXO adjustable coller *halo and cervical fixation* *Florida Manufacturing Co., Daytona, FL*	Conditional 4	1.0	15
Generation 80 Halo System *with Generation 80 Halo Vest and Aluminum Ring* *and Generation 80 Titanium Halo Pins* *OSSUR Reykjavik, Iceland, OSSUR AMERICAS, Aliso Viejo, CA*	Unsafe 1	3	114
Guilford cervical orthosis, modified *halo and cervical fixation* *Guilford & Son, Ltd., Cleveland, OH*	Safe	1.0	15
Guilford cervical orthosis *halo and cervical fixation* *Guilford & Son, Ltd., Cleveland, OH*	Conditional 4	1.0	15
J-Tongs *OSSUR Reykjavik, Iceland, OSSUR AMERICAS, Aliso Viejo, CA*	Unsafe 1	1.5	
JTO Cervico-Thoracic Extension *OSSUR Reykjavik, Iceland, OSSUR AMERICAS, Aliso Viejo, CA*	Safe	3	
'LiL Angel Pediatric Halo System *with Jerome Halo Vest and Resolve Glass-composite Halo Ring* *and Resolve Ceramic-tipped Skull Pins* *OSSUR Reykjavik, Iceland, OSSUR AMERICAS, Aliso Viejo, CA*	Conditional 6	3	114
'LiL Angel Pediatric Halo System *with Resolve Halo Vest and Resolve Glass-composite Halo Ring* *and Resolve Ceramic-tipped Skull Pins* *OSSUR Reykjavik, Iceland, OSSUR AMERICAS, Aliso Viejo, CA*	Conditional 6	3	114
Mark III halo vest *aluminum superstructure, SS rivets, Titanium bolts* *DePuy ACE Medical Co., El Segundo, CA*	Safe	1.5	16
Mark IV halo vest *aluminum superstructure and Titanium bolts* *DePuy ACE Medical Co., El Segundo, CA*	Safe	1.5	16
Miami J Cervical Collar *OSSUR Reykjavik, Iceland, OSSUR AMERICAS, Aliso Viejo, CA*	Safe	3	
MR-compatible halo vest and cervical fixation *Lerman & Son Co., Beverly Hills, CA*	Safe	1.5	

Object	Status	Field Strength (T)	Reference
NecLoc Extrication Collar	Safe	3	
OSSUR Reykjavik, Iceland, OSSUR AMERICAS, Aliso Viejo, CA			
Occian Collar Back	Safe	3	
OSSUR Reykjavik, Iceland, OSSUR AMERICAS, Aliso Viejo, CA			
Open-back halo, aluminum	Safe	1.5	16
DePuy ACE Medical Co., El Segundo, CA			
Open-back halo with Delrin inserts for skull pins	Safe	1.5	16
aluminum and Delrin			
DePuy ACE Medical Co., El Segundo, CA			
Papoos Infant Spinal Immobilization Device	Safe	3	
OSSUR Reykjavik, Iceland, OSSUR AMERICAS, Aliso Viejo, CA			
Patriot Extrication Collar	Safe	3	
OSSUR Reykjavik, Iceland, OSSUR AMERICAS, Aliso Viejo, CA			
Philadelphia Cervical Collar	Safe	3	
OSSUR Reykjavik, Iceland, OSSUR AMERICAS, Aliso Viejo, CA			
Philadelphia coller	Safe	1.0	15
Philadelphia Coller Co., Westville, NJ			
PMT halo cervical orthosis	Safe	1.0	15
PMT Corp., Chanhassen, MN			
PMT halo cervical orthosis with graphite rods and halo ring	Safe	1.0	15
PMT Corp., Chanhassen, MN			
PMT Halo System with Carbon Graphite Open Back Ring	Conditional 5	3	
and Titanium Skull Pins			
PMT Corp., Chanhassen, MN			
Resolve Halo System with Jerome Halo Vest	Conditional 6	3	114
and Resolve Glass-composite Halo Ring			
and Resolve Ceramic-tipped Skull Pins			
OSSUR Reykjavik, Iceland, OSSUR AMERICAS, Aliso Viejo, CA			
Resolve Halo System with Resolve Halo Vest	Conditional 6	3	114
and Resolve Glass-composite Halo Ring			
and Resolve Ceramic-tipped Skull Pins			
OSSUR Reykjavik, Iceland, OSSUR AMERICAS, Aliso Viejo, CA			
S.O.M.I. cervical orthosis	Conditional 4	1.0	15
U.S. Manufacturing Co., Pasadena, CA			
Trippi-Wells tong, Titanium	Safe	1.5	16
DePuy ACE Medical Co., El Segundo, CA			
V1 Halo System with V1 Halo Vest	Conditional 6	3	114
and V1 Halo Ring and V1 Titanium Halo Pins			
OSSUR Reykjavik, Iceland, OSSUR AMERICAS, Aliso Viejo, CA			
V2	Unsafe 1	1.5	
OSSUR Reykjavik, Iceland, OSSUR AMERICAS, Aliso Viejo, CA			

Object	Status	Field Strength (T)	Reference

Heart Valve Prostheses and Annuloplasty Rings

Object	Status	Field Strength (T)	Reference
AAV-2 Heart Valve, Aortic heart valve prosthesis *Arbor Surgical Technologies, Inc., Irvine, CA*	Conditional 6	3	
AHK 7700, Model 7700 heart valve *Medtronic, www.medtronic.com*	Conditional 5	3	
Annuloflex Annuloplasty Ring, Size 26-mm *Sulzer Carbomedics, Inc., Austin, TX*	Safe	1.5, 3	
Annuloflex Annuloplasty RingSize 36-mm *Sulzer Carbomedics, Inc., Austin, TX*	Safe	1.5, 3	
Annuloflo Annuloplasty Ring, Size 26-mm *Sulzer Carbomedics, Inc., Austin, TX*	Safe	1.5, 3	
Annuloflo Annuloplasty Ring, Size 36-mm *Sulzer Carbomedics, Inc., Austin, TX*	Safe	1.5, 3	
AnnuloFlo Mitral Annuloplasty Device *Size 36, Model AR-736* *Sulzer Carbomedics, Inc., Austin, TX*	Safe	1.5, 3	83
Annuloplasty Ring, Models RNG5 and RNG7 *Dynamic Annuloplasty Ring System* *MiCardia, www.micardia.com*	Conditional 6	3	
Annuloplasty ring, Titanium *Sulzer Medica and Sulzer Carbomedics*	Safe	1.5	
Attune Flexible Annuloplasty Ring *St. Jude Medical, www.sjmprofessional.com*	Conditional 5	3	
AorTech Aortic, Model 3800 heart valve *Aortech Ltd., Strathclyde, U.K.*	Conditional 1	1.5	75
AorTech Mitral, Model 4800 heart valve *Aortech Ltd., Strathclyde, U.K.*	Conditional 1	1.5	75
Aortic Mitroflow Synergy PC Aortic Pericardial Heart Valve *Size 19-mm* *Sulzer Carbomedics, Inc., Austin, TX*	Safe	1.5, 3	
Aortic Mitroflow Synergy PC Aortic Pericardial Heart Valve *Size 29-mm* *Sulzer Carbomedics, Inc., Austin, TX*	Safe	1.5, 3	
Aortic SJM Regent Valve Mechanical Heart Valve *Size 27-mm, Rotatable Aortic* *Standard Cuff-Polyester, AGN* *St. Jude Medical, www.sjmprofessional.com*	Conditional 5	3	
Aortic Valve, Size 16-mm *Sulzer Carbomedics, Inc., Austin, TX*	Safe	1.5, 3	
Apical Connector, Model 174A, heart valve *Medtronic, Inc., www.Medtronic.com*	Safe	1.5, 3	84
ATS Medical Open Pivot Aortic Valved Graft *Model # XX denotes size, 502AGxx* *ATS Medical, Minneapolis, MN*	Conditional 6	3	
ATS Medical Open Pivot Bileaflet Heart Valve *AP 360 Aortic, Model # XX denotes size, 505DAxx* *ATS Medical, Minneapolis, MN*	Conditional 6	3	
ATS Medical Open Pivot Bileaflet Heart Valve *AP 360 Mitral, Model # XX denotes size, 505DMxx* *ATS Medical, Minneapolis, MN*	Conditional 6	3	

Object	Status	Field Strength (T)	Reference
ATS Medical Open Pivot, Bileaflet Heart Valve *AP Aortic, Model # XX denotes size, 501DAxx* *ATS Medical, Minneapolis, MN*	Conditional 6	3	
ATS Medical Open Pivot, Bileaflet Heart Valve *AP Mitral, Model # XX denotes size, 501DMxx* *ATS Medical, Minneapolis, MN*	Conditional 6	3	
ATS Medical Open Pivot, Bileaflet Heart Valve *Apex Aortic, Model # XX denotes size, 503DAxx* *ATS Medical, Minneapolis, MN*	Conditional 6	3	
ATS Medical Open Pivot, Bileaflet Heart Valve *Apex Mitral, Model # XX denotes size, 503DMxx* *ATS Medical, Minneapolis, MN*	Conditional 6	3	
ATS Medical Open Pivot, Bileaflet Heart Valve *Standard Aortic, Model # XX denotes size, 500FAxx* *ATS Medical, Minneapolis, MN*	Conditional 6	3	
ATS Medical Open Pivot, Bileaflet Heart Valve *Standard Mitral, Model # XX denotes size, 500DMxx* *ATS Medical, Minneapolis, MN*	Conditional 6	3	
ATS Medical Open Pivot, BiLeaflet Heart Valve *Mitral, Model 500DM29* *Standard Valve, pyrolytic carbon heart valve* *ATS Medical, Minneapolis, MN*	Conditional 1	1.5	75
ATS Medical Open Pivot, BiLeaflet Heart Valve *Aortic, Model 501DA18* *Advanced Performance (AP) pyrolytic carbon heart valve* *ATS Medical, Minneapolis, MN*	Conditional 1	1.5	75
Autogenics Autologous *Model APHV, Eligoy, heart valve* *Autogenics Europe Ltd, Glasgow, Scotland*	Safe	1.5	75
Autogenics Autologous *Model ATCV, Eligoy, heart valve* *Autogenics Europe Ltd, Glasgow, Scotland*	Safe	1.5	75
Beall heart valve *Coratomic Inc., Indiana, PA*	Conditional 1	2.35	17
Beall Mitral pyrolitic carbon *heart valve* *Coratomic Inc., Indianapolis, IN*	Conditional 1	1.5	75
Bileaflet, Model A7760, 29-mm, heart valve *Medtronic, Inc., www.Medtronic.com*	Safe	1.5	
Bicarbon Fitline Mechanical Mitral Valve *Sorin Biomedica Cardio, www.sorin.com*	Conditional 6	3	
Bicarbon Slimline Aortic Mechanical Heart Valve *Sorin Biomedica Cardio, www.sorin.com*	Conditional 6	3	
Biocor Valve, Aortic *Model H3636, heart valve* *St. Jude Medical, www.sjmprofessional.com*	Conditional 5	3	
Biocor Valve, Mitral *Size 35-mm, Model B10-35M,* *Heart Valves and Annuloplasty Rings* *St. Jude Medical, www.sjmprofessional.com*	Conditional 5	3	
Bjork-Shiley (convexo/concave) heart valve *Shiley Inc., Irvine, CA*	Safe	1.5	3

Object	Status	Field Strength (T)	Reference
Bjork-Shiley (universal/spherical) heart valve *Shiley Inc., Irvine, CA*	Conditional 1	1.5	3
Bjork-Shiley, Model 22 MBRC 11030 *heart valve* *Shiley Inc., Irvine, CA*	Conditional 1	2.35	18
Bjork-Shiley, Model MBC *heart valve* *Shiley Inc., Irvine, CA*	Conditional 1	2.35	18
Bjork Shiley Monostrut, Aortic *Model ABMS, heart valve* *Pfizer, Inc., Cincinnati, OH*	Safe	1.5	75
Bjork Shiley Monostrut, Mitral *Model MBRMS, heart valve* *Pfizer, Inc., Cincinnati, OH*	Safe	1.5	75
Bjork Shiley Monostrut, Mitral *Model MBUM, heart valve* *Pfizer, Inc., Cincinnati, OH*	Conditional 1	1.5	75
Bjork Shiley Pyrolitic Carbon Conical Disc *Mitral, Model MBRP, heart valve* *Pfizer, Inc., Cincinnati, OH*	Conditional 1	1.5	75
Bjork Shiley Pyrolitic Carbon Conical Disc *Mitral, Model MBUP, heart valve* *Pfizer, Inc., Cincinnati, OH*	Safe	1.5	75
Bovine Pericardial Patch *Edwards Lifesciences, www.Edwards.com*	Safe	1.5, 3	
Carbomedics CarboSeal *Conduit with Mechanical Valve* *Sorin Biomedica Cardio, www.sorin.com*	Conditional 6	3	
Carbomedics Heart Valve Prosthesis *Annuloflo Annuloplasty Ring, Size 26* *Carbomedics, Austin, TX*	Safe	1.5	
Carbomedics Heart Valve Prosthesis *Annuloflo Annuloplasty Ring, Size 36* *Carbomedics, Austin, TX*	Safe	1.5	
CarboMedics Heart Valve Prosthesis *Aortic Reduced, Model R500, Size 19* *Carbomedics, Austin, TX*	Safe	1.5	19
CarboMedics Heart Valve Prosthesis *Aortic Reduced, Model R500, Size 21* *Carbomedics, Austin, TX*	Safe	1.5	19
CarboMedics Heart Valve Prosthesis *Aortic Reduced, Model R500, Size 23* *Carbomedics, Austin, TX*	Safe	1.5	19
CarboMedics Heart Valve Prosthesis *Aortic Reduced, Model R500, Size 25* *Carbomedics, Austin, TX*	Safe	1.5	19
CarboMedics Heart Valve Prosthesis *Aortic Reduced, Model R500, Size 27* *Carbomedics, Austin, TX*	Safe	1.5	19
CarboMedics Heart Valve Prosthesis *Aortic Reduced, Model R500, Size 29* *Carbomedics, Austin, TX*	Safe	1.5	19

Object	Status	Field Strength (T)	Reference
CarboMedics Heart Valve Prosthesis *Aortic Standard, Model 500, Size 31* *Carbomedics, Austin, TX*	Safe	1.5	19
Carbomedics Heart Valve Prosthesis *Aortic Valve, Size 16* *Carbomedics, Austin, TX*	Safe	1.5	
Carbomedics Heart Valve Prosthesis *Carboseal, Size 31* *Carbomedics, Austin, TX*	Safe	1.5	
CarboMedics Heart Valve Prosthesis *Mitral Standard, Model 700, Size 23* *Carbomedics, Austin, TX*	Safe	1.5	19
CarboMedics Heart Valve Prosthesis *Mitral Standard, Model 700, Size 25* *Carbomedics, Austin, TX*	Safe	1.5	19
CarboMedics Heart Valve Prosthesis *Mitral Standard, Model 700, Size 27* *Carbomedics, Austin, TX*	Safe	1.5	19
CarboMedics Heart Valve Prosthesis *Mitral Standard, Model 700, Size 29* *Carbomedics, Austin, TX*	Safe	1.5	19
CarboMedics Heart Valve Prosthesis *Mitral Standard, Model 700, Size 31* *Carbomedics, Austin, TX*	Safe	1.5	19
CarboMedics Heart Valve Prosthesis *Mitral Standard, Model 700, Size 33* *Carbomedics, Austin, TX*	Safe	1.5	19
Carbomedics Heart Valve Prosthesis *Mitral Valve, Size 33* *Carbomedics, Austin, TX*	Safe	1.5	
Carboseal *Ascending Aortic Prosthesis, Size 33-mm, Model AP 33* *Sulzer Carbomedics, Inc., Austin, TX*	Safe	1.5, 3	
Carboseal *Ascending Aortic Valve Conduit* *Size 33-mm, Model AP-033, Nitinol* *Sulzer Carbomedics, Inc., Austin, TX*	Safe	1.5, 3	83
Carboseal *Ascending Aortic Valve Conduit,* *Size 33-mm, Model AP-033, Titanium* *Sulzer Carbomedics, Inc., Austin, TX*	Safe	1.5, 3	83
Carbomedics Synergy PC *Aortic Pericardial Heart Valve* *Sorin Biomedica Cardio, www.sorin.com*	Conditional 6	3	
Carpentier-Edwards aortic and mitral bioprostheses *Models 2625, 6625* *Edwards Lifesciences, www.Edwards.com*	Conditional 5	1.5, 3	
Carpentie-Edwards BioPhysio Heart Valve Prosthesis *Model 3100, 29M, Nitinol, Silicone* *Edwards Lifesciences, www.Edwards.com*	Safe	1.5, 3	

Object	Status	Field Strength (T)	Reference
Carpentier-Edwards bioprosthetic valved conduit *Model 4300* *Edwards Lifesciences, www.Edwards.com*	Conditional 5	1.5, 3	
Carpentier-Edwards *Classic Annuloplasty Ring, Mitral Model 4400, size 40-mm* *Edwards Lifesciences, www.Edwards.com*	Safe	1.5, 3	77, 83
Carpentier-Edwards Classic annuloplasty mitral and *tricuspid rings with Duraflo treatment, Models 4425, 4525* *Edwards Lifesciences, www.Edwards.com*	Safe	1.5, 3	
Carpentier-Edwards Classic annuloplasty *mitral and tricuspid rings, Models 4400, 4500* *Edwards Lifesciences, www.Edwards.com*	Safe	1.5, 3	
Carpentier-Edwards (porcine) heart valve *American Edwards Laboratories* *Santa Ana, CA*	Conditional 1	2.35	18
Carpentier-Edwards, Annuloplasty Ring, Model 4400 *Baxter Healthcare Corporation, Santa Ana, CA*	Safe	1.5, 3	
Carpentier-Edwards, Annuloplasty Ring, Model 4500 *Baxter Healthcare Corporation, Santa Ana, CA*	Safe	1.5, 3	
Carpentier-Edwards, Annuloplasty Ring, Model 4600 *Baxter Healthcare Corporation Santa Ana, CA*	Safe	1.5, 3	
Carpentier-Edwards, Bioprosthesis *Model 2625, heart valve* *Baxter Healthcare Corporation, Santa Ana, CA*	Safe	1.5, 3	
Carpentier-Edwards, Bioprosthesis *Model 6625, heart valve* *Baxter Healthcare Corporation, Santa Ana, CA*	Safe	1.5, 3	
Carpentier-Edwards Duraflex low pressure porcine *mitral bioprosthesis with extended sewing ring, 6625-ESR-LP* *Edwards Lifesciences, www.Edwards.com*	Conditional 5	1.5, 3	
Carpentier-Edwards Duraflex low pressure *porcine mitral bioprosthesis, Model 6625LP* *Edwards Lifesciences, www.Edwards.com*	Conditional 5	1.5, 3	
Carpentier-Edwards Low Pressure Bioprosthesis *Porcine, Mitral Model 6625-LP, size 35-mm, heart valve* *Edwards Lifesciences, www.Edwards.com*	Safe	1.5, 3	77, 83
Carpentier-Edwards Magna II Pericardial *Aortic Heart Valve Prosthesis, Model 3300/3300TFX* *Edwards Lifesciences, www.Edwards.com*	Conditional 6	3	
Carpentier-Edwards Pericardial Bioprosthesis *Model 2700, heart valve* *Baxter Healthcare Corporation, Santa Ana, CA*	Safe	1.5	
Carpentier-Edwards PERIMOUNT Pericardial Bioprosthesis *Mitral Model 6900, size 33-mm, heart valve* *Edwards Lifesciences, www.Edwards.com*	Conditional 1	1.5, 3	77, 83
Carpentier-Edwards PERIMOUNT Magna *Mitral Ease pericardial bioprosthesis, Model 7200TFX* *Edwards Lifesciences, www.Edwards.com*	Conditional 6	3	
Carpentier-Edwards PERIMOUNT Magna *Mitral Ease pericardial bioprosthesis, Model 7300TFX* *Edwards Lifesciences, www.Edwards.com*	Conditional 6	3	

Object	Status	Field Strength (T)	Reference
Carpentier-Edwards PERIMOUNT Magna *mitral pericardial bioprosthesis, Models 7000, 7000TFX* *Edwards Lifesciences, www.Edwards.com*	Conditional 6	3	
Carpentier-Edwards PERIMOUNT Magna *pericardial aortic bioprostheses, Models 3000, 3000TFX* *Edwards Lifesciences, www.Edwards.com*	Conditional 6	3	
Carpentier-Edwards PERIMOUNT Plus *mitral pericardial bioprosthesis, Model 6900P* *Edwards Lifesciences, www.Edwards.com*	Conditional 5	3	
Carpentier-Edwards PERIMOUNT Theon *pericardial aortic bioprostheses, Models 2700TFX, 2800TFX* *Edwards Lifesciences, www.Edwards.com*	Conditional 5	3	
Carpentier-Edwards PERIMOUNT *pericardial aortic bioprostheses, Models 2700, 2800* *Edwards Lifesciences, www.Edwards.com*	Conditional 5	3	
Carpentier-Edwards Physio Annuloplasty Ring *Mitral Model 4450, size 40-mm* *Edwards Lifesciences, www.Edwards.com*	Conditional 1	1.5, 3	77, 83
Carpentier-Edwards Physio Annuloplasty Ring *Model 4450* *Baxter Healthcare Corporation, Santa Ana, CA*	Safe	1.5	77
Carpentier-Edwards *Physio Annuloplasty Ring, Model 4450, Elgiloy alloy* *Edwards Lifesciences, www.Edwards.com*	Conditional 6	3	
Carpentier-Edwards Physio II Mitral Annuloplasty Ring *Model 5200* *Edwards Lifesciences, www.Edwards.com*	Conditional 6	3	
Carpentier-Edwards *Model 2650, heart valve* *American Edwards Laboratories, Santa Ana, CA*	Conditional 1	2.35	18
Carpentier-Edwards S.A.V. aortic bioprosthesis *Model 2650* *Edwards Lifesciences, www.Edwards.com*	Conditional 5	1.5, 3	
CG Future Annuloplasty ring *Colvin-Galloway Future Band 638B, 638B Band & 638R Ring* *Medtronic, Inc., www.Medtronic.com*	Conditional 5	3	
Colvin-Galloway Future Band 638B *annuloplasty device* *Medtronic, Inc., www.Medtronic.com*	Safe	1.5, 3	84
Contegra 200 heart valve *Medtronic, Inc., www.Medtronic.com*	Safe	1.5, 3	84
Contegra 200S, heart valve *Medtronic, Inc., www.Medtronic.com*	Safe	1.5, 3	84
CoreValve *Medtronic, Inc., www.Medtronic.com*	Conditional 5	3	
Cosgrove-Edwards Annuloplasty Ring *Model 4600* *Baxter Healthcare Corporation, Santa Ana, CA*	Safe	1.5	
Cosgrove-Edwards Annuloplasty *mitral and tricuspid band, Model 4600* *Edwards Lifesciences, www.Edwards.com*	Safe	1.5, 3	

Object	Status	Field Strength (T)	Reference
Cosgrove-Edwards Annuloplasty *mitral and tricuspid band with Duraflo treatment, Model 4625* *Edwards Lifesciences, www.Edwards.com*	Safe	1.5, 3	
CPHV Annuloplasty Ring *pyrolytic carbon, Titanium* *Sulzer Medica and Sulzer Carbomedics*	Safe	1.5	
Cribier Aortic Bioprosthesis *Percutaneous Heart Valve, 316LVM SS* *Edwards Lifesciences, www.Edwards.com*	Safe	3	
Cribier-Edwards Aortic Bioprosthesis *Model 9000 (PHV1A-26) combined with Carpentier-Edwards* *Porcine Bioprosthesis, Model 6650, 31-mm heart valve prostheses* *Edwards Lifesciences, www.Edwards.com*	Conditional 6	3	
Cribier-Edwards aortic bioprosthesis (PHV) *Models 9000, 9000PHV* *Edwards Lifesciences, www.Edwards.com*	Conditional 6	3	
dETlogix mitral annuloplasty ring *Edwards Lifesciences, www.Edwards.com*	Conditional 6	3	
Durafic, Aortic, Model AD *size 33-mm, heart valve*	Conditional 1	1.5	75
Durafic, Model MD, Mitral *heart valve*	Conditional 1	1.5	75
Duraflex Low Pressure Bioprosthesis *Model 6625E6R-LP, heart valve* *Baxter Healthcare Corporation, Santa Ana, CA*	Safe	1.5	
Duraflex Low Pressure Bioprosthesis *Model 6625LP heart valve* *Baxter Healthcare Corporation, Santa Ana, CA*	Safe	1.5	
Duran AnCore, Models 620B, 620R *620RG & 620BG* *Medtronic, Inc., www.Medtronic.com*	Conditional 5	3	
Duran Ring *Model H601H annuloplasty device* *Medtronic, Inc., www.Medtronic.com*	Safe	1.5, 3	84
Duran Ring *Model H608H annuloplasty device* *Medtronic, Inc., www.Medtronic.com*	Safe	1.5, 3	84
Duran Ring *Model 610R annuloplasty device* *Medtronic, Inc., www.Medtronic.com*	Safe	1.5, 3	84
Duran Annuloplasty Ring *Model H601H, 35-mm* *Medtronic, Inc., www.Medtronic.com*	Safe	1.5	
Dynamic Remodeller Annuloplasty Ring *MiCardia Corporation, Irvine, CA*	Conditional 6	3	
Dynaplasty MiCardia Annuloplasty Device *Annuloplasty Ring* *MiCardia Corporation, Irvine, CA*	Conditional 6	3	
Edwards-Duromedics Aortic and Mitral Bileaflet Prosthesis *Models 3160, 9120* *Edwards Lifesciences, www.Edwards.com*	Safe	1.5	

Object	Status	Field Strength (T)	Reference
Edwards MC3 Tricuspid Annuloplasty Ring *Model 4900* *Edwards Lifesciences, www.Edwards.com*	Safe	1.5, 3	
Edwards MIRA Aortic and Mitral Mechanical Valves *Models 3600, 3600f, 3600u, 9600* *Edwards Lifesciences, www.Edwards.com*	Safe	1.5, 3	
Edwards MIRA Mechanical Valve *Mitral, Model 9600, Size 27-mm* *Edwards Lifesciences, www.Edwards.com*	Safe	1.5, 3	83
Edwards MIRAMechanical Valve *Mitral, Model 9600, size 33-mm* *Edwards Lifesciences, www.Edwards.com*	Safe	1.5	
Edwards Myxo ETlogix Annuloplasty Ring *Model 5100, Titanium alloy* *Edwards Lifesciences, www.Edwards.com*	Conditional 6	3	
Edwards Prima aortic stentless bioprosthesis *Model 2500* *Edwards Lifesciences, www.Edwards.com*	Safe	1.5, 3	
Edwards Prima Plus aortic stentless bioprosthesis *Model 2500P* *Edwards Lifesciences, www.Edwards.com*	Safe	1.5, 3	
Edwards SAPIEN *Transcatheter Heart Valve* *Edwards Lifesciences, www.Edwards.com*	Conditional 6	3	
Edwards TEKNA Bileaflet Valve *Model 3200, heart valve* *Baxter Healthcare Corporation, Santa Ana, CA*	Safe	1.5	
Edwards TEKNA Bileaflet Valve *Model 9200, heart valve* *Baxter Healthcare Corporation, Santa Ana, CA*	Safe	1.5	
Edwards-Duromedics Bileaflet Valve *Model 3160, heart valve* *Baxter Healthcare Corporation, Santa Ana, CA*	Safe	1.5	
Edwards-Duromedics Bileaflet Valve *Model 9120, heart valve* *Baxter Healthcare Corporation, Santa Ana, CA*	Safe	1.5	
Freestyle Aortic Root *Model 995, heart valve* *Medtronic, Inc., www.Medtronic.com*	Safe	1.5, 3	84
Freestyle Model 995 *27-mm, heart valve* *Medtronic, Inc., www.Medtronic.com*	Safe	1.5	
HAART Aortic Annuloplasty Ring *BioStable Science & Engineering, Inc., www.biostable-s-e.com*	Conditional 6	3	
Hall-Kaster, Model A7700, heart valve *Medtronic, Inc., www.Medtronic.com*	Conditional 1	1.5	3
Hancock Apical Connector *Left Ventricular Connector, Model 174A* *Medtronic, Inc., www.Medtronic.com*	Conditional 5	3	
Hancock Low Porosity Conduit, Model 150 *Medtronic, Inc., www.Medtronic.com*	Conditional 5	3	

Object	Status	Field Strength (T)	Reference
Hancock, Model 100 *Pulmonic Conduit, heart valve* *Medtronic, Inc., www.Medtronic.com*	Safe	1.5, 3	84
Hancock, Model 105 *Low Porosity Conduit, heart valve* *Medtronic, Inc., www.Medtronic.com*	Safe	1.5, 3	84
Hancock, Model 150 *Pulmonic Conduit, heart valve* *Medtronic, Inc., www.Medtronic.com*	Safe	1.5, 3	84
Hancock, Model 242 *Aortic Valve, heart valve* *Medtronic, Inc., www.Medtronic.com*	Safe	1.5, 3	84
Hancock, Model 342 *Mitral Valve, heart valve* *Medtronic, Inc., www.Medtronic.com*	Safe	1.5, 3	84
Hancock 342, 35-mm, Model 342 *heart valve* *Medtronic, Inc., www.Medtronic.com*	Safe	1.5	
Hancock Conduit *Model 100, 30-mm, heart valve* *Medtronic, Inc., www.Medtronic.com*	Safe	1.5	
Hancock extracorporeal *Model 242R, heart valve* *Johnson & Johnson, Anaheim, CA*	Conditional 1	2.35	19
Hancock extracorporeal *Model M 4365-33, heart valve* *Johnson & Johnson, Anaheim, CA*	Conditional 1	2.35	19
Hancock I (porcine) heart valve *Johnson & Johnson, Anaheim, CA*	Conditional 1	1.5	3
Hancock II (porcine) heart valve *Johnson & Johnson, Anaheim, CA*	Conditional 1	1.5	3
Hancock II, Model T505 *Aortic Valve, heart valve* *Medtronic, Inc., www.Medtronic.com*	Safe	1.5, 3	84
Hancock II, Model T510 *Mitral Valve, heart valve* *Medtronic, Inc., www.Medtronic.com*	Safe	1.5, 3	84
Hancock II, Model T510, 33-mm *heart valve* *Medtronic, Inc., www.Medtronic.com*	Safe	1.5	
Hancock MO II, Model 250 *Aortic Valve, heart valve* *Medtronic, Inc., www.Medtronic.com*	Safe	1.5, 3	84
Hancock MO II, Model 250B *Aortic Valve, heart valve* *Medtronic, Inc., www.Medtronic.com*	Safe	1.5, 3	84
Hancock MO II, Model 250C *Aortic Valve, heart valve* *Medtronic, Inc., www.Medtronic.com*	Safe	1.5, 3	84
Hancock MO II, Model 250D *Aortic Valve, heart valve* *Medtronic, Inc., www.Medtronic.com*	Safe	1.5, 3	84

Object	Status	Field Strength (T)	Reference
Hancock MO II, Model 250E *Aortic Valve, heart valve* *Medtronic, Inc., www.Medtronic.com*	Safe	1.5, 3	84
Hancock MO II, Model 250H *Aortic Valve, heart valve* *Medtronic, Inc., www.Medtronic.com*	Safe	1.5, 3	84
Hancock Pericardial Mitral *Model T410, Haynes alloy, heart valve* *Medtronic Inc., www.Medtronic.com*	Safe	1.5	75
Hancock Pericardial Patch *Models 710, 710L* *Medtronic, Inc., www.Medtronic.com*	Conditional 5	3	
Hancock Pulmonic Conduit, Model 105 *Medtronic, Inc., www.Medtronic.com*	Conditional 5	3	
Hancock Vascor, Model 505 *heart valve* *Johnson & Johnson, Anaheim, CA*	Safe	2.35	19
HLT Transcatheter Aortic Heart Valve *Heart Leaflet Technologies, Inc (HLT), Maple Grove, MN*	Conditional 6	3	
IMR Annuloplasty Ring, Model 4100 *Edwards Lifesciences, www.edwards.com*	Conditional 6	3	
Inonescu-Shiley, Universal ISM *heart valve*	Conditional 1	2.35	19
Intact Aortic, Model A805 *size 19-mm, heart valve* *Medtronic, Inc., www.Medtronic.com*	Safe	1.5	75
Intact Model 705 *Mitral Valve, heart valve* *Medtronic, Inc., www.Medtronic.com*	Safe	1.5, 3	84
Intact Model 750 *Mitral Valve, heart valve* *Medtronic, Inc., www.medtronic.com*	Safe	1.5, 3	
Intact Model 805 *Aortic Valve, heart valve* *Medtronic, Inc., www.Medtronic.com*	Safe	1.5, 3	84
Intact Mitral, Model M705 *size 25-mm, heart valve* *Medtronic Inc., www.Medtronic.com*	Safe	1.5	75
JenaValve Transapical Prosthesis *JenaValve Technology GmbH*	Conditional 6	3	
Jyros Aortic, Model J1A *carbon alloy, heart valve* *Axion Medical Ltd.*	Safe	1.5	75
Jyros Mitral, Model J1M *carbon alloy, heart valve* *Axion Medical Ltd.*	Safe	1.5	75
Lillehi-Kaster, Model 300S heart valve *Medical Inc., Inver Grove Heights, MN*	Conditional 1	2.35	17
Lillehi-Kaster, Model 5009 heart valve *Medical Inc., Inver Grove Heights, MN*	Conditional 1	2.35	19

Object	Status	Field Strength (T)	Reference
Liotta *Aortic, Model MA783, Delrin, heart valve* *St. Jude Medical, www.sjmprofessional.com*	Conditional 5	3	
Magna Mitral, Model 7000 *Bioprosthetic tissue valve, Heart Valve* *Bovine pericardium, PTFE fabric, Elgiloy frame, polyester support* *Edwards Lifesciences, www.Edwards.com*	Conditional 6	3	
Med Hall Conduit, Model R7700 *33-mm, heart valve* *Medtronic, Inc., www.Medtronic.com*	Safe	1.5	
Medtronic Advantage, Model A7760 *Aortic Valve, heart valve* *Medtronic, Inc., www.Medtronic.com*	Safe	1.5, 3	84
Medtronic Advantage, Model M7760 *Mitral Valve, heart valve* *Medtronic, Inc., www.Medtronic.com*	Safe	1.5, 3	84
Medtronic Hall, heart valve *Medtronic, Inc., www.Medtronic.com*	Conditional 1	2.35	18
Medtronic Hall, Model 7700 *33-mm, heart valve* *Medtronic, Inc., www.Medtronic.com*	Safe	1.5	
Medtronic Hall, Model A7700 *Aortic Valve, heart valve* *Medtronic, Inc., www.Medtronic.com*	Safe	1.5, 3	84
Medtronic Hall, Model A7700-D-16 *heart valve* *Medtronic, Inc., www.Medtronic.com*	Conditional 1	2.35	18
Medtronic Hall, Model C7700 *Valved Conduit, heart valve* *Medtronic, Inc., www.Medtronic.com*	Safe	1.5, 3	84
Medtronic Hall, Model M7700 *Mitral Valve, heart valve* *Medtronic, Inc., www.Medtronic.com*	Safe	1.5, 3	84
Medtronic Hall, Model R7700 *Low Porosity Valved Conduit, heart valve* *Medtronic, Inc., www.Medtronic.com*	Safe	1.5, 3	84
Medtronic Hall, Model Z7700 *Low Porosity Valved Conduit, heart valve* *Medtronic, Inc., www.Medtronic.com*	Safe	1.5, 3	84
Melody Transcatheter Pulmonary Valve *Medtronic, Inc., www.medtronic.com*	Conditional 5	3	
MEMO 3D Semirigid Annuloplasty Ring *Used for mitral valve repair* *CarboMedics, a Sorin Group Co., Austin, TX*	Conditional 6	3	
MiCardia Annuloplasty Device *Annuloplasty Ring* *MiCardia Corporation, Irvine, CA*	Conditional 6	3	
Mitral Prosthetic Heart Valve *Model 2100 heart valve* *TRI Technologies, Brazil*	Safe	1.5	70
Mitral Valve, Size 33-mm, A307504F *Sulzer Carbomedics, Inc., Austin, TX*	Safe	1.5, 3	

Object	Status	Field Strength (T)	Reference

Mitroflow, Aortic, Model 11A
   Delrin, heart valve
   Mitroflow Sulzer CarboMedics, U.K.
	Safe	1.5	75

Mitroflow, Aortic, Model 14A
   Delrin, heart valve
   Mitroflow Sulzer CarboMedics, U.K.
	Safe	1.5	75

Mitroflow, Mitral, Model 11M
   Delrin, heart valve
   Mitroflow Sulzer CarboMedics, U.K.
	Safe	1.5	75

Mitroflow Pericardial Heart Valve, Model 12 *Sulzer-Medica and Mitroflow International*	Safe	1.5	70

Mosaic, Model 305, Aortic Valve
   heart valve
   Medtronic, Inc., www.Medtronic.com
	Safe	1.5, 3	84

Mosaic, Model 310, Mitral Valve
   heart valve
   Medtronic, Inc., www.Medtronic.com
	Safe	1.5, 3	84

Mosaic, Model 310, 33-mm
   heart valve
   Medtronic, Inc., www.Medtronic.com
	Safe	1.5, 3	

Mosaic, All Models, heart valve *Medtronic, Inc., www.Medtronic.com*	Conditional 5	1.5, 3	
Mosaic Ultra, heart valve *Medtronic, www.medtronic.com*	Conditional 5	3	

Omnicarbon, Model 35231029
   heart valve
   Medical Inc., Inver Grove Heights, MN
	Conditional 1	2.35	18

Omniscience, Model 6522
   heart valve
   Medical Inc., Inver Grove Heights, MN
	Conditional 1	2.35	18

On-X Valve, Model 6816
   heart valve
   Medical Carbon Research Institute, Austin, TX
	Safe	1.5	

On-X Prosthetic Heart Valve, Aortic
   Aortic with Conform-X Sewing Ring,
   Mitral, Mitral with Conform-X Sewing Cuff, Sizes 25-33
   On-X Life Technologies, Inc., Austin, TX
	Conditional 6	3	

On-X Prosthetic Heart Valve
   Conform-X Mitral Heart Valve Prosthesis, Sizes 25-33
   On-X Life Technologies, Inc., Austin, TX
	Conditional 6	3	

Open Pivot Heart Valve, Mitral (Model 500) *ATS Medical, Inc., Lake Forest, CA*	Conditional 6	3	
Open Pivot Heart Valve, Aortic AP 360 (Model 505) *ATS Medical, Inc., Lake Forest, CA*	Conditional 6	3	
Perceval S Sutureless Aortic Heart Valve *Sorin Biomedica Cardio, www.sorin.com*	Conditional 6	3	
Percutaneous Heart Valve, 316LMV SS *Percutaneous Valve Technologies, Ltd., Israel*	Safe	1.5, 3	

Percutaneous Mitral Annuloplasty Device (PMAD)
   Nitinol, Titanium
   Cardiac Dimensions, Inc., Kirkland, WA
	Safe	3	

Object	Status	Field Strength (T)	Reference
Pericarbon MORE Stented Heart Valve *Sorin Biomedica Cardio, www.sorin.com*	Conditional 6	3	
Physio II Annuloplasty Ring *Edwards Lifesciences, www.Edwards.com*	Conditional 6	3	
Porcine Synergy ST, Aortic, Size 19-mm *Sulzer Carbomedics, Inc., Austin, TX*	Safe	1.5, 3	
Porcine Synergy ST, Mitral, Size 33-mm *Sulzer Carbomedics, Inc., Austin, TX*	Safe	1.5, 3	
Posterior Annuloplasty Band *annuloplasty device, Model H607* *Medtronic, Inc., www.Medtronic.com*	Safe	1.5, 3	84
Posterior Annuloplasty Band *Model 610B, annuloplasty device* *Medtronic, Inc., www.Medtronic.com*	Safe	1.5, 3	84
Profile 3D Annuloplasty Ring *Medtronic, Inc., www.Medtronic.com*	Conditional 5	3	
Pulmonic Bioprosthesis *9000TFXP Cribier-Edwards Pulmonic Bioprosthesis* *and Palmaz XL P3110 Combined prostheses* *Edwards Lifesciences, www.Edwards.com*	Conditional 6	3	
Reduced Aortic CPHV *Carbomedics Prosthetic, Model R5-029, Size 29-mm,* *heart valve, Nitinol* *Sulzer Carbomedics, Inc., Austin, TX*	Safe	1.5, 3	83
Reduced Aortic CPHV *Carbomedics Prosthetic, Model R5-029, Size 29-mm* *heart valve, Titanium* *Sulzer Carbomedics, Inc., Austin, TX*	Safe	1.5, 3	83
Regent Mechanical Heart Valve *Model 27AG-701, 27-mm* *St. Jude Medical, www.sjmprofessional.com*	Conditional 5	3	
Rigid Tilting Disc Aortic/Mitral TTK, Chitra Heart Valve Substitute *Models TC1, TC2, Heart Valve Prosthesis* *TTK Healthcare Limited, www.ttkhealthcare.com*	Conditional 6	3	
Sculptor Ring *Model 605M, annuloplasty device* *Medtronic, Inc., www.Medtronic.com*	Safe	1.5, 3	84
Sculptor Ring Model 605T *annuloplasty device* *Medtronic, Inc., www.Medtronic.com*	Safe	1.5, 3	84
Sculptor Annuloplasty Ring *Model 605M, 35-mm* *Medtronic, Inc., www.Medtronic.com*	Safe	1.5	
SIMULUS Semi-Rigid Annuloplasty Ring *ATS Medical, Inc., Lake Forest, CA*	Conditional 6	3	
Simplici-T Model 670 *Medtronic, Inc., www.Medtronic.com*	Conditional 5	3	
SJM Masters Series Valve *Mitral, Size 37-mm, Model 37 MJ-501, heart valve* *St. Jude Medical, www.sjmprofessional.com*	Conditional 5	3	

Object	Status	Field Strength (T)	Reference
SJM Regent Heart Valve *Aortic, Size 29-mm, Model 29AGN-751, heart valve* *St. Jude Medical, www.sjmprofessional.com*	Conditional 5	3	
SJM Regent Heart Valve *Rotatable, Aortic Standard Cuff-Polyester, Model 25AGN-751-IDE* *St. Jude Medical, www.sjmprofessional.com*	Conditional 5	3	
SJM, St. Jude Medical Tissue Valves *Epic stented tissue valves, Epic Models include EL-xxA and EL-* *xxM for aortic and mitral valves ELS-xxA ELS-xxM for the silicon* *coated variety, EPIC valve product numbers are listed at* *www.sjm.com/devices/modelNumbers.aspx* *Note: "-xx" denotes different sizes available* *St. Jude Medical, www.sjmprofessional.com*	Conditional 5	3	
SJM Tailor Annuloplasty Ring *Size 35-mm, Model TARP-35* *St. Jude Medical, www.sjmprofessional.com*	Conditional 5	3	
Smelloff Cutter, Aortic *Titanium, heart valve* *Sorin Biomedica, Italy*	Conditional 1	1.5	75
Smeloff-Cutter, heart valve *Cutter Laboratories, Berkeley, CA*	Conditional 1	2.35	18
Split Ring, Posterior Band *Model H607* *Medtronic, Inc., www.Medtronic.com*	Conditional 5	3	
Sorin Allcarbon, AS *Model MTR-29AS, 29-mm, pyrolitic carbon, heart valve* *Sorin Biomedica Cardio S.p.A., Saluggia, Italy*	Conditional 1	1.5	75
Sorin, No. 23 *heart valve*	Conditional 1	1.5	20
Sorin Pericarbon (stented) *Mitral, pyrolytic carbon, heart valve* *Sorin Biomedica, Italy*	Conditional 1	1.5	75
St. Jude Medical *Mechanical Heart Valve, SJM Masters Series Rotatable, Aortic* *Model 25AJ-501, heart valve* *St. Jude Medical, www.sjmprofessional.com*	Conditional 5	3	
St. Jude Medical *Mechanical Heart Valve, Model 33MECS-602, 33-mm* *St. Jude Medical, www.sjmprofessional.com*	Conditional 5	3	
St. Jude, Model A 100 *heart valve* *St. Jude Medical Inc., www.SJM.com*	Conditional 1	2.35	19
St. Jude, Model M 101 *heart valve* *St. Jude Medical Inc., www.SJM.com*	Conditional 5	3	
St. Jude Medical, Annuloplasty Rings *Models include AFR-xx, RSAR-xx, SARP-xx, TARP-xx, TAB-xx* *Note: "xx" denotes different sizes available (e.g. 23A-101)* *St. Jude Medical, www.sjmprofessional.com*	Conditional 5	3	

Object	Status	Field Strength (T)	Reference
St. Jude Medical, Mechanical Heart Valves *Models include xxAGN-751, xxAGFN-756, xxAHPJ-505 or* *xxMHPJ-505, xxAEHPJ-505, xxAFHPJ-505, xxAJ-501 or* *xxMJ-501, xxAECJ-502 or xxMECJ-502, xxATJ-503 or xxMTJ-503* *xxMETJ-504, xxA-101 or xxM-101, xxVAVGJ-515, xxCAVGJ-514* **Note: "xx" denotes different sizes available (e.g. 23A-101)* *St. Jude Medical, www.sjmprofessional.com*	Conditional 5	3	
St. Jude Medical, Tissue Valves *Models include E100-xxA-00 or E100-xxM-00, ESP100-xx-00,* *B100-xxA-00 or B100-xxM-00, BSP100-xx,* *B10-xxA-00 or B10-xxM-00, B10SP-xx, TF-xxA** *Note: "xx" denotes different sizes available (e.g. 23A-101)* *St. Jude Medical, www.sjmprofessional.com*	Conditional 5	3	
Standard Mitral CPHV *Carbomedics Prosthetic, Model R5-029, Size 29-mm* *heart valve, Nitinol* *Sulzer Carbomedics, Inc., Austin, TX*	Safe	1.5, 3	83
Standard Mitral CPHV *Carbomedics Prosthetic, Model M7-033, Size 33-mm* *Heart Valve, Titanium* *Sulzer Carbomedics, Inc., Austin, TX*	Safe	1.5, 3	83
Starr-Edwards aortic and mitral prostheses *Models 1000, 1200, 2300, 2310, 2400,* *6000, 6120, 6300, 6310, 6320, 6400* *Edwards Lifesciences, www.Edwards.com*	Safe	2.35	
Starr-Edwards, Model 1000 *heart valve* *Baxter Healthcare Corporation, Santa Ana, CA*	Conditional 1	1.5	
Starr-Edwards, Model 1200 *heart valve* *Baxter Healthcare Corporation, Santa Ana, CA*	Conditional 1	1.5	
Starr-Edwards, Model 1260 *heart valve* *American Edwards Laboratories* *Baxter Healthcare Corporation, Santa Ana, CA*	Conditional 1	2.35	17
Starr-Edwards, Model 2300 *heart valve* *Baxter Healthcare Corporation, Santa Ana, CA*	Conditional 1	1.5	
Starr-Edwards, Model 2310 *heart valve* *Baxter Healthcare Corporation, Santa Ana, CA*	Conditional 1	1.5	
Starr-Edwards, Model 2320 *heart valve* *American Edwards Laboratories* *Baxter Healthcare Corporation, Santa Ana, CA*	Conditional 1	2.35	17
Starr-Edwards, Model 2400 *heart valve* *American Edwards Laboratories* *Baxter Healthcare Corporation, Santa Ana, CA*	Safe	1.5	3
Starr-Edwards, Model 6000 *heart valve* *Baxter Healthcare Corporation, Santa Ana, CA*	Conditional 1	1.5	

Object	Status	Field Strength (T)	Reference
Starr-Edwards, Model 6120 *heart valve* *Baxter Healthcare Corporation, Santa Ana, CA*	Conditional 1	1.5	
Starr-Edwards, Model 6300 *heart valve* *Baxter Healthcare Corporation, Santa Ana, CA*	Conditional 1	1.5	
Starr-Edwards, Model 6310 *heart valve* *Baxter Healthcare Corporation, Santa Ana, CA*	Conditional 1	1.5	
Starr-Edwards, Model 6320 *heart valve* *Baxter Healthcare Corporation, Santa Ana, CA*	Conditional 1	1.5	
Starr-Edwards, Model 6400 *heart valve* *Baxter Healthcare Corporation, Santa Ana, CA*	Conditional 1	1.5	
Starr-Edwards, Model 6520 *heart valve* *Baxter Healthcare Corporation, Santa Ana, CA*	Conditional 1	2.35	19
Starr-Edwards, Model Pre 6000 *heart valve* *American Edwards Laboratories* *Baxter Healthcare Corporation, Santa Ana, CA*	Conditional 1	2.35	17
Sulzer/Carbomedics Synergy PC *Pericardial Heart Valve* *Sulzer-Medica and Mitroflow International* *Richmond, B.C., Canada*	Safe	1.5	70
Tascon *Aortic, Elgiloy, heart valve* *Medtronic, Inc., www.Medtronic.com*	Safe	1.5	75
THV2, Model 9300TFX-29 *Aortic Heart Valve Prosthesis* *Edwards Lifesciences, www.Edwards.com*	Conditional 6	3	
Toronto SPV Valve *Stentless Porcine, Aortic Model SPA-101-25, heart valve* *St. Jude Medical, www.sjmprofessional.com*	Conditional 5	3	
Tri-AdT, Tricuspid Annuloplasty Ring (Models 900SFC-XX) *Medtronic, Inc., www.Medtronic.com*	Conditional 6	3	
TS 3f Enable Aortic Bioprosthesis *Model 6000* *ATS Medical, Inc., Lake Forest, CA*	Conditional 6	3	
Valtech Cardinal Annuloplasty Ring, Mitral *Valtech Cardio LTD*	Conditional 6	3	
Wessex *Aortic, Model WAV10, heart valve* *Sorin Biomedica, Italy*	Safe	1.5	75
Wessex *Mitral, Model WMV20, heart valve* *Sorin Biomedica, Italy*	Safe	1.5	75
Xenofic *Aortic, Model AP80, size 23, SS, heart valve*	Safe	1.5	75

Object	Status	Field Strength (T)	Reference

Hemostatic Clips, Other Clips, Fasteners, and Staples

Object	Status	Field Strength (T)	Reference
Absolok Plus *large, hemostatic clip, polydioxanone* *Ethicon Endo-Surgery, www.ees.com*	Safe	1.5	71
Absolok Plus *medium, hemostatic clip, polydioxanone* *Ethicon Endo-Surgery, www.ees.com*	Safe	1.5	71
Absolok Plus *small, hemostatic clip, polydioxanone* *Ethicon Endo-Surgery, www.ees.com*	Safe	1.5	71
AC2 System Clip *Anastomotic Clip System, Nitinol* *Rox Medical, San Clemente, CA*	Conditional 6	3	
AcuClip *C.P. Titanium, hemostatic clip* *Origin Medsystems, Menlo Park, CA*	Safe	1.5	71
Cosgrove-Gillinov Vascular Occlusion Clip *Nitinol, Titanium* *AtriCure, Inc., West Chester, OH*	Conditional 6	3	
CONTOUR Curved Cutter Staplers *staple, CR40B, CR40G, CS40B, CS40G, STR5G, OUS only* *Ethicon Endo-Surgery Inc., www.ees.com*	Conditional 5	3	
ECHELON (45 and 60) ENDOPATH *Linear Cutter Staplers, staple* *ECR60G, ECR60W, ECR60B, ECR60D, ECR45W,* *ECR45B, ECR45D, ECR45G, ECR45M* *Ethicon Endo-Surgery Inc., www.ees.com*	Conditional 5	3	
ENDOPATH EMS Endoscopic Multifeed Stapler *EMS* *Ethicon Endo-Surgery Inc., www.ees.com*	Conditional 5	3	
ENDOPATH Endoscopic Curved Intraluminal *Circular Staplers, staple, ECS21, ECS25, ECS29, ECS33* *Ethicon Endo-Surgery Inc., www.ees.com*	Conditional 5	3	
ENDOPATH Endoscopic Linear Cutters *and Staplers, staple* *ATB45, TSB45, SCB45, ZR45B, ATG45,* *TR45B, TR45G, TSG45, SCG45, ZR45G,* *NK45B, NAB45, NSG45, NK45G* *Ethicon Endo-Surgery Inc., www.ees.com*	Conditional 5	3	
ENDOPATH Endoscopic Linear Cutters *and Staplers, staple* *TR60W, TR60B,TR60G, 6R45M, 6R45B,* *6SB45, 6CB45, 6TB45, ATW35, TSW35,* *TSB35, TR35W, TR35B, ET45B, EZ45B* *Ethicon Endo-Surgery Inc., www.ees.com*	Conditional 5	3	
ENDOPATH Endoscopic Linear Cutters *and Staplers, staple* *ZR45B, ZR45G, ATW45, TSW45, SCW45, TR45W* *Ethicon Endo-Surgery Inc., www.ees.com*	Conditional 5	3	
Endostaple *Surgical Fastener, MP35N* *MedSource Technologies, Newton, MA*	Safe	1.5, 3	83

Object	Status	Field Strength (T)	Reference
Endostaple	Safe	1.5, 3	83
Surgical Fastener, Nitinol			
MedSource Technologies, Newton, MA			
ES-830 Microcutter Green Staple	Conditional 6	3	
Cardica, Inc., Redwood City, CA			
EVALVE clip	Safe	3	
Cardiovascular Valve Repair System, Elgiloy			
EVALVE, Redwood City, CA			
EVS Vascular Closure Staple	Safe	3	
Titanium alloy, Misc.			
AngioLINK Corporation, Tauton, MA			
EZ Clip	Unsafe 1	1.5	
E Z Clip			
www.olympus-europa.com/endoscopy			
Fascia staple	Safe	1.5, 3	83
316L SS			
United States Surgical, North Haven, CT			
Filshie Clip	Safe	1.5	
Avalon Medical Corporation, Williston, VT			
Gastrointestinal anastomosis clip	Safe	1.5	3
Auto Suture SGIA, SS, hemostatic clip			
United States Surgical Corp., Norwalk, CT			
GIA 4.8 staple	Safe	1.5, 3	83
Titanium			
United States Surgical, North Haven, CT			
GIA 4.8 Formed Titanium Staple	Conditional 6	3	
Multifire Endo GIA 60 - 4.8			
Covidien, www.covidien.com			
Hemoclip, #10	Safe	1.5	3
316L SS, hemostatic clip			
Edward Weck, Triangle Park, NJ			
Hemoclip, Hemostatic Clip	Conditional 6	3	
Teleflex Medical, www.teleflex.com			
Hemoclip, tantalum, hemostatic clip	Safe	1.5	3
Edward Weck, Triangle Park, NJ			
Hem-o-lok Polymer Clip(s)	Safe	1.5, 3	
nonmetallic, Teleflex Medical			
www.teleflexmedical.com			
Hemostasis Clip, DHC-7-230	Conditional 6	3	
Hemostatic Clip			
Cook Medical, www.cookmedical.com			
Hulka Clip	Conditional 6	3	
Richard Wolf Medical Instruments			
Vernon Hills, IL			
IVC venous clip	Safe	1.5	
Teflon			
Pilling Weck Co.			
Ligaclip, Extra Ligating Clips	Conditional 5	3	
LT100, LT200, LT300, LT400			
Ethicon Endo-Surgery Inc., www.ees.com			

Object	Status	Field Strength (T)	Reference
LIGACLIP ERCA *ER320, ER420* *Ethicon Endo-Surgery Inc., www.ees.com*	Conditional 5	3	
LIGACLIP Extra Ligating Clips *LS400, LS100, LS200, LS300* *Ethicon Endo-Surgery Inc., www.ees.com*	Conditional 5	3	
Ligaclip Extra LT 100 *C.P. Titanium, hemostatic clip* *Ethicon Endo-Surgery, www.ees.com*	Safe	1.5	71
Ligaclip Extra LT 200 *C.P. Titanium, hemostatic clip* *Ethicon Endo-Surgery, www.ees.com*	Safe	1.5	71
Ligaclip Extra LT 300 *C.P. Titanium, hemostatic clip* *Ethicon Endo-Surgery, www.ees.com*	Safe	1.5	71
Ligaclip Extra LT 400 *C.P. Titanium, hemostatic clip* *Ethicon Endo-Surgery, www.ees.com*	Safe	1.5	71
LIGACLIP Extra, Ligating Clip, Hemostatic Clip *Ethicon Endo-Surgery, Inc., www.ees.com*	Conditional 6	3	
LIGACLIP, MCA Multiple Clip Applier *MCS20, MCM20, MCL20* *Ethicon Endo-Surgery Inc., www.ees.com*	Conditional 5	3	
Ligaclip, tantalum, hemostatic clip *Ethicon, Inc., Sommerville, NJ*	Safe	1.5	3
Ligaclip, #6, 316L SS *hemostatic clip* *Ethicon, Inc., Sommerville, NJ*	Safe	1.5	3
LIGAMAX, Endoscopic Multiple Clip Applier *Ethicon Endo-Surgery Inc., www.ees.com*	Conditional 5	3	
Ligating clip, small *C.P. Titanium, hemostatic clip* *Horizon Surgical, Evergreen, CO*	Safe	1.5	71
Ligating clip, medium *C.P. Titanium, hemostatic clip* *Horizon Surgical, Evergreen, CO*	Safe	1.5	71
Long Clip HX-600-090L *Olympus Medical Systems Corporation, Japan*	Unsafe 1	1.5	
MCM 20, C.P. Titanium *hemostatic clip* *Ethicon Endo-Surgery, www.ees.com*	Safe	1.5	71
MSM 20, C.P. Titanium *hemostatic clip* *Ethicon Endo-Surgery, www.ees.com*	Safe	1.5	71
MCS 20, C.P. Titanium *hemostatic clip* *Ethicon Endo-Surgery, www.ees.com*	Safe	1.5	71
Micro SurgiClips *Titanium* *U.S. Surgical Corporation, North Haven, CT*	Safe	1.5	

Object	Status	Field Strength (T)	Reference
MultApplier clip	Safe	1.5, 3	83
Titanium			
United States Surgical, North Haven, CT			
Multapplier Titanium Clip	Conditional 6	3	
500-28 Endoclip Multapplier			
Covidien, www.covidien.com			
Ogden Suture Anchor	Safe	1.5, 3	83
Titanium			
United States Surgical, North Haven, CT			
OTSC Clip	Conditional 6	3	
Over The Scope Clip, Nitinol			
Ovesco Endoscopy GmbH, Germany			
Premium SurgiClip, L-13	Safe	1.5	71
C.P. Titanium, hemostatic clip			
United States Surgical, North Haven, CT			
Premium SurgiClip, M-11	Safe	1.5	71
C.P. Titanium, hemostatic clip			
United States Surgical, North Haven, CT			
Premium SurgiClip, S-9	Safe	1.5	71
C.P. Titanium, hemostatic clip			
United States Surgical, North Haven, CT			
PROXIMATE Curved and Straight	Conditional 5	3	
Intraluminal Staplers, staple			
CDH21, SDH21, CDH25, SDH25, CDH29,			
SDH29, CDH33, SDH33			
Ethicon Endo-Surgery Inc., www.ees.com			
PROXIMATE HCS Hemorrhoidal	Conditional 5	3	
Circular Stapler, PPH01, STR10			
Ethicon Endo-Surgery Inc., www.ees.com			
PROXIMATE Linear Cutters	Conditional 5	3	
clip, staple, TLC10, TRT10,			
TLC55, TRT55, TCT55, TRC55, TVC55,			
TRV55, TCT75, TRT75, TCD75,			
TRD75, TLC75, TCR75, TCT10, TCR10			
Ethicon Endo-Surgery Inc., www.ees.com			
PROXIMATE Linear Stapler	Conditional 5	3	
staple, AX55B, AX55G, TLV30, TRV30,			
TL30, TR30, TL60, TR60, TL90,			
TR90, TLH30, TRH30, TLH60, TRH60,			
TLH90, TRH90, TX30V, XR30V,			
TX30B, XR30B, TX30G, XR30G,			
TX60B, XR60B, TX60G, XR60G			
Ethicon Endo-Surgery Inc., www.ees.com			
PROXIMATE PPH	Conditional 5	3	
Hemorrhoidal Circular Stapler, staple, PPH03			
Ethicon Endo-Surgery Inc., www.ees.com			
PROXIMATE Skin Staplers	Conditional 5	3	
staple, PXW35, PRR35, PRW35,			
PMR35, PMW35, PMW55, PXR35			
Ethicon Endo-Surgery Inc., www.ees.com			
QuickClip2 Long	Unsafe 1	1.5	
HX-201LR-135L			
Olympus Medical Systems Corporation, Japan			

Object	Status	Field Strength (T)	Reference
QuickClip2 Long *HX-201UR-135L* *Olympus Medical Systems Corporation, Japan*	Unsafe 1	1.5	
Resolution Clip *304 SS, 17-7PH SS, 304V SS* *Boston Scientific, www.bostonscientific.com*	Unsafe 1	1.5	
Royal staple *316L SS* *United States Surgical, North Haven, CT*	Safe	1.5, 3	83
Staple Commercial, Hemostatic Clip *Teleflex Medical, www.teleflex.com*	Conditional 6	3	
StarClose Clip *Abbott Vascular, www.abbottvascular.com*	Conditional 5	3	
Starclose Surgical Clip *Nitinol* *Abbott Vascular, Santa Clara, CA*	Conditional 6	3	
Surgiclip, M-9.5 *C.P. Titanium, hemostatic clip* *United States Surgical, North Haven, CT*	Safe	1.5	71
Surgiclip, M-11 *C.P. Titanium, hemostatic clip* *United States Surgical, North Haven, CT*	Safe	1.5	71
Surgiclip, Auto Suture M-9.5 *SS, hemostatic clip* *United States Surgical, North Haven, CT*	Safe	1.5	3
Suture Anchor *with Titanium Nitride Coating, Herculon soft tissue anchor* *Covidien, www.covidien.com*	Conditional 6	3	
T-Bar Assembly *T-Fastener* *Kimberly-Clark Health Care, Roswell, GA*	Conditional 6	3	
TA 90-4.8 directional staples *Titanium* *United States Surgical, North Haven, CT*	Safe	1.5, 3	83
Tacker helical fastener *Titanium* *United States Surgical, North Haven, CT*	Safe	1.5, 3	83
Tacker Titanium Helical Clip *Tacker 5-mm Mesh Fixation Device* *Covidien, www.covidien.com*	Conditional 6	3	
Titanium Ligation Clip *Vesocclude Medical, Inc., www.vesoccludemedical.com*	Conditional 6	3	
TriClip Endoscopic Clipping Device *Wilson-Cook Medical Inc., Winston-Salem, NC*	Unsafe 1	1.5	118
U-CLIP *(B180)* *represents largest version of following U-CLIP products:* *S15, S18, S20, S25, S35, S50, S60, V45, V50, V60, V100D, S70,* *S90, S105, S120, B140, B160, B180* *Medtronic Cardiac Surgery, Brooklyn Park, MN*	Conditional 6	3	

Object	Status	Field Strength (T)	Reference
Ultraclip *316 SS* *INRAD, Inc., Grand Rapids, MI*	Safe	1.5	
Ultraclip *Titanium alloy* *INRAD, Inc., Grand Rapids, MI*	Safe	1.5	
Vesocclude Ligating Clip *Vesocclude Medical, LLC* *Mebane, NC*	Conditional 6	3	
Visistat Skin Stapler (Staple) *Hemostatic Clip* *Teleflex Medical, www.teleflex.com*	Conditional 6	3	
Weck Horizon, Titanium Clip, Large *Teleflex Medical, www.teleflex.com*	Conditional 6	3	
Weck Horizon, Titanium Clip, Medium *Teleflex Medical, www.teleflex.com*	Conditional 6	3	

Object	Status	Field Strength (T)	Reference
Miscellaneous			
"J" Hook Bracket *816* *Amerex Corporation, Trussville, AL*	Conditional 7	3	
3/4" Socket Wrench *3/4"*41-mm* *Newmatic Sound, www.newmaticmedical.com*	Conditional 7	3	
357 Magnum Revolver *Model 66-3* *Smith and Wesson, Springfield, MA*	Unsafe 1	1.5	46
4-Leg Base IV Stand, Stainless Steel *Pryor Products* *Oceanside, CA*	Conditional 7	3	
5-Leg Base IV Stand, Aluminum *Pryor Products* *Oceanside, CA*	Conditional 7	3	
AB5000 Ventricle *with In-Flow Cannula and Out-Flow Cannula,* *Cardiac assist device* *Abiomed, Inc., Danvers MA*	Conditional 6	3	113
Accusite pH *Enteral Feeding System pH Site Locator, 10 Fr.* *Zinetics Medical, Salt Lake City, UT*	Unsafe 2	1.5	
ActiFlo Indwelling Bowel Catheter System *also known as Zassi Bowel Management System* *Hollister Incorporated, Libertyville, IL*	Conditional 5	3	
ActiPatch *Drug delivery patch* *BioElectronics Corporation, Frederick, MD*	Unsafe 1	1.5	
Acuvance Jelco (FEP Radiopaque) *intravenous (I.V.) catheter* *Smiths Medical, Southington, CT*	Safe	3	
Acuvance Plus (PUR Radiopaque) *intravenous (I.V.) catheter* *Smiths Medical, Southington, CT*	Safe	3	
Acuvance Plus W (PUR Radiopaque) *intravenous (I.V.) catheter* *Smiths Medical, Southington, CT*	Safe	3	
Adapter used for ICP *Aesculap, Inc., www.aesculapusa.com*	Safe	1.5, 3	
Adiana Radiopaque Implant *Adiana Permanent Contraception System* *Hologic, Inc., www.hologic.com*	Conditional 6	3	
Adiana Silicone Implant *permanent female contraception device* *Adiana, Inc., Redwood City, CA*	Safe	3	
Adjustable Combination Pliers *152-mm* *Newmatic Sound, www.newmaticmedical.com*	Conditional 7	3	

Object	Status	Field Strength (T)	Reference
Adjustable Combination Pliers *P-30* *Ampco Safety Tools, Garland, TX*	Conditional 7	3	
Adjustable-End Wrench, 3/4" *NGK Metals Corporation, Sweetwater, TN*	Conditional 7	3	
Adjustable-End Wrench, 1 1/8" *NGK Metals Corporation, Sweetwater, TN*	Conditional 7	3	
Adjustable Pipe Wrench *W-212AL* *Ampco Safety Tools, Garland, TX*	Conditional 7	3	
Adjustable Pipe Wrench 10" *NGK Metals Corporation, Sweetwater, TN*	Conditional 7	3	
Adjustable Wrench, 24*200-mm *Newmatic Sound, www.newmaticmedical.com*	Conditional 7	3	
Adjustable Wrench, W-70 *Ampco Safety Tools, Garland, TX*	Conditional 7	3	
Adson Tissue Forcep, Ti6Al4V *Johnson & Johnson, www.depuy.com*	Safe	1.5	62
Advance Implant System, Model 10403 *Aspire Medical, Sunnyvale, CA*	Conditional 6	3	
AdVance Male Sling System *AMS, American Medical Systems, www.americanmedicalsystems.com*	Safe	1.5, 3	
Advantiv (PUR Radiopaque) *intravenous (I.V.) catheter* *Smiths Medical, Southington, CT*	Safe	3	
Agile Patency System, Capsule Device *Given Imaging, www.givenimaging.com*	Unsafe 1	1.5	
AirLife Bypass HME *Cardinal Health, Yorba Linda, CA*	Conditional 6	3	
Air-Q Disposable Masked Laryngeal Airway *Mercury Medical, www.mercurymed.com*	Conditional 5	3	
Allen Wrench, WH-1/4 *Ampco Safety Tools, Garland, TX*	Conditional 7	3	
AltaSeal Tubal Occlusion Implant (TOI) *Alta Science, www.altascience.ie*	Conditional 6	3	
Ambu Disposable PEEP Valve *Ambu, Xiamen, China*	Conditional 7	3	
Ambu SPUR II Infant Resuscitator *Ambu, Xiamen, China*	Conditional 7	3	
AMS 800 Urinary Control System *American Medical Systems Inc., www.americanmedicalsystems.com*	Conditional 6	3	
AMS Acticon Neosphincter Prosthesis *AMS, American Medical Systems, www.americanmedicalsystems.com*	Safe	1.5, 3	
AMS Artificial Urinary Sphincter 791 *AMS, American Medical Systems, www.americanmedicalsystems.com*	Safe	1.5, 3	

Object	Status	Field Strength (T)	Reference
AMS Mainstay Urologic Soft-Tissue Anchor *AMS, American Medical Systems, www.americanmedicalsystems.com*	Safe	1.5, 3	
AMS Sphincter 800 *Urinary Control System AMS, American Medical Systems, www.americanmedicalsystems.com*	Safe	1.5, 3	3
Anesthesia Machine MR Magellan-2200 *Model 1 Pneumatically Powered Anesthesia Machine Oceanic Medical Products, Inc., Atchison, KS*	Conditional 7	3	
Anesthesia Machine MR Magellan-2200 *Model-3 Pneumatically Powered Anesthesia Machine Oceanic Medical Products, Inc., Atchison, KS*	Conditional 7	3	
Annular Occlusion Device *AOD AtriCure, Inc., West Chester, OH*	Safe	3	
Annular Occlusion Device *AOD1, 50-mm, Nitinol, Titanium, Polyurethane, Polyester AtriCure, Inc., West Chester, OH*	Conditional 6	3	
Apogee Vaginal Vault Prolapse Repair System *AMS, American Medical Systems, www.americanmedicalsystems.com*	Safe	1.5, 3	
AQUACEL Ag Foam Dressing *ConvaTec Wound Therapeutics, www.convatec.com*	Safe	1.5, 3	
AQUACEL Ag Foam Dressing, Non Adhesive *ConvaTec Wound Therapeutics, www.convatec.com*	Safe	1.5, 3	
Aquacel Ag Dressing *AQUACEL AG Hydrofiber Wound Dressing with Ionic Silver ConvaTec Wound Therapeutics, www.convatec.com*	Safe	1.5, 3	115
AQUACEL Ag Surgical Dressing *ConvaTec Wound Therapeutics, www.convatec.com*	Safe	1.5, 3	
Arctic Sun, Energy Transfer Pad *No metallic components Medivance, Inc., Louisville, CO*	Safe	3	
ARGOS 11-mm Restrictor *Pulmonx, Palo Alto, CA*	Conditional 6	3	
Aria MRI Drill System *Stryker, www.stryker.com*	Conditional 5	3	
Aris Trans-obturator Tape *product for urinary incontinence Coloplast A/S, Humlebaek, Denmark*	Safe	3	
Armboard, Dale, #650 Large *Dale Medical Products, Inc., www.dalemed.com*	Conditional 6	3	
Asept Drainage Catheter System *PFM Medical, Inc.*	Safe	3	
Aspire Medical Advance Implant System *Aspire Medical, Sunnyvale, CA*	Conditional 6	3	
Atrostim Phrenic Nerve Stimulator *Neurostimulation System ATROTECH OY, Tampere, Finland*	Unsafe 1	1.5	

Object	Status	Field Strength (T)	Reference
Autoflush Device *Ref 5897.01, LOT 08 10 02 EA 2007* *Vygon, Paris, France*	Safe	1.5	
Azure, AZ500, Positioning/Comfort Pad *Trulife, Ireland, www.Trulife.com*	Safe	1.5, 3	
B. Braun PERIFIX FX *Epidural Springwound Catheter* *B. Braun Medical Inc.*	Unsafe 1	1.5	
babyPac 100 Ventilator *Smiths Medical PM Inc., Waukesha, WI*	Conditional 5	3	
BACTISEAL Antimicrobial Catheter System *Codman, www.depuy.com*	Safe	3	
Ball Peen Hammer H-00FG *Ampco Safety Tools, Garland, TX*	Conditional 7	3	
BandIt Clip *AtriCure Inc., West Chester, OH*	Conditional 6	3	
Bard Urinary Drainage Bag *C.R. Bard, www.crbard.com*	Conditional 5	5	
Bard Edwards Outflow Tract Fabric *Bard Peripheral Vascular, www.bardpv.com*	Safe	1.5	
Bard Kugal Patch *polypropylene* *Davol, A Bard Company, www.davol.com*	Safe	1.5	
Bard Mesh *Davol, A Bard Company, www.davol.com*	Safe	1.5	
Bard Sauvage Filamentous Fabric *Bard Peripheral Vascular, www.bardpv.com*	Safe	1.5	
Bard Soft Mesh *Davol, A Bard Company, www.davol.com*	Safe	1.5	
Barricaid ARD, Annular Reconstruction Device *Intrinsic Therapeutics, Inc., Woburn, MA*	Conditional 6	3	
Battery, lithium, 3.9 Volt *304 SS and 316L SS, nickle* *Greatbatch Scientific, Clarence, NY*	Conditional 1	1.5	
Battery *Low Magnetic Signature, "C" sized* *Spiral Wound Lithium- Bromine Chloride Cell* *Wilson Greatbatch Technologies, Inc., Clarence NY*	Conditional 7	3	
B-D PosiFlow *needleless IV access connector* *Becton Dickinson, Sandy, Utah*	Safe	1.5	
Beacon Transponder *Calypso Medical Technologies, Inc., Seattle, WA*	Safe	3	
BioArc SP Sling System *AMS, American Medical Systems,* *www.americanmedicalsystems.com*	Safe	1.5, 3	
BioArc TO Subfascial Hammock *AMS, American Medical Systems,* *www.americanmedicalsystems.com*	Safe	1.5, 3	

Object	Status	Field Strength (T)	Reference
BioClip, neurosurgery fixation *Codman, www.depuy.com*	Safe	1.5	
Bioclip, neurosurgical implant *Titanium alloy* *Bioplate, Inc., Los Angeles, CA*	Conditional 6	3	
BioMesh, neurosurgery fixation *C.P. Titanium* *Codman, www.depuy.com*	Safe	1.5	
BioMesh, neurosurgical implant *Titanium* *Bioplate, Inc., Los Angeles, CA*	Conditional 6	3	
Bionector Device *Ref 5897.01, LOT 08 10 02 EA 2007* *Vygon, Paris, France*	Safe	1.5	
Biosearch endo-feeding tube	Safe	1.5	
Bipolar Coagulation Forceps *For use in intraoperative MRI systems* *Aesculap AG & CO.KG, Tuttlingen, Germany*	Safe	1.5, 3	83
Blip Implanted Fiducial Marker *Platinum/Iridium* *Navotek Medical Ltd., Yokneam, Israel*	Conditional 6	3	
Blood Collection Set *SS* *United States Surgical, North Haven, CT*	Safe	1.5, 3	83
Bovine Pericardial Patch, Model 4700 *Edwards Lifesciences, www.edwards.com*	Safe	1.5, 3	
BrachySource *radioactive seed* *Bard Brachytherapy, Inc., Carol Stream, IL*	Conditional 6	3	
Bracket, Model 801 NM 17737 *Amerex Corporation, Trussville, AL*	Conditional 7	3	
Bracket, Model 810 NM 06572 *Amerex Corporation, Trussville, AL*	Conditional 7	3	
Bracket, Model 816 NM 14315 *Amerex Corporation, Trussville, AL*	Conditional 7	3	
Bravo pH Monitoring System *Given Imaging, www.givenimaging.com*	Unsafe 1	1.5	
Bung wrench W-56 *Ampco Safety Tools, Garland, TX*	Conditional 7	3	
Burr Hole Cover *neurosurgery fixation, C.P. Titanium* *Codman, www.depuy.com*	Safe	1.5	
Burr hole cover *neurosurgical implant, Titanium* *Bioplate, Inc., Los Angeles, CA*	Conditional 6	3	
B.Y. Fix Anastomotic Device *Phynox* *HDH Medical Ltd, Israel*	Conditional 6	3	

Object	Status	Field Strength (T)	Reference
B.Y. Fix Anastomotic Device *Stainless Steel* *HDH Medical Ltd, Israel*	Conditional 6	3	
Cannon Catheter II *Chronic Hemodialysis Catheter* *Arrow International, www.arrowintl.com*	Safe	1.5, 3	
CardioBand *Valtech Cardio Ltd., Israel*	Conditional 6	1.5, 3	
Caresite Luer Access Device *B. Braun Medical Inc., Allentown, PA*	Conditional 6	3	
CAREvent MRI *ventilator* *O-Two Medical Technologies, Inc., www.otwo.com*	Conditional 5	3	
Carillon Implant *Mitral Contour System* *Cardiac Dimensions Inc., Kirkland, WA*	Conditional 6	3	
Cart *6 Drawer Breakaway Locking MR Cart with Emergency Cart Package, Model: MR6B-EMG* *The Harloff Company, Colorado Springs, CO*	Conditional 7	3	
Cart *7 Drawer Keylocking MR Cart with Anesthesia Accessory Package, Model: MR7K-MAN* *The Harloff Company, Colorado Springs, CO*	Conditional 7	3	
Cart *7 Drawer Narrow Body Keylocking MR Cart with Emergency Cart, Model: MRN7K-EMG* *The Harloff Company, Colorado Springs, CO*	Conditional 7	3	
Celsius Control Accutrol Catheter *10.7 Fr.* *INNERCOOL Therapies, San Diego, CA*	Conditional 5	1.5	
Celsius Control Accutrol Catheter *14 Fr.* *INNERCOOL Therapies, San Diego, CA*	Conditional 5	1.5	
Celsius Control Standard Catheter *10.7 Fr.* *INNERCOOL Therapies, San Diego, CA*	Conditional 5	1.5	
Celsius Control Standard Catheter *14 Fr.* *INNERCOOL Therapies, San Diego, CA*	Conditional 5	1.5	
CGA 870 Regulator *The Respiratory Group, www.respiratorygroup.com*	Conditional 7	3	
Claw Hammer, 1 lb head, 13" handle *NGK Metals Corporation, Sweetwater, TN*	Conditional 7	3	
Claw Hammer with Handle *680-g* *Newmatic Sound, www.newmaticmedical.com*	Conditional 7	3	
Claw Hammer, H-19FG Ampco Safety Tools, Garland, TX	Conditional 7	3	
CleanScene MRI Fixture *4 x 4 LED, CSMRI44* *Kenall Lighting, Gurnee, IL*	Conditional 7	3	

Object	Status	Field Strength (T)	Reference
ClearCount RFID Tag *ClearCount Medical Solutions, www.clearcount.com*	Conditional 5	3	
Clip Board *Newmatic Sound, www.newmaticmedical.com*	Conditional 7	3	
Codman EDS 3, CSF External Drainage System *Codman, www.depuy.com*	Conditional 6	3	
Codman MicroSensor Skull Bolt *Skull Bolt* *Codman, a Johnson and Johnson Company, Raynham, MA*	Safe	3	
Combination Pliers, slip joint *NGK Metals Corporation, Sweetwater, TN*	Conditional 7	3	
Combination wrench *1304* *Ampco Safety Tools, Garland, TX*	Conditional 7	3	
Common Knife *K-1* *Ampco Safety Tools, Garland, TX*	Conditional 7	3	
COMPASS Headframe (Complete) *using fixation, carbon fiber pin, Delrin Sleeve, Carbon Fiber Pin,* *Delrin Collet w/Nut* *COMPASS International, Inc., Rochester, MN*	Conditional 8	1.5, 3	
COMPASS Headframe (Complete) *using fixation, sharp pin, Delrin Sleeve w/Titanium Tip Insert and* *Delrin Collet w/Nut* *COMPASS International, Inc., Rochester, MN*	Conditional 8	1.5, 3	
Complete Care Urine Collection Bag *C.R. Bard, www.crbard.com*	Conditional 5	3	
Concealed Sprinkler *Model VK462* *The Viking Corporation, Hastings, MI*	Conditional 7	3	
Contraceptive diaphragm *All Flex* *Ortho Pharmaceutical, Raritan, NJ*	Conditional 1	1.5	3
Contraceptive diaphragm *Flat Spring* *Ortho Pharmaceutical, Raritan, NJ*	Conditional 1	1.5	3
Contraceptive diaphragm *Gyne T*	Safe	1.5	47
Contraceptive diaphragm *Koroflex* *Young Drug Products, Piscataway, NJ*	Conditional 1	1.5	3
Contraceptive IUD/IUS *MIRENA, intrauterine system (IUS)* *Berlex Laboratories, Montville, NJ*	Safe	1.5, 3	
Contraceptive IUD *Multiload Cu375, copper, silver*	Safe	1.5	47
Contraceptive IUD *Nova T, copper, silver*	Safe	1.5	47
COOK-SWARTZ Doppler Flow Probe *Cook Medical, www.cookmedical.com, Vandergrift, PA*	Unsafe 1	1.5	
Cool Line Catheter *Alsius Heat Exchange Catheter, ww.zoll.com*	Conditional 5	1.5	

Object	Status	Field Strength (T)	Reference
CoolGuard 3000 Thermoregulation System *Alsius Heat Exchange Catheter, ww.zoll.com*	Unsafe 1	1.5	
Core Temperature Ingestible Capsule *Temperature Device* *VitalSense Integrated Physiological Monitoring System* *Mini Mitter Company, Inc., Bend, OR*	Unsafe 1	1.5	
CORFLO Ultra *Non-weighted, Feeding Tube, Stylet Removed, Polyurethange* *Viasys Healthcard Systems, Wheeling, IL*	Conditional 6	3	
CORFLO, ULTRA 7 *Enteral Feeding Tube* *Viasys MedSystems, Wheeling, IL*	Conditional 6	3	
CORolla TAA Device *CorAssist Cardiovascular Ltd., www.corassist.com*	Conditional 8	1.5, 3	
Coronary Vein Marker *Med-Edge, Inc., www.med-edge.info*	Conditional 6	3	
CO-Set Room Temperature Injectate Kit *Edwards Lifesciences, www.edwards.com*	Conditional 7	3	
CPR Infant Patient Valve, Infant/Child *Patient Valve w/Pop-Off & PEEP Adapter* *Mercury Medical, www.mercurymed.com*	Conditional 5	3	
Craftsman's Knife, 4 1/4" blade *NGK Metals Corporation, Sweetwater, TN*	Conditional 7	3	
Cranial Ceramic Drill bit *ceramic* *MicroSurgical Techniques Inc., Fort Collins, CO*	Safe	1.5	48
Cranial Screw *neurosurgery fixation, size 1.9 x 4.5-mm, Titanium alloy* *Codman, www.depuy.com*	Safe	1.5	
Cranial Screw *neurosurgery fixation, size, 1.5 x 4.5-mm, Titanium alloy* *Codman, www.depuy.com*	Safe	1.5	
CranioFix, Bone Flap Fixation System *Titanium alloy* *Aesculap, Inc., www.aesculapusa.com*	Safe	1.5	50
CranioFix, Burr Hole Clamp *FF0997, 20-mm, Titanium* *Aesculap, Inc., www.aesculapusa.com*	Safe	1.5, 3	83
CranioFix, Burr Hole Clamp *FF100T, 11-mm, Titanium* *Aesculap, Inc., www.aesculapusa.com*	Safe	1.5, 3	83
CranioFix, Burr Hole Clamp *FF101T, 16-mm, Titanium* *Aesculap, Inc., www.aesculapusa.com*	Safe	1.5, 3	83
CranioFix Titanium Clamps *Models including FF099T, FF100T,* *FF101T, FF490T, FF491T, FF492T* *Aesculap, Inc., www.aesculapusa.com*	Safe	3	
CrainioFix 2 *Aesculap, Inc., www.aesculapusa.com*	Safe	1.5	

Object	Status	Field Strength (T)	Reference
CranioFix 2 Titanium Clamps *Models including FF099T, FF100T,* *FF101T, FF490T, FF491T, FF492T* *Aesculap, Inc., www.aesculapusa.com*	Safe	3	
CrainioFix Absorbable *Aesculap, Inc., www.aesculapusa.com*	Safe	1.5, 3	
Crate Opener *70*230-mm* *Newmatic Sound, www.newmaticmedical.com*	Conditional 7	3	
Crate Opener *CJ-1-ST* *Ampco Safety Tools, Garland, TX*	Conditional 7	3	
CV-1 CapsoCam *Pill Camera* *Capso Vision, Inc., Saratoga, CA*	Unsafe 1	1.5	
Cytocan Needle *B. Braun, www.bbraunusa.com*	Conditional 5	1.5, 3	
CYTOGUARD Closed Male Luer Connector *B. Braun, www.bbraunusa.com*	Safe	1.5, 3	
Deck Scraper *45*300-mm* *Newmatic Sound, www.newmaticmedical.com*	Conditional 7	3	
Deck Scraper *S-11G* *Ampco Safety Tools, Garland, TX*	Conditional 7	3	
Deponit, nitroglycerin *transdermal delivery system, aluminized plastic* *Schwarz Pharma, Milwaukee, WI*	Conditional 3	1.5	
Diagonal Cutting Pliers *200-mm* *Newmatic Sound, www.newmaticmedical.com*	Conditional 7	3	
Disetronic Pumps *Disetronic Medical Systems, Inc.* *St. Paul, MN*	Unsafe 1	1.5	
Disposable Sterile, Non-magnetic scalpel #11, MRDS11 *Newmatic Sound, www.newmaticmedical.com*	Conditional 7	3	
Disposable Sterile, Non-magnetic scalpel #21, MRDS21 *Newmatic Sound, www.newmaticmedical.com*	Conditional 7	3	
DISTFLO MINI-CUFF Bypass Graft *Bard Peripheral Vascular, www.bardpv.com*	Safe	1.5	
DOBBHOFF Gastro-Jejunal System *COVIDIEN, www.covidien.com*	Conditional 6	3	
DOBBHOFF Jejunal Feeding/ *Naso-Jejunal/Gastric Decompression System* *COVIDIEN, www.covidien.com*	Conditional 6	3	
DOBBHOFF Nasogastric *Feeding Tube* *COVIDIEN, www.covidien.com*	Conditional 6	3	
DOBBHOFF Naso-Jejunal/ *Gastric Decompression System* *COVIDIEN, www.covidien.com*	Conditional 6	3	

Object	Status	Field Strength (T)	Reference
Double Box End Wrench *W-3130* *Ampco Safety Tools, Garland, TX*	Conditional 7	3	
Double Box Ended Wrench *14*15-mm* *Newmatic Sound, www.newmaticmedical.com*	Conditional 7	3	
Double Open Ended Wrench *18*19-mm* *Newmatic Sound, www.newmaticmedical.com*	Conditional 7	3	
Double Open Ended Wrench *5.5*7-mm* *Newmatic Sound, www.newmaticmedical.com*	Conditional 7	3	
Double Open-end wrench *WO-17X19* *Ampco Safety Tools, Garland, TX*	Conditional 7	3	
Double Step Stool *Newmatic Sound, www.newmaticmedical.com*	Conditional 7	3	
Dressing, PriMatrix Ag Antimicrobial *Dressing, 25-cm x 13-cm* *TEI Biosciences Inc., Boston, MA*	Safe	1.5, 3	
Dry Pad 9 x 9 with Silver Antimicrobial Agent *Newmatic Sound, www.newmaticmedical.com*	Conditional 7	3	
Duet External Drainage System *Model 46914* *Medtronic, Inc., www.medtronic.com*	Conditional 7	3	
Dura-Guard Dural Repair Patch *Synovis Surgical Innovations, www.synovissurgical.com*	Safe	1.5, 3	
DVS, Dose Verification System *implantable radiation dosimeter* *Sicel Technologies, Inc., Morrisville, NC*	Conditional 5	1.5, 3	
E Cylinder Aluminum Construction *Newmatic Sound, www.newmaticmedical.com*	Conditional 7	3	
E/D Cylinder Rack 6 *Newmatic Sound, www.newmaticmedical.com*	Conditional 7	3	
E/D Dual Cylinder Hand Cart *Newmatic Sound, www.newmaticmedical.com*	Conditional 7	3	
EEG electrodes, Adult E-6-GH *gold plated silver* *Grass Co., Quincy, MA*	Safe	0.3	51
EEG electrodes, Pediatric E-5-GH *gold plated silver* *Grass Co., Quincy, MA*	Safe	0.3	51
Elana Ring *Platinum, ELANA BV* *Utrecht, The Netherlands*	Safe	3	
Elevate Female Prolapse Systems *AMS, American Medical Systems,* *www.americanmedicalsystems.com*	Safe	1.5, 3	
Emergency Medical Cot *Model 30-NM* *Ferno-Washington, Inc., Wilmington, OH*	Conditional 7	3	

Object	Status	Field Strength (T)	Reference
Emergency Medical Cot *Model 33-NM* *Ferno-Washington, Inc., Wilmington, OH*	Conditional 7	3	
Emergency Medical Cot *Model 35-ANM* *Ferno Washington Inc., Wilmington, OH*	Conditional 7	3	
EmpowerMR Contrast Injector System *Product Number: 102901* *Bracco Diagnostics, Inc., Princeton, NJ*	Conditional 7	7	
EndoBarrier, EndoBarrier Gastrointestinal Liner *GI Dynamics, Lexington, MA*	Conditional 6	3	
Endo Capsule, Capsule Endoscope System *Olympus Medical Systems Corporation, Japan*	Unsafe 1	1.5	
Endobronchial Valve, EBV-6.5 *Emphasys Medical Inc., Redwood City, CA*	Safe	3	
Endoluminal Occlusion System and Implant Scaffold *Medical Murray, www.medicalmurray.com*	Conditional 6	3	
Endoscope, 30000-10 Endoscope *Shakani Malleable Endoscopic Stylet,* *Clarus Medical, Golden Valley, MN*	Conditional 7	3	
Endoscope, 30000-GLS Scope *Levitan Endoscope* *Clarus Medical, Golden Valley, MN*	Conditional 7	3	
Endoscope, 30001-10 Endoscope *Malleable Pediatric Endoscopic Stylet* *Clarus Medical, Golden Valley, MN*	Conditional 7	3	
Endoscope, rigid, 2.7-mm (Sinuscope) *Greatbatch Scientific, Clarence, NY*	Safe	1.5	59
Endoscope, rigid, 8.0-mm (Laryngoscope) *Greatbatch Scientific, Clarence, NY*	Safe	1.5	59
EndoSure s2 Wireless AAA *(Abdominal Aortic Aneurysm) Pressure Sensor* *CardioMEMS, Inc., Atlanta, GA*	Conditional 5	1.5, 3	
EndoSure Wireless AAA *(Abdominal Aortic Aneurysm) Pressure Sensor* *CardioMEMS, Inc., Atlanta, GA*	Conditional 5	1.5, 3	
Endotracheal (ET) Tube *polyurethane coating with silver* *C.R. Bard, Inc., Covington, GA*	Safe	1.5	
Endotracheal tube with metal ring marker *Trachmate*	Safe	1.5	
Endotracheal Tube *Agento IC, Silver Coated Endotracheal Tube* *Bard Medical Division, Covington, GA*	Conditional 6	3	
ENDO-TUBE *Naso-Jejunal Feeding Tube* *COVIDIEN, www.covidien.com*	Conditional 6	3	
Engineer Hammer, H-14FG *Ampco Safety Tools, Garland, TX*	Conditional 7	3	
ENTRI-FLEX *Nasogastric (NG) Feeding Tube* *COVIDIEN, www.covidien.com*	Conditional 6	3	

Object	Status	Field Strength (T)	Reference
Equine Pericardial Patch, Model XAG *Edwards Lifesciences, www.edwards.com*	Safe	1.5, 3	
ESTRING *Estradiol Vaginal Ring* *Pfizer, www.pfizer.com*	Safe	1.5	
ENTRISTAR *Jejunum Feeding Tube/Gastric Depression Tube* *COVIDIEN, www.covidien.com*	Conditional 6	3	
ESSURE Device *316L SS, Platinum, iridium, nickel, Titanium* *Conceptus, San Marcos, CA*	Safe	1.5, 3	76, 83
ESSURE Device *Nickel-Titanium outer and inner coils* *Conceptus, Inc., Mountain View, CA*	Conditional 6	3	
ESSURE Device *Nickel-Titanium outer coil with a SS inner coil* *Conceptus, Inc., Mountain View, CA*	Conditional 6	3	
Essure Micro-insert *Permanent contraception device* *Conceptus, Inc., Mountain View, CA*	Conditional 6	3	
Esteem *hearing implant* *Envoy Medical, www.envoymedical.com*	Unsafe 1	1.5	
eSVS Mesh *Kips Bay Medical, Plymouth, MN*	Conditional 8	1.5, 3	
EVAHEART *Left Ventricular Assist Device (LVAD)* *www.evaheart-usa.com*	Unsafe 1	1.5	
Extension Set with Caresite Luer Access Device and Spin-Lock Connector *B. Braun Medical Inc., Allentown, PA*	Conditional 6	3	
Extension Set with ULTRASITE Injection Site and Spin-Lock Connector *B. Braun Medical Inc., Allentown, PA*	Conditional 6	3	
Extinguisher *Model B270NM 6-Liter Water Mist Extinguisher* *Amerex Corporation, Trussville, AL*	Conditional 7	7	
Extinguisher *Model B272NM 2.5-Gallon Water Mist Extinguisher* *Amerex Corporation, Trussville, AL*	Conditional 7	7	
Extinguisher *Model 322NM 5.0-LB CO2 Extinguisher* *Amerex Corporation, Trussville, AL*	Conditional 7	7	
Eyelid weight, gold	Safe	1.5	52
EZ Huber Safety Infusion Set *PFM Medical, Inc., Oceanside, CA*	Conditional 6	3	
Fastrac Device *long-term enteral feeding management device* *316LVM SS, Silicone* *Bard Access Systems, www.bardaccess.com*	Conditional 6	3	
Fastrac Gastric Access Port *Silicone, 316LVM SS* *Bard Endoscopic Technologies, Billerica, MA*	Safe	1.5	

Object	Status	Field Strength (T)	Reference
Feeding Tube *C-FMT-8.0-120, Frederick Miller Feeding Tube, Misc.* *Cook Medical, Inc., www.cookmedical.com*	Safe	3	
Feeding Tube *C-FMT-8.0-70, Frederick Miller Feeding Tube, Misc.* *Cook Medical, Inc., www.cookmedical.com*	Safe	3	
Feeding Tube *Gastrostomy Feeding Tube, jejunal* *Kimberly-Clark, Draper, UT*	Safe	3	
Feeding Tube *McClean-Ring Feeding Tube* *Cook Medical, Inc., www.cookmedical.com*	Unsafe 1	1.5	
Fiber-Optic Cardiac Pacing Lead *photonic device* *Biophan Technologies, Inc., Rochester, NY*	Safe	1.5, 3	81
Fiber-optic Intubating *Laryngoscope Blade* *Greatbatch Scientific, Clarence, NY*	Safe	1.5	
Fiber-optic Intubating *Laryngoscope Handle* *Greatbatch Scientific, Clarence, NY*	Safe	1.5	
Fiber-Optic Laryngoscope Blade *Stainless Steel* *PriMedCo, St. Petersburg, FL*	Conditional 7	3	
Fiber-Optic Laryngoscope Handle *Stainless Steel with Battery from Electrohem* *PriMedCo, St. Petersburg, FL*	Conditional 7	3	
Fire Extinguisher *Model 322, 5.0 lb. CO2* *Amerex Corporation, Trussville, AL*	Safe	3	
Fire Extinguisher *Model B270NM, 1 3/4 gallon Water Mist* *Amerex Corporation, Trussville, AL*	Safe	3	
Fire Extinguisher *Model B272NM, 2 1/2 gallon Water Mist* *Amerex Corporation, Trussville, AL*	Safe	3	
Firestar *9-mm semiautomatic* *Star Bonifacio Echeverria, Eibar, Spain*	Unsafe 1	1.5	46
Flex-tip Plus Epidural Catheter *304V SS* *Arrow International Inc., Reading, PA*	Unsafe 2	1.5	
FloTrac Sensor *Edwards Lifesciences, www.edwards.com*	Conditional 5	3	
Flow-Safe CPAP System with Large *Adult Deluxe Contoured Mask* *Mercury Medical, www.mercurymed.com*	Conditional 5	3	
Flowmeter *Quick Click, CFMXXX-XX* *Western Scott Fetzer, Inc., Westlake, OH*	Conditional 7	3	

Object	Status	Field Strength (T)	Reference
Flowmeter *Slim-Line Flowmeter, FMAX0X* *Western Scott Fetzer, Inc., Westlake, OH*	Conditional 7	3	
Flowmeter *Slim-Line Flowmeter, FMEX0X* *Western Scott Fetzer, Inc., Westlake, OH*	Conditional 7	3	
Flowmeter *Slim-Line Flowmeter, FMR100* *Western Scott Fetzer, Inc., Westlake, OH*	Conditional 7	3	
Forceps, ceramic *MicroSurgical Techniques Inc., Fort Collins, CO*	Safe	1.5	48
Forceps, Titanium	Safe	1.39	1
Fortius Catheter *Alsius Heat Exchange Catheter, ww.zoll.com*	Conditional 5	1.5	
FREEHAND System *Implantable Functional Neurostimulator (FNS)* *NeuroControl Corporation, Cleveland, OH*	Conditional 5	1.5	
FREKA Intestinal Tube *Long term intestinal feeding* *Animech Technologies AB, Uppsala, Sweden*	Conditional 6	3	
Fusion, FP801, Positioning/Comfort Pad *Trulife, Ireland, www.Trulife.com*	Safe	1.5, 3	
Gabriel Feeding Tube *Magnetically-Guided Feeding Tube, 12-Fr, GFT112* *Neo-dymium magnets imbedded in distal tip of the tube* *Syncro Medical Innovations, Inc., Canton, OH*	Unsafe 1	3	
Gel pad *various shapes* *AADCO Medical, Inc., Randolph, VT*	Conditional 7	3	
GORE ACUSEAL Cardiovascular Patch *W.L. Gore & Associates, www.goremedical.com*	Safe	1.5, 3	
GORE BIO-A Fistula Plug *W.L. Gore & Associates, www.goremedical.com*	Safe	1.5, 3	
GORE BIO-A Hernia Plug *W.L. Gore & Associates, www.goremedical.com*	Safe	1.5, 3	
GORE BIO-A Tissue Reinforcement *W.L. Gore & Associates, www.goremedical.com*	Safe	1.5, 3	
GORE DUALMESH Biomaterial *W.L. Gore & Associates, www.goremedical.com*	Safe	1.5, 3	
GORE DUALMESH PLUS Biomaterial *DUALMESH PLUS Biomaterial with Holes* *W.L. Gore & Associates, www.goremedical.com*	Safe	1.5, 3	
GORE INFINIT Mesh *W.L. Gore & Associates, www.goremedical.com*	Safe	1.5, 3	
GORE PRECLUDE Peritoneal Membrane *W.L. Gore & Associates, www.goremedical.com*	Safe	1.5, 3	
GORE RESOLUT ADAPT *Regenerative Membrane* *W.L. Gore & Associates, www.goremedical.com*	Safe	1.5, 3	

Object	Status	Field Strength (T)	Reference
GORE RESOLUT ADAPT LT *Regenerative Membrane (bioabsorbable)* *W.L. Gore & Associates, www.goremedical.com*	Safe	1.5, 3	
GORE RESOLUT XT *Regenerative Membrane* *W.L. Gore & Associates, www.goremedical.com*	Safe	1.5, 3	
GORE SEAMGUARD Staple Line Reinforcement *W.L. Gore & Associates, www.goremedical.com*	Safe	1.5, 3	
GORE-TEX Regenerative Membrane *W.L. Gore & Associates, www.goremedical.com*	Safe	1.5, 3	
Grab 'n Go Heliox *portable medical heliox system, aluminum cylinder* *CAUTION: DO NOT USE STEEL CYLINDERS* *Praxair Healthcare Services, Burr Ridge, IL*	Conditional 7	3	
Grab 'n Go Vantage *portable oxygen system, aluminum D cylinder* *CAUTION: DO NOT USE STEEL CYLINDERS* *Praxair Healthcare Services, Burr Ridge, IL*	Conditional 7	3	
Grab 'n Go Vantage *portable oxygen system, aluminum E cylinder* *CAUTION: DO NOT USE STEEL CYLINDERS* *Praxair Healthcare Services, Burr Ridge, IL*	Conditional 7	3	
Grab 'n Go Vantage *regulator/pressure gauge* *CAUTION: DO NOT USE STEEL CYLINDERS* *Praxair Healthcare Services, Burr Ridge, IL*	Conditional 7	3	
Grab 'n Go Vantage *D cylinder, oxygen tank* *CAUTION: DO NOT USE STEEL CYLINDERS* *Praxair Healthcare Services, Burr Ridge, IL*	Conditional 7	3	
Grab 'n Go Vantage *E cylinder, oxygen tank* *CAUTION: DO NOT USE STEEL CYLINDERS* *Praxair Healthcare Services, Burr Ridge, IL*	Conditional 7	3	
Groove Joint Pliers, 2 1/2" *NGK Metals Corporation, Sweetwater, TN*	Conditional 7	3	
Groove Joint Pliers, 10" *Newmatic Sound, www.newmaticmedical.com*	Conditional 7	3	
Groove Joint Pliers, 300-mm *Newmatic Sound, www.newmaticmedical.com*	Conditional 7	3	
Groove Joint Pliers, P-39 *Ampco Safety Tools, Garland, TX*	Conditional 7	3	
Gurney with IV Pole *Newmatic Sound, www.newmaticmedical.com*	Conditional 7	3	
Gurney *Newmatic Sound, www.newmaticmedical.com*	Conditional 7	3	
Hamper *HAMPF* *Newmatic Sound, www.newmaticmedical.com*	Conditional 7	3	

Object	Status	Field Strength (T)	Reference
Hand Tool Kit *six piece, NF-240, Standard screw driver, Philips screw driver,* *Wrench, Pliers, Adjustable pliers, Crate opener* *AADCO Medical, Inc., Randolph, VT*	Conditional 7	3	
Heine Gamma Sphygmomanometer *Newmatic Sound, www.newmaticmedical.com*	Conditional 7	3	
Hemashield Finesse *Ultra-Thin, Knitted, Cardiovascular Patch, vascular graft, Polyester* *Boston Scientific Corporation, Quincy, MA*	Safe	3	
Hemashield Gold Microvel *Knitted Double Velour, Vascular Graft, Polyester* *Boston Scientific Corporation, Quincy, MA*	Safe	3	
Hex Key Wrench, 1.5-mm *Newmatic Sound, www.newmaticmedical.com*	Conditional 7	3	
Hex Key Wrench, 1-1/16" *Newmatic Sound, www.newmaticmedical.com*	Conditional 7	3	
HoverMatt, HM34DC - 34"x78" *heat-sealed air mattress, nylon twill with polyurethane coating* *HoverTech International, Bethlehem, PA*	Conditional 6	3	
HoverMatt, HM34HS - 34"x78" *heat-sealed air mattress, nylon twill* *HoverTech International, Bethlehem, PA*	Conditional 6	3	
Hummingbird Parenchyma, ICP Monitoring *InnerSpace, www.innerspacemedical.com*	Conditional 5	1.5, 3	
Hyperinflation System, Hyperinflation Valve Assembly *with Pop-Off Valve and Manometer* *Mercury Medical, www.mercurymed.com*	Conditional 5	3	
IBV Valve, Nitinol *Spiration Inc., Redmond, WA*	Conditional 6	3	
Icy Catheter *Alsius Heat Exchange Catheter* *ww.zoll.com*	Conditional 5	1.5	
IMPLANON *etonogestrel implant, contraceptive implant, flexible plastic rod* *Organon USA Inc., Roseland, NJ*	Safe	1.5	109
Implantable Spinal Fusion Stimulator *Bone Fusion Stimulator, Model SpF-100* *Electro-Biology, Inc. (EBI), Parsippany, NJ*	Conditional 5	1.5	63
Implantable Spinal Fusion Stimulator *Bone Fusion Stimulator* *Electro-Biology, Inc. (EBI), Parsippany, NJ*	Conditional 5	1.5	
In-Fast Bone Screw *Titanium alloy* *AMS, American Medical Systems,* *www.americanmedicalsystems.com*	Safe	3	
In-Fast Loop Screw *Titanium alloy* *AMS, American Medical Systems,* *www.americanmedicalsystems.com*	Safe	3	
In-Fast Sling System *AMS, American Medical Systems,* *www.americanmedicalsystems.com*	Safe	1.5, 3	

Object	Status	Field Strength (T)	Reference
In-Fast Swivel Screw *Titanium alloy* *AMS, American Medical Systems,* *www.americanmedicalsystems.com*	Safe	3	
In-Fast Ultra Sling System *AMS, American Medical Systems,* *www.americanmedicalsystems.com*	Safe	1.5, 3	
Infusion Set, MMT-11X *Medtronic MiniMed Inc., Northridge, CA*	Safe	1.5	
Infusion Set, MMT-31X *Medtronic MiniMed Inc., Northridge, CA*	Safe	1.5	
Infusion Set, MMT-32X *Medtronic MiniMed Inc., Northridge, CA*	Safe	1.5	
Infusion Set, MMT-37X *Medtronic MiniMed Inc., Northridge, CA*	Safe	1.5	
Infusion Set, MMT-39X *Medtronic MiniMed Inc., Northridge, CA*	Safe	1.5	
Infusion Set, Polyfin, MMT-106 *Medtronic MiniMed Inc., Northridge, CA*	Unsafe 1	1.5	
Infusion Set, Polyfin, MMT-107 *Medtronic MiniMed Inc., Northridge, CA*	Unsafe 1	1.5	
Infusion Set, Polyfin, MMT-16X *Medtronic MiniMed Inc., Northridge, CA*	Unsafe 1	1.5	
Infusion Set, Polyfin, MMT-30X *Medtronic MiniMed Inc., Northridge, CA*	Unsafe 1	1.5	
Infusion Set, Polyfin, MMT-36X *Medtronic MiniMed Inc., Northridge, CA*	Unsafe 1	1.5	
Insulin Pump *Animas 2020 Insulin Pump* *Animas Corporation, www.animascorp.com*	Unsafe 1	1.5	
Insulin Pump *IR 1000 Insulin Pump* *Animas Corporation, www.animascorp.com*	Unsafe 1	1.5	
Insulin Pump *IR 1100 Insulin Pump* *Animas Corporation, www.animascorp.com*	Unsafe 1	1.5	
Insulin Pump *IR 1200 Insulin Pump* *Animas Corporation, www.animascorp.com*	Unsafe 1	1.5	
Insulin Pump *IR Animas 1200* *Animas Corporation, www.animascorp.com*	Unsafe 1	1.5	
Intima-II I.V. Catheter System *BD Medical Systems, Becton Dickinson, Sandy, Utah*	Safe	1.5	
Intracranial depth electrodes *for EEG recordings, nickle-chromium alloy* *Superior Tube Company, Norristown, NY*	Safe	1.5	53
Intracranial Pressure Monitor (ICP) *Pressio ICP Monitoring Device* *SOPHYSA, France*	Unsafe 1	1.5	

Object	Status	Field Strength (T)	Reference
Intraflex Feeding Tube *tungstun weight, plastic*	Safe	1.5	
Intrauterine contraceptive device (IUD) *Copper T, copper* *Searle Pharmaceuticals, Chicago, IL*	Safe	1.5	54
Intrauterine Contraceptive Device *Copper T 380A, ParaGard* *FEI, North Tanawanda, NY*	Conditional 5	3	111
Intrauterine contraceptive device (IUD) *Lippey loop, plastic*	Safe	1.5	
Intrauterine contraceptive device (IUD) *Perigard* *Gyne Pharmaceuticals*	Safe	1.5	
InVance Male Sling System *AMS, American Medical Systems,* *www.americanmedicalsystems.com*	Safe	1.5, 3	
IsoMed *implantable drug infusion system* *Medtronic, Inc., www.Medtronic.com*	Conditional 5	1.5	
IUD, LCS, Ultra Low Dose Levonorgestrel *Contraceptive System* *Bayer Schering Pharma Oy, Turku, Finland*	Conditional 6	3	
IV Pole, HD NM *Model 513-10* *Ferno Washington Inc., Wilmington, Ohio*	Conditional 7	3	
IV Pole, PN R&D#0556 *Pryor Products, Oceanside, CA*	Conditional 7	3	
IV Stand 4 Hook with Casters, Aluminum *Newmatic Sound, www.newmaticmedical.com*	Conditional 7	3	
IV Stand 4 Hook with Casters *Newmatic Sound, www.newmaticmedical.com*	Conditional 7	3	
Janitorial Cleaning Cart *Continental Commercial Products, Bridgeton, MO*	Conditional 7	3	
Jelco (FEP Radiopaque) *intravenous (I.V.) catheter* *Smiths Medical, Southington, CT*	Safe	3	
Jelco (FEP) *intravenous (I.V.) catheter* *Smiths Medical, Southington, CT*	Safe	3	
Jelco 2 (FEP) *intravenous (I.V.) catheter* *Smiths Medical, Southington, CT*	Safe	3	
Jelco W (FEP) *intravenous (I.V.) catheter* *Smiths Medical, Southington, CT*	Safe	3	
KimVent Multi Access Port *Closed Suction Catheter* *Kimberly Clark, Roswell, GA*	Conditional 6	3	
KimVent Percutaneous Dilatational *Tracheostomy Tube* *Kimberly Clark, Roswell, GA*	Conditional 6	3	

Object	Status	Field Strength (T)	Reference
Ladder 8-foot *Newmatic Sound, www.newmaticmedical.com*	Conditional 7	3	
Ladder, Aluminum TIA 6-ft, Twin Front *Cuprum S.A. de C.V.*	Conditional 7	3	
Ladder, Fiberglass TIA 6-ft, Twin Front *Cuprum S.A. de C.V.*	Conditional 7	3	
Langenbeck Periosteal Elevator *304 SS* *Johnson & Johnson Professional, Inc., www.depuy.com*	Safe	1.5	62
Laparoscopic Graspers *Greatbatch Scientific, Clarence, NY*	Safe	1.5	
LAP-BAND (LAPBAND) *adjustable gastric band* *INAMED, Goleta, CA*	Safe	3	
LAP-BAND (LAPBAND) AP System *Adjustable Gastric Banding System with OMNIFORM Design* *Allergan, Inc., www.allergan.com*	Conditional 5	3	
LAP-BAND (Lapband) AP Adjustable Gastric *Banding System with OMNIFORM Design* *Allergan, www.allergan.com*	Conditional 5	3	
Large Flexible Burr Hole Cover *neurosurgery fixation, C.P. Titanium* *Codman, www.depuy.com*	Safe	1.5	
Large Rigid Burr Hole Cover *neurosurgery fixation, C.P. Titanium* *Codman, www.depuy.com*	Safe	1.5	
Laryngoscope Blade, Fiber-Optic *Sun-Flex, MAC 4, 304 SS* *PriMedCo*	Conditional 7	3	
Laryngoscope Blade, Fiber-Optic *Straight, 304 SS* *PriMedCo*	Conditional 7	3	
Laryngoscope Blade Miller 00, LRYM00 *Newmatic Sound, www.newmaticmedical.com*	Conditional 7	3	
Laryngoscope Blade Miller 04, LRYM4 *Newmatic Sound, www.newmaticmedical.com*	Conditional 7	3	
Laryngoscope Fiber Optic Blade *Size Mac 2* *Scope Medical, India*	Conditional 7	3	
Laryngoscope Fiber Optic Blade *Size Mac 3* *Scope Medical, India*	Conditional 7	3	
Laryngoscope Fiber Optic Blade *Size Mac 4* *Scope Medical, India*	Conditional 7	3	
Laryngoscope Fiber Optic Blade *Size Mill 1* *Scope Medical, India*	Conditional 7	3	
Laryngoscope Fiber Optic Blade *Size Mill 2* *Scope Medical, India*	Conditional 7	3	

Object	Status	Field Strength (T)	Reference
Laryngoscope Fiber Optic Blade *Size Mill 3* *Scope Medical, India*	Conditional 7	3	
Laryngoscope Fiber Optic *Handle Medium Size* *Scope Medical, India*	Conditional 7	3	
Laryngoscope Handle *Model 15-MRI-HMED-1, Blade - Mac 3, Model 15-MRI-MAC3* *Lithium Battery, Model 15-MRI-L1* *NovaMed, LLC, Rye, New York*	Conditional 7	3	
Laryngoscope Handle Standard, LRYH *Newmatic Sound, www.newmaticmedical.com*	Conditional 7	3	
LED Downlight Fixture *MRIDL6VL* *Kenall Lighting, Gurnee, Illinois*	Conditional 7	3	
Licox CC1.P1 Oxygen and Temperature Probe *Brain Tissue Oxygen Monitoring System* *Integra NeuroSciences, Plainsboro, NJ*	Conditional 5	1.5	
LifeGuard Safety Infusion Set *ANGIODYNAMICS Inc., Manchester, GA*	Conditional 6	3	
Light Source *for Malleable Pediatric Endoscopic Stylet,* *Malleable Pediatric Endoscopic Stylet, and Levitan Endoscope* *5197-201 Turbo LED Light Source* *nonmagnetic power source is needed* *Clarus Medical, Golden Valley, MN*	Conditional 7	3	
Lightweight Aluminum Gurney *Newmatic Sound, www.newmaticmedical.com*	Conditional 7	3	
Lineman Pliers, 200-mm *Newmatic Sound, www.newmaticmedical.com*	Conditional 7	3	
Lineman's pliers, P-35 *Ampco Safety Tools, Garland, TX*	Conditional 7	3	
Linen Hamper 18-inch D-Casters *Newmatic Sound, www.newmaticmedical.com*	Conditional 7	3	
LINX Reflux Management System *Torax Medical, www.toraxmedical.com*	Unsafe 1	1.5	
LMA Fastrach, ETT Size 8 *The Laryngeal Mask Company, Singapore*	Conditional 5	3	
LMA Fastrach Endotracheal Tube *size 8-mm, endotracheal tube* *LMA North America, Inc., San Diego, CA*	Conditional 5	1.5	
LMA-Classic *size 5, large adult, laryngeal mask airway* *LMA North America, Inc., San Diego, CA*	Conditional 5	1.5	
LMA Flexible, Size 6 *The Laryngeal Mask Company, Singapore*	Conditional 5	3	
LMA-Flexible *size 2, larygeal mask airway* *LMA North America, Inc., San Diego, CA*	Conditional 5	1.5	
LMA ProSeal, Size 5 *The Laryngeal Mask Company, Singapore*	Conditional 5	3	

Object	Status	Field Strength (T)	Reference
LMA-ProSeal, endotracheal tube *LMA North America, Inc., San Diego, CA*	Conditional 5	1.5	
LMA Supreme, Size 5 *The Laryngeal Mask Company, Singapore*	Conditional 5	3	
Long nose side cut pliers, P-326 *Ampco Safety Tools, Garland, TX*	Conditional 7	3	
Low Magnetic Signature, Lithium Battery (C size) *Greatbatch Scientific, Clarence, NY*	Safe	1.5	
Low magnetic Signature Lithium Battery, Part # BTRY *Newmatic Sound, www.newmaticmedical.com*	Conditional 7	3	
LUNA PVO *NFOCUS Neuromedical, Palo Alto, CA*	Conditional 6	3	
LVIS Device, Intraluminal Support Device *Microvention, www.microvention.com*	Conditional 5	3	
Mac 4, 15-MRI-FOD-Mac 4, Plastic *Laryngoscope part* *NovaMed, LLC, Rye, New York*	Conditional 7	3	
Mac 5, 15-MRI-Mac 5, SS *Laryngoscope part* *NovaMed, LLC, Rye, New York*	Conditional 7	3	
Maestro Neuroregulator *Model 1002, Neurostimulator, Obesity Treatment* *EnteroMedics Inc., St. Paul, MN*	Unsafe 1	1.5	
Manometer, Disposable Manometer Assembly *Mercury Medical, www.mercurymed.com*	Conditional 5	3	
Manometer, NF-121 *for mounting on IV pole* *AADCO Medical, Inc., Randolph, VT*	Conditional 7	3	
Manual Jet Ventilator (P/N 00-325-MRI) *Anesthesia Associates, Inc., San Marcos, CA*	Conditional 7	3	
May Hegar Needle, Holder, Ti6Al-4V *Johnson & Johnson Professional, Inc., www.depuy.com*	Safe	1.5	62
Mayo Stand 16-inch x 21-inch *Newmatic Sound, www.newmaticmedical.com*	Conditional 7	3	
Mechanical Ventilator, MR Magellan *Pneumatically Powered, Mechanical Ventilator* *Oceanic Medical Products, Inc., Atchison, KS*	Conditional 7	3	
Medex 3000 Series MRI Syringe Infusion Pump *Medex, Dublin, OH*	Conditional 5	1.5	
Medfusion 3500 Syringe Pump *Smiths Medical, www.smiths-medical.com*	Conditional 5	3	
Medical M Cylinder Hand Cart *Newmatic Sound, www.newmaticmedical.com*	Conditional 7	3	
Medium Handle, 15-MRI-HMED-2 *Laryngoscope part* *NovaMed, LLC, Rye, New York*	Conditional 7	3	
Medium Handle, 15-MRI-HMED-3 *Laryngoscope part* *NovaMed, LLC, Rye, New York*	Conditional 7	3	

Object	Status	Field Strength (T)	Reference

Medivance Nasogastric Sump Tube
    with YSI Series 400 Temperature Sensor
    Medivance, Inc., Louisville, CO
	Conditional 5	3	

MEDRAD Continuum MR Infusion System *MEDRAD, Inc., Indianola, PA*	Conditional 5	1.5, 3	
Mercury Duotube-feeding, feeding tube	Safe	1.5	
Micro Needle Holder *Greatbatch Scientific, Clarence, NY*	Safe	1.5	
Micro Round Handled Scissors *Greatbatch Scientific, Clarence, NY*	Safe	1.5	
Micro Tissue Forceps *Greatbatch Scientific, Clarence, NY*	Safe	1.5	
Micro Tying Forceps *Greatbatch Scientific, Clarence, NY*	Safe	1.5	

Mil 4, 15-MRI-FOMD-Mil 4
    SS, plastic, Laryngoscope part
    NovaMed, LLC, Rye, New York
	Conditional 7	3	

MiniArc Precise Single-Incision Sling System
    AMS, American Medical Systems,
    www.americanmedicalsystems.com
	Safe	1.5, 3	

MiniMed 2007, Implantable Insulin Pump *Medtronic MiniMed Inc., Northridge, CA*	Unsafe 1	1.5	
MiniMed 407C, Infusion Pump *Medtronic MiniMed Inc., Northridge, CA*	Unsafe 1	1.5	
MiniMed 508, Insulin Pump *Medtronic MiniMed Inc., Northridge, CA*	Unsafe 1	1.5	
Mitek anchor *Miteck Products, Westood, MA*	Safe	1.5	
Mitroflow Valsalva Conduit *Sorin Group, www.sorin.com*	Conditional 6	3	

Mobile lead acrylic barrier
    S-602 NF, for use in MRI and Image Guided Therapy
    AADCO Medical, Inc., Randolph, VT
	Conditional 7	3	

Monarc Subfascial Hammock
    AMS, American Medical Systems,
    www.americanmedicalsystems.com
	Safe	1.5, 3	

MONARC System
    Edwards Lifesciences
    www.Edwards.com
	Conditional 5	3	

Monkey Wrench, 58 x 305-mm *Newmatic Sound, www.newmaticmedical.com*	Conditional 7	3	
MR Bone Punch, Dismantalable *Aesculap, Inc., www.aesculapusa.com*	Safe	1.5	74

MR Compatible Laryngoscope Handle
    short size handle
    MINRAD INC., Buffalo, NY
	Conditional 7	3	

MR Compatible Laryngoscope Handle
    standard size handle
    MINRAD INC., Buffalo, NY
	Conditional 7	3	

Object	Status	Field Strength (T)	Reference
MR Compatible WISCONSIN 4 Laryngoscope Blade *short size handle* *MINRAD INC., Buffalo, NY*	Conditional 7	3	
MR Currette, Curved, 90 degree Blunt Ring *Aesculap, Inc., www.aesculapusa.com*	Safe	1.5	74
MR Suction Cannula, with Suction Stop *Aesculap, Inc., www.aesculapusa.com*	Safe	1.5	74
MR-Brain Spatula with Silicone *Model FF408K* *Aesculap AG & CO.KG, Tuttlingen, Germany*	Safe	1.5, 3	83
MRI Conditional Flashlight, FLSH *Newmatic Sound, www.newmaticmedical.com*	Conditional 7	3	
MRI Conditional Pen, Part # MRPEN2 *Newmatic Sound, www.newmaticmedical.com*	Conditional 7	3	
MRI Conditional Roller Ball Pen, Part # MRPEN1 *Newmatic Sound, www.newmaticmedical.com*	Conditional 7	3	
MRI Disposable Scalpel *Titanium* *QSUM Biopsy Disposables LLC, Boulder, CO*	Conditional 7	3	
MRidium 3850 MRI IV Pump *MRidium Corporation, www.iradimed.com*	Conditional 5	3	
MRidium 3860 MRI IV Pump *MRidium Corporation, www.iradimed.com*	Conditional 5	3	
MRI FastSystem Retractor System *Omni-Tract Surgical, Minneapolis, MN*	Safe	1.5	83
MRI IV Pole, adjustable *NF-110* *AADCO Medical, Inc., Randolph, VT*	Conditional 7	3	
MRI Laryngoscope LED Handle *Newmatic Sound, www.newmaticmedical.com*	Conditional 7	3	
MRI Needle, Inconel *QSUM Biopsy Disposables LLC, Boulder, CO*	Conditional 7	3	
MRI Non-Magnetic 1.5v Dry Cell Battery *Newmatic Sound, www.newmaticmedical.com*	Conditional 7	3	
MRI Walk-O2-Bout Regulator *The Respiratory Group, www.respiratorygroup.com*	Conditional 7	3	
MRI Wheelchair 18" wide *NF-500* *AADCO Medical, Inc., Randolph, VT*	Conditional 7	3	
MR-Kocher-Langenbeck Retractor *70 X 14-mm* *Aesculap, Inc., www.aesculapusa.com*	Safe	1.5	74
MR-Mallet with Alloy Handle *50 grams* *Aesculap, Inc., www.aesculapusa.com*	Safe	1.5	74
MR IV Pole *MRidium Corporation, www.iradimed.com*	Conditional 5	3	
MR-Septum Speculum *Aesculap, Inc., www.aesculapusa.com*	Safe	1.5	74
MR-Weil-Blakesley Ethmoid Forceps *Aesculap, Inc., www.aesculapusa.com*	Safe	1.5	74

Object	Status	Field Strength (T)	Reference
MR Wheelchair, 26 x 20 DP *Gendron, www.gendroninc.com*	Conditional 7	1.5, 3	
Neo-Fit Neonatal Endotracheal Tube Grip/Holder *Cooper Surgical, www.coopersurgical.com*	Conditional 6	3	
Neo-Tee Infant T-Piece Resuscitator *Mercury Medical, www.mercurymed.com*	Conditional 5	3	
NephroMax High Pressure *Nephrostomy Balloon Catheter* *Boston Scientific, www.bostonscientific.com*	Safe	1.5, 3	
Neuro Arch *Pulsar Vascular, www.pulsarvascular.com*	Conditional 6	3	
Neurostimulation System *Activa PC Deep Brain Neurostimulator (Model 37601)* *DBS System* *Medtronic, Inc., www.Medtronic.com*	Conditional 5	1.5	
Neurostimulation System *Activa RC Deep Brain Neurostimulator (Model 37612)* *DBS System* *Medtronic, Inc., www.Medtronic.com*	Conditional 5	1.5	
Neurostimulation System *Activa SC Deep Brain Neurostimulator (Model 37602)* *DBS System* *Medtronic, Inc., www.Medtronic.com*	Conditional 5	1.5	
Neurostimulation System *Activa SC Deep Brain Neurostimulator (Model 37603)* *DBS System* *Medtronic, Inc., www.Medtronic.com*	Conditional 5	1.5	
Neurostimulation System *deep brain stimulation, Activa System* *includes Model 7426 Soletra and Model 7424 Itrel II* *neurostimulators, Model 3387 and Model 3389 DBS leads* *Medtronic, Inc., www.Medtronic.com*	Conditional 5	1.5	79, 80, 100
Neurostimulation system *deep brain stimulation* *Itrel II* *Medtronic, Inc., www.Medtronic.com*	Conditional 5	1.5	99, 101
Neurostimulation system *deep brain stimulation* *Kinetra* *Medtronic, Inc., www.Medtronic.com*	Conditional 5	1.5	99, 100
Neurostimulation system *deep brain stimulation* *Soletra* *Medtronic, Inc., www.Medtronic.com*	Conditional 5	1.5	92, 99
Neurostimulation System *Enterra Therapy, Gastric Electrical Stimulation (GES) System* *Medtronic, Inc., www.Medtronic.com*	Unsafe 1	1.5	
Neurostimulation System *Eon (IPG), Spinal Cord Stimulation* *St. Jude Medical, www.sjmprofessional.com*	Unsafe 1	1.5	
Neurostimulation System *Eon C, Spinal Cord Stimulation* *St. Jude Medical, www.sjmprofessional.com*	Unsafe 1	1.5	

Object	Status	Field Strength (T)	Reference
Neurostimulation System *Eon Mini, Spinal Cord Stimulation* *St. Jude Medical, www.sjmprofessional.com*	Unsafe 1	1.5	
Neurostimulation System *Genesis, Spinal Cord Stimulation* *St. Jude Medical, www.sjmprofessional.com*	Unsafe 1	1.5	
Neurostimulation System *GenesisRC, Spinal Cord Stimulation* *St. Jude Medical, www.sjmprofessional.com*	Unsafe 1	1.5	
Neurostimulation System *GenesisXP, Spinal Cord Stimulation* *St. Jude Medical, www.sjmprofessional.com*	Unsafe 1	1.5	
Neurostimulation System *InterStim Therapy, Sacral Nerve Stimulation for Urinary Control* *Medtronic, Inc., www.Medtronic.com*	Unsafe 1	1.5	99
Neurostimulation System *Neurostep* *Neurostream Technologies, www.neurostream-technologies.com*	Unsafe 1	1.5	
Neurostimulation System *NeuRx Diaphragm Pacing System DPS* *Synapse Biomedical, www.synapsebiomedical.com*	Unsafe 1	1.5	
Neurostimulation System *PrimeAdvanced Spinal Cord Neurostimulator* *PrimeAdvanced, Model 37702* *Medtronic, Inc., www.Medtronic.com*	Conditional 5	1.5	
Neurostimulation System *Reclaim Deep Brain Neurostimulator, Model 3760* *DBS System* *Medtronic, Inc., www.Medtronic.com*	Conditional 5	1.5	
Neurostimulation System *Renew, Spinal Cord Stimulation* *St. Jude Medical, www.sjmprofessional.com*	Unsafe 1	1.5	
Neurostimulation System *Renova Cortical Stimulation System* *Northstar Neuroscience, Seattle, WA*	Unsafe 1	1.5	
Neurostimulation System *RestoreAdvanced Spinal Cord Neurostimulator* *·RestoreAdvanced, Model 37713* *Medtronic, Inc., www.Medtronic.com*	Conditional 5	1.5	
Neurostimulation System *RestoreUltra Spinal Cord Neurostimulator* *RestoreUltra, Model 37712* *Medtronic, Inc., www.Medtronic.com*	Conditional 5	1.5	
Neurostimulation system *spinal cord stimulation, chronic pain, Itrel 3* *Medtronic, Inc., www.Medtronic.com*	Conditional 5	1.5	99
Neurostimulation system *spinal cord stimulation, chronic pain, Mattrix* *Medtronic, Inc., www.Medtronic.com*	Unsafe 1	1.5	99
Neurostimulation system *spinal cord stimulation, chronic pain, Restore* *Medtronic, Inc., www.Medtronic.com*	Conditional 5	1.5	99

Object	Status	Field Strength (T)	Reference
Neurostimulation system *spinal cord stimulation, chronic pain, Synergy* *Medtronic, Inc., www.Medtronic.com*	Conditional 5	1.5	99
Neurostimulation system *spinal cord stimulation, chronic pain, SynergyCompact* *Medtronic, Inc., www.Medtronic.com*	Conditional 5	1.5	99
Neurostimulation system *spinal cord stimulation, chronic pain, SynergyPlus* *Medtronic, Inc., www.Medtronic.com*	Conditional 5	1.5	99
Neurostimulation system *spinal cord stimulation, chronic pain, Versitrel* *Medtronic, Inc., www.Medtronic.com*	Conditional 5	1.5	99
Neurotimulation System *Targeted Hypoglossal Neurostimulation (THN) Sleep Therapy* *aura6000 system* *ImThera Medical Inc. www.imtheramedical.com*	Unsafe 1	1.5	
Neurostimulation system *Vagus Nerve Stimulation, Vagal Nerve Stimulator* *VNS Therapy, NeuroCybernetic Prosthesis (NCP) System* *Cyberonics, Inc., www.vnstherapy.com*	Conditional 5	1.5, 3	
NeuroVentriClear *Ventricular Drainage Catheter Set* *Cook Neurological, Inc., Leechburg, PA*	Safe	3	
Nextus/Raz Soft Tissue Anchor *Straight, Titanium alloy* *AMS, American Medical Systems,* *www.americanmedicalsystems.com*	Safe	3	
Nextus/Raz Soft Tissue Anchor, Curved *Titanium alloy* *AMS, American Medical Systems,* *www.americanmedicalsystems.com*	Safe	3	
Nit-Occlud ASD-R *PFM S.R.L., www.pfmsrl.com*	Conditional 6	3	
Non-Magnetic Adjustable Chair *Newmatic Sound, www.newmaticmedical.com*	Conditional 7	3	
Non-Magnetic Cylinder Cart *Newmatic Sound, www.newmaticmedical.com*	Conditional 7	3	
Non-magnetic Floor Sweeper, SWPR *Newmatic Sound, www.newmaticmedical.com*	Conditional 7	3	
Non-Magnetic Prism Glasses *Newmatic Sound, www.newmaticmedical.com*	Conditional 7	3	
Non-Magnetic Sprague Rappaport Stethoscope *Newmatic Sound, www.newmaticmedical.com*	Conditional 7	3	
NovaSilk, synthetic mesh *Coloplast A/S, Humlebaek, Denmark*	Safe	3	
NuvaRing, Contraceptive device *Schering Corporation, Kenilworth, NJ*	Safe	1.5	
Oasis Elite, EL218, Positioning/Comfort Pad *Trulife, Ireland, www.Trulife.com*	Safe	1.5, 3	
Oasis, OA053, Positioning/Comfort Pad *Trulife, Ireland, www.Trulife.com*	Safe	1.5, 3	

Object	Status	Field Strength (T)	Reference
OmniPod Insulin Management System *Controlling device must be removed* *Insulet Corporation, www.myomnipod.com*	Unsafe 1	1.5	
ON-Q SilverDressing *I-Flow Corporation, www.iflo.com*	Conditional 6	3	
Onyx HD-500 Liquid Embolic System *ev3 Inc., www.ev3.net*	Conditional 8	1.5, 3	
Onyx Liquid Embolic System *ev3 Inc., www.ev3.net*	Conditional 8	1.5, 3	
Opti-Flo Tube Attachment Device (T.A.D.) *ConvaTec Wound Therapeutics, United Kingdom*	Conditional 6	3	
Optistar MR Contrast Delivery System *Mallinckrodt, St. Louis, MO*	Safe	1.5	
Optiva (PUR Radiopaque) *intravenous (I.V.) catheter* *Smiths Medical, Southington, CT*	Safe	3	
Optiva 2 (PUR Radiopaque) *intravenous (I.V.) catheter* *Smiths Medical, Southington, CT*	Safe	3	
Optiva W (PUR Radiopaque) *intravenous (I.V.) catheter* *Smiths Medical, Southington, CT*	Safe	3	
OxyTOTE NG, All In One System *Western MNS-603* *Western Enterprises, Westlake, OH*	Conditional 7	3	
P140 System Implant, HeartNet *Paracor Medical, Inc., Sunnyvale, CA*	Conditional 6	3	
P150 System Implant, HeartNet *Paracor Medical, Inc., Sunnyvale, CA*	Conditional 6	3	
Palatal System Implant Assembly *Pavad Medical, Inc., Fremont, CA*	Conditional 5	1.5	
PAS-Port Proximal, Anastomosis System Implant *Cardica, Redwood City, CA*	Conditional 6	3	
Patient Scoop, Model 65 EXL *Ferno-Washington, Inc., Wilmington, OH*	Conditional 7	3	
Pediatric Tracheostomy Tube *Smiths Medical, www.smiths-medical.com*	Conditional 5	3	
PEDI-TUBE *Pediatric Nasogastric (NG) Feeding Tube* *COVIDIEN, www.covidien.com*	Conditional 6	3	
Peep Valve *Mercury Medical, www.mercurymed.com*	Conditional 5	3	
Peep Valve with Filter *Mercury Medical, www.mercurymed.com*	Conditional 5	3	
Penfield Dissector *304 SS* *Johnson & Johnson Professional, Inc., www.depuy.com*	Safe	1.5	62
Percutaneous Intraspinal Catheter *Model 8516* *Medtronic, Inc., www.medtronic.com*	Unsafe 2	1.5	

Object	Status	Field Strength (T)	Reference
Pericardial Patch, Hancock, Model 710 *Medtronic, Inc., www.medtronic.com*	Safe	1.5, 3	84
Pericardial Patch, Hancock, Model 710L *Medtronic, Inc., www.medtronic.com*	Safe	1.5, 3	84
Perigee Transobturator Anterior Prolapse Repair System *AMS, American Medical Systems,* *www.americanmedicalsystems.com*	Safe	1.5, 3	
Peri-Guard Repair Patch *Synovis Surgical Innovations, www.synovissurgical.com*	Safe	1.5, 3	
Peripheral Nerve Stimulator *MR-STIM, Model GN-013* *Greatbatch Scientific, Clarence, NY*	Safe	1.5	
Peri-Strips Dry with Veritas Collagen Matrix *Synovis Surgical Innovations, www.synovissurgical.com*	Safe	1.5, 3	
Phillips Screwdriver, 200-mm *Newmatic Sound, www.newmaticmedical.com*	Conditional 7	3	
PillCam, All models *Given Imaging, www.givenimaging.com*	Unsafe 1	1.5	
PillCam COLON 2 capsule endoscopy *Given Imaging, www.givenimaging.com*	Unsafe 1	1.5	
PillCam M2A Capsule Endoscopy Device *Ingestible Capsule* *Given Imaging Inc., www.givenimaging.com*	Unsafe 1	1.5	
PillCam ESO Capsule Endoscopy Device *Ingestible Capsule* *Given Imaging Inc., www.givenimaging.com*	Unsafe 1	1.5	
PillCam ESO2 Capsule Endoscopy Device *Ingestible Capsule* *Given Imaging Inc., www.givenimaging.com*	Unsafe 1	1.5	
PillCam SB Capsule Endoscopy Device *Ingestible Capsule* *Given Imaging Inc., www.givenimaging.com*	Unsafe 1	1.5	
Pinnacle Pelvic Floor Repair (PFR) Kit *Boston Scientific, www.bostonscientific.com*	Safe	1.5	
Pipe Wrench, 50-mm *Newmatic Sound, www.newmaticmedical.com*	Conditional 7	3	
PneumRx Lung Volume Reduction Coil (LVRC) *PneumRx, Inc., www.pneumrx.com*	Conditional 6	3	
Polyform Mesh, Polypropylene *Boston Scientific, www.bostonscientific.com*	Safe	1.5	
Polyform Synthetic Mesh *Boston Scientific, www.bostonscientific.com*	Safe	1.5	
Polyurethane Flange *Biodesign Enterocutaneous Fistula Plug* *Cook Medical, Inc., www.cookmedical.com*	Conditional 6	3	
Ponto Wide Implant, Used With *Bone Conduction Hearing System* *Oticon Medical, www.oticonmedical.com*	Conditional 6	3	
Port Delivery System (PDS) Implant *Forsight Vision, Menlo Park, CA*	Conditional 6	3	

Object	Status	Field Strength (T)	Reference
Portex Bivona Flextend Tracheostomy Tube *All similar products, Tracheostomy* *Smiths Medical International, England*	Conditional 6	3	
Portex Bivona Laryngectomy Tube, All similar products *Laryngectomy Tube* *Smiths Medical International, England*	Safe	3	
Portex Bivona Non-Wire *Reinforced Cuffed Tracheostomy Tube* *All similar products, Tracheostomy* *Smiths Medical International, England*	Conditional 6	3	
Portex Bivona Neonatal Tracheostomy Tube *Smiths Medical, www.smiths-medical.com*	Conditional 5	3	
Portex Bivona Sleep Apoea (Apnea) Tube *All similar products, Sleep Apoea (Apnea) Tube* *Smiths Medical International, England*	Safe	3	
Portex Bivona Uncuffed *Non-Reinforced Endotracheal Tube* *All similar products* *Smiths Medical International, England*	Safe	3	
Portex Bivona Uncuffed *Non-Wire Reinforced Tracheostomy Tube* *All similar products, Tracheostomy* *Smiths Medical International, England*	Safe	3	
Portex Bivona Wire, Reinforced Endotracheal Tube *All similar products, Endotracheal* *Smiths Medical International, England*	Conditional 6	3	
Portex Bivona Wire, Reinforced *Tracheostomy Tube, All similar products, Tracheostomy* *Smiths Medical International, England*	Conditional 6	3	
Portex Cricothyroidotomy Tube *Cricothyroidotomy* *Smiths Medical International, England*	Conditional 6	3	
Portex Cuffed Endotracheal Tube *All similar products* *Smiths Medical International, England*	Conditional 6	3	
Portex Guedel Airway *Airway, All similar products* *Smiths Medical International, England*	Safe	3	
Portex Heat and Moisture Exchanger *All similar products* *Smiths Medical International, England*	Safe	3	
Portex Mini-Trach, Tracheostomy *Smiths Medical International, England*	Safe	3	
Portex Nasal Oxygen Set *All similar products, Nasal Oxygen Set* *Smiths Medical International, England*	Safe	3	
Portex Non-Wire *Reinforced Cuffed Tracheostomy Tube,* *All similar products, Tracheostomy* *Smiths Medical International, England*	Conditional 6	3	

Object	Status	Field Strength (T)	Reference
Portex Orator Speaking Valve *All similar products, Speaking Valve* *Smiths Medical International, England*	Safe	3	
Portex Tracheal Tube Holder *All similar products, Endotracheal Tube Holder* *Smiths Medical International, England*	Safe	3	
Portex Uncuffed Non-Wire *Reinforced Endotracheal Tube, All similar products, Endotracheal* *Smiths Medical International, England*	Safe	3	
Portex Uncuffed *Non-reinforced Tracheostomy Tube* *All similar products, Tracheostomy* *Smiths Medical International, England*	Safe	3	
Portex, UniPerc Tracheostomy Tube *Tracheostomy* *Smiths Medical, www.smiths-medical.com*	Conditional 5	3	
Portex Wire Reinforced Endotracheal Tube *All similar products* *Smiths Medical International, England*	Conditional 6	3	
Post Valve and Aluminum E Cylinder *PX-8703-1CW* *Western Scott Fetzer, Inc., Westlake, OH*	Conditional 7	3	
Post Valve, MPV-5870 *Western Scott Fetzer, Inc., Westlake, OH*	Conditional 7	3	
PPS Quick Safety Huber Needle *Perouse Medical.com, www.perousemedical.com*	Conditional 6	3	
Precision Spinal Cord Stimulation System *Neurostimulation System* *Boston Scientific Corporation, www.bostonscientific.com*	Unsafe 1	1.5	
PREVAIL Paragastric Implant System *Vibrynt Inc., www.vibrynt.com*	Conditional 6	3	
ProAct, Male Adjustable Continence Therapy *Uromedica Inc., Plymouth, MN*	Conditional 6	3	
Protectiv (FEP Radiopaque) *intravenous (I.V.) catheter* *Smiths Medical, Southington, CT*	Safe	3	
Protectiv Acuvance 2 (PUR Radiopaque) *intravenous (I.V.) catheter* *Smiths Medical, Southington, CT*	Safe	3	
Protectiv Jelco (FEP Radiopaque) *intravenous (I.V.) catheter* *Smiths Medical, Southington, CT*	Safe	3	
Protectiv Plus (PUR Radiopaque) *intravenous (I.V.) catheter* *Smiths Medical, Southington, CT*	Safe	3	
Protectiv Plus W (PUR Radiopaque) *intravenous (I.V.) catheter* *Smiths Medical, Southington, CT*	Safe	3	
Protectiv W (FEP Radiopaque) *intravenous (I.V.) catheter* *Smiths Medical, Southington, CT*	Safe	3	

Object	Status	Field Strength (T)	Reference
Putty Knife, 40 x 200-mm *Newmatic Sound, www.newmaticmedical.com*	Conditional 7	3	
Putty Knife, K-20 *Ampco Safety Tools, Garland, TX*	Conditional 7	3	
Putty Knife, Wooden Handle *NGK Metals Corporation, Sweetwater, TN*	Conditional 7	3	
PVC Sling Bariatric Gurney *Newmatic Sound, www.newmaticmedical.com*	Conditional 7	3	
RapidFlap LS *Resorbable Cranial Flap Fixation, Biomet Microfixation* *www. www.lorenzsurgical.com*	Safe	1.5, 3	
Ratchet Wrench *3/4" x 320-mm* *Newmatic Sound, www.newmaticmedical.com*	Conditional 7	3	
Realize Adjustable Gastric Band *also known as Swedish Adjustable Gastric Band* *Ethicon Endosurgery, Inc., www.e-ifu.com*	Conditional 5	3	
REALIZE Adjustable Gastric Band-C *Ethicon Endo-Surgery, Inc., www.ees.com*	Conditional 5	3	
Rebound HRD, Hernia Repair Device *Nitinol* *Minnesota Medical, Plymouth, MN*	Conditional 6	3	
Regulator and Aluminum Cylinder System *AirTOTE, MTS-303* *Western Scott Fetzer, Inc., Westlake, OH*	Conditional 7	3	
Regulator and Aluminum Cylinder System *OxyTOTE, MTS-603* *Western Scott Fetzer, Inc., Westlake, OH*	Conditional 7	3	
Regulator and Aluminum Cylinder System *OxyTOTE, MTS-803* *Western Scott Fetzer, Inc., Westlake, OH*	Conditional 7	3	
Regulator and Aluminum Cylinder System *PediaTOTE, MTS-103* *Western Scott Fetzer, Inc., Westlake, OH*	Conditional 7	3	
Regulator, NMR-540-15FM *Western Scott Fetzer, Inc., Westlake, OH*	Conditional 7	3	
Regulator, NMR-870-15FM *Western Scott Fetzer, Inc., Westlake, OH*	Conditional 7	3	
Regulator, NMR-870-P *Western Scott Fetzer, Inc., Westlake, OH*	Conditional 7	3	
Regulator, Western NMR-870-15FM *MR Conditional Regulator on Aluminum M6A cylinder* *Western Enterprises, Westlake, OH*	Conditional 7	3	
Regulator, Western NMR-870-15FM *MR Conditional Regulator with non-conforming G-2-4000N inlet* *gauge on Aluminum M6A cylinder* *Western Enterprises, Westlake, OH*	Conditional 7	3	
Regulator *Western NMR-540-15FM* *MR Conditional Regulator with non-conforming G-2-4000N inlet* *gauge on Aluminum M6A cylinder* *Western Enterprises, Westlake, OH*	Conditional 7	3	

Object	Status	Field Strength (T)	Reference
Relieva Stratus Microflow Spacer *Acclarent, Inc., Menlo Park, CA*	Conditional 6	3	
Repliform Tissue Regeneration Matrix *Boston Scientific, www.bostonscientific.com*	Safe	1.5, 3	
RespiCardia System *neurostimulation system, phrenic nerve stimulator* *Cardiac Concepts, Inc., www.cardiacconcepts.com*	Unsafe 1	1.5	
RF BION Microstimulator *Neurostimulation System* *Alfred E. Mann Foundation for Scientific Research, Valencia, CA*	Conditional 5	1.5	89
Rheos Baroreflex System *Rheos Hypertension (HT) Therapy* *CVRx Inc., Minneapolis, MN*	Unsafe 1	1.5	
Robotic Radiosurgery Tumor Marking Seed *Tumor marking device, Gold, Silver* *RADONTEK LTD., Ankara, Turkey*	Conditional 6	3	
Round Wire Brush *B-399* *Ampco Safety Tools, Garland, TX*	Conditional 7	3	
Rusch Larygoscope Handle *brass head, aluminum barrel, arbon-zinc battery, SS* *Teleflex Medical, Durham, NC*	Conditional 7	3	
Rusch Macintosh Size 4 *Fiber-optic Laryngoscope Blade* *Teleflex Medical, Durham, NC*	Conditional 7	3	
SAM Sling *SAM Medical Products, Portland, OR*	Conditional 6	3	
Sancuso (Granisetron Transdermal System, Transdermal Patch) *ProStrakan*	Safe	1.5	
Sand bag *12 pound, Vinyl Silica Sand Bag* *Newmatic Sound Systems, Inc.*	Conditional 7	3	
Scalpel, Microsharp Ceramic Scalpels, *sizes #10, #11, #11c, #15, ceramic* *MicroSurgical Techniques, Inc., Fort Collins, CO*	Safe	1.5	48
Scalpel, SS	Unsafe 1	1.5	
Scissors, Ceramic *Microsurgical Techniques, Inc., Fort Collins, CO*	Safe	1.5	48
Scissors, 225-mm *Newmatic Sound, www.newmaticmedical.com*	Conditional 7	3	
Scraper, S-10G *Ampco Safety Tools, Garland, TX*	Conditional 7	3	
Screw driver, Phillips *S-1099A* *Ampco Safety Tools, Garland, TX*	Conditional 7	3	
Screwdriver, Slot, Flat Head *NGK Metals Corporation, Sweetwater, TN*	Conditional 7	3	
Screw driver, standard *S-49* *Ampco Safety Tools, Garland, TX*	Conditional 7	3	

Object	Status	Field Strength (T)	Reference
Screw *Titanium alloy* *Bioplate, Inc., Los Angeles, CA*	Conditional 6	3	
SecurAcath Universal Version *Interrad Medical, Inc., St. Paul, MN*	Conditional 6	3	
SecurAcath Universal Version 1.1 *Interrad Medical, Inc., St. Paul, MN*	Conditional 6	3	
SERVO-i Ventilator, MRI Version *MAQUET, Inc., www.maquet.com*	Conditional 5	1.5, 3	
Seven System *Continuous Glucose Monitoring System* *DexCom, Inc., San Diego, CA*	Unsafe 1	1.5	
ShapeLoc Soft Tissue Fastener *MedShape Solutions, Inc., Atlanta, GA*	Conditional 6	3	
Shelhigh Injectable Pulmonic Valve *pulmonic valve replacement prosthesis, Nitinol, bovine pericardium* *Shelhigh Inc., Union, NJ*	Conditional 6	3	
Sherwood post-valve *Praxair, Inc., Tonawanda, NY*	Conditional 7	3	
Shoe Handle Wire-brush, 4 x 17 rows *NGK Metals Corporation, Sweetwater, TN*	Conditional 7	3	
Side Cutting Pliers, P-36 *Ampco Safety Tools, Garland, TX*	Conditional 7	3	
SilverSite Access Site Dressing *4-mm opening* *Tri-State Hospital Supply Corporation, Howell, MI*	Conditional 6	3	
Single PVC Hamper Cart *Newmatic Sound, www.newmaticmedical.com*	Conditional 7	3	
Sleuth *Implantable ECG Monitoring System, Model 2010 Sleuth IMD* *6.5-cm version* *Transoma Medical, St. Paul, MN*	Conditional 5	1.5	
Sleuth AT Implantable Monitoring System *Models 9006/9008* *Transoma Medical, St. Paul, MN*	Conditional 5	1.5	
Slot Screwdriver, 11 x 300-mm *Newmatic Sound, www.newmaticmedical.com*	Conditional 7	3	
Slot Screwdriver, 3 x 50-mm *Newmatic Sound, www.newmaticmedical.com*	Conditional 7	3	
Solyx SIS, Single Incision Sling System *Boston Scientific, www.bostonscientific.com*	Safe	1.5, 3	
SPARC Sling System *AMS, American Medical Systems,* *www.americanmedicalsystems.com*	Safe	1.5, 3	
Spectris MR Injection System *Medrad, Inc., Indianola, PA*	Safe	1.5	
Spiegelberg System Bolt *SS* *Aesculap, Inc., www.aesculapusa.com*	Safe	1.5, 3	83
Spine Fusion Stimulator, SpF PLUS-Mini *Biomet Spine, www.biomet.com*	Conditional 5	1.5	

Object	Status	Field Strength (T)	Reference
Spine Fusion Stimulator, SpF-XL IIb *Biomet Spine* *www.biomet.com*	Conditional 5	1.5	
Sponge Forcep *Ti6Al-4V* *Johnson & Johnson Professional, Inc., www.depuy.com*	Safe	1.5	62
SPRINKER *Model F4FR-NF, Non-Ferrous Quick Response Concealed* *Automatic Sprinkler for MRI Type Applications* *The Reliable Automatic Sprinkler Co., Inc., Elmsford, NY*	Conditional 7	3	
StarClose SE Vascular Closure System *Abbott Vascular, www.abbottvascular.com*	Conditional 5	3	
StarClose Vascular Closure System *Abbott Vascular, www.abbottvascular.com*	Conditional 5	3	
Step Stool with Handrail *Newmatic Sound, www.newmaticmedical.com*	Conditional 7	3	
Stereotactic headframe with removable mouthpiece *aluminum, 8-18 SS Delrin, Titanium* *Compass International, Inc., Rochester, MN*	Safe	1.5	
Straight-In Sacral Colpopexy System *AMS, American Medical Systems,* *www.americanmedicalsystems.com*	Safe	1.5, 3	
Stretcher, 1000 MR *Gendron, Inc., Archbold, OH*	Conditional 7	3	
Stryker PainPump 2 *Infusion Pump* *Stryker Instruments, Kalamazoo, MI*	Unsafe 1	1.5	
Stryker PainPump *Infusion Pump* *Stryker Instruments, Kalamazoo, MI*	Unsafe 1	1.5	
Subcutaneous Evacuating Port System, SEPS *Medtronic, Inc., www.Medtronic.com*	Unsafe 1	1.5	
Suction/Irrigation Handle for Sinuscope *Greatbatch Scientific, Clarence, NY*	Safe	1.5	
Suction Regulator, Model Number 881VR *Genstar Technologies Co., Inc., Chino, CA*	Conditional 7	3	
Super ArrowFlex PSI *10 Fr. x 65-cm, 304V SS* *Arrow International Inc., Reading, PA*	Unsafe 2	1.5	
Super ArrowFlex PSI *9 Fr. x 11-cm, 304 V SS* *Arrow International Inc., Reading, PA*	Unsafe 2	1.5	
Supple Peri-Guard Repair Patch *Synovis Surgical Innovations* *www.synovissurgical.com*	Safe	1.5, 3	
SUPPRELIN LA Implant *Histrelin acetate subcutaneous implant* *Endo Pharmaceuticals, www.supprelinla.com*	Safe	1.5	
Supris *Suprapubic mesh sling* *Coloplast A/S, Humlebaek, Denmark*	Safe	3	

Object	Status	Field Strength (T)	Reference
SureConnect Patient Connector *Baxa Corporation, Englewood, CO*	Conditional 5	3	
Surecan Needle *B. Braun, www.bbraunusa.com*	Conditional 5	1.5, 3	
Surecan Safety II, Safety Needle *B. Braun, www.bbraunusa.com*	Conditional 6	3	
Swedish Adjustable Gastric Band (SAGB) *Titanium, Silicone* *Ethicon Endo-Surgery, Inc., www.ees.com*	Safe	1.5, 3	
Symphony, A Counter Pulsation *Device for Heart Failure Patient* *Abiomed, Inc., Danvers, MA*	Conditional 5	3	
SynchroMed EL *implantable drug infusion system* *Medtronic, Inc., www.Medtronic.com*	Conditional 5	1.5, 3	
SynchroMed II *implantable drug infusion system* *Medtronic, Inc., www.Medtronic.com*	Conditional 5	1.5, 3	
SynchroMed *implantable drug infusion system* *Medtronic, Inc., www.Medtronic.com*	Conditional 5	1.5, 3	
Table Model Mercury Blood Pressure Manometer *Table model, NF-120* *AADCO Medical, Inc., Randolph, VT*	Conditional 7	3	
Tantalum powder	Safe	1.39	1
Tape Mechanical Occlusive Device (TMOD) *implantable artificial urinary sphincter* *GT Urological, LLC, Minneapolis, MN*	Conditional 7	3	
Tears Naturale Port Punctal Occluder *Alcon Research, Ltd., Fort Worth, Texas*	Safe	1.5	
Telemetric ICP (Intracranial Pressure) Sensor Probe *Neckarate GmbH & Co KG, www.neckarate.com*	Unsafe 1	1.5	
Testicular prosthesis or implant *gel-filled* *Coloplast A/S, Humlebaek, Denmark*	Safe	3	
Testicular prosthesis or implant *saline-filled* *Coloplast A/S, Humlebaek, Denmark MR safe*	Safe	3	
Testicular prosthesis or implant *Torosa* *Coloplast A/S, Humlebaek, Denmark*	Safe	3	
TheraCath, 304 V SS *Arrow International Inc., Reading, PA*	Unsafe 2	1.5	
TheraSeed Radioactive Seed Implant *Titanium, graphite, lead* *Theragenics Corporation, Buford, GA*	Safe	1.5, 3	
Tin Snips *S-1144, W-212AL* *Ampco Safety Tools, Garland, TX*	Conditional 7	3	
Titanium Adjustable Wrench *Newmatic Sound, www.newmaticmedical.com*	Conditional 7	3	

Object	Status	Field Strength (T)	Reference
Titanium Bengolea Haemostatic Forceps *Curved* *Newmatic Sound, www.newmaticmedical.com*	Conditional 7	3	
Titanium Gerald Dissecting Forceps *Newmatic Sound, www.newmaticmedical.com*	Conditional 7	3	
Titanium Knot *LSI Solutions Inc., Victor, NY*	Conditional 6	3	
Titanium Potts Micro Scissors *angulated 60 degrees* *Newmatic Sound Systems, www.newmaticsound.com*	Conditional 7	3	
Transport Chair 20-inch *Newmatic Sound, www.newmaticmedical.com*	Conditional 7	3	
TransWarmer Infant Transport Mattress *Cooper Surgical, www.coopersurgical.com*	Conditional 6	3	
TruWave Disposable Pressure Transducer *Edwards Lifesciences, www.edwards.com*	Conditional 5	3	
TS System Arterial Closure Device *Arterial Closure Device (ACD)* *Vasorum Ltd, Ireland*	Conditional 6	3	
TVFMI, Titanium Vocal Fold Medializing Implant (Friedrich) *Titanium (ASTM Grade F67 Medical Grade)* *Kurz Medical, Inc., Norcross, GA*	Safe	3	
Tweezers, Ceramic *prototype, ceramic* *MicroSurgical Techniques, Inc., Fort Collins, CO*	Safe	1.5	48
Tweezers, 8340 *Ampco Safety Tools, Garland, TX*	Conditional 7	3	
ULT - Drainage Catheter *Cook Medical, www.cookmedical.com*	Conditional 6	3	
ULTRASITE Valve *B. Braun Medical Inc., Allentown, PA*	Conditional 6	3	
UroLift Anchor *316L SS, SS* *NeoTract, Pleasanton, CA*	Conditional 5	3	
Urolume Endoprosthesis *AMS, American Medical Systems,* *www.americanmedicalsystems.com*	Safe	1.5, 3	
V-Chordal Surgical *Valtech Cardio Ltd., Israel*	Conditional 6	3	
V.A.C. GranuFoam Silver *Dressing* *KCI USA, Inc., San Antonio, TX*	Conditional 6	3	
VANTAS Implant *Histrelin Implant* *Endo Pharmaceuticals, www.vantasimplant.com*	Safe	1.5	
Vascu-Guard Vascular Patch *Peripheral Vascular Patch* *Synovis Surgical Innovations, www.synovissurgical.com*	Safe	1.5, 3	
Vascular marker, O-ring washer *302 SS* *PIC Design, Middlebury, CT*	Conditional 1	1.5	

Object	Status	Field Strength (T)	Reference
Vectra Vascular Access Graft (VAG) *Bard Peripheral Vascular, www.bardpv.com*	Safe	1.5	
Vehicle Bracket *810NM* *Amerex Corporation, Trussville, AL*	Conditional 7	3	
Venaflo II Vascular Graft *Bard Peripheral Vascular, www.bardpv.com*	Safe	1.5	
Ventricular Partitioning Implant *VPD* *CardioKinetix Inc., Redwood City, CA*	Conditional 6	3	
VeriChip *Microtransponder,* *miniaturized radio frequency identification device* *VeriChip Corporation, Palm Beach, FL*	Conditional 5	7	
Veritas Collagen Matrix *Synovis Surgical Innovations, www.synovissurgical.com*	Safe	1.5, 3	
Viadur *leuprolide acetate implant, Titanium* *Bayer HealthCare Pharmaceuticals, West Haven, CT*	Safe	1.5	
Vitallium implant	Safe	1.5	
V-Link Luer Activated Device *with VitalShield Protective Coating, Non-DEHP Y-Type Catheter* *Extension Set, Non-DEHP Y-Type, Catheter Extension Set* *Baxter Healthcare, Round Lake, IL*	Conditional 6	3	
VOCARE Bladder System *Implantable Functional Neuromuscular Stimulator (FNS)* *Neurostimulation System* *NeuroControl Corporation, Valley View, OH*	Conditional 5	1.5	
VPASS Implant *316L SS* *Percardia Inc., Merrimack, NH*	Safe	3	
Vygon AutoFlush *Plastic, 316L SS* *Vygon Coporation, Norristown, PA*	Conditional 6	3	
Vygon Bionector *Needle Access Device, Plastic, 316L SS* *Vygon Corporation, Norristown, PA*	Conditional 6	3	
Wall Bracket *17737 (801)* *Amerex Corporation, Trussville, AL*	Conditional 7	3	
Watchman Gen 4 Implant *Atritech Inc., Plymouth, MN*	Conditional 6	3	
WATCHMAN Left Atrial Appendage Closure Device *Nitinol, Titanium* *Atritech Inc., Plymouth, MN*	Conditional 6	3	
WayPoint Anchor *FHC, Inc., Bowdoin, ME*	Conditional 6	3	
WedgeLoc Suture Anchor *MedShape Solutions, Inc., Atlanta, GA*	Conditional 6	3	
Western EZ-OX Plus System *ALQ-2342 on an Aluminum D cylinder* *Western Enterprises, Westlake, OH*	Conditional 7	3	

Object	Status	Field Strength (T)	Reference
Western EZ-OX Plus System *ALQ-2342 on an Aluminum D cylinder* *Western Enterprises, Westlake, OH*	Conditional 7	3	
Wheelchair 18-inch Detachable Foot Rest *Newmatic Sound, www.newmaticmedical.com*	Conditional 7	3	
Wheelchair 22-inch Detachable Foot Rest *Newmatic Sound, www.newmaticmedical.com*	Conditional 7	3	
Wheelchair 26-inch Detachable Foot Rest *Newmatic Sound, www.newmaticmedical.com*	Conditional 7	3	
Wheelchair IV/Oxygen Tank Holder *Newmatic Sound, www.newmaticmedical.com*	Conditional 7	3	
Wheelchair, 20" SS Heavy *Duty Folding Aquatic Wheelchair* *Aqua Creek Products, LLC, Missoula, MT*	Conditional 7	3	
Wheelchair, Merlexi Craft Liberty *MRI Synthetic Resin Manual Wheelchair* *Turbo Wheelchair Co., Beaufort, SC*	Conditional 7	3	
Wheelchair, MR 18, 4000 MR *SPORTLITE* *Gendron, Inc., Archbold, OH*	Conditional 7	3	
Winged infusion set, MRI compatible *E-Z-EM, Inc., Westbury, NY*	Safe	1.5	58
Woodson Elevator, 304 SS *Johnson & Johnson Professional, Inc., www.depuy.com*	Safe	1.5	62
Wristband, Soft Infant Wristband *Zebra Technologies, Vernon Hills, IL*	Safe	1.5, 3	
Wristband, Z-Band 4000 *Zebra Technologies, Vernon Hills, IL*	Safe	1.5, 3	
Wristband, Z-Band Comfort *Zebra Technologies, Vernon Hills, IL*	Safe	1.5, 3	
Wristband, Z-Band Direct (no color) *Zebra Technologies, Vernon Hills, IL*	Safe	1.5, 3	
Wristband, Z-Band Direct with Color (Red) *Zebra Technologies, Vernon Hills, IL*	Safe	1.5, 3	
Wristband, Z Band Quick Clip & Red Clip *Zebra Technologies, Vernon Hills, IL*	Safe	1.5, 3	
Xenform Soft Tissue Repair Matrix *Boston Scientific, www.bostonscientific.com*	Safe	1.5, 3	
Xseal *Essential Medical, Wayne, PA*	Conditional 6	3	
YD post-valve *Praxair, Inc., Tonawanda, NY*	Conditional 7	3	
Zephyr Transcopic Endobronchial Valve *Emphasys Medical Inc., Redwood City, CA*	Conditional 6	3	
Zip Implant Device *Titanium alloy* *Bioplate, Inc., Los Angeles, CA*	Conditional 6	3	

Object	Status	Field Strength (T)	Reference

Ocular Implants, Lens Implants, and Devices

Object	Status	Field Strength (T)	Reference
Ahmed glaucoma valve *glaucoma drainage implant, nonmetallic* *New World Medical, Rancho Cucamonga, CA*	Safe	3	105
ARGOS-IO, Eye Implant, Ocular Implant *Implandata Ophthalmic Products GmbH, www.implandata.com*	Conditional 6	3	
Baerveldt glaucoma drainage implant *glaucoma drainage implant, nonmetallic* *Pharmacia Co., Kalamazoo, MI*	Safe	3	
Clip 250, double tantalum clip *tantalum, ocular* *Mira Inc.*	Safe	1.5	29
Clip 50, double tantalum clip *tantalum, ocular* *Mira Inc.*	Safe	1.5	29
Clip 51, single tantalum clip *tantalum, ocular* *Mira Inc.*	Safe	1.5	29
Clip 52, single tantalum clip *tantalum, ocular* *Mira Inc.*	Safe	1.5	29
Double tantalum clip *tantalum, ocular* *Storz Instrument Co.*	Safe	1.5	29
Double tantalum clip style 250 *tantalum, ocular* *Storz Instrument Co.*	Safe	1.5	29
DuraPlug, Temporary Canalicular Insert *EagleVision, Memphis, TN*	Safe	3	
EaglePlug *Punctum Plug* *EagleVision, Memphis, TN*	Safe	3	
Eagle FlexPlug *Punctum Plug* *EagleVision, Memphis, TN*	Safe	3	
Ex-PRESS Mini Glaucoma Shunt, 316LVM *Optonol Ltd., Israel*	Conditional 6	3	117
Fatio eyelid spring/wire, ocular	Unsafe 1	1.5	30
Gelansert *Temporary Canalicular Insert* *EagleVision, Memphis, TN*	Safe	3	
Gold eyelid spring, ocular	Safe	1.5	
Hydrus Aqueous Implant, Ocular Implant *Ivantis, Inc. www.ivantisinc.com*	Conditional 6	3	
Intraocular Lens, Models 12A, 12P, 12S, 24P, 31P, 42P, 61P, 71, 71B, 71M, 71P, 71PC, 71R, 75M, 75P, EXP D *Bausch & Lomb, www.bausch.com*	Unsafe 1	1.5	
Implantable Miniature Telescope *VisionCare Ophthalmic Technologies, Inc., www.visioncareinc.net*	Conditional 6	3	
Intraocular Lens Implant, Binkhorst, iridocapsular lense *Platinum-iridium loop, ocular*	Safe	1.0	

Object	Status	Field Strength (T)	Reference
Intraocular Lens Implant, Binkhorst, iridocapsular lense *Platinum-iridium loop, ocular*	Safe	1.5	31
Intraocular Lens Implant, Binkhorst, iridocapsular lense *Titanium loop, ocular*	Safe	1.0	31
Intraocular Lens Implant, Worst, Platinum clip lense *ocular*	Safe	1.0	31
Joseph valve, glaucoma drainage implant *Valve Implants Limited, Hertford, England*	Safe	3	31
Krupin-Denver eye valve to disc implant *glaucoma drainage implant, nonmetallic* *E. Benson Hood Laboratories, Pembroke, MA*	Safe	3	
Lens Implant, CR5BUO *Alcon Laboratories, Inc., Fort Worth, TX*	Safe	3	
Lens Implant, CZ60BD *Alcon Laboratories, Inc., Fort Worth, TX*	Safe	3	
Lens Implant, CZ70BD *Alcon Laboratories, Inc., Fort Worth, TX*	Safe	3	
Lens Implant, LC80BD *Alcon Laboratories, Inc., Fort Worth, TX*	Safe	3	
Lens Implant, LX10BD *Alcon Laboratories, Inc., Fort Worth, TX*	Safe	3	
Lens Implant, LX90BD *Alcon Laboratories, Inc., Fort Worth, TX*	Safe	3	
Lens Implant, MA30AC *Alcon Laboratories, Inc., Fort Worth, TX*	Safe	3	
Lens Implant, MA60AC *Alcon Laboratories, Inc., Fort Worth, TX*	Safe	3	
Lens Implant, MA30BA *Alcon Laboratories, Inc., Fort Worth, TX*	Safe	3	
Lens Implant, MA50BM *Alcon Laboratories, Inc., Fort Worth, TX*	Safe	3	
Lens Implant, MA60BM *Alcon Laboratories, Inc., Fort Worth, TX*	Safe	3	
Lens Implant, MA60MA *Alcon Laboratories, Inc., Fort Worth, TX*	Safe	3	
Lens Implant, MC30BA *Alcon Laboratories, Inc., Fort Worth, TX*	Safe	3	
Lens Implant, MA40BD *Alcon Laboratories, Inc., Fort Worth, TX*	Safe	3	
Lens Implant, MC50BD *Alcon Laboratories, Inc., Fort Worth, TX*	Safe	3	
Lens Implant, MC60BD *Alcon Laboratories, Inc., Fort Worth, TX*	Safe	3	
Lens Implant, MC50BM *Alcon Laboratories, Inc., Fort Worth, TX*	Safe	3	
Lens Implant, MC51BM *Alcon Laboratories, Inc., Fort Worth, TX*	Safe	3	
Lens Implant, MC60BM *Alcon Laboratories, Inc., Fort Worth, TX*	Safe	3	

Object	Status	Field Strength (T)	Reference
Lens Implant, MC61BM *Alcon Laboratories, Inc., Fort Worth, TX*	Safe	3	
Lens Implant, MC60CM *Alcon Laboratories, Inc., Fort Worth, TX*	Safe	3	
Lens Implant, MC61CM *Alcon Laboratories, Inc., Fort Worth, TX*	Safe	3	
Lens Implant, MC70CM *Alcon Laboratories, Inc., Fort Worth, TX*	Safe	3	
Lens Implant, MC71CM *Alcon Laboratories, Inc., Fort Worth, TX*	Safe	3	
Lens Implant, MN20BD *Alcon Laboratories, Inc., Fort Worth, TX*	Safe	3	
Lens Implant, MN30BD *Alcon Laboratories, Inc., Fort Worth, TX*	Safe	3	
Lens Implant, MN40BD *Alcon Laboratories, Inc., Fort Worth, TX*	Safe	3	
Lens Implant, MN60BD *Alcon Laboratories, Inc., Fort Worth, TX*	Safe	3	
Lens Implant, MN60D3 *Alcon Laboratories, Inc., Fort Worth, TX*	Safe	3	
Lens Implant, MTA2UO *Alcon Laboratories, Inc., Fort Worth, TX*	Safe	3	
Lens Implant, MTA3UO *Alcon Laboratories, Inc., Fort Worth, TX*	Safe	3	
Lens Implant, MTA4UO *Alcon Laboratories, Inc., Fort Worth, TX*	Safe	3	
Lens Implant, MTA5UO *Alcon Laboratories, Inc., Fort Worth, TX*	Safe	3	
Lens Implant, MTA6UO *Alcon Laboratories, Inc., Fort Worth, TX*	Safe	3	
Lens Implant, MZ20BD *Alcon Laboratories, Inc., Fort Worth, TX*	Safe	3	
Lens Implant, MZ30BD *Alcon Laboratories, Inc., Fort Worth, TX*	Safe	3	
Lens Implant, MZ40BD *Alcon Laboratories, Inc., Fort Worth, TX*	Safe	3	
Lens Implant, MZ60BD *Alcon Laboratories, Inc., Fort Worth, TX*	Safe	3	
Lens Implant, MZ70BD *Alcon Laboratories, Inc., Fort Worth, TX*	Safe	3	
Lens Implant, MZ20CD *Alcon Laboratories, Inc., Fort Worth, TX*	Safe	3	
Lens Implant, MZ60CD *Alcon Laboratories, Inc., Fort Worth, TX*	Safe	3	
Lens Implant, MZ60MD *Alcon Laboratories, Inc., Fort Worth, TX*	Safe	3	
Lens Implant, MZ60PD *Alcon Laboratories, Inc., Fort Worth, TX*	Safe	3	
Lens Implant, SA30AL *Alcon Laboratories, Inc., Fort Worth, TX*	Safe	3	

Object	Status	Field Strength (T)	Reference
Lens Implant, SA30AT *Alcon Laboratories, Inc., Fort Worth, TX*	Safe	3	
Lens Implant, SA60AT *Alcon Laboratories, Inc., Fort Worth, TX*	Safe	3	
Lens Implant, SN60AT *Alcon Laboratories, Inc., Fort Worth, TX*	Safe	3	
Lens Implant, SA60D3 *Alcon Laboratories, Inc., Fort Worth, TX*	Safe	3	
Lens Implant, SN60D3 *Alcon Laboratories, Inc., Fort Worth, TX*	Safe	3	
Lens Implant, SN60T3 *Alcon Laboratories, Inc., Fort Worth, TX*	Safe	3	
Lens Implant, SN60T4 *Alcon Laboratories, Inc., Fort Worth, TX*	Safe	3	
Lens Implant, SN60T5 *Alcon Laboratories, Inc., Fort Worth, TX*	Safe	3	
Lens Implant, SN60WF *Alcon Laboratories, Inc., Fort Worth, TX*	Safe	3	
Lens Implant, SN6AD3 *Alcon Laboratories, Inc., Fort Worth, TX*	Safe	3	
Lens Implant, SN60WS *Alcon Laboratories, Inc., Fort Worth, TX*	Safe	3	
Molteno drainage device *glaucoma drainage implant, nonmetallic* *Molteno Ophthalmic Ltd., Dunedin, New Zealand*	Safe	3	
OZURDEX Implant, dexamethasone intravitreal implant *Allergan, Inc., www.allergan.com*	Safe	1.5	
Retinal tack, 303 SS, ocular *Bascom Palmer Eye Institute*	Safe	1.5	32
Retinal tack, 303 SS, ocular *Duke*	Safe	1.5	32
Retinal tack, aluminum textraoxide *ocular, ruby*	Safe	1.5	32
Retinal tack, cobalt, nickel, ocular *Greishaber, Fallsington, PA*	Safe	1.5	32
Retinal tack, martensitic SS, ocular *Western European*	Unsafe 1	1.5	32
Retinal tack, Titanium alloy, ocular *Coopervision, Irvine, CA*	Safe	1.5	32
Retinal tack, Norton staple *Platinum, rhodium, ocular* *Norton*	Safe	1.5	32
Single tantalum clip *tantalum, ocular*	Safe	1.5	29
SuperEagle Punctum Plug *EagleVision, Memphis, TN*	Safe	3	
SuperFlex Punctum Plug *EagleVision, Memphis, TN*	Safe	3	
Tapered Shaft Flow Controller *EagleVision, Memphis, TN*	Safe	3	

Object	Status	Field Strength (T)	Reference
Troutman magnetic ocular implant	Unsafe 1	1.5	
Unitech round wire eye spring, ocular	Unsafe 1	1.5	
Wide Angle Implantable Miniature Telescope	Conditional 6	3	
Lens Implant, VisionCare Ophthalmic Technologies, Inc., Saratoga, CA			

Object	Status	Field Strength (T)	Reference

Orthopedic Implants, Materials, and Devices

Object	Status	Field Strength (T)	Reference
Absolute Absorbable Interference Screw	Safe	1.5, 3	
Ace-Fischer External Fixation System *DePuy, www.depuy.com*	Unsafe 1	1.5	
Adjustable External Fixation Device *external fixation device, carbon composite, SS* *Biomet, Inc., Warsaw, IN*	Conditional 5	3	
Advent Cervical Disc *Blackstone Medical, Inc., Wayne, NJ*	Conditional 8	1.5, 3	
Aequalis Humeral Plate *and component parts, 120-mm plate* *4.0-mm x 60-mm length self tapping cancellous locking screw* *3.5-mm x 50-mm length self tapping cortical compression screw* *3.5-mm x 40-mm length self tapping cortical locking screw* *19-gauge cerclage wire* *Tornier, Inc., Stafford, TX*	Conditional 6	3	
Agility Total Ankle *Titanium alloy tibial, CoCrMo alloy talus* *DePuy, www.depuy.com*	Conditional 6	3	
AML Hip Stem *CoCrMo alloy with CoCrMo alloy head* *DePuy Orthopaedics, Warsaw, IN*	Conditional 6	3	
AML femoral component bipolar hip prosthesis *orthopedic implant* *Zimmer, Warsaw, IN*	Safe	1.5	3
A-MAV Spinal Arthroplasty System *cobalt chromium alloy* *Medtronic, www.medtronic.com*	Safe	1.5	
APERIUS PercLID System *Medtronic, www.medtronic.com*	Conditional 5	3	
ASR-Surface Replacement Hip *CoCrMo alloy acetabulum and head* *DePuy, www.depuy.com*	Conditional 6	3	
ATLANTIS Anterior Cervical Plate System *Medtronic, Inc., www.Medtronic.com*	Conditional 6	3	
ATLAS Cable System *Medtronic, Inc., www.Medtronic.com*	Conditional 6	3	
AVN Cage *DePuy, www.DePuy.com*	Conditional 6	3	
Biocomposite Interference Screw, Cannulated, Delta Tapered *Arthrex, www.Arthrex.com*	Safe	1.5, 3	
BIOCRYL INTERFERENCE SCREW *Nonmetallic* *DePuy, www.DePuy.com*	Safe	1.5, 3	
Bio-Intrafix Tapered Screw *Nonmetallic* *DePuy, www.DePuy.com*	Safe	1.5, 3	
Bio-Intrafix Tibial Sheath *Nonmetallic* *DePuy, www.DePuy.com*	Safe	1.5, 3	

Object	Status	Field Strength (T)	Reference
BioKnotless Anchor w/Ethibond *Nonmetallic* *DePuy, www.DePuy.com*	Safe	1.5, 3	
BioKnotless Anchor w/Panacryl *Nonmetallic* *DePuy, www.DePuy.com*	Safe	1.5, 3	
BioKnotless BR Anchor w/Orthocord *Nonmetallic* *DePuy, www.DePuy.com*	Safe	1.5, 3	
BioKnotless BR Anchor w/Panacryl *Nonmetallic* *DePuy, www.DePuy.com*	Safe	1.5, 3	
BioKnotless Plus Anchor w/Ethibond *Nonmetallic* *DePuy, www.DePuy.com*	Safe	1.5, 3	
BioKnotless Plus Anchor w/Orthocord *Nonmetallic* *DePuy, www.DePuy.com*	Safe	1.5, 3	
BioKnotless Plus Anchor w/Panacryl *Nonmetallic* *DePuy, www.DePuy.com*	Safe	1.5, 3	
BioKnotless RC Anchor w/Ethibond *Nonmetallic* *DePuy, www.DePuy.com*	Safe	1.5, 3	
BioKnotless RC Anchor w/Panacryl *Nonmetallic* *DePuy, www.DePuy.com*	Safe	1.5, 3	
Biomet Bio-Modular Reverse Shoulder Products *Biomet, www.Biomet.com*	Conditional 5	1.5, 3	
Biomet Metal on Metal Hip Device *Biomet, www.Biomet.com*	Conditional 5	1.5, 3	
Biomet Oxford Partial Knee Implants *Biomet, www.Biomet.com*	Conditional 5	1.5, 3	
Biomet Sports Medicine JuggerKnot Mini Soft Anchor *Biomet, www.Biomet.com*	Safe	1.5, 3	
Biomet Sports Medicine Sternal Fixation Device *Biomet, www.Biomet.com*	Conditional 5	1.5, 3	
Biomet Upper Extremity Fixation Devices *Biomet, www.Biomet.com*	Conditional 5	1.5, 3	
Bio-Modular Shoulder System Reverse Conversion Option *Biomet, www.Biomet.com*	Conditional 5	1.5, 3	
Biomet Plating Systems *Biomet, www.Biomet.com*	Conditional 5	1.5, 3	
Biomet Vanguard Knee Joint Replacement Prostheses *Biomet, www.Biomet.com*	Conditional 5	1.5, 3	
BioROC EZ, Nonmetallic *DePuy, www.DePuy.com*	Safe	1.5, 3	
BioPro Great Toe M-P Joint, Cobalt Chrome *BioPro, Inc., Port Huron, MI*	Safe	1.5	

Object	Status	Field Strength (T)	Reference
Biosymetric P.P. (Finger) Fixator *external fixation device, 316 SS, carbon composite* *Biomet, Inc., Warsaw, IN*	Conditional 6	3	
Biomet Ziploop *Biomet, www.Biomet.com*	Conditional 5	1.5, 3	
Bone Tendon Bio-TransFix *Arthrex, www.Arthrex.com*	Safe	1.5, 3	
BOOMERANG II PEEK Body Spacer *Medtronic, Inc., www.medtronic.com*	Conditional 6	3	
Bryan Cervical Disc System *Medtronic, Inc., www.medtronic.com*	Conditional 8	1.5, 3	
BTB Cross Pins, 2.7mm x 42mm BIOCRYL (TCP/PLA) *Nonmetallic* *DePuy, www.DePuy.com*	Safe	1.5, 3	
BRYAN Cervical Disc System *Medtronic, Inc., www.Medtronic.com*	Conditional 6	3	
CADISC-C, Artificial Disc *Ranier Technology Limited, www.ranier.co.uk*	Conditional 6	3	
CAISKIT, Nonmetallic *DePuy, www.DePuy.com*	Safe	1.5, 3	
CAIS Scaffold *DePuy Mitek, www.depuy.com*	Safe	1.5, 3	
CAIS Staple *DePuy Mitek, www.depuy.com*	Safe	1.5, 3	
CAPSTONE PEEK System *Medtronic, Inc., www.medtronic.com*	Conditional 6	3	
CD HORIZON BalanC *Medtronic, Inc., www.medtronic.com*	Conditional 5	1.5, 3	
CD HORIZON ENGAGE *Medtronic, Inc., www.medtronic.com*	Conditional 5	3	
CD HORIZON Engage Rod System *Medtronic, Inc., www.medtronic.com*	Conditional 5	1.5, 3	
CD HORIZON SOLERA Posterior Stabilization System *Medtronic, Inc., www.medtronic.com*	Conditional 5	3	
C-Stem with CoCrMo Head *CoCrMo, high strength SS* *DePuy Orthopaedics, Warsaw, IN*	Conditional 6	3	
Cannulated cancellous screw, 6.5 x 50-mm *Titanium alloy, orthopedic implant* *DePuy ACE Medical Co., El Segundo, CA*	Safe	1.5	
Captured screw assembly, 100-mm *Titanium alloy, orthopedic implant* *DePuy ACE Medical Co., El Segundo, CA*	Safe	1.5	
CD HORIZON LEGACY 6.35-mm Stainless Steel Spinal System *75-mm long spinal construct, unilateral* *Medtronic, Inc., www.Medtronic.com*	Conditional 8	1.5, 3	
CD HORIZON LEGACY 6.35-mm Stainless Steel Spinal System *175-mm long spinal construct, bilateral* *Medtronic, Inc., www.medtronic.com*	Conditional 8	1.5, 3	

Object	Status	Field Strength (T)	Reference
CD HORIZON LEGACY MAS *Multi Axial Screw (MAS), Spinal System, spinal construct* *Medtronic, www.medtronic.com*	Conditional 5	3	
CD HORIZON SOLERA Spinal System *Medtronic, www.medtronic.com*	Conditional 5	3	
CD HORIZON Spinal System *Medtronic Rod Connector (MRC)* *Medtronic, www.medtronic.com*	Conditional 5	3	
Cervical wire, 18 gauge *316L SS, orthopedic implant*	Safe	0.3	33
CerviCore Intervertebral Disc *Stryker Spine-Summit, Summit, NJ*	Conditional 6	3	
Charite Artificial Disc *DePuy Spine, www.depuy.com*	Safe	3	
Charnley-Muller hip prosthesis, Protasyl-10 alloy *orthopedic implant*	Safe	0.3	
Clearfix Meniscal PLA Absorbable Screw, Nonmetallic *DePuy, www.DePuy.com*	Safe	1.5, 3	
Clearfix Meniscal Screw Driver, Nonmetallic *DePuy, www.DePuy.com*	Safe	1.5, 3	
CLYDESDALE PEEK (polyetheretherketone) *Vertebral Body Spacer* *Medtronic, www.medtronic.com*	Conditional 5	3	
Cobalt Chrome Staple, Cobalt Chrome, ASTM F75 *Smith & Nephew, Inc., Memphis, TN*	Safe	1.5, 3	83
Compression Hip Screw Plate *and Lag Screw (tested as assembly), 316L SS* *Smith & Nephew, Inc., Memphis, TN*	Safe	1.5, 3	83
CORNERSTONE PSR Implant *Medtronic, Inc., www.medtronic.com*	Conditional 5	3	
Cortical bone screw, 4.5 x 36-mm *Titanium alloy* *DePuy ACE Medical Co., El Segundo, CA*	Safe	1.5	
Cortical bone screw, large, Titanium alloy *Zimmer, Warsaw, IN*	Safe	1.5	34
Cortical bone screw, small, Titanium alloy *Zimmer, Warsaw, IN*	Safe	1.5	34
Cotrel rod, SS-ASTM, grade 2, orthopedic implant	Safe	1.5	
Cotrel rods, with hooks, 316L SS, orthopedic implant	Safe	0.3	33
Cougar Lateral Cage System *DePuy, www.DePuy.com*	Conditional 5	3	
CUFF LINK Bone Tunnel Device, Nonmetallic *DePuy, www.DePuy.com*	Safe	1.5, 3	
Delta Tapered PEEK Interference Screw *Arthrex, www.Arthrex.com*	Safe	1.5, 3	
Delta Total Shoulder, SS *DePuy, www.depuy.com*	Conditional 6	3	
DePuy Mitek Metal Anchors *DePuy Mitek, www.DePuy.com*	Conditional 5	3	

Object	Status	Field Strength (T)	Reference
Disposable Titanium Skull Pin *polymer body, titanium alloy pin-point* *Integra LifeSciences, Cincinnati, Ohio*	Conditional 6	3	
Divide Absorbable Adhesion Barrier, Nonmetallic *DePuy, www.DePuy.com*	Safe	1.5, 3	
Drummond wire, 316L SS *orthopedic implant*	Safe	0.3	33
DTT, device for transverse traction *316L SS, orthopedic implant*	Safe	0.3	33
E1 Implant(s) ultra-high molecular weigh *polyethylene (UHMWPE)and dl-alpha-Tocopherol (vitamin E)* *Biomet Inc., www.biomet.com*	Safe	1.5, 3	
Emergency Bone Screw *Titanium alloy* *Biomet, Inc., Warsaw, IN*	Conditional 6	3	
Endoscopic noncannulated *interference screw, Titanium, orthopedic implant* *Acufex Microsurgical, Norwood, MA*	Safe	1.5	34
EOI Spinal System EPPS (Expanding Polyaxial Pedicle Screw) *Expanding Orthopedics Inc., Israel*	Conditional 8	1.5, 3	
Expedium Implant System *DePuy, www.DePuy.com*	Conditional 5	1.5, 3	
External Fixation Device, Hoffman II MRI *External Fixation System* *Stryker Trauma AG, Switzerland*	Conditional 5	1.5, 3	
External Fixation Device, Hoffman II (Standard) *External Fixation System* *Stryker Trauma AG, Switzerland*	Unsafe 1, 2	1.5, 3	
External Fixation Device, JET-X Fixator *Smith & Nephew, Memphis, TN*	Conditional 5	1.5	
Facet Screw *Medtronic, www.medtronic.com*	Conditional 5	3	
Femoral Intrafix, Hard *Nonmetallic* *DePuy, www.DePuy.com*	Safe	1.5, 3	
Femoral Intrafix, Standard *Nonmetallic* *DePuy, www.DePuy.com*	Safe	1.5, 3	
FlexiCore Intervertebral Disc *Stryker Spine-Summit, Summit, NJ*	Conditional 6	3	
Fixation staple *cobalt-chromium alloy, orthopedic implant* *Richards Medical Co., Memphis, TN*	Safe	1.5	34
FD Tibial Intramedullary Nail, 316 SS *Biomet, Inc., Warsaw, IN*	Conditional 6	3	
Femoral Head Implant *cobalt chromium* *Biomet, Inc., Warsaw, IN*	Conditional 6	3	
Focal Femoral Condyle Resurfacing System *HemiCAP* *Arthrosurface, Inc., www.arthrosurface.com*	Conditional 8	1.5, 3	

Object	Status	Field Strength (T)	Reference
Furlong H-AC THR System *Joint Replacement Instrumentation Limited (JRI Ltd), Sheffield, U.K.*	Conditional 6	3	
Furlong Modular Revision System Hemiarthroplasty *Joint Replacement Instrumentation Limited (JRI Ltd), Sheffield, U.K.*	Conditional 6	3	
GII Titanium Anchor, Titanium *Mitek Products, Norwood, MA*	Safe	1.5	
Global Total Shoulder, CoCrMo head and *stem/poly bearing component* *DePuy, www.depuy.com*	Conditional 6	3	
Gryphon P BR Anchor w/Orthocord *Nonmetallic* *DePuy, www.DePuy.com*	Safe	1.5, 3	
Gryphon P BR DS Anchor w/Orthocord *Nonmetallic* *DePuy, www.DePuy.com*	Safe	1.5, 3	
Gryphon T BR Anchor w/Orthocord *Nonmetallic* *DePuy, www.DePuy.com*	Safe	1.5, 3	
Gryphon T BR DS Anchor w/ Orthocord *Nonmetallic* *DePuy, www.DePuy.com*	Safe	1.5, 3	
Halifax clamps, orthopedic implant *American Medical Electronics Richardson, TX*	Safe	1.5	
Hallmark Anterior Cervical Plate System *Blackstone Medical, Inc., Wayne, NJ*	Conditional 8	1.5, 3	
Harrington compression rod *with hooks and nuts, 316L SS, orthopedic implant*	Safe	0.3	33
Harrington distraction rod with hooks *316L SS, orthopedic implant*	Safe	0.3	33
Harris hip prosthesis *Zimmer, Warsaw, IN*	Safe	1.5	3
Healix BR 3-Suture Anchor w/Orthocord *Nonmetallic, Depuy* *www.Depuy.co*	Safe	1.5, 3	
Healix BR Anchor w/Ethibond *Nonmetallic* *DePuy, www.DePuy.com*	Safe	1.5, 3	
Healix BR Anchor w/Orthocord *Nonmetallic* *DePuy, www.DePuy.com*	Safe	1.5, 3	
Healix BR Anchor w/Orthocord and Needles *Nonmetallic* *DePuy, www.DePuy.com*	Safe	1.5, 3	
Healix BR Anchor w/Panacryl *Nonmetallic* *DePuy, www.DePuy.com*	Safe	1.5, 3	
Healix PEEK 3-Suture Anchor w/Orthocord *Nonmetallic* *DePuy, www.DePuy.com*	Safe	1.5, 3	

Object	Status	Field Strength (T)	Reference
Healix PEEK Anchor w/Orthocord *Nonmetallic* *DePuy, www.DePuy.com*	Safe	1.5, 3	
Healix PEEK Anchor w/Panacryl *Nonmetallic* *DePuy, www.DePuy.com*	Safe	1.5, 3	
Hip implant, austenitic SS *orthopedic implant* *DePuy Inc., Warsaw, IN*	Safe	1.5, 3	83
iForma, orthopedic implant *CONFORMIS, Inc., Lexington, MA*	Conditional 6	3	
IMF Wire, 316 SS *Biomet, Inc., Warsaw, IN*	Conditional 6	3	
Ilizarov-Taylor Spatial Frame *metal version* *Smith and Nephew, Memphis, TN*	Unsafe 1	1.5	
Implantable Titanium Fixation Plate *Micro, Mini, Fracture, Threadlock and Sternal* *KLS Martin, www.klsmartinusa.com*	Conditional 8	1.5, 3	
Intrafix Tapered Screw, Nonmetallic *DePuy, www.DePuy.com*	Safe	1.5, 3	
Intrafix Tibial Sheath, Nonmetallic *DePuy, www.DePuy.com*	Safe	1.5, 3	
Intramedullary Nail *Titanium nail and polymer composite* *Smith and Nephew*	Conditional 8	1.5, 3	
Ionic Spine Spacer System, Titanium alloy *EBI, L.P., Parsippany, NJ*	Safe	1.5	
Jewett nail, orthopedic implant *Zimmer, Warsaw, IN*	Safe	1.5	3
JuggerKnot Soft Anchor *Biomet, www.Biomet.com*	Safe	1.5, 3	
Kirschner intermedullary rod *Kirschner Medical, Timonium, MD*	Safe	1.5	3
KneeSpring Knee Implant System *Moximed, Inc., www.moximed.com*	Conditional 8	1.5, 3	
Large External Fixation System *Identified as MR Conditional, only* *Synthes, www.synthes.com*	Conditional 5	1.5, 3	
LimiFlex Spinal Stabilization System *Simpirica Spine, Inc., www.simpirica.com*	Conditional 8	1.5, 3	
Linx HT Ligament Fastener, Nonmetallic *DePuy, www.DePuy.com*	Safe	1.5, 3	
L plate, 6-hole, Titanium alloy *orthopedic implant* *DePuy ACE Medical Co., El Segundo, CA*	Safe	1.5	
L Rod, cobalt-nickel alloy *orthopedic implant* *Richards Medical Co., Memphis, TN*	Safe	1.5	
LT-CAGE Lumbar Tapered Fusion Device Implant *Medtronic, Inc., www.Medtronic.com*	Conditional 6	3	

Object	Status	Field Strength (T)	Reference
Low Profile MTP Plate *Arthrex, www.Arthrex.com*	Conditional 8	1.5, 3	
Low Profile Screw, Cannulated, SS *Arthrex, www.Arthrex.com*	Conditional 8	1.5, 3	
Low Profile Screw, Cannulated, Titanium *Arthrex, www.Arthrex.com*	Conditional 8	1.5, 3	
LUPINE Loop Anchor, Nonmetallic *DePuy, www.DePuy.com*	Safe	1.5, 3	
Lupine Loop BR Anchor w/DS Orthocord *Nonmetallic* *DePuy, www.DePuy.com*	Safe	1.5, 3	
LUPINE Loop Dual Suture (DS) Anchor *Nonmetallic* *DePuy, www.DePuy.com*	Safe	1.5, 3	
Lupine Loop Plus Anchor w/Ethibond *Nonmetallic* *DePuy, www.DePuy.com*	Safe	1.5, 3	
Lupine Loop Plus Anchor w/Orthocord *Nonmetallic* *DePuy, www.DePuy.com*	Safe	1.5, 3	
Lupine Loop Plus Anchor w/Panacryl *Nonmetallic* *DePuy, www.DePuy.com*	Safe	1.5, 3	
Lupine Loop Plus Dual Suture (DS) *Anchor w/Orthocord, Nonmetallic* *DePuy, www.DePuy.com*	Safe	1.5, 3	
Luque Wire *orthopedic implant*	Safe	0.3	33
M. KUROSAKA ADVANTAGE CANNULATED FIXATION SCREW *DePuy Mitek A Johnson & Johnson Company, Raynham, MA*	Conditional 6	3	
M. KUROSAKA ADVANTAGE *Cannulated Fixation Screw* *MRI information applies to many other similar implants* *DePuy, www.DePuy.com*	Conditional 6	3	
Mandibular Locking Bone Plate *316 SS* *Biomet, Inc., Warsaw, IN*	Conditional 6	3	
MAVERICK Disc Replacement System *Medtronic, Inc., www.Medtronic.com*	Conditional 6	3	
MEDPOR ATTRACTOR Screw, 17-4 SS *Porex Surgical, Newnan, GA*	Unsafe 1	1.5	
MENISCAL FASTENER, Nonmetallic *DePuy, www.DePuy.com*	Safe	1.5, 3	
Meta-Lock Suture Anchor System *Tarsus Medical, Inc., www.tarsusmedical.com*	Conditional 6	3	
MICROFIX QUICKANCHOR Plus, Nonmetallic *DePuy, www.DePuy.com*	Safe	1.5, 3	
MILAGRO Interference Screw, Nonmetallic *DePuy, www.DePuy.com*	Safe	1.5, 3	
MiniLok QUICKANCHOR Plus, Nonmetallic *DePuy, www.DePuy.com*	Safe	1.5, 3	

Object	Status	Field Strength (T)	Reference
MR Safe Clamps *for use with Large External Fixation System* *Synthes, www.synthes.com*	Conditional 5	1.5, 3	
MOBIS Spinal Implant, PEEK, Tantalum Pins *SIGNUS Medizintechnik GmbH, www.signus-med.de*	Conditional 6	3	
MOBIS Spinal Implant, PEEK, Titanium Pins *SIGNUS Medizintechnik GmbH, www. www.signus-med.de*	Conditional 6	3	
Moe spinal instrumentation *Zimmer, Warsaw, IN*	Safe	1.5	
Monoblock Neolif Intersomatic Cage *Tantalum* *Biomet, Inc., Warsaw, IN*	Conditional 6	3	
NGage Surgical Mesh System *Blackstone Medical, Inc.* *Wayne, NJ*	Conditional 8	1.5, 3	
NOVAL Spinal Implant *SIGNUS Medizintechnik GmbH, www.signus-med.de*	Conditional 6	3	
NUBIC Spinal Implant, PEEK, Titanium Pins *SIGNUS Medizintechnik GmbH, www.signus-med.de*	Conditional 6	3	
NUBIC XL Spinal Implant, PEEK, Titanium Pins *SIGNUS Medizintechnik GmbH, www.signus-med.de*	Conditional 6	3	
Panalok Anchor *clear PLA polymer anchor* *Mitek Products, Norwood, MA*	Safe	1.5	
Pectus Bar Implant *Part# 01-3707* *Biomet, Jacksonville, FL*	Conditional 8	1.5, 3	
Pectus Bar Implant *Part# 01-3717* *Biomet, Jacksonville, FL*	Conditional 8	1.5, 3	
Pedicle Screw and Locking Clip *for use in the Elaspine Implant System* *SpineLab AG, Switzerland*	Conditional 6	3	
PEEK PREVAIL Cervical Interbody Device *Medtronic, www.medtronic.com*	Conditional 5	3	
Piccolo Composite Femoral and Tibial Nailing System *N.M.B. Medical Applications Ltd., Israel*	Conditional 8	1.5, 3	
Piccolo Composite Plate System *N.M.B. Medical Applications Ltd., Israel*	Conditional 8	1.5, 3	
PRESTIGE LP Cervical Disc System *Medtronic, Inc., www.Medtronic.com*	Conditional 5	3	
PRESTIGE ST Cervical Disc System *Medtronic, Inc., www.Medtronic.com*	Conditional 5	3	
Propio Foot *OSSUR Reykjavik, Iceland, OSSUR AMERICAS, Aliso Viejo, CA*	Unsafe 1	1.5	
PYRAMID Anterior Lumbar Plate and Screws *Medtronic, Inc., www.Medtronic.com*	Conditional 6	3	
Opus Magnum Implant *ArthroCare, ArthroCare.com*	Conditional 5	1.5, 3	
OPUS SpeedFix *ArthroCare, ArthroCare.com*	Safe	1.5, 3	

Object	Status	Field Strength (T)	Reference
OPUS SpeedLock Knotless Fixation Device *ArthroCare, ArthroCare.com*	Safe	1.5, 3	
OPUS SpeedScrew Device *ArthroCare, ArthroCare.com*	Safe	1.5, 3	
Orthocord, Nonmetallic *DePuy, www.DePuy.com*	Safe	1.5, 3	
Orthocord Suture, Size #2 *DePuy Mitek, www.depuy.com*	Safe	1.5, 3	
OSS Distal Femoral Replacement Prosthesis *Titanium alloy, cobalt chrome moly, 316 SS* *Biomet, Inc., Warsaw, IN*	Conditional 6	3	
OsseoFix, Titanium *Alphatec Spine Inc., Carlsbad, CA*	Conditional 6	3	
Osseotite Dental Post Implant *Titanium alloy* *Biomet, Inc., Warsaw, IN*	Conditional 6	3	
OsteoGen Implantable Bone Growth Stimulator *No MRI Info* *Biomet, www.Biomet.com*	Unsafe 1	1.5	
Otto Bock Microprocessor Knee *Otto Bock HealthCare, Minneapolis, MN*	Unsafe 1	1.5	
Oxidized Zirconium Knee, Femoral Component *Smith & Nephew, Inc., Memphis, TN*	Safe	1.5, 3	83
PANALOK #2 ETHIBOND, Nonmetallic *DePuy, www.DePuy.com*	Safe	1.5, 3	
Panalok Absorbable Anchor, Nonmetallic *DePuy, www.DePuy.com*	Safe	1.5, 3	
Panalok Loop Anchor, Nonmetallic *DePuy, www.DePuy.com*	Safe	1.5, 3	
Panalok RC Loop Anchor, Nonmetallic *DePuy, www.DePuy.com*	Safe	1.5, 3	
Panalok RC QA+DS Suture Orthocord *Nonmetallic* *DePuy, www.DePuy.com*	Safe	1.5, 3	
Panalok RC QuickAnchor Plus *Nonmetallic* *DePuy, www.DePuy.com*	Safe	1.5, 3	
Perfix interence screw, 17-4 SS *orthopedic implant* *Instrument Makar, Okemos, MI*	Conditional 1	1.5	34
PERIMETER C Spinal System *Medtronic, Inc., www.medtronic.com*	Conditional 5	3	
PERIMETER PEEK Vertebral Body Spacer *Medtronic, Inc., www.medtronic.com*	Conditional 5	3	
Piccolo Composite Femoral Nailing System *N.M.B. Medical Applications Ltd., www.carbo-fix.com*	Conditional 8	1.5, 3	
Piccolo Composite Tibial Nailing System *N.M.B. Medical Applications Ltd., www.carbo-fix.com*	Conditional 8	1.5, 3	
Pinnacle MOM Acetabular Cup System *Titanium alloy shell, CoCrMo insert* *DePuy, www.depuy.com*	Conditional 6	3	

Object	Status	Field Strength (T)	Reference
Profile Plate System *DePuy, www.DePuy.com*	Conditional 8	1.5, 3	
Propeller Head Small Cannulated Screw *Biomet, www.Biomet.com*	Conditional 5	1.5, 3	
Pyrocarbon Implant *Replacement (PIR) System* *Moirai Orthopaedics, Inc., Metairie, LA*	Conditional 6	3	
PyroTitan Humeral Resurfacing *Arthroplasty Implant* *Ascension Humeral Resurfacing Arthroplasty (HRA) System* *Ascension Orthopedics, Inc., Austin, TX*	Conditional 6	3	
Quantum Composite Nailing System *N.M.B. Medical Applications Ltd., Israel*	Conditional 8	1.5, 3	
RABEA Cervical Cage, Titanium *SIGNUS Medizintechnik GmbH, www.signus-med.de*	Conditional 6	3	
RABEA Cervical Cage, PEEK, Titanium Pins *SIGNUS Medizintechnik GmbH, www.signus-med.de*	Conditional 6	3	
RapidFlap *Biomet, www.Biomet.com*	Safe	1.5, 3	
RapidLoc Meniscal Repair-PLA Tophat *Nonmetallic* *DePuy, www.DePuy.com*	Safe	1.5, 3	
RapidLoc PDS Meniscal Repair System *Nonmetallic* *DePuy, www.DePuy.com*	Safe	1.5, 3	
Reconstruction Plate With Screws *KLS Martin L.P., Jacksonville, FL*	Conditional 8	1.5, 3	
Restoration Modular Hip System *Stryker Orthopaedics, Mahwah, NJ*	Conditional 8	1.5, 3	
Reusable Titanium Skull Pin *titanium alloy coated in titanium nitride* *Integra LifeSciences, Cincinnati, OH*	Conditional 6	3	
RigidFix Biocry Tibial ST Cross Pin Kit *Nonmetallic* *DePuy, www.DePuy.com*	Safe	1.5, 3	
RigidFix Biocryl Femoral ST Cross Pin Kit *Nonmetallic* *DePuy, www.DePuy.com*	Safe	1.5, 3	
RigidFix BTB Cross Pin Kit *Nonmetallic* *DePuy, www.DePuy.com*	Safe	1.5, 3	
RigidFix FEM/TIB BTB Cross Pin Kit *Nonmetallic* *DePuy, www.DePuy.com*	Safe	1.5, 3	
RigidFix Femoral ST Cross Pin Kit *Nonmetallic* *DePuy, www.DePuy.com*	Safe	1.5, 3	
RigidFix Kit, Nonmetallic *DePuy, www.DePuy.com*	Safe	1.5, 3	
RigidFix Tibial ST Cross Pin Kit *Nonmetallic* *DePuy, www.DePuy.com*	Safe	1.5, 3	

Object	Status	Field Strength (T)	Reference
ROC XS, Nonmetallic *DePuy, www.DePuy.com*	Safe	1.5, 3	
Rod-To-Rod Clamp *Biomet, www.Biomet.com*	Safe	1.5	
SLM Pin-To-Rod Clamp *Biomet, www.Biomet.com*	Safe	1.5	
Rusch Rod, orthopedic implant	Safe	1.5	
SEMIAL Spinal Implant *PEEK, Titanium Pins* *SIGNUS Medizintechnik GmbH, www.signus-med.de*	Conditional 6	3	
Side plate, 6-hole, Titanium alloy *DePuy ACE Co., El Segundo, CA*	Safe	1.5	
Sigma RP Total Knee *CoCrMo alloy and polyethylene* *DePuy, www.depuy.com*	Conditional 6	3	
SKELITE Ceramic Bone Graft *Medtronic, www.medtronic.com*	Safe	1.5, 3	
SMA Staple *Medtronic, Inc., www.Medtronic.com*	Conditional 6	3	
Small External Fixator *external fixation device,* *carbon composite, Titanium alloy, aluminum, SS* *Biomet, Inc., Warsaw, IN*	Conditional 5	3	
Soteira Kyphoplasty System, Cement Director *Soteira, Inc., Natick, MA*	Conditional 6	3	
SOVEREIGN Spinal Interbody System *Medtronic, Inc., www.medtronic.com*	Conditional 5	3	
SOVEREIGN Spinal System *Medtronic, www.medtronic.com*	Conditional 5	3	
SpineAlign, orthopedic implant *Nitinol* *SpineWorks, Santa Clara, CA*	Conditional 6	3	
Spinal L-Rod, orthopedic implant *DePuy, www.depuy.com*	Safe	1.5	
Spiralok w/o Needles - Ethibond, Nonmetallic *DePuy, www.DePuy.com*	Safe	1.5, 3	
Spiralok w/o Needles - Panacryl, Nonmetallic *DePuy, www.DePuy.com*	Safe	1.5, 3	
Spiralok w/Orthocord, Nonmetallic *DePuy, www.DePuy.com*	Safe	1.5, 3	
Spiralok with Needles - Ethibond, Nonmetallic *DePuy, www.DePuy.com*	Safe	1.5	
Spiralok with Needles - Panacryl, Nonmetallic *DePuy, www.DePuy.com*	Safe	1.5, 3	
Stainless steel mesh, orthopedic implant *Zimmer, Warsaw, IN*	Safe	1.5	3
Stainless steel plate, orthopedic implant *Zimmer, Warsaw, IN*	Safe	1.5	3
Stainless steel screw, orthopedic implant *Zimmer, Warsaw, IN*	Safe	1.5	3

Object	Status	Field Strength (T)	Reference
Stainless steel wire, orthopedic implant *Zimmer, Warsaw, IN*	Safe	1.5	3
Staple plate, large, Zimaloy *orthopedic implant* *Zimmer, Warsaw, IN*	Safe	1.5	3
Sternal Talon, all versions *KLS Martin L.P., Jacksonville, FL*	Conditional 6	3	
Summit Basic, orthopedic implant *DePuy, www.depuy.com*	Conditional 6	3	
Summit Hip Stem *Titanium alloy with CoCrMo alloy head* *DePuy, www.depuy.com*	Conditional 6	3	
SuperAnchor, MRI information applies to *many other similar implants* *DePuy, www.DePuy.com*	Conditional 6	3	
Synde-Lock Fixation Device *Tarsus Medical, Inc., www.tarsusmedical.com*	Conditional 6	3	
Synthes AO DCP 2, 3, 4, 5 hole plate *orthopedic implant*	Safe	1.5	
T2 ALTITUDE Expandable Corpectomy System *with 25 mm expandable centerpiece with 15 degree endcaps* *Medtronic, www.medtronic.com*	Conditional 5	1.5, 3	
T2 XVBR Spinal System, Expandable Centerpiece Device *with T2 Spinal System 25 mm Extended Endcaps, 8 Degree* *Medtronic, Inc., www.Medtronic.com*	Conditional 6	3	
T2 XVBR Spinal System *generation 1.5, with 25 mm expandable* *centerpiece with 15 degree endcaps* *Medtronic, www.medtronic.com*	Conditional 5	1.5, 3	
Tapered Hip Stem *Arthrex, www.Arthrex.com*	Conditional 8	1.5, 3	
Taylor Spatial Frame, metal version *Smith and Nephew, Memphis, TN*	Unsafe 1	1	
Teno Fix Tendon Repair System *Ortheon Medical, LLC, Winter Park, FL*	Safe	1.5	
TETRIS Round Shape, Spinal Implant *PEEK, Tantalum Pins* *SIGNUS Medizintechnik GmbH, www.signus-med.de*	Conditional 6	3	
TETRIS Spinal Implant, PEEK *SIGNUS Medizintechnik GmbH, www.signus-med.de*	Conditional 6	3	
TETRIS Spinal Implant, Titanium *SIGNUS Medizintechnik GmbH, www.signus-med.de*	Conditional 6	3	
TETRIS II Spinal Implant, PEEK, Tantalum Pins *SIGNUS Medizintechnik GmbH, www.signus-med.de*	Conditional 6	3	
TETRIS II Spinal Implant, Titanium *SIGNUS Medizintechnik GmbH, www.signus-med.de*	Conditional 6	3	
ThreadLock Transport Distractor *KLS Martin L.P., Jacksonville, FL*	Conditional 8	1.5, 3	
TiMesh Cranial Plating System *Medtronic, Inc., www.medtronic.com*	Safe	1.5	

Object	Status	Field Strength (T)	Reference
Tibial Intramedullary Nail *with Transfixation Screws, Titanium alloy* *DePuy, www.depuy.com*	Conditional 6	3	
Tibial nail, 9-mm *Titanium alloy* *DePuy ACE Medical Co., El Segundo, CA*	Safe	1.5	
Titanium 3D Mesh *1.5-mm, 200-mm x 200-mm* *KLS Martin L.P., Jacksonville, FL*	Conditional 8	1.5, 3	
Titanium Femoral Reconstruction Nail, Titanium alloy *Biomet, Inc., Warsaw, IN*	Conditional 6	3	
Titanium Intramedullary Nail, Titanium alloy *Smith & Nephew, Inc., Memphis, TN*	Safe	1.5, 3	83
Titanium Vertebral Body Spacer *Medtronic, Inc., www.medtronic.com*	Conditional 6	3	
Toe Joint, All Models *Biopro, Inc., www.bioproimplants.com*	Conditional 6	3	
TOPS (Total Posterior Arthroplasty System) and VersaLink System *Impliant Ltd.*	Conditional 6	3	
TSRH Spinal System *Medtronic, Inc., www.medtronic.com*	Conditional 5	1.5, 3	
TunneLoc Tibial Fixation Device *Biomet, www.Biomet.com*	Safe	1.5	
Ultima Tri-Flange *Acetabulum Cage, Titanium alloy* *DePuy, www.depuy.com*	Conditional 6	3	
UltraFix RC Suture Anchor *316L SS* *Linvatec Corporation*	Safe	1.5	
Universal Reconstruction Ribbon *Titanium, orthopedic implant* *DePuy ACE Medical Co., El Segundo, CA*	Safe	1.5	
Variable Angle Compression Hip Screw *316L SS* *Biomet, Inc., Warsaw, IN*	Conditional 6	3	
VERTE-STACK VBS IMPLANT BOOMERANG *Medtronic, Inc., www.Medtronic.com*	Conditional 6	3	
VERTEX SELECT Reconstruction System *Full and 60-mm versions* *Medtronic, www.medtronic.com*	Conditional 8	1.5, 3	
VSP Implant System *DePuy, www.DePuy.com*	Conditional 5	1.5, 3	
WedgeLoc Suture Anchor with Opti-Fiber Sutures *MedShape Solutions* *Atlanta, GA*	Conditional 6	3	
Wristore Distal Radius Fracture Fixator *external fixation device* *Zimmer, Inc., Warsaw, IN*	Conditional 5	3	
X10 CROSSLINK Plate *Medtronic, Inc., www.medtronic.com*	Conditional 5	3	

Object	Status	Field Strength (T)	Reference
X-Mesh Expandable Cage System *DePuy, www.DePuy.com*	Conditional 8	1.5, 3	
X STOP Interspinous Process *Decompression (IPD) Implant* *Medtronic, Inc., www.Medtronic.com*	Conditional 6	3	
Zielke rod with screw, washer and nut, 316L SS	Safe	0.3	33

Object	Status	Field Strength (T)	Reference

Otologic and Cochlear Implants

Object	Status	Field Strength (T)	Reference
Adjustable Length Titanium Ossicular (ALTO) Partial Prostheses *Grace Medical, www.gracemedical.com/mri.htm*	Conditional 5	1.5	
Adjustable Micron PORP *Otologic implant, Titanium* *Gyrus ACMI, Inc., www.gyrusacmi.com*	Conditional 5	3	
Adjustable Micron TORP *Otologic implant, Titanium* *Gyrus ACMI, Inc., www.gyrusacmi.com*	Conditional 5	3	
Aerial Total Dusseldorf Titanium, 0.2 x 7.0-mm *middle ear implant, Otologic implant* *Kurz Medical, Inc., Norcross, GA*	Safe	3	
Aerial Total Tuebingen Titanium *0.2 x 7.0-mm, middle ear implant, Otologic implant* *Kurz Medical, Inc., Norcross, GA*	Safe	3	
ALTO Partial and Total Prosthesis *Device Family, ALTO Partial and Total Prosthesis;* *Family Product Number(s), 6XX;* *Device Material(s), Titanium, HA (hydroxyapatite), Silicone* *Grace Medical, www.gracemedical.com*	Conditional 6	3	
Austin Tytan Piston *Titanium, Otologic implant* *Treace Medical, Nashville, TN*	Safe	1.5	35
Baha, Bone Conduction Implant *Cochlear Americas, Englewood, CO*	Conditional 5	1.5	
Bell Partial Dusseldorf Titanium, 0.2 x 4.5-mm *Otologic implant* *Kurz Medical, Inc., Norcross, GA*	Safe	3	
Bell Partial Tuebingen Titanium, 0.2 x 3.5-mm *Otologic implant* *Kurz Medical, Inc., Norcross, GA*	Safe	3	
Berger V Bobbin, Ventilation tube *Titanium, Otologic implant* *Richards Medical Co., Memphis, TN*	Safe	1.5	35
Berger V Bobbin VT, Ventilation tube *Otologic implant, Titanium* *Gyrus ACMI, Inc., www.gyrusacmi.com*	Conditional 5	3	
Blue Bobbin VT, Ventilation tube *Otologic implant, Titanium* *Gyrus ACMI, Inc., www.gyrusacmi.com*	Conditional 5	3	
Bobbin VT, Ventilation tube *Otologic implant, Titanium* *Gyrus ACMI, Inc., www.gyrusacmi.com*	Conditional 5	3	
Bucket Handle, Stapes Prosthesis *Otologic implant, Titanium* *Gyrus ACMI, Inc., www.gyrusacmi.com*	Conditional 5	3	
Causse Flex H/A, partial ossicular prosthesis *Titanium, Otologic implant* *Microtek Medical, Inc., Memphis, TN*	Safe	1.5	36

Object	Status	Field Strength (T)	Reference
Causse Flex H/A, total ossicular prosthesis *Titanium, Otologic implant* *Microtek Medical Inc., Memphis, TN*	Safe	1.5	36
Chicago Bucket Handle *Stapes Prosthesis, Otologic implant, Titanium* *Gyrus ACMI, Inc., www.gyrusacmi.com*	Conditional 5	3	
Classic SS, Otologic Implant, 316L SS *Gyrus ACMI, Inc., www.gyrusacmi.com*	Conditional 5	3	
Classic Stapes Prosthesis *Otologic implant, Titanium* *Gyrus ACMI, Inc., www.gyrusacmi.com*	Conditional 5	3	
Classic Stapes Prostheses *Otologic Implant, Titanium* *Gyrus ACMI, Inc., www.gyrusacmi.com*	Conditional 5	3	
CliP Partial Prosthesis Titanium *(Dresden type), 0.2 x 3.5-mm, Otologic implant* *Kurz Medical, Inc., Norcross, GA*	Safe	3	
CliP Piston Wengen Titanium *0.6 x 5.5-mm, Otologic implant* *Kurz Medical, Inc., Norcross, GA*	Safe	3	
Cochlear Implant, HiRes 90K Cochlear Implant *Advanced Bionics Corporation, Sylmar, CA*	Conditional 5	0.3, 1.5	
Cochlear implant, Nucleus 24 ABI Cochlear Implant System *Cochlear Corporation, Engelwood, CO*	Conditional 5	1.5	
Cochlear implant, Nucleus Mini 20-channel *Cochlear Corporation, Engelwood, CO*	Unsafe 1	1.5	38
Cochlear implant *3M/House*	Unsafe 1	0.6	37
Cochlear implant *3M/Vienna*	Unsafe 1	0.6	37
Cody tack *Otologic implant*	Safe	0.6	37
Collar Bobbin VT, Ventilation tube *Otologic implant, Titanium* *Gyrus ACMI, Inc., www.gyrusacmi.com*	Conditional 5	3	
Custom Classic Stapes, Otologic Implant, 316L SS *Gyrus ACMI, Inc., www.gyrusacmi.com*	Conditional 5	3	
De La Cruz, Fluoroplastic *Platinum, Piston* *Medtronic Xomed, Jacksonville, TN*	Conditional 5	1.5	
Dornhoffer Footplate Shoe *Otologic implant, Titanium* *Gyrus ACMI, Inc., www.gyrusacmi.com*	Conditional 5	3	
Dornhoffer Malleable PORP *Otologic Implant, 316L SS* *Gyrus ACMI, Inc., www.gyrusacmi.com*	Conditional 5	3	
Dornhoffer Titanium *Otologic implant, Titanium* *Gyrus ACMI, Inc., www.gyrusacmi.com*	Conditional 5	3	
Ehmke hook stapes prosthesis *Platinum, Otologic implant* *Richards Medical Co., Memphis, TN*	Safe	1.5	35

Object	Status	Field Strength (T)	Reference
Fisch Piston *Teflon, SS, Otologic implant* *Richards Medical Co., Memphis, TN*	Safe	1.5	38
Fisch Piston *Otologic Implant, 316L SS* *Gyrus ACMI, Inc., www.gyrusacmi.com*	Conditional 5	3	
Fisch Teflon Piston *Otologic Implant, 316L SS* *Gyrus ACMI, Inc., www.gyrusacmi.com*	Conditional 5	3	
Flex H/A notched *offset total ossicular prosthesis, 316L SS, Otologic implant* *Microtek Medical, Inc., Memphis, TN*	Safe	1.5	36
Flex H/A offset partial ossicular prosthesis *316L SS, Otologic implant* *Microtek Medical, Inc., Memphis, TN*	Safe	1.5	36
FLPL Malleable Piston *Otologic Implant, 316L SS* *Gyrus ACMI, Inc., www.gyrusacmi.com*	Conditional 5	3	
FLPL/Titanium VT, Ventilation tube *Otologic implant, Titanium* *Gyrus ACMI, Inc., www.gyrusacmi.com*	Conditional 5	3	
Goldenberg Mal Porp *Otologic Implant, 316L SS* *Gyrus ACMI, Inc., www.gyrusacmi.com*	Conditional 5	3	
Gyrus All Titanium Centered PORP *partial ossicular replacement prosthesis, Titanium* *Gyrus ACMI, Inc., wwwgyrusacmi.com*	Safe	3	106
Gyrus All Titanium Monolithic Centered TORP *total ossicular replacement prosthesis, Titanium* *Gyrus ACMI, Inc., wwwgyrusacmi.com*	Safe	3	106
Gyrus, PORP, partial ossicular replacement prosthesis *Titanium* *Gyrus ACMI, Inc., wwwgyrusacmi.com*	Safe	3	106
Gyrus, TORP, total ossicular replacement prosthesis *Titanium* *Gyrus ACMI, Inc., wwwgyrusacmi.com*	Safe	3	106
Gyrus SMart Stapes Piston, Titanium *Gyrus ACMI, Inc., wwwgyrusacmi.com*	Safe	3	106
House double loop *ASTM-318-76 Grade 2 SS, Otologic implant* *Storz, St. Louis, MO*	Safe	1.5	35
House double loop *tantalum, Otologic implant* *Storz, St. Louis, MO*	Safe	1.5	35
House single loop *ASTM-318-76, Grade 2 SS, Otologic implant* *Storz, St. Louis, MO*	Safe	1.5	31
House single loop *tantalum, Otologic implant* *Storz, St. Louis, MO*	Safe	1.5	35

Object	Status	Field Strength (T)	Reference
House Wire Loop *Otologic Implant, 316LVM SS* *Gyrus ACMI, Inc., www.gyrusacmi.com*	Conditional 5	3	
House wire *SS, Otologic implant* *Otomed*	Safe	0.5	39
House wire *tantalum, Otologic implant* *Otomed*	Safe	0.5	39
House-type incus prosthesis *Otologic implant*	Safe	0.6	
House-type SS, piston and wire *ASTM-318-76 Grade 2 SS, Otologic implant* *Xomed-Treace Inc., A Bristol-Myers Squibb Co.*	Safe	1.5	35
House-type wire loop *stapes prosthesis, 316L SS, Otologic implant* *Richards Medical Co., Memphis, TN*	Safe	1.5	35
InSound XT Series *InSound Medical, Newark, CA*	Unsafe 1	1.5	
K-Helix Prosthesis *Device Family, K-Helix Prosthesis;* *Family Product Number(s) 756-XXX, 757-XXX;* *Device Material(s), Titanium* *Grace Medical, www.gracemedical.com*	Conditional 6	3	
K Piston Titanium *0.6 x 10.0-mm, middle ear implant, Otologic implant* *Kurz Medical, Inc., Norcross, GA*	Safe	3	
Kurz Aerial *Titanium* *Kurz Medical*	Safe	3	106
Kurz Aerial-Total-Dusseldorf-Titanium *TORP, total ossicular replacement prosthesis* *Kurz Medical*	Safe	3	106
Kurz Bell *Titanium* *Kurz Medical*	Safe	3	106
Kurz Bell-Partial-Dusseldorf-Titanium *PORP, partial ossicular replacement prosthesis, Titanium* *Kurz Medical*	Safe	3	106
Kurz Piston, Titanium *Kurz Medical*	Safe	3	106
Kurz Piston-Titanium *stapes, Titanium* *Kurz Medical*	Safe	3	106
Lippy Modified Bucket Handle *Stapes Prosthesis, Otologic implant, Titanium* *Gyrus ACMI, Inc., www.gyrusacmi.com*	Conditional 5	3	
Lippy Modified Stapes Prostheses *Otologic Implant, Titanium* *Gyrus ACMI, Inc., www.gyrusacmi.com*	Conditional 5	3	
Lyric Hearing Device *InSound Medical, Newark, CA*	Unsafe 1	1.5	

Object	Status	Field Strength (T)	Reference
McGee Piston *Otologic Implant, 316LVM SS* *Gyrus ACMI, Inc., www.gyrusacmi.com*	Conditional 5	3	
McGee piston stapes prosthesis *316L, SS, Otologic implant* *Richards Medical Co., Memphis, TN*	Safe	1.5	35
McGee piston stapes prosthesis *Platinum, 316L SS, Otologic implant* *Richards Medical Co., Memphis, TN*	Safe	1.5	35
McGee piston stapes prosthesis *Platinum, chromium-nickel alloy, SS, Otologic implant* *Richards Medical Co., Memphis, TN*	Unsafe 1	1.5	38
McGee Shepard's Crook Piston *Otologic Implant, SS* *Gyrus ACMI, Inc., www.gyrusacmi.com*	Conditional 5	3	
McGee Sheperd's Crook stapes prosthesis *316L SS, Otologic implant* *Richards Medical Co., Memphis, TN*	Safe	1.5	35
MED-EL COMBI 40+, MED-EL Cochlear Implant System *MED-EL Corporation* *COMBI 40+ is MRI safe at 0.2, 1.0 and 1.5 Tesla depending on* *regulatory approval in different countries. Contact MED-EL prior to* *MRI examination for important guidelines, www.medel.com*	Conditional 5	0.2, 1, 1.5	98
MED-EL CONCERT Cochlear Implant *Med-El, www.medel.com*	Conditional 5	0.2	
MED-EL SONATA Cochlear Implant *Med-El, www.medel.com*	Conditional 5	0.2	
Medtronic-Xomed *PORP, partial ossicular replacement prosthesis, Titanium* *Medtronic-Xomed, Jacksonville, FL*	Safe	3	106
Medtronic-Xomed *TORP, total ossicular replacement prosthesis, Titanium* *Medtronic-Xomed, Jacksonville, FL*	Safe	3	106
MEY Modified Lippy *Otologic Implant, 316L SS* *Gyrus ACMI, Inc., www.gyrusacmi.com*	Conditional 5	3	
Micron Bobbin Blue VT, Ventilation tube *Otologic implant, Titanium* *Gyrus ACMI, Inc., www.gyrusacmi.com*	Conditional 5	3	
Micron Bobbin VT, Ventilation tube *Otologic implant, Titanium* *Gyrus ACMI, Inc., www.gyrusacmi.com*	Conditional 5	3	
Micron II Modular, PORP *Otologic implant, Titanium* *Gyrus ACMI, Inc., www.gyrusacmi.com*	Conditional 5	3	
Micron II Modular, TORP *Otologic implant, Titanium* *Gyrus ACMI, Inc., www.gyrusacmi.com*	Conditional 5	3	
Micron II Monolithic, PORP *Otologic implant, Titanium* *Gyrus ACMI, Inc., www.gyrusacmi.com*	Conditional 5	3	

Object	Status	Field Strength (T)	Reference
Micron II Monolithic, TORP *Otologic implant, Titanium* *Gyrus ACMI, Inc., www.gyrusacmi.com*	Conditional 5	3	
Micron Plus VT, Ventilation tube *Otologic implant, Titanium* *Gyrus ACMI, Inc., www.gyrusacmi.com*	Conditional 5	3	
Micron Spoon Bobbin VT, Ventilation tube *Otologic implant, Titanium* *Gyrus ACMI, Inc., www.gyrusacmi.com*	Conditional 5	3	
Minimal Type Ventilation Tube, Gold Coated SS *Kurz, www.kurzmed.de*	Unsafe 1	1.5	
Modified Lippy, Otologic Implant, 316L SS *Gyrus ACMI, Inc., www.gyrusacmi.com*	Conditional 5	3	
Moretz Type VT, Ventilation tube *Otologic implant, Titanium* *Gyrus ACMI, Inc., www.gyrusacmi.com*	Conditional 5	3	
NitiBOND Stapes Prosthesis *Heinz Kurz GmbH* *Dusslingen, Germany*	Conditional 6	3	
Nucleus 22, Cochlear Implant *Without removable magnet* *Cochlear LTD* *http://professionals.cochlearamericas.com*	Unsafe 1	1.5	
Nucleus 22, Cochlear Implant *With removable magnet* *Cochlear LTD, http://professionals.cochlearamericas.com*	Conditional 5	1.5	
Nucleus 24 Series, Cochlear Implant *Cochlear LTD, http://professionals.cochlearamericas.com*	Conditional 5	1.5	
Nucleus Freedom, Cochlear Implant *Cochlear LTD, http://professionals.cochlearamericas.com*	Conditional 5	1.5	
Offset ALTO Total Prosthesis *MRI information applies to Pistons* *SS/Teflon, P/N 410-600;* *Titanium/Teflon, P/N 409-XXX, 417-XXX;* *Platinum/Titanium, P/N 418-XXX, 419-XXX;* *Grace Medical, Memphis, TN*	Conditional 6	3	
Offset ALTO Total Prosthesis *MRI information applies to Pistons* *SS/Teflon, P/N 410-600;* *Titanium/Teflon, P/N 409-XXX, 417-XXX;* *Platinum/Titanium, P/N 418-XXX, 419-XXX;* *Grace Medical, Memphis, TN*	Conditional 6	3	
Offset ALTO Total Prosthesis *MRI information applies to* *Platinum/Teflon, P/N 411-XXX, 412-XXX,* *415-XXX, 452-XXX, 453-XXX;* *Nitinol/Teflon, P/N 465-XXX, 466-XXX,* *467-XXX, 468-XXX, 469-XXX;* *Grace Medical, Memphis, TN*	Conditional 6	3	

Object	Status	Field Strength (T)	Reference
Offset ALTO Total Prosthesis *MRI information applies to Buckets* *Titanium, CP2 & CP4* *P/N 420-XXX through 430-XXX* *OCR's, Middle Ear Implants, Titanium CP2,* *other materials HA and Silicone* *ALTO 600 Series, Titanium CP2* *Fixed Length 700 Series* *Grace Medical, Memphis, TN*	Conditional 6	3	
Partial and Total Prosthesis *Device Family, Partial and Total Prosthesis;* *Family Product Number(s), 1XX, 190-XXX;* *Device Material(s), HA, hydroxyapatite* *Grace Medical, www.gracemedical.com/mri.htm* *www.gracemedical.com*	Safe	3	
Partial and Total Prosthesis *Device Family, Partial and Total Prosthesis;* *Family Product Number(s), 2XX, 193;* *Device Material(s), HA (hydroxyapatite), Silicone* *Grace Medical, www.gracemedical.com/mri.htm* *www.gracemedical.com*	Safe	3	
Pediatric VT *Ventilation tube, Otologic implant, Titanium* *Gyrus ACMI, Inc., www.gyrusacmi.com*	Conditional 5	3	
Piston Teflon Wire *Otologic Implant, 316L SS* *Gyrus ACMI, Inc., www.gyrusacmi.com*	Conditional 5	3	
Plasti-pore piston *316L SS, Plasti-pore material, Otologic implant* *Richards Medical Co., Memphis, TN*	Safe	1.5	35
Platinum ribbon loop stapes prosthesis *Platinum, Otologic implant* *Richards Medical Co., Memphis, TN*	Safe	1.5	35
Precise Prosthesis *Device Family, Precise Prosthesis;* *Family Product Number(s),* *700-XXX, 705-XXX, 720-XXX, 750-XXX, 765-XXX, 770-XXX;* *Device Material(s), Titanium, HA (hydroxyapatite)* *Grace Medical, www.gracemedical.com/mri.htm* *www.gracemedical.com*	Conditional 6	3	
Pulsar Cochlear Implant, PULSARCI100 *MedEl Corporation, Durham, NC*	Conditional 5	0.2	98
Reuter Bobbin, Ventilation tube *316L SS, Ctologic implant* *Richards Medical Co., Memphis, TN*	Safe	1.5	35
Reuter Bobbin VT *Ventilation tube, Otologic implant, Titanium* *Gyrus ACMI, Inc., www.gyrusacmi.com*	Conditional 5	3	
Reuter Bobbin Vent Tube *Ventilation tube, Otologic Implant, 316L SS* *Gyrus ACMI, Inc., www.gyrusacmi.com*	Conditional 5	3	
Reuter drain tube *Otologic implant*	Safe	1.5	35

Object	Status	Field Strength (T)	Reference
Richards bucket handle stapes prosthesis *316L SS, Otologic implant* *Richards Medical Co., Memphis, TN*	Safe	1.5	35
Richard's Bucket Handle *Otologic Implant, Tantalum* *Gyrus ACMI, Inc., www.gyrusacmi.com*	Conditional 5	3	
Richards piston stapes prosthesis *Platinum, fluoroplastic, Otologic implant* *Richards Medical Co., Memphis, TN*	Safe	1.5	35
Richards Plasti-pore with Armstrong-style *Platinum ribbon, Platinum, Otologic implant* *Richards Medical Co., Memphis, TN*	Safe	1.5	35
Richards Platinum Teflon piston *0.6-mm, Teflon, Platinum, Otologic implant* *Richards Medical Co., Memphis, TN*	Safe	1.5	38
Richards Platinum Teflon piston *0.8-mm, Teflon, Platinum, Otologic implant* *Richards Medical Co., Memphis, TN*	Safe	1.5	38
Richards Shepherd's crook *Platinum, Otologic implant* *Richards Medical Co., Memphis, TN*	Safe	0.5	39
Richards Teflon piston *Teflon, Otologic implant* *Richards Medical Co., Memphis, TN*	Safe	1.5	38
Roberson Stapes Prosthesis *Titanium* *Medtronic Xomed, Inc.*	Safe	3	
Roberts Universal Prosthesis *PORP, Otologic implant, Titanium* *Gyrus ACMI, Inc., www.gyrusacmi.com*	Conditional 5	3	
Roberts Universal Prosthesis *TORP, Otologic implant, Titanium* *Gyrus ACMI, Inc., www.gyrusacmi.com*	Conditional 5	3	
Robinson incus replacement prosthesis *ASTM-318-76 Grade 2 SS, Otologic implant* *Storz, St. Louis, MO*	Safe	1.5	35
Robinson stapes prosthesis *ASTM-318-76 Grade 2 SS, Otologic implant* *Storz, St. Louis, MO*	Safe	1.5	35
Robinson-Moon offset *stapes prosthesis, ASTM-318-76 Grade 2 SS, Otologic implant* *Storz, St. Louis, MO*	Safe	1.5	35
Robinson-Moon-Lippy offset *stapes prosthesis, ASTM- 318-76 Grade 2 SS, Otologic implant* *Storz, St. Louis, MO*	Safe	1.5	35
Ronis Piston *Stapes prosthesis, 316L SS, fluoroplastic, Otologic implant* *Richards Medical Co., Memphis, TN*	Safe	1.5	35
Ronis Piston *Otologic Implant, 316L SS* *Gyrus ACMI, Inc., www.gyrusacmi.com*	Conditional 5	3	

Object	Status	Field Strength (T)	Reference
Ronis Wire Piston *Otologic Implant, 316L SS* *Gyrus ACMI, Inc., www.gyrusacmi.com*	Conditional 5	3	
Shea cup piston stapes prosthesis *Platinum, fluoroplastic, Otologic implant* *Richards Medical Co., Memphis, TN*	Safe	1.5	35
Shea malleus attachment piston *Teflon, Otologic implant* *Richards Medical Co., Memphis, TN*	Safe	1.5	38
Shea SS *and Teflon wire prosthesis, Teflon, 316L SS, Otologic implant* *Richards Medical Co., Memphis, TN*	Safe	1.5	38
Scheer FLPL Wire *Otologic Implant, 316L SS* *Gyrus ACMI, Inc., www.gyrusacmi.com*	Conditional 5	3	
Scheer piston *Teflon, 316L SS, Otologic implant* *Richards Medical Co., Memphis, TN*	Safe	1.5	33
Scheer piston stapes prosthesis *316L SS, fluoroplastic, Otologic implant* *Richards Medical Co., Memphis, TN*	Safe	1.5	35
Schuk Wire Piston *Otologic Implant, 316L SS* *Gyrus ACMI, Inc., www.gyrusacmi.com*	Conditional 5	3	
Schuknecht gelfoam and wire *prosthesis, Armstrong style, 316L SS, Otologic implant* *Richards Medical Co., Memphis, TN*	Safe	1.5	40
Schuknecht piston stapes prosthesis *316L SS, fluoroplastic, Otologic implant* *Richards Medical Co., Memphis, TN*	Safe	1.5	35
Schuknecht Tef-wire incus attachment *ASTM-318-76 Grade 2 SS, Otologic implant* *Storz, St. Louis, MO*	Safe	1.5	35
Schuknecht Tef-wire malleus attachment *ASTM-318-76 Grade 2 SS, Otologic implant* *Storz, St. Louis, MO*	Safe	1.5	35
Schuknecht Teflon wire piston *0.6-mm, Teflon, 316L SS, Otologic implant* *Richards Medical Co., Memphis, TN*	Safe	1.5	38
Schuknecht Teflon wire piston *0.8-mm, Teflon, 316L SS, Otologic implant* *Richards Medical Co., Memphis, TN*	Safe	1.5	38
Sheehy incus replacement *ASTM-318-76 Grade 2 SS, Otologic implant* *Storz, St. Louis, MO*	Safe	1.5	35
Sheehy incus strut *316L SS, Otologic implant* *Richards Medical Co., Memphis, TN*	Safe	1.5	38
Sheehy Stapes Replacement strut *Otologic Implant, 316L SS* *Gyrus ACMI, Inc., www.gyrusacmi.com*	Conditional 5	3	

Object	Status	Field Strength (T)	Reference
Sheehy-Type Incus Replacement strut *Teflon, 316L SS, Otologic implant* *Richards Medical Co., Memphis, TN*	Safe	1.5	35
Sheehy-Type Incus *Replacement strut, Otologic Implant, 316L SS* *Gyrus ACMI, Inc., www.gyrusacmi.com*	Conditional 5	3	
Shepherd Crook Piston *Otologic Implant, 316L SS* *Gyrus ACMI, Inc., www.gyrusacmi.com*	Conditional 5	3	
Shipp Modified Berger VT, Ventilation tube *Otologic implant, Titanium* *Gyrus ACMI, Inc., www.gyrusacmi.com*	Conditional 5	3	
Silverstein malleus clip, Ventilation Tube *Teflon, 316L SS, Otologic implant* *Richards Medical Co., Memphis, TN*	Safe	1.5	38
SMart De La Cruz Piston *Otologic Implant, Nitinol/Fluoroplastic* *Gyrus ACMI, Inc., www.gyrusacmi.com*	Conditional 5	3	
SMart Malleus Piston *Otologic Implant, Nitinol/Fluoroplastic* *Gyrus ACMI, Inc., www.gyrusacmi.com*	Conditional 5	3	
SMart Piston *Otologic Implant, Fluoroplastic/Nitinol* *Gyrus ACMI, Inc., www.gyrusacmi.com*	Conditional 5	3	
SOUNDTEC Direct Drive Hearing System *SOUNDTEC, Inc., Oklahoma City, OK*	Unsafe 1	1.5	
Spoon Bobbin Ventilation tube *316L SS, Otologic implant* *Richards Medical Co., Memphis, TN*	Safe	1.5	35
Spoon-Bobbin Vent Tube *Ventilation tube, Otologic Implant, 316L SS* *Gyrus ACMI, Inc., www.gyrusacmi.com*	Conditional 5	3	
Stainless Steel/Fluoroplastic *Sanna-Type Piston* *MRI information applies to Pistons* *SS/Teflon, P/N 410 600;* *Titanium/Teflon, P/N 409-XXX, 417-XXX;* *Platinum/Titanium, P/N 418-XXX, 419-XXX;* *Grace Medical, Memphis, TN*	Conditional 6	3	
Stainless Steel/Fluoroplastic *Sanna-Type Piston* *MRI information applies to Platinum/Teflon,* *P/N 411-XXX, 412-XXX, 415-XXX, 452-XXX, 453-XXX;* *Nitinol/Teflon, P/N 465-XXX, 466-XXX,* *467-XXX, 468-XXX, 469-XXX;* *Grace Medical, Memphis, TN*	Conditional 6	3	

Object	Status	Field Strength (T)	Reference
Stainless Steel/Fluoroplastic *Sanna-Type Piston* *MRI information applies to Buckets* *Titanium, CP2 & CP4, P/N 420-XXX through 430-XXX* *OCR's, Middle Ear Implants* *Titanium CP2, other materials HA and Silicone* *ALTO 600 Series* *Titanium CP2* *Fixed Length 700 Series* *Grace Medical, Memphis, TN*	Conditional 6	3	
Stainless Steel Vent Tube & Stainless Steel Wire *VT-1400-0, because the size of the metallic mass associated with* *this product, the MRI test findings apply to all of the following* *products from Micromedics, Inc.* *VT-0205-, Fluoroplastic with stainless steel wire* *VT-0702-, Silicone with stainless steel wire* *VT-1402-, Stainless Steel with stainless steel wire* *VT-1412-, Titanium with stainless steel wire* *VT-1505-, Polyethylene with stainless steel wire* *Micromedics, Inc., Eagan, MN*	Conditional 6	3	
Stapes, fluoroplastic/Platinum, piston *Otologic implant* *Microtek Medical, Inc., Memphis, TN*	Safe	1.5	36
Stapes, fluoroplastic/SS piston *316L SS, Otologic implant* *Microtek Medical, Inc., Memphis, TN*	Safe	1.5	36
Stapes Grommet *Replacement strut, Otologic Implant, 316L SS* *Gyrus ACMI, Inc., www.gyrusacmi.com*	Conditional 5	3	
Stapes Prosthesis, Bucket *Device Family,* *Stapes Prosthesis, Bucket;* *Family Product Number(s),* *420-XXX, 421-XXX, 422-XXX, 423-XXX, 424-XXX, 425-XXX,* *426-XXX, 427-XXX, 428-XXX, 429-XXX, 430-XXX;* *Device Material(s), Titanium, Nitinol* *Grace Medical, www.gracemedical.com/mri.htm* *www.gracemedical.com*	Conditional 6	3	
Stapes Prosthesis, Piston *Device Family,* *Stapes Prosthesis, Piston;* *Family Product Number(s),* *409-XXX, 410-XXX, 411-XXX, 412-XXX, 413-XXX,* *415-XXX, 417-XXX, 418-XXX,* *Device Material(s), Titanium, Platinum, Stainless Steel, Nitinol,* *Fluroplastic,* *Grace Medical, www.gracemedical.com/mri.htm* *www.gracemedical.com*	Conditional 6	3	

Object	Status	Field Strength (T)	Reference
Stapes Prosthesis, Piston *Device Family,* *Stapes Prosthesis, Piston;* *Family Product Number(s),* *419-XXX, 452-XXX, 453-XXX, 465-XXX, 466-XXX, 467-XXX,* *468-XXX, 469-XXX;* *Device Material(s),* *Titanium, Platinum, Stainless Steel, Nitinol, Fluroplastic* *Grace Medical, www.gracemedical.com/mri.htm* *www.gracemedical.com*	Conditional 6	3	
Stapes Prostheses, Piston *Device Family,* *Stapes Prostheses, Pistons;* *Family Product Number(s), 401-XXX, 402-XXX, 403-XXX, 404-* *XXX, 405-XXX, 406-XXX, 408-XXX;* *Device Material(s), Fluoroplastic* *Grace Medical, www.gracemedical.com/mri.htm* *www.gracemedical.com*	Safe	3	
Strasnick Prosthesis *Device Family, Strasnick Prosthesis;* *Family Product Number(s), 220-XXX, 270-XXX;* *Device Material(s), Titanium, Silicone* *Grace Medical, www.gracemedical.com/mri.htm* *www.gracemedical.com*	Conditional 6	3	
Tantalum Wire Loop *Otologic Implant, Tantalum* *Gyrus ACMI, Inc., www.gyrusacmi.com*	Conditional 5	3	
Tantalum wire loop *Stapes prosthesis, Tantalum, Otologic implant* *Richards Medical Co., Memphis, TN*	Safe	1.5	35
Teflon Malleable Piston *Otologic Implant, 316L SS* *Gyrus ACMI, Inc., www.gyrusacmi.com*	Conditional 5	3	
Teflon Piston *Otologic Implant, 316L SS* *Gyrus ACMI, Inc., www.gyrusacmi.com*	Conditional 5	3	
Teflon Wire Piston *Otologic Implant, 316L SS* *Gyrus ACMI, Inc., www.gyrusacmi.com*	Conditional 5	3	
Tef-Platinum piston *Platinum, Otologic implant* *Xomed-Treace Inc., A Bristol-Myers Squibb Co.*	Safe	1.5	35
Touma Modified Crook Piston *Otologic Implant, 316L SS* *Gyrus ACMI, Inc., www.gyrusacmi.com*	Conditional 5	3	
The Big Easy Piston, Stapes Prosthesis *Otologic Implant* *www.angelmedex.com*	Safe	1.5, 3	
Total ossicular replacement prosthesis (TORP) *316L SS, Otologic implant* *Richards Medical Co., Memphis, TN*	Safe	1.5	38

Object	Status	Field Strength (T)	Reference
Trapeze ribbon loop stapes prosthesis *Platinum, Otologic implant* *Richards Medical Co., Memphis, TN*	Safe	1.5	35
Trocar with Wire *Kurz, www.kurzmed.de*	Unsafe 1	1.5	
TTP Aerial Vario Titanium *0.2 x 7.0-mm, middle ear implant, Otologic implant* *Kurz Medical, Inc., Norcross, GA*	Safe	3	
TTP Bell Vario Titanium *0.2 x 4.5-mm, middle ear implant, Otologic implant* *Kurz Medical, Inc., Norcross, GA*	Safe	3	
Tuebingen Type Ventilation Tubes with Wire, Gold, SS *Kurz, www.kurzmed.de*	Unsafe 1	1.5	
Tuebingen Type Ventilation Tubes with Wire, Silver, SS *Kurz, www.kurzmed.de*	Unsafe 1	1.5	
Tuebingen Type Ventilation Tubes with Wire, Titanium, SS *Kurz, www.kurzmed.de*	Unsafe 1	1.5	
UniBobbin VT, Ventilation tube *Otologic implant, Titanium* *Gyrus ACMI, Inc., www.gyrusacmi.com*	Conditional 5	3	
Venturi Plus VT, Ventilation tube *Otologic implant, Titanium* *Gyrus ACMI, Inc., www.gyrusacmi.com*	Conditional 5	3	
Venturi VT, Ventilation tube *Otologic implant, Titanium* *Gyrus ACMI, Inc., www.gyrusacmi.com*	Conditional 5	3	
Vibrant Soundbridge *Symphonix Devices, Inc., San Jose, CA*	Unsafe 1	1.5	
Wehrs Incus Prosthesis, Otologic Implant *Gyrus ACMI, www.gyrusacmi.com*	Conditional 5	3	
Williams Microclip *316L SS, Otologic implant* *Richards Medical Co., Memphis, TN*	Safe	1.5	35
Williams Microclip *Wire clip, Otologic Implant, 316L SS* *Gyrus ACMI, Inc., www.gyrusacmi.com*	Conditional 5	3	
Winkel Partial Plester Titanium *0.2 x 3.5-mm, Otologic implant* *Kurz Medical, Inc., Norcross, GA*	Safe	3	
Xomed Baily stapes implant *Otologic implant*	Safe	1.5	35
Xomed ceravital *partial ossicular prosthesis* *Otologic implant*	Safe	1.5	
Xomed stapes prosthesis *Robinson-style, Otologic implant* *Richard's Co., Nashville, TN*	Safe	1.5	35
Xomed stapes *ASTM-318-76 Grade 2 SS, Otologic implant* *Xomed-Treace Inc., A Bristol-Myers Squibb Co.*	Safe	1.5	35

Object	Status	Field Strength (T)	Reference

Patent Ductus Arteriosus (PDA), Atrial Septal Defect (ASD), Ventricular Septal Defect (VSD) Occluders, and Patent Foramen Ovale (PFO) Closure Devices

Object	Status	Field Strength (T)	Reference
AMPLATZER Cardiac Plug *(also known as ACP device), Nitinol, SS, Platinum/iridium, Polyester AGA Medical Corporation, www.sjm.com/aga-medical*	Conditional 6	3	
AMPLATZER Duct Occluder II *AGA Medical Corporation, www.sjm.com/aga-medical*	Conditional 6	3	
AMPLATZER Multifenestrated *Septal Occluder, Cribriform AGA Medical Corporation, www.sjm.com/aga-medical*	Conditional 6	3	
AMPLATZER Muscular VSD Occluder *AGA Medical Corporation, www.sjm.com/aga-medical*	Conditional 6	3	
AMPLATZER Muscular VSD PI Occluder *AGA Medical Corporation, www.sjm.com/aga-medical*	Conditional 6	3	
AMPLATZER PFO Occluder *Nitinol, SS, Platinum/iridium, Polyester AGA Medical Corporation, www.sjm.com/aga-medical*	Conditional 6	3	
AMPLATZER Post Infarction *Muscular Ventricular Septal Device Nitinol, SS, Platinum/iridium, Polyester AGA Medical Corporation, www.sjm.com/aga-medical*	Conditional 6	3	
AMPLATZER Septal Occluder *Nitinol, SS, Platinum/iridium, Polyester AGA Medical Corporation, www.sjm.com/aga-medical*	Conditional 6	3	
AMPLATZER Transcatheter Occlusion Device *AGA Medical Corporation, www.sjm.com/aga-medical*	Conditional 6	3	
AMPLATZER Vascular Plug Device *AGA Medical Corporation, www.sjm.com/aga-medical*	Conditional 6	3	
AMPLATZER Vascular Plug 4 *AVP4 device AGA Medical Corporation, www.sjm.com/aga-medical*	Conditional 6	3	
Atrial Septal Defect Occluder, Guardian Angel *12-mm, occluder Microvena Corporation, White Bear Lake, MN*	Safe	1.5	
Atrial Septal Defect Occluder, Guardian Angel *40-mm, occluder Microvena Corporation, White Bear Lake, MN*	Safe	1.5	
Atriasept Closure Device *Cardia, Inc., Eagan, MN*	Conditional 6	3	
Bard Clamshell Septal Umbrella *17-mm, occluder C.R. Bard, Inc., Billerica, MA*	Safe	1.5	41
Bard Clamshell Septal Umbrella *23-mm, occluder C.R. Bard, Inc., Billerica, MA*	Safe	1.5	41
Bard Clamshell Septal Umbrella *28-mm, occluder C.R. Bard, Inc., Billerica, MA*	Safe	1.5	41

Object	Status	Field Strength (T)	Reference
Bard Clamshell Septal Umbrella *33-mm, occluder* *C.R. Bard, Inc., Billerica, MA*	Safe	1.5	41
Bard Clamshell Septal Umbrella *40-mm, occluder* *C.R. Bard, Inc., Bellerica, MA*	Safe	1.5	41
BioSTAR Septal Repair Implant *NMT Medical, Inc., Boston, MA*	Safe	3	
BioTREK *patent foramen ovale (PFO) closure device* *NMT Medical, Boston, MA*	Safe	3	
CardioSEAL Septal Occluder *17-mm, MP35N* *NMT Medical, Inc., Boston, MA*	Safe	1.5	
CardioSEAL Septal Occluder *23-mm, MP35N* *NMT Medical, Inc., Boston, MA*	Safe	1.5	
CardioSEAL Septal Occluder *28-mm, MP35N* *NMT Medical, Inc., Boston, MA*	Safe	1.5	
CardioSEAL Septal Occluder *33-mm, MP35N* *NMT Medical, Inc., Boston, MA*	Safe	1.5	
CardioSEAL Septal Occluder *40-mm, MP35N* *NMT Medical, Inc., Boston, MA*	Safe	1.5	
CardioSEAL Septal Repair Implant, MP35N *NMT Medical, Inc., Boston, MA*	Safe	3	107
CardioSEAL Septal Repair Implant *NMT Medical, Inc., Boston, MA*	Conditional 6	3	
Celt ACD Vascular Closure Device *Vasorum, www.vasorum.ie*	Conditional 6	3	
Cocoon Septal Occluder *Nitinol, Platinum* *Vascular Innovations Co. Ltd, Nonthaburi, Thailand*	Conditional 6	3	
GORE HELEX Septal Occluder *W.L. Gore & Associates, www.goremedical.com*	Conditional 6	3	
HELEX *ASD closure device, occluder, size 15-mm, Nitinol* *W. L. Gore and Associates, Inc.,www.goremedical.com*	Conditional 5	3	
HELEX *ASD closure device, occluder, size 35-mm, Nitinol* *W. L. Gore and Associates, Inc.,www.goremedical.com*	Conditional 5	3	
HELEX Septal Occluder *Nitinol* *W.L. Gore and Associates, Inc., www.goremedical.com*	Conditional 5	3	
Intrasept *patent foramen ovale (PFO) closure device, Nitinol, Titanium* *Cardia Inc., Burnsville, MN*	Conditional 6	3	
Lock Clamshell Septal Occlusion Implant *17-mm, occluder, 304 V SS* *C.R. Bard, Inc., Billerica, MA*	Conditional 2	1.5	41

Object	Status	Field Strength (T)	Reference
Lock Clamshell Septal Occlusion Implant *23-mm, occluder, 304 V SS* *C.R. Bard, Inc., Billerica, MA*	Conditional 2	1.5	41
Lock Clamshell Septal Occlusion Implant *28-mm, occluder, 304 V SS* *C.R. Bard, Inc., Billerica, MA*	Conditional 2	1.5	41
Lock Clamshell Septal Occlusion Implant *33-mm, occluder, 304 V SS* *C.R. Bard, Inc., Billerica, MA*	Conditional 2	1.5	41
Lock Clamshell Septal Occlusion Implant *40-mm, occluder, 304 V SS* *C.R. Bard, Inc., Billerica, MA*	Conditional 2	1.5	41
Nit-Occlud PDA-R Occluder *PFM s.r.l*	Conditional 6	3	
Nit-Occlud Spiral Coil *PFM Medical, Inc., Oceanside, CA*	Conditional 6	3	
Premere PFO Closure System *patent foramen ovale (PFO) closure device* *St. Jude Medical, www.sjmprofessional.com*	Conditional 5	3	
Rashkind PDA Occlusion Implant *12-mm, occluder, 304V SS* *C.R. Bard, Inc., Billerica, MA*	Conditional 2	1.5	41
Rashkind PDA Occlusion Implant *17-mm, occluder, 304 V SS* *C.R. Bard, Inc., Billerica, MA*	Conditional 2	1.5	41
STARFlex Septal Repair Implant *MP35N, Nitinol* *NMT Medical, Inc., Boston, MA*	Safe	3	
Ultrasept PFO Occluder *Cardia, Inc., www.cardiainc.com*	Conditional 6	3	

Object	Status	Field Strength (T)	Reference

Pellets and Bullets

Object	Status	Field Strength (T)	Reference
BBs (Crosman)	Unsafe 1	1.5	
BBs (Daisy)	Unsafe 1	1.5	
Bullet, .357 inch, aluminum, lead *pellets and bullets* *Winchester*	Safe	1.5	42
Bullet, .357 inch, bronze, plastic *pellets and bullets* *Patton-Morgan*	Safe	1.5	42
Bullet, .357 inch, copper, lead *pellets and bullets* *Cascade*	Safe	1.5	42
Bullet, .357 inch, copper, lead *pellets and bullets* *Hornady*	Safe	1.5	42
Bullet, .357 inch, copper, lead *pellets and bullets* *Patton-Morgan*	Safe	1.5	42
Bullet, .357 inch, lead *pellets and bullets* *Remington*	Safe	1.5	42
Bullet, .357 inch, nickel, copper, lead *pellets and bullets* *Winchester*	Safe	1.5	42
Bullet, .357 inch, nylon, lead *pellets and bullets* *Smith & Wesson*	Safe	1.5	42
Bullet, .357 inch, steel, lead *pellets and bullets* *Fiocchi*	Safe	1.5	42
Bullet, .380 inch, copper, nickel, lead *pellets and bullets* *Winchester*	Unsafe 1	1.5	42
Bullet, .380 inch, copper, plastic, lead *pellets and bullets* *Glaser*	Safe	1.5	42
Bullet, .44 inch, Teflon, bronze *pellets and bullets* *North American Ordinance*	Safe	1.5	42
Bullet, .45 inch, copper, lead *pellets and bullets* *Samson*	Safe	1.5	42
Bullet, .45 inch, steel, lead *pellets and bullets* *Evansville Ordinance*	Unsafe 1	1.5	42
Bullet, 7.62 x 39-mm, copper, steel *pellets and bullets* *Norinco*	Unsafe 1	1.5	42
Bullet, 9-mm, copper, lead *pellets and bullets* *Norma*	Unsafe 1	1.5	42

Object	Status	Field Strength (T)	Reference
Bullet, 9-mm, copper, lead *pellets and bullets* *Remington*	Safe	1.5	42
Shot, 00 buckshot, lead *pellets and bullets*	Safe	1.5	42
Shot, 12 gauge, size: 00, copper, lead *pellets and bullets* *Federal*	Safe	1.5	42
Shot, 4, lead *pellets and bullets*	Safe	1.5	42
Shot, 7 1/2, lead *pellets and bullets*	Safe	1.5	42

Object	Status	Field Strength (T)	Reference

Penile Implants

Object	Status	Field Strength (T)	Reference
Penile implant, 700 Ultrex Plus *AMS, American Medical Systems,* *www.americanmedicalsystems.com*	Safe	1.5, 3	
Penile implant, AMS 700 Ultrex Preconnected *AMS, American Medical Systems,* *www.americanmedicalsystems.com*	Safe	1.5, 3	
Penile implant, AMS 700 CX Inflatable *AMS, American Medical Systems,* *www.americanmedicalsystems.com*	Safe	1.5	43
Penile implant, AMS 700 CX/CXM *AMS, American Medical Systems,* *www.americanmedicalsystems.com*	Safe	1.5, 3	
Penile implant, AMS 700CXR *AMS, American Medical Systems,* *www.americanmedicalsystems.com*	Safe	3	
Penile implant, AMS 700 Inflate/Deflated Pump *AMS, American Medical Systems,* *www.americanmedicalsystems.com*	Safe	3	
Penile implant, AMS Tactile Pump *AMS, American Medical Systems,* *www.americanmedicalsystems.com*	Safe	3	
Penile implant, AMS 700 Ultrex *AMS, American Medical Systems,* *www.americanmedicalsystems.com*	Safe	1.5, 3	
Penile implant, AMS Ambicor *AMS, American Medical Systems,* *www.americanmedicalsystems.com*	Safe	1.5, 3	
Penile implant, AMS Dynaflex *AMS, American Medical Systems,* *www.americanmedicalsystems.com*	Safe	1.5, 3	
Penile implant, AMS Hydroflex *AMS, American Medical Systems,* *www.americanmedicalsystems.com*	Safe	1.5, 3	
Penile implant, AMS Malleable 600 *AMS, American Medical Systems,* *www.americanmedicalsystems.com*	Safe	1.5, 3	43
Penile implant, AMS Malleable 600M *AMS, American Medical Systems,* *www.americanmedicalsystems.com*	Safe	1.5, 3	
Penile implant, AMS Malleable 650 *AMS, American Medical Systems,* *www.americanmedicalsystems.com*	Safe	1.5, 3	
Penile Implant, AMS 700 Series *3-Piece Inflatable Penile Implant* *American Medical Systems Inc.,* *www.americanmedicalsystems.com*	Conditional 6	3	
Penile Implant, DURA II Penile Prosthesis *AMS, American Medical Systems,* *www.americanmedicalsystems.com*	Safe	1.5, 3	

Object	Status	Field Strength (T)	Reference
Penile implant, Duraphase	Unsafe 1	1.5	
Penile Implant, Excel Inflatable Penile Prosthesis *Model 90-95XXSC, MP35N, Urethane, Silicone, Polysulfone* *Coloplast Corporation, Minneapolis, MN*	Conditional 6	3	
Penile implant, Flex-Rod II (Firm) *Surgitek, Medical Engineering Corp., Racine, WI*	Safe	1.5	43
Penile implant, Flexi-Flate *Surgitek, Medical Engineering Corp., Racine, WI*	Safe	1.5	43
Penile implant, Flexi-Rod (Standard) *Surgitek, Medical Engineering Corp., Racine, WI*	Safe	1.5	43
Penile Implant, Genesis Malleable Penile Implant *Coloplast, UCC - Surgical Urology, Minneapolis, MN*	Conditional 6	3	
Penile implant, Jonas *Dacomed Corp., Minneapolis, MN*	Safe	1.5	43
Penile implant, Mentor Flexible *Mentor Corp, Minneapolis, MN*	Safe	1.5	43
Penile implant, Mentor Inflatable *Mentor Corp., Minneapolis, MN*	Safe	1.5	43
Penile implant, OmniPhase *Dacomed Corp., Minneapolis, MN*	Unsafe 1	1.5	43
Penile implant, Osmond, external	Safe	1.5	
Penile Implant, Spectra Penile Implant *AMS, American Medical Systems,* *www.americanmedicalsystems.com*	Conditional 6	3	
Penile Implant, Titan Inflatable Penile Prosthesis *Model 90-98XXIC* *Coloplast Corporation, Minneapolis, MN*	Conditional 6	3	
Penile Implant, Titan Inflatable Penile Prosthesis *Model 90-98XXIC* *Coloplast Corporation, Minneapolis, MN*	Conditional 6	3	
Penile Implant, Titan Inflatable Penile Prosthesis *Model 90-98XXIC* *Coloplast Corporation, Minneapolis, MN*	Conditional 6	3	
Penile Implant, Titan Inflatable Penile Prosthesis *Model 90-98ICOTR* *Coloplast Corporation, Minneapolis, MN*	Conditional 6	3	
Penile Implant, Titan Inflatable Penile Prosthesis *Model 90-99SCOTR* *Coloplast Corporation, Minneapolis, MN*	Conditional 6	3	
Penile implant, Uniflex 1000	Safe	1.5	

Object	Status	Field Strength (T)	Reference

Pessaries

Object	Status	Field Strength (T)	Reference
95% Rigid Siliconem, Pessary *CooperSurgical, Inc., Trumbull, CT*	Safe	3	
Cube (with drainage holes) Pessary *CooperSurgical, Inc., Trumbull, CT*	Safe	3	
Cube with Drainm EvaCare Pessary, Silicone *Coloplast Corporation, Minneapolis, MN*	Safe	3	
Cube EvaCare Pessary, Silicone *Coloplast Corporation, Minneapolis, MN, MN*	Safe	3	
Cube Pessary CooperSurgical, Inc., Trumbull, CT	Safe	3	
Cube Pessary, Silicone *Bioteque America, Inc., Fremont, CA*	Safe	3	
Cup Pessary EvaCare, Silicone *Coloplast Corporation, Minneapolis, MN*	Safe	3	
Cup Pessary, Silicone *Bioteque America, Inc., Fremont, CA*	Safe	3	
Dish Pessary with Support, EvaCare, Silicone *Coloplast Corporation, Minneapolis, MN*	Safe	3	
Dish Pessary, Silicone *Bioteque America, Inc., Fremont, CA*	Safe	3	
Donut, EvaCare Pessary, Silicone *Coloplast Corporation, Minneapolis, MN*	Safe	3	
Donut Pessary *CooperSurgical, Inc., Trumbull, CT*	Safe	3	
Donut Pessary, Silicone *Bioteque America, Inc., Fremont, CA*	Safe	3	
Gehrung with Support, EvaCare Pessary, Silicone *Coloplast Corporation, Minneapolis, MN*	Safe	3	
Gelhorn Pessary, Silicone *Bioteque America, Inc., Fremont, CA*	Safe	3	
Gellhorn with Drain EvaCare Pessary, Silicone *Coloplast Corporation, Minneapolis, MN*	Safe	3	
Gellhorn/95% Rigid Pessary *CooperSurgical, Inc., Trumbull, CT*	Safe	3	
Gellhorn/Flexible - Short Stem Pessary *CooperSurgical, Inc., Trumbull, CT*	Safe	3	
Gellhorn/Flexible Pessary *CooperSurgical, Inc., Trumbull, CT*	Safe	3	
Gellhorn/Flexible Pessary *CooperSurgical, Inc., Trumbull, CT*	Safe	3	
Hodge with Support EvaCare Pessary, Silicone *Coloplast Corporation, Minneapolis, MN*	Safe	3	
Hodge EvaCare Pessary, Silicone *Coloplast Corporation, Minneapolis, MN*	Safe	3	
Incontinence Dish With Support/Folding Pessary *CooperSurgical, Inc., Trumbull, CT*	Safe	3	
Incontinence Dish/Folding Pessary *CooperSurgical, Inc., Trumbull, CT*	Safe	3	

Object	Status	Field Strength (T)	Reference
Inflatoball Pessary *CooperSurgical, Inc., Trumbull, CT*	Safe	3	
Marland Pessary, Silicone *Bioteque America, Inc., Fremont, CA*	Safe	3	
Marland with Support EvaCare Pessary, Silicone *Coloplast Corporation, Minneapolis, MN*	Safe	3	
Marland EvaCare Pessary, Silicone *Coloplast Corporation, Minneapolis, MN*	Safe	3	
Oval with Support EvaCare Pessary, Silicone *Coloplast Corporation, Minneapolis, MN*	Safe	3	
Oval Pessary, Silicone *Bioteque America, Inc., Fremont, CA*	Safe	3	
Regular/Folding Pessary *CooperSurgical, Inc., Trumbull, CT*	Safe	3	
Rigid Acrylic Gelhorn Pessary *CooperSurgical, Inc., Trumbull, CT*	Safe	3	
Ring Pessary with Knob EvaCare Pessary, Silicone *Coloplast Corporation, Minneapolis, MN*	Safe	3	
Ring With Knob/Folding Pessary *CooperSurgical, Inc., Trumbull, CT*	Safe	3	
Ring with Knob Pessary *also known as Knobbed Ring, Silicone* *Bioteque America, Inc., Fremont, CA*	Safe	3	
Ring With Nylon Pegs Pessary *CooperSurgical, Inc., Trumbull, CT*	Safe	3	
Ring With Support With Knob *Pessary* *CooperSurgical, Inc., Trumbull, CT*	Safe	3	
Ring With Support and Knob/Folding Pessary *CooperSurgical, Inc., Trumbull, CT*	Safe	3	
Ring with Support EvaCare Pessary, Silicone *Coloplast Corporation, Minneapolis, MN*	Safe	3	
Ring EvaCare Pessary, Silicone *Coloplast Corporation, Minneapolis, MN*	Safe	3	
Ring Pessary, Silicone *Bioteque America, Inc., Fremont, CA*	Safe	3	
Schatz/Folding Pessary *CooperSurgical, Inc., Trumbull, CT*	Safe	3	
Shaatz EvaCare Pessary, Silicone *Coloplast Corporation, Minneapolis, MN*	Safe	3	
Shaatz Pessary, Silicone *Bioteque America, Inc., Fremont, CA*	Safe	3	
Silicone Flexible Gelhorn Pessary *CooperSurgical, Inc., Trumbull, CT*	Safe	3	
Tandem-Cube Pessary *CooperSurgical, Inc., Trumbull, CT*	Safe	3	

Sutures

Object	Status	Field Strength (T)	Reference
Suture, Biosyn, Needle removed *glycomer 631* *United States Surgical, North Haven, CT*	Safe	1.5, 3	83
Suture, Chromic gut, Needle removed, gut *United States Surgical, North Haven, CT*	Safe	1.5, 3	83
Suture, Flexon, Needle removed *SS coated with FEP* *United States Surgical, North Haven, CT*	Safe	1.5, 3	83
Suture, Flexon, Needle removed *Stainless Braid with Teflon Coating* *Flexon Multifilament Stainless Steel, Needle removed* *Covidien, www.covidien.com*	Conditional 6	3	
Suture, Maxon, Needle removed *polyglyconate* *United States Surgical, North Haven, CT*	Safe	1.5, 3	83
Suture, Monosof, Needle removed *nylon, lead weight, with latex bolster* *United States Surgical, North Haven, CT*	Safe	1.5, 3	83
Suture, Novafil, Needle removed, polybutester *United States Surgical, North Haven, CT*	Safe	1.5, 3	83
Suture, Plain gut, Needle removed *United States Surgical, North Haven, CT*	Safe	1.5, 3	83
Suture, Polysorb, Needle removed *lactomer 9-1* *United States Surgical, North Haven, CT*	Safe	1.5, 3	83
Suture, SecureStrand, Needle removed *UHMW polyethylene* *United States Surgical, North Haven, CT*	Safe	1.5, 3	83
Suture, Sofsilk, Needle removed *United States Surgical, North Haven, CT*	Safe	1.5, 3	83
Suture, Steel, Needle removed, 316L SS *United States Surgical, North Haven, CT*	Safe	1.5, 3	83
Suture, Steel Suture, Needle removed *Size 7 Metric, 316L SS Suture* *Covidien, www.covidien.com*	Conditional 6	3	
Suture, Surgilon, Needle removed, braided nylon *United States Surgical, North Haven, CT*	Safe	1.5, 3	83
Suture, Surgipro, Needle removed, polypropylene *United States Surgical, North Haven, CT*	Safe	1.5, 3	83

Object	Status	Field Strength (T)	Reference
Vascular Access Ports, Infusion Pumps, and Catheters			
A Port Implantable Access System, Titanium *Therex Corporation, Walpole, MA*	Safe	1.5	44
Access Implantable, Titanium, plastic *Celsa, Cedex, France*	Safe	1.5	44
ACCU-CHEK Spirit Insulin Pump *ACCU-CHEK, www.ACCU-CHEK.com*	Unsafe 1	1.5	
AccuRx Constant Flow Implantable Pump *Titanium, Silicone* *Advanced Neuromodulation Systems, Plano, TX*	Safe	1.5	
Acuvance Jelco, FEP Radiopaque *Intravenous (I.V.) catheter, Silicone* *Smiths Medical ASD, Inc., Southington, CT*	Conditional 6	3	
Acuvance Plus, PUR Radiopaque *Intravenous (I.V.) catheter, Silicone* *Smiths Medical ASD, Inc., Southington, CT*	Conditional 6	3	
Acuvance Plus-W, PUR Radiopaque *Intravenous (I.V.) catheter, Silicone* *Smiths Medical ASD, Inc., Southington, CT*	Conditional 6	3	
AdvantIV, PUR Radiopaque *Intravenous (I.V.) catheter, Silicone* *Smiths Medical ASD, Inc., Southington, CT*	Conditional 6	3	
Ambulatory Infusion System, CADD - 1 *Ambulatory Infusion Pump* *Smiths Medical, St. Paul, MN*	Unsafe 1	1.5	
Ambulatory Infusion System, CADD - Legacy 1 *Ambulatory Infusion Pump* *Smiths Medical, St. Paul, MN*	Unsafe 1	1.5	
Ambulatory Infusion System, CADD - Legacy PCA *Ambulatory Infusion Pump* *Smiths Medical, St. Paul, MN*	Unsafe 1	1.5	
Ambulatory Infusion System, CADD - Legacy PLUS *Ambulatory Infusion Pump* *Smiths Medical, St. Paul, MN*	Unsafe 1	1.5	
Ambulatory Infusion System, CADD - Legacy *Ambulatory Infusion Pump* *Smiths Medical, St. Paul, MN*	Unsafe 1	1.5	
Ambulatory Infusion System, CADD - Micro *Ambulatory Infusion Pump* *Smiths Medical, St. Paul, MN*	Unsafe 1	1.5	
Ambulatory Infusion System, CADD - MS 3 *Ambulatory Infusion Pump* *Smiths Medical, St. Paul, MN*	Unsafe 1	1.5	
Ambulatory Infusion System, CADD - PCA *Ambulatory Infusion Pump* *Smiths Medical, St. Paul, MN*	Unsafe 1	1.5	
Ambulatory Infusion System, CADD - PLUS *Ambulatory Infusion Pump* *Smiths Medical, St. Paul, MN*	Unsafe 1	1.5	

Object	Status	Field Strength (T)	Reference
Ambulatory Infusion System, CADD - Prizm PCS II *Ambulatory Infusion Pump* *Smiths Medical, St. Paul, MN*	Unsafe 1	1.5	
Ambulatory Infusion System, CADD - Prizm PCS *Ambulatory Infusion Pump* *Smiths Medical, St. Paul, MN*	Unsafe 1	1.5	
Ambulatory Infusion System, CADD - Prizm VIP *Ambulatory Infusion Pump* *Smiths Medical, St. Paul, MN*	Unsafe 1	1.5	
Ambulatory Infusion System, CADD - Solis *Ambulatory Infusion Pump* *Smiths Medical, St. Paul, MN*	Unsafe 1	1.5	
Ambulatory Infusion System, CADD - TPN *Ambulatory Infusion Pump* *Smiths Medical, St. Paul, MN*	Unsafe 1	1.5	
ambIT Epidural Pump *external pump, Model 22028* *Medtronic, Inc. and Sorensen Medical, Inc.*	Unsafe 1	1.5	
Broviac catheter single lumen *Silicone, barium sulfate* *Bard Access Systems, Salt Lake City, UT*	Safe	1.5	
Button Vascular Access Port *polysulfone polymer, Silicone* *Infusaid Inc., Norwood, MA and Angiodynamics, Inc.*	Safe	1.5	45
CathLink LP, Titanium *Bard Access Systems, www.bardaccess.com*	Safe	1.5	44
CathLink SP, Titanium *Bard Access Systems, www.bardaccess.com*	Safe	1.5	45
Cathlon FEP Intravenous (I.V.) Catheter *Silicone* *Smiths Medical ASD, Inc., Southington, CT*	Conditional 6	3	
Celsite Port and Catheter, Titanium *B. Braun Medical* *Bethlehem, PA*	Safe	1.5	45
Celsite Access Port, Vascular Access Port *B. Braun, www.bbraunusa.com*	Conditional 5	1.5, 3	
Central Venous Port, Vascular Access Port *Covidien, www.covidien.com*	Conditional 6	1.5, 3	
Certainty Port, Implantable Vascular Access Port *MedComp* *Harleysville, PA*	Conditional 6	3	
Chemosite Port I, Low Profile, Single Lumen Vascular Access Port *Covidien, www.covidien.com*	Conditional 6	3	
CODMAN 3000 Implantable Infusion Pump *Codman, www.depuy.com*	Conditional 5	3	
Cozmo Pump, Insulin Pump *Deltec Diabetes Division, St. Paul, MN*	Unsafe	1.5	
Dana Diabecare IISG Insulin Pump *Sooil, www.sooilusa.com*	Unsafe 1	1.5	
Deltec 3000, Large Volume Infusion Pump *Smiths Medical, St. Paul, MN*	Unsafe 1	1.5	

Object	Status	Field Strength (T)	Reference
Deltec Micro 3100, Large Volume Infusion Pump *Smiths Medical, St. Paul, MN*	Unsafe 1	1.5	
Dome Port, Vascular Access Port, Titanium *Davol Inc., Subsidiary of C.R. Bard, Inc.*	Safe	1.5	
Dual MacroPort, polysulfone polymer, Silicone *Infusaid Inc., Norwood, MA and Angiodynamics, Inc.*	Safe	1.5	44
Dual MicroPort, polysulfone polymer, Silicone *Infusaid Inc., Norwood, MA and Angiodynamics, Inc.*	Safe	1.5	44
Dual-Lumen PORT-A-CATH *Portal and Wing-Lock Connector, Vascular Access Port* *Smiths Medical MD, Inc., St. Paul, MN*	Safe	1.5	44
DuraCath Intraspinal Catheter *316L SS, Silicone* *Advanced Neuromodulation Systems, Plano, TX*	Conditional 6	3	
GRIPPER PLUS Needle, SS needle, 19 gauge, 1 ¼ inch *Smiths Medical MD, Inc., St. Paul, MN*	Conditional 5	3	
GRIPPER PLUS Safety Needle *Deltec, Inc., www.smiths-medical.com/brands/deltec*	Conditional 5	3	
GRIPPER PLUS Safety Needle *Smiths Medical MD, Inc., St. Paul, MN*	Safe	3	
Groshong Catheter	Conditional 1	1.5	
Groshong Catheter, dual lumen, 9.5 Fr. *Silicone, barium sulfate, tungsten* *Bard Access Systems, www.bardaccess.com*	Safe	1.5	45
Groshong Catheter, single lumen, 8 Fr. *Silicone, barium sulfate, tungsten* *Bard Access Systems, www.bardaccess.com*	Safe	1.5	45
Healthport ETI Spinal, Model ETI *Implantable Intracorporeal Access System* *Plan 1 Health s.r.l.*	Conditional 6	3	
Healthport PLP, Access Port *Plan 1 Health s.r.l.*	Conditional 6	3	
Healthport Focus Access Port *Plan 1 Health s.r.l.*	Conditional 6	3	
HeRO Vascular Access Device *HeRO Graft Component, HeRO Outflow Catheter Component* *GRAFTcath, Inc., Eden Prairie, MN*	Conditional 6	3	
Hickman Catheter, dual lumen, 10.0 Fr. *Silicone, barium sulfate* *Bard Access Systems, www.bardaccess.com*	Safe	1.5	45
Hickman Catheter, single lumen, 3.0 Fr. *Bard Access Systems, www.bardaccess.com*	Safe	1.5	45
Hickman Port, Pediatric, Vascular Access Port, Titanium *Davol, Inc., Subsidiary of C.R. Bard, Inc., Salt Lake City, UT*	Safe	1.5	44
Hickman Port, Vascular Access Port, 316L SS *Davol Inc., Subsidiary of C.R. Bard, Inc., Salt Lake City, UT*	Conditional 1	1.5	44
Hickman subcutaneous port, Vascular Access Port *SS, Titanium, plastic* *Davol, Inc., Subsidiary of C.R. Bard, Inc.*	Safe	1.5	45

Object	Status	Field Strength (T)	Reference
Hickman subcutaneous port, Vascular Access Port *venous catheter, Titanium* *Davol Inc., Subsidiary of C.R. Bard, Inc., Salt Lake City, UT*	Safe	1.5	44
HMP-Port, Vascular Access Port, plastic *Horizon Medical Products, Atlanta, GA and Angiodynamics, Inc.*	Safe	1.5	44
Implantable Infusion Pump, Model 3000-16 *Titanium* *Codman, www.depuy.com*	Safe	1.5, 3	83
Implantable Infusion Pump, Model 3000-30 *Titanium* *Codman, www.depuy.com*	Safe	1.5, 3	83
Implantable Infusion Pump, Model 3000-50 *Titanium* *Codman, www.depuy.com*	Safe	1.5, 3	83
Implantofix II, Vascular Access Port *polysulfone* *Burron Medical Inc., Bethlehem, PA*	Safe	1.5	44
Infusaid, Model 400, Vascular Access Port, Titanium *Infusaid Inc., Norwood, MA*	Safe	1.5	44
Infusaid, Model 600, Vascular Access Port, Titanium *Infusaid Inc., Norwood, MA*	Safe	1.5	44
Infuse-A-Kit, plastic *Infusaid, Norwood, MA and Angiodynamics, Inc.*	Safe	1.5	44
Jelco 2 FEP Radiopaque Intravenous (I.V.) catheter *Silicone* *Smiths Medical ASD, Inc., Southington, CT*	Conditional 6	3	
Jelco FEP Intravenous (I.V.) catheter, Silicone *Smiths Medical ASD, Inc., Southington, CT*	Conditional 6	3	
Jelco-W FEP Radiopaque *Intravenous (I.V.) catheter, Silicone* *Smiths Medical ASD, Inc., Southington, CT*	Conditional 6	3	
Jet Port Plus Vascular Access Port *Clinical Plastic Products SA* *La Chaux-de-Fonds, Switzerland*	Conditional 6	3	
LifePort Plastic Port(s), Vascular Access Port *Angiodynamics, Inc., www.Angiodynamics.com*	Safe	1.5, 3	
LifePort Titanium Port(s), Vascular Access Port *Angiodynamics, Inc., www.Angiodynamics.com*	Conditional 6	3	
LifePort Vascular Access Port *AngioDynamics, www.angiodynamics.com*	Conditional 6	3	
LifePort Vascular Access System *attachable catheter and bayonet lock ring, plastic* *Strato Medical Group, Beverly, MA and Angiodynamics, Inc.*	Safe	1.5	44
LifePort Vascular Access System *attachable catheter, plastic* *Strato Medical Group, Beverly, MA and Angiodynamics, Inc.*	Safe	1.5	44
LifePort Vortex LVTX 5213 *Dual Titanium Vascular Access Port* *Angiodynamics, Inc.*	Conditional 6	3	
Lifeport, Model 1013 *Vascular Access Port, Titanium* *Strato Medical Corp., Beverly, MA and Angiodynamics, Inc.*	Safe	1.5	44

Object	Status	Field Strength (T)	Reference
LifePort, Model 6013 *Vascular Access Port, Delrin* *Strato Medical Corporation, Beverly, MA and Angiodynamics, Inc.*	Safe	1.5	44
Low Profile MRI Port *Vascular Access Port, Delrin* *Davol, Inc., Subsidiary of C.R. Bard, Inc.*	Safe	1.5	44
Low Profile MRI Port *Vascular Access Port, Titanium* *Davol, Inc. Subsidiary of C.R. Bard, Inc., Salt Lake City, UT*	Safe	1.5	45
Macroport Vascular Access Port *polysulfone, Titanium* *Infusaid Inc., Norwood, MA and Angiodynamics, Inc.*	Safe	1.5	
Mediport Vascular Access Port *Cormed*	Safe	1.5	
MedStream Programmable Infusion Pump *MedStream Programmable Infusion Pump* *Codman, www.DePuy.com*	Conditional 5	3	112
Medtronic MiniMed 2007 *Implantable Insulin Pump System* *Medtronic MiniMed, Northridge, CA*	Unsafe 1	1.5	
MicroPort Vascular Access Port *Infusaid Inc., Norwood, MA and Angiodynamics, Inc.*	Safe	1.5	44
MiniMed Paradigm REAL-Time Insulin Pump *Continuous Glucose Monitoring System* *522 and 722 Insulin Pumps* *Medtronic Minimed, Northridge, CA*	Unsafe 1	1.5	
MRI Hard Base Implanted Port *Vascular Access Port, plastic* *Davol, Inc., Salt Lake City, UT*	Safe	1.5	44
M.R.I. Implantable Port with Suture Plugs *Implantable Vascular Access Port* *Bard Access Systems, www.bardaccess.com*	Conditional 6	3	
M.R.I. isp Implanted PowerPort with Suture Rings *Implantable Vascular Access Port* *Bard Access Systems, www.bardaccess.com*	Conditional 6	3	
MRI Port Vascular Access Port *Delrin, Silicone* *Davol, Inc., Subsidiary of C.R. Bard, Inc.*	Safe	1.5	44
M.R.I. PowerPort Vue, Implantable Vascular Access Port *Bard Access Systems, www.bardaccess.com*	Conditional 6	3	
M.R.I. Vital Port Systems *Standard Size, Vascular Access Port* *Cook Medical, Inc., www.cookmedical.com*	Conditional 5	3	
Non-Coring (Huber) Needle *Medi-tech* *Boston Scientific, www.bostonscientific.com*	Safe	1.5, 3	83
Norport-AC Vascular Access Port *Titanium* *Norfolk Medical, www.norfolkmedical.com*	Safe	1.5	44
Norport-DL Vascular Access Port *316L SS* *Norfolk Medical, www.norfolkmedical.com*	Safe	1.5	44

Object	Status	Field Strength (T)	Reference
Norport-LS Vascular Access Port *316L SS* *Norfolk Medical, www.norfolkmedical.com*	Safe	1.5	44
Norport-LS Vascular Access Port *polysulfone* *Norfolk Medical, www.norfolkmedical.com*	Safe	1.5	44
Norport-LS Vascular Access Port *Titanium* *Norfolk Medical, www.norfolkmedical.com*	Safe	1.5	44
Norport-PT Vascular Access Port *Titanium* *Norfolk Medical, www.norfolkmedical.com*	Safe	1.5	44
NorPort Single Lumen Port System *Vascular Access Port* *Norfolk Medical, www.norfolkmedical.com*	Conditional 6	3	
Norport-SP Vascular Access Port *Norfolk Medical, www.norfolkmedical.com*	Safe	1.5	44
OmegaPort Access System *Vascular Access Port, Titanium, 316L SS* *Norfolk Medical, www.norfolkmedical.com*	Safe	1.5	44
OmegaPort-SR Access System *Vascular Access Port, Titanium, 316L SS* *Norfolk Medical, www.norfolkmedical.com*	Safe	1.5	44
OneTouch Ping Insulin Pump *Animas, www.animas.com*	Unsafe 1	1.5	
Open-ended Catheter, single lumen, 6 Fr. (ChronoFlex) *Davol, Inc., Subsidiary of C.R. Bard, Inc.*	Safe	1.5	45
Open-ended Catheter, single lumen, 8 Fr. (ChronoFlex) *Davol, Inc., Subsidiary of C.R. Bard, Inc.*	Safe	1.5	45
OptiPort Catheter, single lumen *Silicone* *Simms-Deltec, St. Paul, MN*	Safe	1.5	45
Optiva PUR Radiopaque *Intravenous (I.V.) catheter, Silicone* *Smiths Medical ASD, Inc., Southington, CT*	Conditional 6	3	
Optiva-W PUR Radiopaque *Intravenous (I.V.) catheter, Silicone* *Smiths Medical ASD, Inc., Southington, CT*	Conditional 6	3	
Optiva 2 PUR Radiopaque *Intravenous (I.V.) catheter, Silicone* *Smiths Medical ASD, Inc., Southington, CT*	Conditional 6	3	
P.A.S. PORT Elite with *PolyFlow Polyurethane Catheter* *Deltec, Inc., St. Paul, MN*	Safe	1.5, 3	83
Percutaneous Vascular Access System (PVAS) *DermaPort, Santa Clarita, CA*	Conditional 6	3	
PeriPort Vascular Access Port *polysulfone, Titanium* *Infusaid, Inc., Norwood, MA and Angiodynamics, Inc.*	Safe	1.5	44
Phantom Vascular Access Port *Norfolk Medical, www.norfolkmedical.com*	Safe	1.5	44

Object	Status	Field Strength (T)	Reference
Plastic Port Vascular Access Port *polysulfone, Titanium* *Cardial, Saint-Etienne, France*	Safe	1.5	44
POLYSITE Implantable Vascular Access Port *Perouse Medical, www.perousemedical.com*	Conditional 6	3	
PORT-A-CATH GRIPPER Needle *Deltec, Inc., St. Paul, MN*	Safe	1.5, 3	83
PORT-A-CATH I, Standard Portal with Ultra-Lock Connector *Vascular Access Port* *Smiths Medical MD, Inc., St. Paul, MN*	Conditional 6	3	
PORT-A-CATH II Dual-Lumen *Low Profile with PolyFlow, Polyurethane Catheter* *Deltec, Inc., St. Paul, MN*	Safe	1.5, 3	83
PORT-A-CATH II Dual-Lumen *with Silicone Catheter* *Deltec, Inc., St. Paul, MN*	Safe	1.5, 3	83
PORT-A-CATH II Single-Lumen *Low Profile with PolyFlow, Polyurethane Catheter* *Deltec, Inc., St. Paul, MN*	Safe	1.5, 3	83
PORT-A-CATH II Single-Lumen *with PolyFlow Polyurethane Catheter* *Deltec, Inc., St. Paul, MN*	Safe	1.5, 3	83
PORT-A-CATH II Low Profile Intraspinal Portal *Smiths Medical MD, Inc., St. Paul, MN*	Conditional 6	3	
PORT-A-CATH Needle *Deltec, Inc., St. Paul, MN*	Conditional 5	1.5, 3	83
PORT-A-CATH Titanium Dual Lumen Portal *Titanium* *Pharmacia Deltec, St. Paul, MN*	Safe	1.5	44
PORT-A-CATH Titanium Peritoneal Portal *Titanium* *Pharmacia Deltec, St. Paul, MN*	Safe	1.5	44
PORT-A-CATH Titanium *Venous Low Profile Portal, Titanium* *Pharmacia Deltec, St. Paul, MN*	Safe	1.5	44
PORT-A-CATH Titanium *Venous Portal, Titanium* *Pharmacia Deltec, St. Paul, MN*	Safe	1.5	44
PORT-A-CATH, P.S.A. Port Portal *Titanium* *Pharmacia Deltec, St. Paul, MN*	Safe	1.5	44
PORT-A-CATH *Epidural Portal and Cath-Shield Connector* *Vascular Access Port* *Smiths Medical MD, Inc., St. Paul, MN*	Conditional 6	3	
PORT-A-CATH *Metal Hub 90 degree Bent Needle* *Smiths Medical MD, Inc., St. Paul, MN*	Safe	3	
PORT-A-CATH *Metal Hub Straight Needle* *Smiths Medical MD, Inc., St. Paul, MN*	Safe	3	

Object	Status	Field Strength (T)	Reference
PORT-A-CATH *Peritoneal Portal with Ultra-Lock Connector* *Smiths Medical MD, Inc., St. Paul, MN*	Conditional 6	3	
PORT-A-CATH *Plastic Hub 90-degree Bent Needle* *Smiths Medical MD, Inc., St. Paul, MN*	Conditional 5	3	
PORT-A-CATH *Plastic Hub Straight Needle* *Smiths Medical MD, Inc., St. Paul, MN*	Conditional 5	3	
Power Dual Tita Port *Clinical Plastic Products SA, Switzerland*	Conditional 6	3	
PowerPort Duo MRI Port *ChronoFlex Catheter and Cathlock* *Vascular Access Port,* *Bard Access Systems, www.bardaccess.com*	Safe	1.5, 3	
PowerPort Implantable Port With Suture Plugs *Implantable Vascular Access Port* *Bard Access Systems, www.bardaccess.com*	Conditional 6	3	
PowerPort M.R.I., Titanium *Bard Access Systems, www.bardaccess.com*	Conditional 5	3	
PowerPort Vascular Access Port, Titanium *Bard Access Systems, www.bardaccess.com*	Conditional 5	3	
PowerPort isp Implanted Port *Bard Access Systems, www.bardaccess.com*	Conditional 5	3	
PowerPort isp M.R.I. Implanted Port *Bard Access Systems, www.bardaccess.com*	Conditional 5	3	
PowerPort isp Implanted Port with Suture Plugs *Bard Access System, www.bardaccess.com*	Conditional 6	3	
PowerPort M.R.I. Implanted Port *Bard Access Systems, www.bardaccess.com*	Conditional 5	3	
PowerPort Slim Implantable Port with Suture Plugs *Implantable Vascular Access Port* *Bard Access Systems, www.bardaccess.com*	Conditional 6	3	
PowerPort Vue Titanium *Implantable Vascular Access Port* *Bard Access Systems, www.bardaccess.com*	Conditional 6	3	
ProFuse Dignity Infusion Port *Medcomp, Harleysville, PA*	Conditional 6	3	
ProtectIV FEP Radiopaque Intravenous (I.V.) catheter, Silicone *Smiths Medical ASD, Inc., Southington, CT*	Conditional 6	3	
ProtectIV Acuvance 2 PUR Radiopaque *Intravenous (I.V.) catheter, Silicone* *Smiths Medical ASD, Inc., Southington, CT*	Conditional 6	3	
ProtectIV Plus PUR Radiopaque *Intravenous (I.V.) catheter* *Smiths Medical ASD, Inc., Southington, CT*	Conditional 6	3	
ProtectIV Plus-W PUR Radiopaque *Intravenous (I.V.) catheter* *Smiths Medical ASD, Inc., Southington, CT*	Conditional 6	3	
ProtectIV-W FEP Radiopaque *Intravenous (I.V.) catheter* *Smiths Medical ASD, Inc., Southington, CT*	Conditional 6	3	

Object	Status	Field Strength (T)	Reference
Purple JPP-HP Vascular Access Port *Clinical Plastic Products SA, La Chaux-de-Fonds, Switzerland*	Conditional 6	3	
Purple TJL-HP Vascular Access Port *Clinical Plastic Products SA, La Chaux-de-Fonds, Switzerland*	Conditional 6	3	
Q-Port Vascular Access Port, 316L SS *Quinton Instrument Co., Seattle, WA*	Conditional 1	1.5	44
Realize Injection Port, Access Port *Ethicon Endosurgery, Inc., www.ees.com*	Conditional 5	3	
Rhapsody Vascular Access System *GrantAdler Corporation, Naperville, IL*	Conditional 6	3	
R-Port Premier Vascular Access Port *Silicone, plastic, SS* *Boston Scientific, www.bostonscientific.com*	Safe	1.5, 3	83
S.E.A. Vascular Access Port, Titanium *Harbor Medical Devices, Inc., Boston, MA*	Safe	1.5	44
Smart Port CT-Injectable Port *AngioDynamics, www.angiodynamics.com*	Conditional 6	3	
Smart Port(s), Vascular Access Port *Angiodynamics, Inc., www.Angiodynamics.com*	Conditional 6	3	
Snap-Lock Vascular Access Port *Titanium, polysulfone polymer, Silicone* *Infusaid Inc., Norwood, MA and Angiodynamics, Inc.*	Safe	1.5	44
Solo MicroPump Insulin Pump *Medingo US, Inc., www.Medingo.com*	Unsafe 1	1.5	
Standard M.R.I. Single Chamber System *Polysulfone Port, Titanium Connector, Silicone Catheter* *Cook Medical, www.cookmedical.com*	Conditional 6	3	
Standard Titanium Dual Chamber System *Titanium Port, Titanium Connector, Silicone Catheter* *Cook Medical, www.cookmedical.com*	Conditional 6	3	
Stealth Invisiport Vascular Access Port *Medical Murray, Inc., North Barrington, IL*	Conditional 6	3	
Synchromed, Model 8500-1 *Titanium, thermoplastic, Silicone* *Medtronic, Inc., www.Medtronic.com*	Conditional 5	1.5, 3	44
Tesio Catheter, SS, polyurethane *Medcomp, Harleysville, PA*	Conditional 6	3	
Tita Jet Light Arterial II Vascular Access Port *Clinical Plastic Products SA, La Chaux-de-Fonds, Switzerland*	Conditional 6	3	
Tita Jet Light Vascular Access Port *Clinical Plastic Products SA, La Chaux-de-Fonds, Switzerland*	Conditional 6	3	
TitanPort Titanium Vascular Access Port *Norfolk Medical, www.norfolkmedical.com and* *Angiodynamics, Inc.*	Safe	1.5	
TitanPort Vascular Access Port *AngioDynamics, www.angiodynamics.com*	Conditional 6	3	
T-Port Vascular Access Port *Clinical Plastic Products SA, La Chaux-de-Fonds, Switzerland*	Conditional 6	3	
Triple Lumen *Arrow International, www.arrowintl.com*	Safe	1.5	

Object	Status	Field Strength (T)	Reference
Triumph-1 Vascular Access Port, Titanium *AngioDynamics, www.angiodynamics.com*	Conditional 6	3	
Triumph-1 Plastic Port(s), Vascular Access Port *Angiodynamics, Inc., www.Angiodynamics.com*	Safe	1.5, 3	
Vascular Access Catheter With Repair Kit	Safe	1.5	
Vasport Vascular Access Port *Titanium, fluoropolymer* *Gish Biomedical, Inc., Santa Ana, CA*	Safe	1.5	44
Vaxcel Implantable Access System *Plastic Low Profile Port* *Boston Scientific, www.bostonscientific.com*	Safe	3	
Vaxcel Implantable Vascular Access System *with PASV Valve Technology, Titanium Mini Port With PASV valve* *Boston Scientific, Natick, MA*	Safe	3	
Vaxcel Implantable Vascular Access System *with PASV Valve Technology,* *Titanium Standard Port With PASV valve* *Boston Scientific, Natick, MA*	Safe	3	
Vaxess, Titanium Mini-Port with Silicone catheter *Vascular Access Port, Titanium, Silicone* *Boston Scientific, www.bostonscientific.com*	Safe	1.5, 3	83
Vaxess, Titanium, Vascular Access Port *Titanium, polyurethane* *Boston Scientific, www.bostonscientific.com*	Safe	1.5, 3	83
Vaxess Vascular Access Port *19 gauge x 1/2", 90 degree hub* *Medi-tech, Boston Scientific, www.bostonscientific.com*	Safe	1.5, 3	83
Vaxess Vascular Access Port *plastic, polyurethane, Medi-tech* *Boston Scientific, www.bostonscientific.com*	Safe	1.5, 3	83
Vital-Port, Dual, Vascular Access Port *polysulfone, Titanium* *Cook Corp., Leechburg, PA*	Safe	1.5	45
Vital-Port System, Dual Chamber, Titanium Petite *Vascular Access Port* *Cook Medical, Inc., www.cookmedical.com*	Conditional 5	3	
Vital-Port System, Dual Chamber, Titanium Standard *Vascular Access Port* *Cook Medical, Inc., www.cookmedical.com*	Conditional 5	3	
Vital-Port System, MRI Petite *Vascular Access Port* *Cook Medical, Inc., www.cookmedical.com*	Conditional 5	3	
Vital-Port System, MRI Standard *Vascular Access Port* *Cook Medical, Inc., www.cookmedical.com*	Conditional 5	3	
Vital-Port System, Titanium Mini *Vascular Access Port* *Cook Medical, Inc., www.cookmedical.com*	Conditional 5	3	
Vital-Port System, Titanium Petite *Vascular Access Port* *Cook Medical, Inc., www.cookmedical.com*	Conditional 5	3	

Object	Status	Field Strength (T)	Reference
Vital-Port System, Titanium Petite Standard *Vascular Access Port* *Cook Medical, Inc., www.cookmedical.com*	Conditional 5	3	
Vital-Port System *Titanium for Peripheral Placement Mini, Vascular Access Port* *Cook Medical, Inc., www.cookmedical.com*	Conditional 5	3	
Vital-Port Vascular Access Port *Cook Corp., Leechburg, PA*	Safe	1.5	45
Vortex LP Plastic Port(s), Vascular Access Port *Angiodynamics, Inc., www.Angiodynamics.com*	Safe	1.5, 3	
Vortex LP Titanium Port(s), Vascular Access Port *Angiodynamics, Inc., www.Angiodynamics.com*	Conditional 6	3	
Vortex MP Port(s), Vascular Access Port *Angiodynamics, Inc., www.Angiodynamics.com*	Conditional 6	3	
Vortex TR Plastic Port(s) Vascular Access Port *Angiodynamics, Inc., www.Angiodynamics.com*	Safe	1.5, 3	
Vortex TR Titanium Port(s) Vascular Access Port *Angiodynamics, Inc., www.Angiodynamics.com*	Conditional 6	3	
Vortex VX Port(s) Vascular Access Port *Angiodynamics, Inc., www.Angiodynamics.com*	Conditional 6	3	
Vortex Port, Models LP, MP, TR, VX *Vascular Access Port* *AngioDynamics, www.angiodynamics.com*	Conditional 6	3	

THE LIST

REFERENCES

1. New PFJ, et al. Potential hazards and artifacts of ferromagnetic and nonferromagnetic surgical and dental materials and devices in nuclear magnetic resonance imaging. Radiology 1983;147:139-148.

2. Becker RL, Norfray JF, Teitelbaum GP, et al. MR imaging in patients with intracranial aneurysm clips. Am J Roentgenol 1988;9:885-889.

3. Shellock FG, Crues JV. High-field strength MR imaging and metallic biomedical implants: an ex vivo evaluation of deflection forces. Am J Roentgenol 1988;151:389-392.

4. Brown MA, Carden JA, Coleman RE, et al. Magnetic field effects on surgical ligation clips. Magn Reson Imaging 1987;5:443-453.

5. Dujovny M, et al. Aneurysm clip motion during magnetic resonance imaging: in vivo experimental study with metallurgical factor analysis. Neurosurgery 1985;17:543-548.

6. Barrafato D, Henkelman RM. Magnetic resonance imaging and surgical clips. Can J Surg 1984;27:509-512.

7. Moscatel M, Shellock FG, Morisoli S. Biopsy needles and devices: assessment of ferromagnetism and artifacts during exposure to a 1.5 Tesla MR system. J Magn Reson Imaging 1995;5:369-372.

8. Shellock FG, Shellock VJ. Additional information pertaining to the MR-compatibility of biopsy needles and devices. J Magn Reson Imaging 1996;6:441.

9. Hathout G, Lufkin RB, Jabour B, et al. MR-guided aspiration cytology in the head and neck at high field strength. J Magn Reson Imaging 1992;2:93-94.

10. Fagan LL, Shellock FG, Brenner RJ, Rothman B. Ex vivo evaluation of ferromagnetism, heating, and artifacts of breast tissue expanders exposed to a 1.5 T MR system. J Magn Reson Imaging 1995;5:614-616.

11. Teitelbaum GP, et al. Ferromagnetism and MR imaging: safety of carotid vascular clamps. Am J Neuroradiol 1990;11:267-272.

12. Gegauff A, Laurell KA, Thavendrarajah A, et al. A potential MRI hazard: forces on dental magnet keepers. J Oral Rehabil 1990;17:403-410.

13. Shellock FG. Ex vivo assessment of deflection forces and artifacts associated with high-field strength MRI of "mini-magnet" dental prostheses. Magn Reson Imaging 1989;7 (Suppl 1):38.

14. Shellock FG, Slimp G. Halo vest for cervical spine fixation during MR imaging. Am J Roentgenol 1990;154:631-632.

15. Clayman DA, et al. Compatibility of cervical spine braces with MR imaging. A study of nine nonferrous devices. Am J Neuroradiol 1990;11:385-390.

16. Shellock FG. MR imaging and cervical fixation devices: assessment of ferromagnetism, heating, and artifacts. Magn Reson Imaging 1996;14:1093-1098.

17. Soulen RL, Budinger TF, Higgins CB. Magnetic resonance imaging of prosthetic heart valves. Radiology 1985;154:705-707.

18. Shellock FG, Morisoli SM. Ex vivo evaluation of ferromagnetism, heating, and artifacts for heart valve prostheses exposed to a 1.5 Tesla MR system. J Magn Reson Imaging 1994;4:756-758.

19. Hassler M, Le Bas JF, Wolf JE, et al. Effects of magnetic fields used in MRI on 15 prosthetic heart valves. J Radiol 1986;67:661-666.

20. Frank H, Buxbaum P, Huber L, et al. In vitro behavior of mechanical heart valves in 1.5 T superconducting magnet. Eur J Radiol 1992;2:555-558.

21. Teitelbaum GP, et al. MR imaging artifacts, ferromagnetism, and magnetic torque of intravascular filters, stents, and coils. Radiology 1988;166:657-664.

22. Marshall MW, et al. Ferromagnetism and magnetic resonance artifacts of platinum embolization microcoils. Cardiovasc Intervent Radiol 1991;14:163-166.

23. Watanabe AT, Teitelbaum GP, Gomes AS, et al. MR imaging of the bird's nest filter. Radiology 1990;177:578-579.

24. Leibman CE, Messersmith RN, Levin DN, et al. MR imaging of inferior vena caval filter: safety and artifacts. Am J Roentgenol 1988;150:1174-1176.

25. Shellock FG, Detrick MS, Brant-Zawadski M. MR-compatibility of the Guglielmi detachable coils. Radiology 1997;203:568-570.

26. Kiproff PM, et al. Magnetic resonance characteristics of the LGM vena cava filter: technical note. Cardiovasc Intervent Radiol 1991;14:254-255.

27. Teitelbaum GP, Raney M, Carvlin MJ, et al. Evaluation of ferromagnetism and magnetic resonance imaging artifacts of the Strecker tantalum vascular stent. Cardiovasc Intervent Radiol 1989;12:125-127.

28. Girard MJ, et al. Wallstent metallic biliary endoprosthesis: MR imaging characteristics. Radiology 1992;184:874-876.

29. Shellock FG, Myers SM, Schatz CJ. Ex vivo evaluation of ferromagnetism determined for metallic scleral "buckles" exposed to a 1.5 T MR scanner. Radiology 1992;185:288-289.

30. de Keizer RJ, Te Strake L. Intraocular lens implants (pseudophakoi) and steelwire sutures: a contraindication for MRI? Doc Ophthalmol 1984;61:281-284.

31. Albert DW, Olson KR, Parel JM, et al. Magnetic resonance imaging and retinal tacks. Arch Ophthalmol 1990;108:320-321.

32. Joondeph BC, Peyman GA, Mafee MF, et al. Magnetic resonance imaging and retinal tacks [Letter]. Arch Ophthalmol 1987;105:1479-1480.

33. Lyons CJ, Betz RR, Mesgarzadeh M, et al. The effect of magnetic resonance imaging on metal spine implants. Spine 1989;14:670-672.

34. Shellock FG, Mink JH, Curtin S, et al. MRI and orthopedic implants used for anterior cruciate ligament reconstruction: assessment of ferromagnetism and artifacts. J Magn Reson Imaging 1992;2:225-228.

35. Shellock FG, Schatz CJ. High-field strength MR imaging and metallic otologic implants. Am J Neuroradiol 1991;12:279-281.

36. Nogueira M, Shellock FG. Otologic bioimplants: ex vivo assessment of ferromagnetism and artifacts at 1.5 Tesla. Am J Roentgenol 1995;163:1472-1473.

37. Mattucci KF, et al. The effect of nuclear magnetic resonance imaging on metallic middle ear prostheses. Otolaryngol Head Neck Surg 1986;94:441-443.

38. Applebaum EL, Valvassori GE. Further studies on the effects of magnetic resonance fields on middle ear implants. Ann Otol Rhinol Laryngol 1990;99:801-804.

39. White DW. Interaction between magnetic fields and metallic ossicular prostheses. Am J Otol 1987;8:290-292.

40. Leon JA, Gabriele OF. Middle ear prosthesis: significance in magnetic resonance imaging. Magn Reson Imaging 1987;5:405-406.

41. Shellock FG, Morisoli SM. Ex vivo evaluation of ferromagnetism and artifacts for cardiac occluders exposed to a 1.5 Tesla MR system. J Magn Reson Imaging 1994;4:213-215.

42. Teitelbaum GP, Yee CA, Van Horn DD, et al. Metallic ballistic fragments: MR imaging safety and artifacts. Radiology 1990;175:855-859.

43. Shellock FG, Crues JV, Sacks SA. High-field magnetic resonance imaging of penile prostheses: in vitro evaluation of deflection forces and imaging artifacts [Abstract]. In: Book of Abstracts, Society of Magnetic Resonance in Medicine. Berkeley, CA, Society of Magnetic Resonance in Medicine 1987;3:915.

44. Shellock FG, Nogueira M, Morisoli S. MR imaging and vascular access ports: ex vivo evaluation of ferromagnetism, heating, and artifacts at 1.5 T. J Magn Reson Imaging 1995;4:481-484.

45. Shellock FG, Shellock VJ. Vascular access ports and catheters tested for ferromagnetism, heating, and artifacts associated with MR imaging. Magn Reson Imaging 1996;14:443-447.

46. Kanal E, Shaibani A. Firearm safety in the MR imaging environment. Radiology 1994;193:875-876.

47. Hess T, Stepanow B, Knopp MV. Safety of intrauterine contraceptive devices during MR imaging. Eur Radiol 1996;6:66-68.

48. Shellock FG, Shellock VJ. Evaluation of MR compatibility of 38 bioimplants and devices. Radiology 1995;197:174.

49. Shellock FG, Shellock VJ. Ceramic surgical instruments: ex vivo evaluation of compatibility with MR imaging. J Magn Reson Imaging 1996;6:954-956.

50. Shellock FG, Shellock VJ. Evaluation of cranial flap fixation clamps for compatibility with MR imaging. Radiology 1998;822-825.

51. Lufkin R, Jordan S, Lylcyk M. MR imaging with topographic EEG electrodes in place. Am J Neuroradiol 1988;9:953-954.

52. Marra S, et al. Effect of magnetic resonance imaging on implantable eyelid weights. Ann Otol Rhinol Laryngol 1995;104:448-452.

53. Zhang J, et al. Temperature changes in nickel-chromium intracranial depth electrodes during MR scanning. Am J Neuroradiol 1993;14:497-500.

54. Mark AS, Hricak H. Intrauterine contraceptive devices: MR imaging. Radiology 1987;162:311-314.

55. Go KG, et al. Interaction of metallic neurosurgical implants with magnetic resonance imaging at 1.5 Tesla as a cause of image distortion and of hazardous movement of the implant. Clin Neurosurg 1989;91:109-115.

56. Fransen P, Dooms G, Thauvoy. Safety of the adjustable pressure ventricular valve in magnetic resonance imaging: problems and solutions. Neuroradiology 1992;34:508-509.

57. ECRI, Health devices alert. A new MRI complication? May 27, 1988.

58. To SYC, Lufkin RB, Chiu L. MR-compatible winged infusion set. Comput Med Imaging Graph 1989;13:469-472.

59. Shellock FG. MR-compatibility of an endoscope designed for use in interventional MRI procedures. Am J Roentgenol 1998;71:1297-1300.

60. Shellock FG, Shellock VJ. Cardiovascular catheters and accessories: Ex vivo testing of ferromagnetism, heating, and artifacts associated with MRI. J Magn Reson Imaging 1998;8:1338-1342.

61. Shellock FG, Shellock VJ. Metallic marking clips used after stereotactic breast biopsy: ex vivo testing of ferromagnetism, heating, and artifacts associated with MRI. Am J Roentgenol 1999;172:1417-1419.

62. Shellock FG. MRI safety of instruments designed for interventional MRI: assessment of ferromagnetism, heating, and artifacts. Workshop on New Insights into Safety and Compatibility Issues Affecting In Vivo MR, Syllabus 1998; pp. 39.

63. Shellock FG, et al. Implantable spinal fusion stimulator: assessment of MRI safety. J Magn Reson Imaging 2000;12:214-223.

64. Shellock FG, Shellock VJ. Stents: Evaluation of MRI safety. Am J Roentgenol 1999;173:543-546.

65. Teissl C, et al. Cochlear implants: in vitro investigation of electromagnetic interference at MR imaging-compatibility and safety aspects. Radiology 1998;208:700-708.

66. Teissl C, et al. Magnetic resonance imaging and cochlear implants: compatibility and safety aspects. J Magn Reson Imaging 1999;9:26-38.

67. Ortler M, Kostron H, Felber S. Transcutaneous pressure-adjustable valves and magnetic resonance imaging: an ex vivo examination of the Codman-Medos programmable valve and the Sophy adjustable pressure valve. Neurosurgery 1997;40:1050-1057.

68. Shellock FG, Shellock VJ. MR-compatibility evaluation of the Spetzler titanium aneurysm clip. Radiology 1998;206:838-841.

69. Jost C, Kuman V. Are current cardiovascular stents MRI safe? J Invasive Cardiol 1998;10:477-479.

70. Shellock FG, Shellock VJ. MRI Safety of cardiovascular implants: evaluation of ferromagnetism, heating, and artifacts. Radiology 2000;214:P19H.

71. Weishaupt D, et al. Ligating clips for three-dimensional MR angiography at 1.5 T: In vitro evaluation. Radiology 2000;214:902-907.

72. Hug J, et al. Coronary arterial stents: safety and artifacts during MR imaging. Radiology 2000;216:781-787.

73. Taal BG, Muller SH, Boot H, Koop W. Potential risks and artifacts of magnetic resonance imaging of self-expandable esophageal stents. Gastrointestinal Endoscopy 1997;46:424-429.

74. Shellock FG. Metallic surgical instruments for interventional MRI procedures: evaluation of MR safety. J Magn Reson Imaging 2001;13:152-157.

75. Edwards, M-B, Taylor KM, Shellock FG. Prosthetic heart valves: evaluation of magnetic field interactions, heating, and artifacts at 1.5 Tesla. J Magn Reson Imaging 2000;12:363-369.

76. Shellock FG. New metallic implant used for permanent female contraception: evaluation of MR safety. Am J Roentgenol 2002;178:1513-1516.

77. Shellock FG. Prosthetic heart valves and annuloplasty rings: assessment of magnetic field interactions, heating, and artifacts at 1.5-Tesla. Journal of Cardiovascular Magnetic Resonance. 2001;3:159-169.

78. Shellock FG. Metallic neurosurgical implants: evaluation of magnetic field interactions, heating, and artifacts at 1.5 Tesla. J Magn Reson Imaging 2001;14:295-299.

79. Rezai AR, Finelli D, Ruggieri P, Tkach J, Nyenhuis JA, Shellock FG. Neurostimulators: Potential for excessive heating of deep brain stimulation electrodes during MR imaging. J Magn Reson Imaging 2001;14:488-489.

80. Finelli DA, Rezai AR, Ruggieri P, Tkach J, Nyenhuis J, Hridlicka G, Sharan A, Stypulkowski PH, Shellock FG. MR-related heating of deep brain stimulation electrodes: an *in vitro* study of clinical imaging sequences. Am J Neuroradiol 2002;23:1795-1802.

622 References

81. Greatbatch W, Miller V, Shellock FG. Magnetic resonance safety testing of a newly-developed, fiber-optic cardiac pacing lead. J Magn Reson 2002;16:97-103.

82. Shellock FG, et al. Aneurysm clips: evaluation of magnetic field interactions and translational attraction using "long-bore" and "short-bore" 3.0-Tesla MR systems. Am J Neuroradiol 2003;24:463-471.

83. Shellock FG. Biomedical implants and devices: assessment of magnetic field interactions with a 3.0-Tesla MR system. J Magn Reson Imaging 2002;16:721-732.

84. Medtronic Heart Valves, Medtronic, Inc., Minneapolis, MN, Permission to publish 3-Tesla MR testing information for Medtronic Heart Valves provided by Kathryn M. Bayer, Senior Technical Consultant, Medtronic Heart Valves, Technical Service, 1-800-328-2518, extension -42861 or 763-514-2861.

85. Shellock FG, Tkach JA, Ruggieri PM, Masaryk TJ. Cardiac pacemakers, ICDs, and loop recorder: Evaluation of translational attraction using conventional ("long-bore") and "short-bore" 1.5- and 3.0-Tesla MR systems. Journal of Cardiovascular Magnetic Resonance 2003;5:387-397.

86. Product Information, Style 133 Family of Breast Tissue Expanders with Magna-Site Injection Sites, McGhan Medical/INAMED Aesthetics, Santa Barbara, CA.

87. Shellock FG, Gounis M, Wakhloo A, Detachable coil for cerebral aneurysms: *In vitro* evaluation of magnet field interactions, heating, and artifacts at 3-Tesla. American Journal of Neuroradiology 2005;26:363-366.

88. Shellock FG. Forder J. Drug eluting coronary stent: *In vitro* evaluation of magnet resonance safety at 3-Tesla. Journal of Cardiovascular Magnetic Resonance 2005;7:415-419.

89. Shellock FG, et al. Implantable microstimulator: magnetic resonance safety at 1.5-Tesla. Investigative Radiology 2004;39:591-594.

90. Shellock FG. MR safety and the Reveal Insertable Loop Recorder. Signals, No. 49, Issue 3, pp. 8, 2004

91. Reveal Plus Insertable Loop Recorder, http://www.medtronic.com/ physician/reveal/mri.html, Medtronic, Inc., Minneapolis, MN.

92. Kinetra Dual Program Neurostimulator for Deep Brain Simulation, 7428 (Medtronic, Inc.), Kinetra MRI labeling. www.Medtronic.com

93. RF BION Microstimulator, Alfred E. Mann Foundation, Valencia, CA; http://www.aemf.org and Advanced Bionics Corporation, Sylmar, CA; http://www.advancedbionics.com/

94. Codman, a Johnson and Johnson Company, Raynham, MA; Cerebrospinal Fluid Shunt Valves and Accessories, http://www.codmanjnj.com/ CSFshunting.asp

95. Codman, a Johnson and Johnson Company, Raynham, MA; Cerebrospinal Fluid Shunt Valves and Accessories, http://www.codmanjnj.com/PDFs/Prog_ProcedureGuide.pdf

96. Medtronic Neurosurgery, Goleta, CA; Cerebrospinal Fluid Shunt Valves and Accessories, http://www.medtronic.com/neurosurgery/shunts.html

97. Sophysa USA, Inc., Costa Mesa, CA; Cerebrospinal Fluid Shunt Valves and Accessories, http://www.sophysa.com

98. MED-EL Corporation, Durham, NC; http://www.MEDEL.com

99. Medtronic Neurological Technical Services Department, Tech Note. MRI Guidelines for Neurological Products, Issue No. NTN 04-03 Rev 2, July, 2005, Important Note: Before scanning a patient with this implant or device, obtain the latest MRI safety information by contacting Medtronic, Neurological Technical Services Department (800) 707-0933 or visit www.Medtronic.com.

100. Henderson J, Tkach J, Phillips M, Baker K, Shellock FG, Rezai A. Permanent neurological deficit related to magnetic resonance imaging in a patient with implanted deep brain stimulation electrodes for Parkinson's disease: Case report. Neurosurgery 2005;57:E1063.

101. Rezai AR, Baker K, Tkach J, Phillips M, Hrdlicka G, Sharan A, Nyenhuis J, Ruggieri P, Henderson J, Shellock FG. Is magnetic resonance imaging safe for patients with neurostimulation systems used for deep brain stimulation (DBS)? Neurosurgery 2005;57:1056-1062.

102. Shellock FG. MR Safety at 3-Tesla: Bare Metal and Drug Eluting Coronary Artery Stents. Signals No. 53, Issue 2, pp. 26-27, 2005.

103. Shellock FG. MR Safety and Cerebral Spinal Fluid Shunt (CSF) Valves. Signals, No. 51, Issue 4, pp. 10, 2004.

104. Shellock FG, Habibi R, Knebel J. Programmable CSF shunt valve: *In vitro* assessment of MRI safety at 3-Tesla. American Journal of Neuroradiology. 2006;27:661-665.

105. Ceballos EM, Parrish RK. Plain film imaging of Baerveldt glaucoma drainage implants. American Journal of Neuroradiology 2002;23;935-937.

106. Martin AD, et al. Safety evaluation of titanium middle ear prostheses at 3.0 Tesla. Otolaryngol Head Neck Surg 2005;132:537-42.

107. Shellock FG, Valencerina S. Septal repair implants: evaluation of MRI safety at 3-Tesla. Magnetic Resonance Imaging 2005;23:1021-1025.

108. Nehra A, Moran CJ, Cross DT, Derdeyn CP. MR safety and imaging of Neuroform Stents at 3-T. Am J Neuoradiol 2004;25:1476-1478.

109. Westerway SC, et al. Implanon implant detection with ultrasound and magnetic resonance imaging. Aust NZ Obstet Gynaecol 2003;43:346-350.

110. Shellock FG, Wilson SF, Mauge CP. Magnetically programmable shunt valve: MRI at 3-Tesla. Magnetic Resonance Imaging 2007;25:1116-21.

111. Zieman M, Kanal E. Copper T 380A IUD and magnetic resonance imaging. Contraception.2007;75:93-5.

112. Shellock FG, Crivelli R, Venugopalan R. Programmable infusion pump and catheter: evaluation using 3-Tesla MRI. Neuromodulation 2008;11:163-170.

113. Shellock FG, Valencerina S. Ventricular assist implant (AB5000): *In Vitro* assessment of MRI issues at 3-Tesla. Journal of Cardiovascular Magnetic Resonance 2008;10:23-30.

114. Diaz FL, Tweardy L, Shellock FG. Cervical external immobilization devices: evaluation of magnetic resonance imaging issues at 3.0 Tesla. Spine. 2010;35:411-5.

115. Nyenhuis J, Duan L. An evaluation of MRI safety and compatibility of a silver-impregnated antimicrobial wound dressing. J Am Coll Radiol. 2009;6:500-5.

116. Shellock FG. Valencerina S. In vitro evaluation of MR imaging issues at 3-T for aneurysm clips made from MP35N: Findings and information applied to 155 additional aneurysm clips. AJNR Am J Neuroradiol. 2010;31:615-619.

117. Geffen N, et al. Is the Ex-PRESS glaucoma shunt magnetic resonance imaging safe? J Glaucoma. 2009;70:532-6.

118. Gill KR, Pooley RA, Wallace MB. Magnetic resonance imaging compatibility of endoclips. Gastrointest Endosc. 2009;70:532-6.

119. Shellock FG, et al. Assessment of MRI issues for a 3-T "immune" programmable CSF shunt valve. Am J Roentgenol 2011;197:202-207.

APPENDIX I

GUIDANCE FOR INDUSTRY AND FDA STAFF

CRITERIA FOR SIGNIFICANT RISK INVESTIGATIONS OF MAGNETIC RESONANCE DIAGNOSTIC DEVICES

Document issued on: July 14, 2003

This document supersedes "Guidance for Magnetic Resonance Diagnostic Devices – Criteria for Significant Risk Investigations" issued n September 29, 1997

U.S. Department of Health and Human Services
Food and Drug Administration
Center for Devices and Radiological Health
Radiological Devices Branch
Division of Reproductive, Abdominal, and Radiological Devices
Office of Device Evaluation

PREFACE

Public Comment

Written comments and suggestions may be submitted at any time for Agency consideration to Division of Dockets Management, Food and Drug Administration, 5630 Fishers Lane, Room 1061, (HFA-305), Rockville, MD, 20852. When submitting comments, please refer to the exact title of this guidance document. Comments may not be acted upon by the Agency until the document is next revised or updated.

Additional Copies

Additional copies are available from the Internet at: http://www.fda.gov/cdrh/ode/guidance/793.pdf or to receive this document by fax, call the CDRH Facts-On-Demand system at 800-899-0381 or 301-827-0111 from a touch-tone telephone. Press 1 to enter the system. At the second voice prompt, press 1 to order a document. Enter the document number (793) followed by the pound sign (#). Follow the remaining voice prompts to complete your request.

This guidance represents the Food and Drug Administration's (FDA's) current thinking on this topic. It does not create or confer any rights for or on any person and does not operate to bind FDA or the public. You can use an alternative approach if the approach satisfies the requirements of the applicable statutes and regulations. If you want to discuss an alternative approach, contact the FDA staff responsible for implementing this guidance. If you cannot identify the appropriate FDA staff, call the appropriate number listed on the title page of this guidance.

INTRODUCTION

This guidance describes the device operation conditions for magnetic resonance diagnostic devices that FDA considers significant risk for the purposes of determining whether a clinical study requires Agency approval of an Investigation Device Exemption (IDE). Magnetic resonance diagnostic devices are class II devices described under 21 CFR 892.1000. The product codes for these devices are:

LNH Magnetic Resonance Imaging System

LNI Magnetic Resonance Spectroscopic System

This guidance supersedes Guidance for Magnetic Resonance Diagnostic Devices - Criteria for Significant Risk Investigations, issued September 29, 1997. We have revised our recommendation for the main static magnetic field strength, increasing it to 8 Tesla for most populations. This is based on ongoing experience in the field and numerous literature reviews (1, 2).

FDA's guidance documents, including this guidance, do not establish legally enforceable responsibilities. Instead, guidances describe the Agency's current thinking on a topic and should be viewed only as recommendations, unless specific regulatory or statutory requirements are cited. The use of the word should in Agency guidances means that something is suggested or recommended, but not required.

THE LEAST BURDENSOME APPROACH

We believe we should consider the least burdensome approach in all areas of medical device regulation. This guidance reflects our careful review of the relevant scientific and legal requirements and what we believe is the least burdensome way for you to comply with those requirements. However, if you believe that an alternative approach would be less burdensome, please contact us so we can consider your point of view. You may send your written comments to the contact person listed in the preface to this guidance or to the CDRH Ombudsman. Comprehensive information on CDRH's Ombudsman, including ways to contact him, can be found on the Internet at http://www.fda.gov/cdrh/ombudsman/

STUDIES OF MAGNETIC RESONANCE DIAGNOSTIC DEVICES

If a clinical study is needed to demonstrate substantial equivalence, i.e., conducted prior to obtaining 510(k) clearance of the device, the study must be conducted under the IDE regulation (21 CFR Part 812). FDA believes that a magnetic resonance diagnostic device used under any one of the operating conditions listed below is a significant risk device as defined in 21 CFR 812.3(m)(4) and, therefore, that studies involving such a device do not qualify for the abbreviated IDE requirements of 21 CFR 812.2(b). In addition to the requirement of having an FDA-approved IDE, sponsors of significant risk studies must comply with the regulations governing institutional review boards (21 CFR Part 56) and informed consent (21 CFR Part 50).

SIGNIFICANT RISK MAGNETIC RESONANCE DIAGNOSTIC DEVICES

You should consider the following operating conditions when assessing whether a study may be considered significant risk:

- main static magnetic field
- specific absorption rate (SAR)
- gradient fields rate of change
- sound pressure level

Generally, FDA deems magnetic resonance diagnostic devices significant risk when used under any of the operating conditions described below.

Main Static Magnetic Field

Population	Main static magnetic field greater than (Tesla)
adults, children, and infants aged > 1 month	8
neonates i.e., infants aged 1 month or less	4

Specific Absorption Rate (SAR)

Site	Dose	Time (min) equal to or greater than:	SAR (W/kg)
whole body	averaged over	15	4
head	averaged over	10	3
head or torso	per gram of tissue	5	8
extremities	per gram of tissue	5	12

Gradient Fields Rate of Change

Any time rate of change of gradient fields (dB/dt) sufficient to produce severe discomfort or painful nerve stimulation

Sound Pressure Level

Peak unweighted sound pressure level greater than 140 dB.

A-weighted root mean square (rms) sound pressure level greater than 99 dBA with hearing protection in place.

These criteria apply only to device operating conditions. Other aspects of the study may involve significant risks and the study, therefore, may require IDE approval regardless of operating conditions. See Blue Book Memorandum entitled Significant Risk and Non-significant Risk Medical Device Studies, http://www.fda.gov/cdrh/d861.html for further discussion.

After FDA determines that the device is substantially equivalent, clinical studies conducted in accordance with the indications reviewed in the 510(k), including clinical design validation studies conducted in accordance with the quality systems regulation, are exempt from the investigational device exemptions (IDE) requirements. However, such studies must be performed in conformance with 21 CFR 56 and 21 CFR 50.

(1) Kangarlu A, Burgess RE, Zu H, et al. Cognitive, cardiac and physiological studies in ultra high field magnetic resonance imaging. Magnetic Resonance Imaging, 1999;17:1407-1416.

(2) Schenck John F, Safety of strong, static magnetic fields. Journal of Magnetic Resonance Imaging, 2000;12:2-19.

APPENDIX II

WEB SITES FOR MRI SAFETY, BIOEFFECTS, AND PATIENT MANAGEMENT

There are two web sites devoted to MRI safety, bioeffects, and patient management: www.MRIsafety.com and www.IMRSER.org

www.MRIsafety.com

The international information resource for MRI safety, bioeffects, and patient management.®

This web site provides up-to-date information for healthcare providers and patients seeking answers to questions on MRI safety-related topics. The latest information is also provided for screening patients with implants, materials, and medical devices. *This website is updated on a regular basis by Frank G. Shellock, Ph.D.*

Key Features

- The List: A searchable database that contains information for thousands of implants, devices, and other objects tested for MRI issues.
- Safety Information: Concise information that pertains to the latest recommendations and guidelines for patient care and management in the MRI environment.
- Screening Forms: Information and forms for screening patients and other individuals available to imaging facilities in a "downloadable" PDF format.

www.IMRSER.org

The web site of the Institute for Magnetic Resonance Safety, Education, and Research (IMRSER)

The Institute for Magnetic Resonance Safety, Education, and Research (IMRSER) was formed in response to the growing need for information on matters pertaining to magnetic resonance (MR) safety. The IMRSER is the first independent, multidisciplinary, professional organization devoted to promoting awareness, understanding, and communication of MRI safety issues through education and research.

The functions and activities of the IMRSER involve development of MR safety guidelines and dissemination of this information to the MR community. This is accomplished through the efforts of the two Advisory Boards: the Medical, Scientific, and Technology Advisory Board and the Corporate Advisory Board.

The Medical, Scientific, and Technology Advisory Board consists of recognized leaders in the field of MR including diagnostic radiologists, clinicians, research scientists, physicists, MRI technologists, MRI facility managers, and other allied healthcare professionals involved in MR technology and safety. The members of the Medical, Scientific, and Technology Advisory Board represent academic, private, research, and institutional MR facilities utilizing scanners operating at static magnetic field strengths ranging from 0.2-Tesla (including dedicated-extremity and interventional MR systems) to 7-Tesla. In addition, the Food and Drug Administration has assigned a Federal Liaison to the IMRSER.

The Corporate Advisory Board is comprised of representatives from the medical industry including MR system manufacturers, contrast agent pharmaceutical companies, RF coil manufacturers, MR accessory vendors, medical product manufacturers, and other related corporate organizations.

The Institute for Magnetic Resonance Safety, Education, and Research develops MR safety guidelines utilizing the pertinent peer-reviewed literature and by relying on each board member's extensive clinical, research, or other appropriate experience. Notably, documents developed by the IMRSER consider and incorporate MR safety guidelines and recommendations created by the International Society for Magnetic Resonance in Medicine (ISMRM), the American College of Radiology (ACR), the Food and Drug Administration (FDA), the National Electrical Manufacturers Association (NEMA), the Medical Devices Agency (MDA), the International Electrotechnical Commission (IEC), the International Commission on Non-Ionizing Radiation Protection (ICNIRP), and other organizations.

The MR Safety Papers section of this website includes a wide selection of peer-reviewed articles that are available to site visitors as PDF files, posted with permission from the Journal of Magnetic Resonance Imaging, the International Society for Magnetic Resonance in Medicine, Radiology, the Journal of Cardiovascular Magnetic Resonance, the

Institute for Electrical and Electronics Engineers, IEEE Transactions on Magnetics, the Journal of the American College of Cardiology, and Concepts in Magnetic Resonance. Notably, the majority of these papers were published by members of the Medical, Scientific, and Technology Advisory Board of the Institute for Magnetic Resonance Safety, Education, and Research.

APPENDIX III

WEBSITES FOR BIOMEDICAL COMPANIES

3M Healthcare -	www.3m.com
AADCO Medical, Inc. -	www.aadcomed.com
Abbott Vascular Devices -	www.abbott.com
ABIOMED, Inc. -	www.abiomed.com
Acclarent, Inc. -	www.acclarent.com
Advanced Bionics Corporation -	www.bionicear.com
Advanced Neuromodulation Systems -	www.ans-medical.com
Adtech Medical Instrument Corporation –	www.adtechmedical.com
Aesculap, Inc. -	www.aesculap.com
AGA Medical Corporation -	www.amplatzer.com
Alcon Laboratories Inc.-	www.alcon.com
Alcon Research, Ltd. -	www.alconlabs.com
Alphatec Spine -	www.alphatecspine.com
Alveolus, Inc. -	www.alveolus.com
Alsius Corporation -	www.alsius.com
Amerex Corporation -	amerex-fire.com
Ampco Safety Tools -	www.ampcosafetytools.com
American Medical Systems -	www.americanmedicalsystems.com
Angiodynamics, Inc. -	www.angiodynamics.com
Animas Corporation -	www.Animascorp.com
Arbor Surgical Technologies, Inc. -	www.arborsurgical.com
Arthrex -	www.arthrex.com
Applied Medical -	www.appliedmed.com
Aspire Medical -	www.aspiremedical.com
AtriCure, Inc. -	www.atricure.com
Atritech, Inc. -	www.atritech.com
Atrium Medical Corporation -	www.atriummed.com
ATS Medical -	www.atsmedical.com
B. Braun Medical Inc. -	www.bbraunusa.com
Baxa Corporation -	www.baxa.com
Baxter International, Inc.	www.Baxter.com
Becton, Dickinson, and Co. -	www.bd.com
Berlex Laborotories -	www.berlex.com

Biomerix Corporation - www.Biomerix.com
Biomet, Inc. - www.biomet.com
Bioness, Inc. - www.Bioness.com
Bioplate, Inc. - www.bioplate.com
Biosensors International - www.biosensorsintl.com
Biopsy Sciences - www.biopsysciences.com
Biotronik - www.Biotronik.com
BIOTRONIK AG - www.biotronik.ch
Blackstone Medical, Inc. - www.blackstonemedical.com
Bolton Medical, Inc. - www.boltonmedical.com
Boston Scientific Corporation - www.bostonscientific.com
Bracco Diagnostics Inc. - www.Bracco.com
Bronchus Technologies, Inc. - www.bronchus.com
Calypso Medical Technologies - www.calypsomedical.com
Cardia, Inc. - www.cardia.com
Cardica - www.cardica.com
Cardiac Dimensions - www.cardiacdimensions.com
Cardinal Health - www.cardinal.com
CardioKinetix Inc. - www.cardiokinetix.com
CardioMEMS, Inc. - www.cardiomems.com
Cayanne Medical - www.cayennemedical.com
Coaxia, Inc. - www.coaxia.com
Codman, a Johnson and Johnson Company - www.depuy.com
Coherex Medical- www.coherex.com
Coloplast Corporation - www.coloplast.com
Conceptus Inc.- www.conceptus.com
Conor Medsystems - www.conormed.com
ConvaTec Wound Therapeutics - www.convatec.com
Cook Medical - www.cookmedical.com
Corassist Medical - www.corassist.com
Cordis - www.cordis.com
Cornova, Inc. - www.cornova.com
COVIDIEN - www.covidien.com
C.R. Bard, Inc. - www.crbard.com
Crux Biomedical, Inc. - www.cruxbiomedical.com
Cyberkinetics Neurotechnology Systems, Inc. - www.cyberkineticsinc.com
Cyberonics, Inc. - www.cyberonics.com
Datascope Corporation - www.datascope.com
DePuy Products, Inc. - www.depuy.com
DermaPort - www.dermaport.net

DeRoyal Technologies -	www.deroyal.com
Devax, Inc. -	www.devax.net
DexCom, Inc. –	www.dexcom.com
Edwards Lifeciences -	www.edwards.com
Emphasys Medical Inc. -	www.emphasysmedical.com
Endologix, Inc. -	www.endologix.com
EndoMed, Inc. -	www.endomedinc.com
EnteroMedics, Inc. -	www.enteromedics.com
Endotex Interventional Systems, Inc. -	www.endotex.com
ev3, The Endovascular Company -	www.ev3.net
Ethicon Endo-Surgery -	www.eesus.jnj.com
Evalve, Inc. -	www.evalveinc.com
Ferno -	www.ferno.com
Finetech Medical Ltd. -	www.finetech-medical.co.uk
Hitachi Medical Systems America, Inc. -	www.hitachimed.com
Hollister -	www.hollister.com
HoverTech International -	www.hovermatt.com
Gendron, Inc. -	www.gendroninc.com
General Electric Healthcare -	www.gehealthcare.com
Genstar Technologies -	www.genstartech.com
GI Dynamics, Inc. -	www.gidynamics.com
Glaukos Corporation -	www.glaukos.com
GrantAdler Corporation -	www.grantadler.com
GT Urological -	www.gturological.com
Glaukos Corporation -	www.glaukos.com
Gyrus -	www.gyrusacmi.com
Hollister Inc. -	www.hollister.com
Health Beacons Inc. -	www.healthbeacons.com
Hisamitsu Pharmaceutical Co., Inc. -	www.hisamitsu.co.jp/english
Hitachi Medical Systems America -	www. hitachimed.com
Icon Interventional Systems, Inc. -	www.icon-us.com
IDEV Technologies, Inc. -	www.idevtechnologies.com
I-Flow Corporation -	www.iflo.com
Impliant Ltd. -	www.Impliant.com
INAMED -	www.inamed.com
INNERCOOL Therapies -	www.innercool.com
INRAD, Inc. -	www.inrad-inc.com
InSound Medical -	www.insoundmedical.com
Integra Lifesciences Corporation -	www.integralife.com
Interrad Medical, Inc. -	www.interradmedical.com

Intrinsic Therapeutics, Inc. -   www.intrinsic-therapeutics.com
Intuitive Surgical, Inc. -   www.intuitivesurgical.com
Invatec -   www.invatec.com
Ivantis -   www.ivantisinc.com
JenaValve Technology -   www.jenavalve.de
Joint Replacement Instrumentation Limited (JRI Ltd.) - www.jri-ltd.co.uk
Kaneka Corporation -   www.kaneka.co.jp
KCI USA, Inc. -   www.kci1.com
KFx Medical Corporation -   www.kfxmedical.com
Kimberly-Clark Health Care -   www.kimberly-clark.com
Kips Bay Medical, Inc. -   www.kipsbaymedical.com
LeMaitre Vascular -   www.lemaitre.com
LMA North America -   www.lmana.com
LSI Solutions, Inc. -   www.lsisolutions.com
Magmedix -   www.magmedix.com
Medcomp -   www.medcompnet.com
MED-EL -   www.medel.com
Medivance, Inc. -   www.medivance.com
Medline Industries, Inc. -   www.medline.com
Medlogics -   www.medlogicsdc.com
MEDRAD, INC. -   www.medrad.com
Medtronic, Inc. -   www.medtronic.com
Medtronic Xomed -   xomed.com
Mentor Corporation -   www.mentorcorp.com
Micardia Corporation -   www.micardiac.com
Micell Technologies -   www.micell.com
MicroVention -   www.microvention.com
Micrus Endovascular Corporation –   www.micrusendovascular.com
MiniMed, Inc. -   www.minimed.com
Minrad, Inc. -   www.minrad.com
Moximed -   www.moximed.com
Mylan Technologies Inc. -   www.mylantech.com
Navotek Medical Ltd. -   www.navotek.com
NeuroVASx, Inc. -   www.neurovasx.com
Newmatic Sound Systems, Inc. -   www.newmaticsound.com
Nfocus Neuromedical, Inc. -   www.nfocusneuro.com
NGK Metals Corporation -   www.ngkmetals.com
NMT Medical, Inc. -   www.nmtmedical.com
NuVasive, Inc. -   www.nuvasive.com
Optonol Ltd. -   www.optonol.com

OrbusNeich Medical, Inc. -	www.orbusneich.co
Orthofix -	www.orthofix.com
OSSUR AMERICAS -	www.ossur.com
Otto Bock HealthCare –	www.ottobockus.com
Paracor Medical, Inc. -	www.paracor.com
Percardia Inc. -	www.percardia.com
Phoenix Biomedical Corporation -	www.phoenixbiomedical.com
PMT Corporation -	www.pmtcorp.com
Praxair Healthcare Services -	www.praxair.com
Prescient Medical -	www.prescientmedical.com
ProStrakan -	www.prostrakan.com
Pulmonx -	www.pulmonx.com
Pulsar Vascular -	www.pulsarvascular.com
QSUM -	www.qsum.net
Radianse, Inc. -	www.radianse.com
Rafael Medical Technologies, Inc. -	www.rafaelmedical.com
Rex Medical -	www.rexmedical.com
Rhythmlink International, LLC -	www.rhythmlink.com
Rubicor Medical, Inc. -	www.rubicor.com
SAM Medical Products -	www.sammedical.com
Second Sight -	www.2-sight.com
Shelhigh Inc. -	www.shelhigh.com
Sicel Technologies, Inc. -	www.siceltech.com
Siemens Medical Solutions -	www.siemens.com
Smith & Nephew, Inc. -	www.smithnephew.com
Smiths Medical -	www.smiths-medical.com
Sorin Group -	www.sorin.com
Spiration Inc. -	www.spiration.com
St. Jude Medical, Inc. -	www.sjm.com
Stentys -	www.stentys.com
Stryker Instruments -	www.stryker.com
Sulzer Carbomedics, Inc. -	www.sulzercarbomedics.com
SuperDimension -	www.superdimension.com
Svelte Medical Systems, Inc. -	www.sveltemedical.com
Tarsis Biomedical -	www.tarsisbiomedical.com
Tarsus Medical Inc. -	www.tarsusmedical.com
Teleflex Medical -	www.teleflexmedical.com
The Viking Corporation -	www.vikingcorp.com
Theragenics Corporation -	www.theraseed.com
Torax Medical -	www.toraxmedical.com

TriVascular, Inc. -	www.trivascular.com
Uromedica Inc. -	www.uromedica-inc.com
U.S. Surgical Corporation -	www.ussurg.com
ValleyLab/Tyco -	www.tycohealthcare.com
Vascular Architects, Inc. -	www.vasculararchitects.com
Vascutek Ltd. -	www.vascutek.com
Vesocclude Medical -	www.vesoccludemedical.com
VisionCare Ophthalmic Technologies Ltd. -	www.visioncare.co.il
Vygon Ltd. -	www.vygonus.com
Western Enterprises -	www.westernenterprises.com
W.L. Gore and Associates, Inc. -	www.wlgore.com
Wright Medical Technology -	www.WMT.com
Xlumena -	www.xlumena.com
XTENT -	www.xtent.com
Zimmer -	www.zimmer.com

APPENDIX IV

Guidance for Industry and FDA Staff Establishing Safety and Compatibility of Passive Implants in the Magnetic Resonance (MR) Environment

Document issued on: August 21, 2008

For questions regarding this document, contact Terry O. Woods, Ph.D. at 301-796-2503 or by email at terry.woods@fda.hhs.gov

U.S. Department of Health and Human Services
Food and Drug Administration
Center for Devices and Radiological Health
Division of Solid and Fluid Mechanics
Office of Science & Engineering Laboratories

Preface
Public Comment

Written comments and suggestions may be submitted at any time for Agency consideration to the Division of Dockets Management, Food and Drug Administration, 5630 Fishers Lane, Room 1061, (HFA-305), Rockville, MD, 20852.

When submitting comments, please refer to the exact title of this guidance document. Comments may not be acted upon by the Agency until the document is next revised or updated.

Additional Copies

Additional copies are available from the Internet at:
http://www.fda.gov/cdrh/osel/guidance/1685.pdf. You may also send an e-mail request to dsmica@fda.hhs.gov to receive an electronic copy of the guidance or send a fax request to 240-276-3151 to receive a hard

copy. Please use the document number (1685) to identify the guidance you are requesting.

This guidance represents the Food and Drug Administration's (FDA's) current thinking on this topic. It does not create or confer any rights for or on any person and does not operate to bind FDA or the public. You can use an alternative approach if the approach satisfies the requirements of the applicable statutes and regulations. If you want to discuss an alternative approach, contact the FDA staff responsible for implementing this guidance. If you cannot identify the appropriate FDA staff, call the appropriate number listed on the title page of this guidance.

1. Introduction

This guidance addresses testing and labeling of passive implants for safety and compatibility in the magnetic resonance (MR) environment. In preparing a premarket approval application (PMA), Investigational Device Exemption (IDE), and premarket notification (510(k)) submission, this guidance document applies to MR devices that serve their function without the supply of electronic power. Active implants or devices that are not implants do not fall within the scope of this guidance.

The information in this guidance supplements the Agency's related publications on PMA's, IDE's, and 510(k)s and is not intended to describe or substitute the information otherwise required in the following premarket submissions:

-Premarket Approval Application (PMA) Information

For general information about PMA applications, refer to 21 CFR 814 or "Application Methods," at
http://www.fda.gov/cdrh/devadvice/pma/app_methods.html.

-Investigational Device Exemption (IDE) Information

For general IDE information, refer to 21 CFR Part 812 or to the "Introduction IDE Overview," at
http://www.fda.gov/cdrh/devadvice/ide/index.shtml.

-Premarket Notification (510(k)) Information

For general information on 510(k), refer to 21 CFR 807.87, the guidance entitled "Format for Traditional and Abbreviated 510(k)s" and "Premarket Notification 510(k)" in the (Center for Devices and Radiological Health) CDRH Device Advice at
http://www.fda.gov/cdrh/devadvice/314.html.

A manufacturer who intends to market a passive implant must conform to the general controls of the Federal Food, Drug, and Cosmetic Act (the act).

The Least Burdensome Approach

We believe we should consider the least burdensome approach in all areas of medical device regulation. This guidance reflects our careful review of the relevant scientific and legal requirements and what we believe is the least burdensome way for you to comply with those requirements. However, if you believe that an alternative approach would be less burdensome, please contact us so we can consider your point of view. You may send your written comments to the contact person listed in the preface to this guidance or to the CDRH Ombudsman. Comprehensive information on CDRH's Ombudsman, including ways to contact him, can be found on the Internet at http://www.fda.gov/cdrh/ombudsman/.

FDA's guidance documents, including this guidance, do not establish legally enforceable responsibilities. Instead, guidances describe the Agency's current thinking on a topic and should be viewed only as recommendations, unless specific regulatory or statutory requirements are cited. The use of the word should in Agency guidances means that something is suggested or recommended, but not required.

2. MR Testing

The main issues affecting the safety and compatibility of passive implants in the MR environment concern magnetically induced displacement force and torque, radio frequency (RF) heating, and image artifacts. The MR static field induces displacement forces and torques on magnetic materials. Patients have been killed by the projectile effect on devices and by the rotations produced by magnetically induced force and torque (1). RF heating in the body is created by currents induced by the RF excitation pulses applied during MR scanning. Patients have been severely burned as a result during an MR scan (2). The presence of an implant may produce an image artifact that may appear as a void region or as a geometric distortion of the true image. If the image artifact is near the area of interest, the artifact may make the MR scan uninformative or may lead to an inaccurate clinical diagnosis, potentially resulting in inappropriate medical action.

We recommend that you provide the nonclinical testing described below in your PMA, IDE or 510(k) to establish the safety and compatibility of your passive implant in the MR environment. Testing should encompass the range of sizes of the device you intend to market. If you do not test all sizes of the device you intend to market, we recommend you test a size or combination of sizes that represent the worst-case scenario for each test.

We recommend you explain the rationale for determining why the size(s) you selected represent the worst-case scenario for each test.

We suggest you present data in a clear tabular or graphical form. We also recommend you describe all testing protocols. Each protocol description should include:

- test objective
- equipment used
- acceptance criteria
- rationale for test conditions
- rationale for the acceptance criteria
- number of devices tested
- description of devices tested, including device size
- description of any differences between test sample and final product, and justification for why differences would not impact the applicability of the test to the final product
- results (summarized and raw form).

Terminology

Terminology for defining the safety of items in the MR environment is provided in ASTM F2503 Standard Practice for Marking Medical Devices and Other Items for Safety in the Magnetic Resonance Environment. We recognize implementing new terminology may be challenging, but FDA believes this new terminology will help reduce the possibility of injuries involving passive implants related to MRI (Magnetic Resonance Imaging). We recommend using the terminology MR Safe, MR Conditional, and MR Unsafe, defined in ASTM F2503. If you label your device as "MR Safe," your submission should include a scientific rationale or the testing described below. If you label your device as "MR Conditional," your submission should include the testing described below. If you label your device as "MR Unsafe," your submission should include a scientific rationale or the testing described below.

MR Safe based on scientific rationale

A scientifically based rationale rather than test data may be sufficient to support identifying an implant as "MR Safe," for example, a nonconducting or a nonmagnetic item, such as a plastic Petri dish, poses no known hazards in all MR environments.

If you intend to use a scientific rationale to support identifying your device as "MR Safe," we recommend that you provide a scientific rationale that addresses the following issues.

- magnetically induced displacement force
- magnetically induced torque
- heating of your device by RF (radio frequency) fields.

MR Unsafe based on scientific rationale

A scientifically based rationale rather than test data, may be sufficient to support identifying an item as "MR Unsafe."

If you intend to use a scientific rationale to support identifying your device as "MR Unsafe," we recommend that you provide a scientific rationale to address:

- magnetically induced displacement force
- magnetically induced torque
- heating of your device by RF (radio frequency) fields.

MR Conditional, MR Safe, or MR Unsafe based on experimental data

If you identify your device as "MR Conditional," we recommend you provide experimental data as described below. You may also choose to provide experimental data to support identifying your device as "MR Safe" or "MR Unsafe." In each case, we recommend you follow the methods described in the standards below or equivalent methods.

-Magnetically Induced Displacement Force

ASTM F2052, Standard Test Method for Measurement of Magnetically Induced Displacement Force on Medical Devices in the Magnetic Resonance Environment

-Magnetically Induced Torque

ASTM F2213, Standard Test Method for Measurement of Magnetically Induced Torque on Medical Devices in the Magnetic Resonance Environment

-Heating by RF Fields

ASTM F2182, Standard Test Method for Measurement of Radio Frequency Induced Heating Near Passive Implants During Magnetic Resonance Imaging

-Image Artifact

ASTM F2119, Standard Test Method for Evaluation of MR Image Artifacts from Passive Implants

Although commercial 1.5-T MR systems are currently the most common, 3-T MR systems are becoming more common. A medical device that is MR Safe or MR Conditional in a 1.5-T scanner may not be MR Safe or MR Conditional in an MR system with a higher or lower field strength. The amount of RF heating can vary depending on the system geometry, MR system and scan conditions, and the conductive length of the device. The critical length for a specific device during a particular MR scan cannot be calculated precisely, so we recommend you evaluate a range of lengths and conditions to determine the worst case conditions for RF induced heating. To achieve worst-case heating conditions in the phantom, you should pay attention to the local electric and magnetic field distribution near the implant inside the phantom. These fields need to be similar to the local electric and magnetic field distribution near the implant inside the patient so the heating of the implant in the phantom is comparable to the heating inside the patient. Anatomical positioning of the implant in the phantom does not reliably predict the implant heating in the patient. Therefore, we recommend you describe the field conditions and system geometry under which you tested your device and demonstrate that your test conditions are comparable to worst-case clinical conditions. Accurate assessment of the whole body averaged specific absorption rate (WB-SAR) used in your testing is critical to determining whether your testing represents reasonable worst-case heating conditions. Therefore, we recommend that you base WB-SAR assessments upon calorimetry measurements rather than relying on the MR scanner display, which may not have adequate accuracy. See also **3.**

Labeling for the MR Environment

3. Labeling for the MR Environment

General labeling requirements for medical devices are described in 21 CFR Part 801. See CDRH Device Advice (http://www.fda.gov/cdrh/devadvice/33.html) for additional information. In accordance with 21 CFR 814.20(b)(10), you must submit all proposed labeling in a PMA.

A 510(k) must include labeling in sufficient detail to satisfy the requirements of 21 CFR 807.87(e). An IDE must include labeling to satisfy the requirements of 21 CFR 812.5. The following suggestions may assist you in preparing labeling that satisfies the requirements of 21 CFR Part 8013 (3).

MR Labeling

We recommend you consider using the MR terminology in ASTM F2503, Standard Practice for Marking Medical Devices and Other Items for Safety in the Magnetic Resonance Environment. See **Section 2. MR Testing** for information describing the process to determine the appropriate MR safety term for your device.

MR Safe

The following statement may be used in your labeling for a MR Safe device: The (insert device name) is MR Safe.

MR Unsafe

The following statement may be used in your labeling for an MR Unsafe device: The (insert device name) is MR Unsafe.

Labeling for an MR Unsafe implant should recommend that patients register their implant information with the MedicAlert Foundation (www.medicalert.org) or equivalent organization.

MR Conditional

Labeling for MR Conditional devices should indicate the device was tested under non-clinical conditions and list the conditions under which the device can be safely scanned, for example:

Non-clinical testing has demonstrated the (insert device name) is MR Conditional. It can be scanned safely under the following conditions:

- static magnetic field of ___ Tesla
- spatial gradient field of ___ Gauss/cm
- maximum whole body averaged specific absorption rate (SAR) of ___ W/kg for ___ minutes of scanning.

In non-clinical testing, the (insert device name) produced a temperature rise of less than ___ °C at a maximum whole body averaged specific absorption rate (SAR) of ___ W/kg, as assessed by calorimetry for ___ minutes of MR scanning in a (field strength _____) (model _____) (manufacturer _____) (software version _____) MR scanner.

Image Artifact – General

We also recommend your labeling indicate the amount of image artifact and that you acquire MR images using standard sequences (e.g., as described in ASTM F2119) or an equivalent method. We recommend your labeling indicate the extent of the artifact for one or more of the sequences used in your testing. The labeling should also include information about the shape and extent of the artifact. For devices with a lumen, the labeling should indicate whether the lumen is obscured by the artifact. A dimensioned figure showing the implant in its typical implant site and the extent of the artifact in at least one plane may be included. It may be helpful to provide a separate dimensioned drawing of the implant and a figure showing the typical implant site.

Image Artifact – Special Examples

Devices with Slight (1-2-mm) Artifact

The following statement may be used for a device with an image artifact that extends only slightly (1-2 mm) beyond the device:

MR image quality may be compromised if the area of interest is in the same area or relatively close to the position of the device. Therefore, it may be necessary to optimize MR imaging parameters for the presence of this implant.

Devices with a Lumen

For devices with a lumen, we recommend you specify whether the lumen is obscured by the artifact, for example:

The image artifact extends approximately __ mm from the device, both inside and outside the device lumen when scanned in nonclinical testing using the sequence: _____ in a (Field Strength) (Model)(Manufacturer)(software version) MR system with _____ coil.

We also recommend that the device labeling for an MR Conditional implant recommend that patients register the conditions under which the implant can be scanned safely with the MedicAlert Foundation (www.medicalert.org) or equivalent organization.

REFERENCES

(1) Woods, T.O. "MRI Safety" in Wiley Encyclopedia of Biomedical Engineering (Metin Akay, ed.) Hoboken: John Wiley & Sons, Inc., 2006, pp. 2360-2371.

(2) Ibid.

(3) Although final labeling is not required for 510(k) clearance, labeling is reviewed in a 510(k) and the final labeling must comply with the requirements of 21 CFR Part 801 before a medical device is introduced into interstate commerce. In addition, final labeling for prescription medical devices must comply with 21 CFR 801.109. Labeling recommendations in this guidance are consistent with the requirements of Part 801.

Frank G. Shellock, Ph.D. is a physiologist with more than 25 years of experience conducting laboratory and clinical investigations in the field of magnetic resonance imaging. He is an Adjunct Clinical Professor of Radiology and Medicine at the Keck School of Medicine, University of Southern California, Adjunct Professor of Clinical Physical Therapy, Division of Biokinesiology and Physical Therapy, School of Dentistry, University of Southern California and the Director of MRI Studies at the Biomimetic Microelectronic Systems, National Science Foundation (NSF) - Engineering Research Center, University of Southern California, and the Founder of the Institute for Magnetic Resonance Safety, Education, and Research (www.IMRSER.org). As a commitment to the field of MRI safety, bioeffects, and patient management, he created and maintains the internationally popular web site, www.MRIsafety.com.

Dr. Shellock has authored or co-authored more than 220 publications in the peer-reviewed literature. He co-authored the MRI safety section of the Cardiovascular MR Self-Assessment Program (CMR-SAP) for the American College of Cardiology and three of his medical textbooks are considered best sellers - **Reference Manual for Magnetic Resonance Safety, Implants and Devices**; **Magnetic Resonance Procedures: Health Effects and Safety**; and **Kinematic MRI of the Joints: Functional Anatomy, Kinesiology, and Clinical Applications**

Dr. Shellock is a member of the Sub-Committee on MRI safety issues for the American Society for Testing and Materials (ASTM) International. Additionally, he serves in advisory roles to government, industry, and other policy-making organizations. Dr. Shellock is an Associate Editor for the Journal of Magnetic Resonance Imaging and a Reviewing Editor for several medical and scientific journals including Radiology, Investigative Radiology, Magnetic Resonance in Medicine, Magnetic Resonance Imaging, the American Journal of Roentgenology, the Journal of Cardiovascular Magnetic Resonance, Circulation, Neuoradiology, the European Heart Journal, Neurosurgery, and the Journal of the American College of Cardiology.

Memberships in professional societies include the American College of Radiology, the International Society for Magnetic Resonance in Medicine (ISMRM), the Radiological Society of North America, the Hawaii Radiological Society, the Regulatory Affairs Professional Society, and the Society for Cardiovascular Magnetic Resonance. He is also a Fellow and member of the American College of Cardiology and the American College of Sportsmedicine.

In 2004, the International Society for Magnetic Resonance in Medicine recognized the significant contributions Dr. Shellock has made to the scientific and educational mission of the ISMRM by designating him a Fellow of the Society. The American College of Radiology awarded him a Distinguished Committee Service Award for years of dedicated service to the *Practice Guidelines and Technical Standards Committee – Body MRI*.

Dr. Shellock is a recipient of a National Research Service Award from the National Institutes of Health, National Heart, Lung, and Blood Institute and has received numerous grants from governmental agencies and private organizations. He is currently participating in research to define safety for cardiac pacemakers, implantable cardioverter defibrillators, neurostimulation systems, implantable infusion pumps, and other electronically-activated devices.

Dr. Shellock has lectured both nationally and internationally and has provided plenary lectures to numerous organizations including the Radiological Society of North America, the International Society for Magnetic Resonance in Medicine, the American College of Radiology, the American Roentgen Ray Society, the American Society of Neuroradiology, the Environmental Protection Agency, the Oklahoma Heart Institute, the Head and Neck Radiology Society, the Center for Devices and Radiological Health (FDA), the Magnetic Resonance Managers Society, the American Heart Association, the American College of Cardiology, the American Society of Neuroimaging, the Society for Cardiovascular Magnetic Resonance, the Heart Rhythm Society, the Finnish Radiological Society, the International Congress of Radiology, the Japanese Society of Neuroradiology, the British Chapter of the International Society for Magnetic Resonance in Medicine, the Royal Australian and New Zealand College of Radiologists, and the Institute of Physics and Engineering in Medicine.

Dr. Shellock's company, **Magnetic Resonance Safety Testing Services**, specializes in the assessment of MRI issues for implants and devices as well as the evaluation of electromagnetic field-related bioeffects and the development of new clinical MR imaging applications for low-field (0.2-Tesla), high-field, and very-high-field strength MR systems (www.MagneticResonanceSafetyTesting.com).